Atlas of
HEAD AND NECK SURGERY

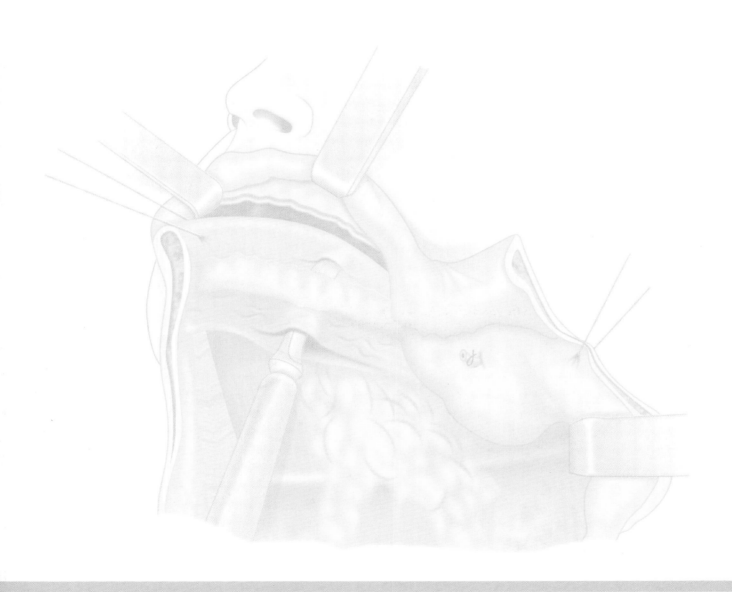

Atlas of
HEAD AND NECK SURGERY

Series Editor

Chris de Souza

Honorary ENT and Skull Base Surgeon
Tata Memorial Hospital, Mumbai
Consultant Otolaryngologist and Head Neck Surgeon
Lilavati Hospital and Holy Family Hospital
Mumbai, Maharashtra, India

Volume Editors

Ziv Gil MD PhD

Professor and Chairman
Department of Otolaryngology, Head and Neck Surgery, and the Laboratory for
Applied Cancer Research, Rambam Medical Center
The Technion, Israel Institute of Technology, Haifa, Israel

Dan M Fliss MD

Professor and Chairman
Department Otolaryngology, Head and Neck Surgery
and Maxillofacial Surgery
Tel Aviv Sourasky Medical Center
6 Weizmann St, Israel

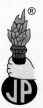

JAYPEE BROTHERS MEDICAL PUBLISHERS (P) LTD

New Delhi • London • Philadelphia • Panama

Jaypee Brothers Medical Publishers (P) Ltd

Headquarters

Jaypee Brothers Medical Publishers (P) Ltd
4838/24, Ansari Road, Daryaganj
New Delhi 110 002, India
Phone: +91-11-43574357
Fax: +91-11-43574314
Email: jaypee@jaypeebrothers.com

Overseas Offices

J.P. Medical Ltd
83, Victoria Street, London
SW1H 0HW (UK)
Phone: +44-2031708910
Fax: +02-03-0086180
Email: info@jpmedpub.com

Jaypee-Highlights Medical Publishers Inc.
City of Knowledge, Bld. 237, Clayton
Panama City, Panama
Phone: +507-301-0496
Fax: +507-301-0499
Email: cservice@jphmedical.com

Jaypee Brothers Medical Publishers Ltd
The Bourse
111 South Independence Mall East
Suite 835, Philadelphia, Pennsylvania, USA
19106, USA
Phone: + 267-519-9789
Email: joe.rusko@jaypeebrothers.com

Jaypee Brothers
Medical Publishers (P) Ltd
17/1-B Babar Road, Block-B
Shaymali, Mohammadpur
Dhaka-1207, Bangladesh
Mobile: +08801912003485
Email: jaypeedhaka@gmail.com

Jaypee Brothers
Medical Publishers (P) Ltd
Shorakhute, Kathmandu
Nepal
Phone: +00977-9841528578
Email: jaypee.nepal@gmail.com

Website: www.jaypeebrothers.com
Website: www.jaypeedigital.com

Inquiries for bulk sales may be solicited at: jaypee@jaypeebrothers.com

This book has been published in good faith that the contents provided by the contributors contained herein are original, and is intended for educational purposes only. While every effort is made to ensure accuracy of information, the publisher and the editors specifically disclaim any damage, liability, or loss incurred, directly or indirectly, from the use or application of any of the contents of this work. If not specifically stated, all figures and tables are courtesy of the editors. Where appropriate, the readers should consult with a specialist or contact the manufacturer of the drug or device.

Atlas of Head and Neck Surgery

First Edition: **2013**

ISBN 978-93-5090-380-3

Printed at: Ajanta Offset & Packagings Ltd., New Delhi

Dedicated to

My parents Ada and Isaac Gil

Ziv Gil

The memory of my parents, Thea and Dr Adolf Fliss who first arouse my interest in
Otolaryngology. Their love, education, dedication and drive have shaped me.
My loving wife Maayana for her insight, wisdom,
patience and support throughout most of my adult life.
My four children, Naomi, Ehud, Ruth and Yael who are a constant source of
joy and pride. I thank each one of you for your love and understanding.

Dan M Fliss

Contributors

Docteur Jean Abitol
Chevalier de la Légion d'Honneur
Adjunct Professor ORL Drexel University
College of Medicine of Pennsylvania
Philadelphia, USA
President of the International Society for
Laser Surgery and Medicine
Chef de Clinique à la Faculté de Médecine
de Paris
Oto-Rhino-Laryngologiste - Chirurgie Laser
- Chirurgie Cervico-Faciale
Scientific Advisory Board of the
International Association of Phono-Surgery
Scientific Advisory Board of the Voice
Foundation (USA)

Docteur Patrick Abitbol
Chef de Clinique à la Faculté de Médecine
de Paris
Oto-Rhino-Laryngologiste - Chirurgie Laser
- Chirurgie Cervico-Faciale
Rue Largillière, Paris, France

Aharon Amir
Department of Plastic and Reconstructive
Surgery,
The Tel-Aviv Sourasky Medical Center,
Tel-Aviv, Israel

Ehud Arad
Department of Plastic and Reconstructive
Surgery,
The Tel-Aviv Sourasky Medical Center,
Tel-Aviv, Israel

Yoav Barnea
Department of Plastic and
Reconstructive Surgery
The Tel-Aviv Sourasky Medical Center,
Tel-Aviv, Israel

Sophie El Bédoui MD
Head and Neck Department
Centre Oscar Lambret
3, rue Combemale
Lille, France

Piero Berti MD
Department of Surgery, University of Pisa
Ospedale Cisanello Ed 30A 2nd Floor
Via Paradisa, Pisa, Italy
Lenine G Brandão MD PhD
Chairman—Department of Head and
Neck Surgery
University of São Paulo Medical School
São Paulo, Brazil

Claudio R Cernea MD PhD
Professor of Surgery
Department of Head and Neck Surgery
University of São Paulo Medical School
São Paulo, Brazil

Francisco J Civantos
Professor of Otolaryngology
Co-chief, Division of Head and Neck
Surgery
Sylvester Cancer Center
University of Miami, USA

Jacob T Cohen MD
Department of Otolaryngology Head and
Neck Surgery
Tel-Aviv Sourasky Medical Center and the
Faculty of
Medicine Tel-Aviv University, Israel

Giovanni Cristalli
Department of Otolaryngology Head and
Neck Surgery
National Cancer Institute Regina Elena
Via E. Chianesi 53
Rome, Italy

Jacqueline Crupi
Department of Otolaryngology Head and
Neck Surgery
National Cancer Institute Regina Elena
Via E. Chianesi 53
Rome, Italy

Ari DeRowe MD
Director—Pediatric Otolaryngology Unit
Department of Otolaryngology Head and
Neck Surgery and Maxillofacial Surgery
Tel-Aviv Sourasky Medical Center
Tel-Aviv University Sackler School of
Medicine, Israel

Fernando Luiz Dias MD PhD FACS
Chief, Head and Neck Service
Brazilian National Cancer Institute
Chairman, Department of Head and Neck
Surgery
Postgraduate School of Medicine
Catholic University of Rio De Janeiro, Brazil

Joshua L Dunklebarger MD
Summit ENT and Hearing Services
Summit Keystone Pavilion
Chambersburg, Pennsylvania, USA

Behfar Eivazi MD
Department of Otolaryngology,
Head and Neck Surgery.
University of Marburg, Germany

Robert L Ferris MD PhD FACS
UPMC Endowed Professor of Head and
Neck Oncologic Surgery
Department of Otolaryngology
University of Pittsburgh
Pittsburgh, Pennsylvania, USA

Dan M Fliss MD
Professor and Chairman
Department Otolaryngology, Head and
Neck Surgery and Maxillofacial Surgery
Tel-Aviv Sourasky Medical Center
6 Weizmann St, Israel

Jeremy L Freeman MD FRCSC FACS
Professor of Otolaryngology—Head and
Neck Surgery
Professor of Surgery
University of Toronto
Temmy Latner/Dynacare
Chairman in Head and Neck Oncology
Mount Sinai Hospital
Toronto, Ontario, Canada

Ziv Gil MD PhD
Professor and Chairman
Department of Otolaryngology
Head and Neck Surgery, and the Laboratory
for Applied Cancer Research
Rambam Medical Center, The Technion,
Israel Institute of Technology, Haifa, Israel

Eyal Gur
Department of Plastic and Reconstructive
Surgery
The Tel-Aviv Sourasky Medical Center
Tel-Aviv, Israel

Ehab Y Hanna MD FACS
Professor and Vice Chairman
Director of Skull Base Surgery
Department of Head and Neck Surgery
Medical Director Head and Neck Center
University of Texas Anderson Cancer Center
Houston, Texas, USA

Sheng-Po Hao MD FACS FICS
Professor and Chairman
Department of Otolaryngology Head and
Neck Surgery
Director
Comprehensive Oral Cancer Center
Shin Kong Wu Ho-Su Memorial Hospital
Professor and Program Director
School of Medicine, Fu-Jen University
Taiwan
Secretary General
Asian Society of Head and Neck Oncology
(ASHNO)

Gady Har-EI MD FACS
Chairman, Department of Otolaryngology
Head and Neck Surgery, Lenox Hill Hospital
Professor of Otolaryngology and
Neurosurgery
SUNY-Downstate Medical Center
New York, USA

Shin Kong Wu Ho-Su
Memorial Hospital
Professor and Program Director
School of Medicine, Fu-Jen University
Taiwan
Secretary General
Asian Society of Head and Neck Oncology
(ASHNO)

N Gopalakrishna Iyer MBBS PhD FRCS
Consultant Head and Neck Surgeon,
Department of Surgical Oncology, National
Cancer Centre Singapore
Assistant Professor, Duke-NUS Graduate
Medical School, Singapore

Adam S Jacobson MD
Assistant Professsor
Albert Einstein College of Medicine
Attending, Department of Otolaryngology -
Head and Neck Surgery
Beth Israel Medical Center
10 Union Square East, Suite 5B
New York, NY, USA

Ilana Kaplan
Director of the Oral Pathology Service
Tel-Aviv Sourasky Medical Center, Tel-Aviv
Senior Lecturer in Pathology, Sackler School
of Medicine, Tel-Aviv University, Israel

Peter J Koltai MD FACS
Professor and Chief
Division of Pediatric Otolaryngology
Stanford University School of Medicine
Lucile Packard Children's Hospital

Moshe Kon
Division of Plastic,
Reconstructive and Hand Surgery,
Utrecht University Medical Center,
Utrecht, The Netherlands

Dennis Kraus
Director,
Center for Head and Neck Oncology
New York Head and neck Institute
North Shore-LIJ Cancer Institute
New York, NY, USA

Shih-Wei Kuo FRACS
Otolaryngology/ Head and Neck Surgeon
Macquarie University Hospital
3 Technology place, Macquarie University,
NSW, Australia

Jean Louis Lefebvre
Head and Neck Department
Centre Oscar Lambret 3, rue Combemale,
Lille, France

David Leshem
Department of Plastic and Reconstructive
Surgery,
The Tel-Aviv Sourasky Medical Center,
Tel-Aviv, Israel

Carol M Lewis MD MPH
Assistant Professor
Department of Head and Neck Surgery
University of Texas, MD Anderson Cancer
Center
1515 Holcombe Blvd, Unit 1445
Houston, Texas, USA

Peter Li MD
Clinical Assistant Professor,
Department of Otolaryngology—Head and
Neck Surgery,
Stanford Hospitals and Clinics

Roberto Araujo Lima MD PhD
Attending Surgeon
Head and Neck Service
Brazilian National Cancer Institute
Associate Professor, Department of Head
and Neck Surgery
Postgraduate School of Medicine
Catholic University of Rio de Janeiro, Brazil

Pavan S Mallur MD
Instructor, Otology and Laryngology
Harvard Medical School
Beth Israel Deaconess Medical Center
110 Francis Street, Suite 6E
Boston, Massachusetts, USA

Valentina Manciocco
Department of Otolaryngology Head and
Neck Surgery
National Cancer Institute Regina Elena
Via E. Chianesi 53
Rome, Italy

Paolo Marchesi
Department of Otolaryngology Head and
Neck Surgery
National Cancer Institute Regina Elena
Via E. Chianesi, Rome, Italy

Nevo Margalit
Vice Chairman and Head of the Skull Base
Service
Neurosurgery, Tel-Aviv Medical Center
Israel

Gabriele Materazzi MD
Department of Surgery, University of Pisa
Ospedale Cisanello Ed 30A 2nd Floor
Via Paradisa 2, Pisa, Italy

Giuseppe Mercante
Department of Otolaryngology Head and
Neck Surgery
National Cancer Institute Regina Elena
Via E. Chianesi
Rome, Italy

Paolo Miccoli MD FACS
Department of Surgery, University of Pisa
Ospedale Cisanello Ed 30A 2nd Floor
Via Paradisa 2, Pisa, Italy

Ehud Miller
Department of Plastic and Reconstructive
Surgery,
The Tel-Aviv Sourasky Medical Center,
Tel-Aviv, Israel

Eugene N Myers MD FACS, FRCS Edn (Hon)
Distinguished Professor and Emeritus Chair
Department of Otolaryngology
University of Pittsburgh
Pittsburgh, Pennsylvania, USA

Oded Nahlieli DMD
Professor and Chairman, Department of
Oral and Maxillofacial Surgery, Barzilai
Medical Center, Ashkelon Israel affiliated
to the Faculty of Medicine Ben Gurion
University of the Negev, Beer Sheba,
ISRAEL. Associate Professor Michigan
University, Michigan, USA

Piero Nicolai MD
Professor and Chief
Department of Otolaryngology—Head and
Neck Surgery
University of Brescia
Spedali Civili of Brescia
Piazza, Spedali Civili 1, Brescia, Italy

Erez Nossek
Young attendings
Neurosurgery
Tel-Aviv Medical Center, Israel

Raul Pellini
Department of Otolaryngology Head and
Neck Surgery
National Cancer Institute Regina Elena
Via E. Chianesi 53
Rome, Italy

Giorgio Peretti
Professor and Chief
Department of Otolaryngology—Head and
Neck Surgery
University of Genoa
Ospedale San Martino
Largo Rosanna Benzi 8
Genoa, Italy

Cesare Piazza
Assistant Professor
Department of Otolaryngology—Head and
Neck Surgery
University of Brescia
Spedali
Civili of Brescia 1, Brescia, Italy

Barbara Pichi
Department of Otolaryngology Head and
Neck Surgery
National Cancer Institute Regina Elena
Via E. Chianesi 53
Rome, Italy

Paolo Ruscito
Department of Otolaryngology Head and
Neck Surgery
National Cancer Institute Regina Elena
Via E. Chianesi 53
Rome, Italy

Mordechai Sela DMD
Professor of Prosthodontics, Department of
Maxillofacial Prosthetics,
Hebrew University Hadassah Medical
Center, Jerusalem, Israel

Jatin P Shah MD PhD FACS Hon FRCS(Edin)
Hon FDSRCS(Lon) HonFRACS
Professor of Surgery
Elliot W Strong Chair in Head and Neck
Oncology,
Chief, Head and Neck Program,
Memorial Sloan Kettering Cancer Center,
New York, NY, USA

Manish D Shah MD MPhil FRCSC
Assistant Professor
Department of Otolaryngology Head and
Neck Surgery
University of Toronto
Toronto, Canada

Ashok R Shaha MD
Professor of Surgery
Jatin P. Shah Chairman in Head and Neck
Surgery,
Memorial Sloan Kettering Cancer Center,
New York, USA

Tal Shahar
Young Attendings
Neurosurgery
Tel-Aviv Medical Center, Israel

Yuval Shapira
Young attendings
Neurosurgery
Tel-Aviv Medical Center, Israel

Anat Buller Sharon DMD MSc
Clinical Lecturer
Department of Maxillofacial Prosthetics,
Hebrew University Hadassah Medical
Center, Jerusalem, Israel

Benjamin Shlomi DMD
Head of Oral and Maxillofacial Surgery Unit
Department of Otolaryngoloy Head and
Neck surgery, Tel-Aviv Sourasky Medical
Center
Israel

Giuseppe Spriano
Professor and Chief
Department of Otolaryngology Head and
Neck Surgery
National Cancer Institute Regina Elena
Via E. Chianesi 53
Rome, Italy

Amir Szold MD
Medical Director
Assia Medical Group,
Tel-Aviv, Israel

Valentina Terenzi MD
Department of Otolaryngology Head and
Neck Surgery
National Cancer Institute Regina Elena
Via E. Chianesi 53
Rome, Italy

Mark L Urken MD
Professor of Otolaryngology Albert Einstein
College of Medicine
Director of Head and Neck Surgery
Continuum Cancer Center
CoDirector Institute Head and Neck and
Thyroid Cancer
Beth Israel Medical Center
10 Union Square East, Suite 5B
New York, New York, USA

Fernando Walder MD PhD
Assistant Professor -
ENT and Head and Neck Department
Federal University of São Paulo

Oshri Wasserzug MD
Department of Pediatric Otolaryngology
UT Southwestern Medical Center
Children's Medical Center,
Dallas, Texas, USA

Randal S Weber MD
Professor and Chairman
Department of Head and Neck Surgery,
University of Texas, USA MD
Anderson Cancer Center
Holcombe Blvd, Houston, Texas, USA

Fu Chan Wei
Department of Plastic and Reconstructive
Surgery,
Chang Gung Memorial Hospital, Taipei,
Chang Gung University Medical College,
Taoyuan, Taiwan, Japan

William Ignace Wei MS FRCS FRCSE FRACS
(Hon) FACS(Hon)
FHKAM(ORL)(Surg)
Head Department of Surgery
Director Li Shu Pui ENT Head and Neck
Surgery Centre
Hong Kong Sanatorium & Hospital
Hong Kong SAR China

Jochen A Werner MD
Department of Otolaryngology,
Head and Neck Surgery
University of Marburg, Germany

Jochen A Werner
Professor and Chairman
Department of Otolaryngology, Head and
Neck Surgery
Philipps University of Marburg
Baldingerstraße, Marburg

Arik Zaretzki
Department of Plastic and
Reconstructive Surgery,
The Tel-Aviv Sourasky Medical Center,
Tel-Aviv, Israel

Jose P Zevallos MD
University of Medicine and Dentistry
New Jersey, USA

Daniel Zikk MD
Otolaryngology Head and Neck Surgery
Deputy Director
Department of Otolaryngology Head and
Neck and Maxillofacial Surgery.
Tel-Aviv Medical Center,
Tel-Aviv University, Israel

Ron Zuker MD FRCS(C) FACS FAAP
The Hospital for Sick Children
Toronto, Canada

Preface

A picture is worth a thousand words. This wonderfully illustrated *Atlas of Head and Neck Surgery* aptly brings this statement to life. This atlas serves as an introduction to those about to embark on this wonderful journey of learning head and neck surgery. Since the book is written and illustrated by all the very eminent personalities in this field, it serves all those who are in the field, right from the novice all the way up to the accomplished surgeon. For the novice, this is a baptismal introduction. While for the accomplished specialist, it provides valuable insights into the various advances that have blossomed in this area. The editors and authors have worked hard and unselfishly to teach through this atlas.

As the series editor, I thank and congratulate the eminent editors and all the very eminent authors for all their efforts, time and expertize they have given to this project. I am sure all those who read this atlas will understand better all the various dimensions that go into head and neck surgery. It is the goal of every physician to serve his patient better. This book is directed at helping that physician accomplish this goal.

Chris de Souza
Series Editor

Preface

The head and neck is located in a confluence of vital structures. It is also one of the last zones to be explored surgically. It is unique not only because of its complex anatomy but also due to the large variety of tumors, which originate in this region. Recently with the welcome infusion of new surgical approaches and radiology techniques, we have witnessed a significant improvement not only in survival of patients with head and neck tumors, but also with the preservation and improvement of their quality of life.

As more clinicians from different disciplines are entering the field of head and neck oncology, there is a need for systemic illustration of the surgical techniques used for treatment of patients with benign and malignant neoplasms, and for those with inflammatory and infectious diseases located in this region. This surgical atlas was contemplated to provide accessible and comprehensive knowledge of state of the art surgical techniques used for extirpation of head and neck tumors, and it requires no prior knowledge in the field. The atlas also presents contemporary reconstruction and rehabilitation techniques, which are frequently used in head and neck cancer patients.

Although the emphasis is on the surgical techniques, we have tried to introduce all the major ideas that a physician involved in treating these patients would be expected to know—with the highlight of important anatomical and technical issue in head and neck surgery.

While some books give an excellent introduction to head and neck surgery, they use either intraoperative pictures or cartoons for elimination of technical issues related to either resection of reconstruction of head and neck tumors. On the other hand, this atlas presents step-by-step illustrations of the operation, from preparation and incision to the last step of reconstruction. The *cook-book* format of this atlas also utilizes alongside intraoperative pictures and cartoons, to facilitate learning and understanding of the techniques. Finally, major classical and contemporary references are given at the end of each chapter allowing guidance for those who are interested in further reading.

Many of our renowned teachers and colleagues contributed to the development of this book, which is the result of years of training and treating patients. Some of the chapters are written by experts who designed and established the techniques themselves. This book too owes much to the physicians, nurses and paramedical team which are committed to the multidisciplinary team spirit management of head and neck patients.

Ziv Gil
Dan M Fliss
Volume Editors

Acknowledgments

We express our deep appreciation for the editorial assistance and hardwork of Ms Payal Bharti and the creative drawings of Mr Hoshank. The editors express their gratitude to M/s Jaypee Brothers Medical Publishers (P) Ltd, New Delhi, India, for without their dedication, this book would not have been completed.

Contents

Chapter 1

The Midfacial Degloving Approach

Pavan S Mallur, Gady Har-El

INTRODUCTION

The concept of midfacial degloving was first introduced by Portmann and Retrouvey in 1927, when they described an intraoral sublabial approach to the maxillary sinus.[1] Converse latera later expanded this approach in 1950, when he reported on the use of a sublabial incision for unilateral reconstruction of the midfacial skeleton.[2] Despite these advances in midfacial surgery, it was not until 1974 that Casson et al. combined the sublabial incision with the intranasal, intercartilaginous, and full transfixion incisions to perform a full midfacial degloving.[3] Since the 1970s, the modern version of this technique has been popularized by Conley,[4] Price,[5,6] Maniglia and Phillips.[7]

The midfacial degloving (MFD) approach combines the sublabial incision used in external approaches to sinus surgery with intranasal incisions used in cosmetic rhinologic surgery. It should be emphasized that this is an approach, not an isolated surgical procedure, that results in a wide exposure of the nasal cavity, all paranasal sinuses, midfacial skeleton and the anterior cranial base. Obvious advantages of this approach over conventional lateral rhinotomy, Weber-Ferguson or transpalatal incisions, include avoidance of disfiguring facial incisions, extensive bilateral exposure and preservation of functional oral cavity and oropharyngeal anatomy. The MFD technique, as such provides a cosmetically and functionally superior result in an approach that is useful for both extirpative and reconstructive procedures.[8-11]

Since its advent, the indications have expanded to include a number of procedures for various pathologic entities. Traditionally, the approach has proven useful for benign but locally destructive lesions, such as inverted papilloma,[12,13] juvenile angiofibroma,[10] odontogenic cysts and neoplasms, vascular lesions and benign fibro-osseous lesions.[14-17] Additionally, the approach has been described for the treatment of midfacial trauma, naso-orbitoethmoid (NOE) fractures and orbital floor reconstruction.[18-20] Though less utilized, the MFD approach is also useful for selected sinonasal malignancies, as long as the exposure does not limit the extent of negative margins in resection.[14,15] In the cases of large malignancies that encroach on the skull base or have a large dural interface, combining the MFD approach with subfrontal or frontal craniotomy may provide the necessary exposure for complete en bloc resection of the malignancy. Regions that may be approached with the MFD include frontal and sphenoid sinuses, anterior cranial base, clivus and pterygopalatine space.[8-11]

PREOPERATIVE EVALUATION AND ANESTHESIA

Preoperative work-up prior to planned midfacial degloving is generally dictated by the disease entity. For inflammatory lesions or benign neoplasms, computed tomography (CT) scanning at minimum, helps to delineate the bony extent and the skull base involvement. While soft tissue delineation may be aided with CT scanning with intravenous (IV) contrast, magnetic resonance imaging (MRI) is generally superior to CT in this respect, especially when evaluating benign or malignant neoplasms. Evaluation of soft tissue extent, identification of paranasal sinus secretions or obstruction, perineural invasion, periorbital invasion and dural involvement may all be identified accurately with

MRI scanning. When planning the extent of resection, preoperative biopsy or intraoperative frozen section may help in surgical planning.

Anesthetic technique and patient preparation involve standard precautions for general anesthesia. General orotracheal intubation is typically preferred. After placement of ointment on the cornea, bilateral tarsorrhaphy sutures are placed with 6-0 nylon sutures through the conjunctival edge of the lids. Care is taken to avoid placement of the suture through the external skin aspect to avoid lash inversion and subsequent corneal abrasion.

Local anesthetic should be used extensively prior to the onset of the procedure to induce vasoconstriction and to facilitate dissection. Generally, 30–40 ml of 1:200,000 epinephrine suffices for this. We perform intraoral infiltration of the sublabial region and greater palatine foramen. Similar to rhinoplasty technique, endonasal infiltration through the intercartilaginous space is performed in the area of the nasal bones, nasal dorsum, glabella, nasomaxillary grooves and medial canthal regions. Transcutaneous infiltration of the frontal bones and medial orbital walls is also performed.

SURGICAL TECHNIQUES

The MFD approach begins with the intranasal portion of the procedure. A complete transfixion incision is made and connected bilaterally with a complete intercartilaginous incision. This effectively separates the upper lateral cartilages from the lower lateral cartilages, the latter of which will be included with the superiorly retracted flap. Extensive undermining through the intercartilaginous incision should be performed bilaterally over the anterior wall of the maxillary sinus and superiorly over the frontal bone, releasing the soft tissue envelope from the nasal skeleton and septal angle. The intercartilaginous incision is then continued caudally and medially through the periosteum of the nasal floor and pyriform aperture and connected to the transfixion incision (Fig. 1). This will complete the circumvestibular incisions of the procedure.

The next part of the procedure involves "degloving" of the facial soft tissues from the nasal skeleton and maxilla. A sublabial incision is made 4–6 mm above the teeth from first molar to first molar. Additional exposure may be attained by extending the incision ipsilaterally to the third molar. In addition to wider exposure, this may facilitate ligation of the internal maxillary artery, if this is planned. Dissection proceeds in the subperiosteal plane over the alveolus and maxilla, connecting with the previous plane of dissection through the intercartilaginous incision. Care must be taken to preserve each infraorbital bundle during this dissection. This effectively separates the skin envelope, lower lateral cartilages and upper lip from the bony midface. Additional dissection may proceed laterally over each zygoma and superiorly over the frontal bone. Superior retraction is obtained by placing two Penrose drains, one through each nostril and around the upper lip. This should be released periodically, every 20–30 minutes to allow reperfusion of the central lip. At this point, the degloving portion is complete and any remaining procedure may proceed with this wide exposure as in Figure 2.

The authors have described one modification of the original procedure with the aim of preventing postoperative vestibular stenosis. After completion of the degloving

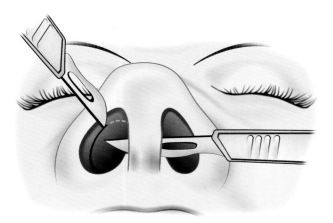

Fig. 1: Circumvestibular intranasal incisions. Note transfixion incision combined with intercartilaginous and caudal/nasal floor incisions

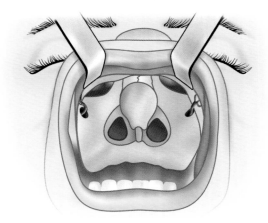

Fig. 2: Completed midfacial degloving approach. Note wide exposure to bilateral anterior maxillary walls, zygoma, nasal bones and glabella. Note preservation of the infraorbital neurovascular bundle

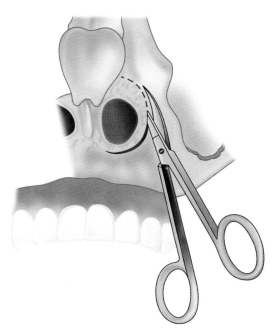

Fig. 3: Creation of the bipedicled vestibular skin flap caudal to the upper lateral cartilages and at the edge of the bony nasal aperture

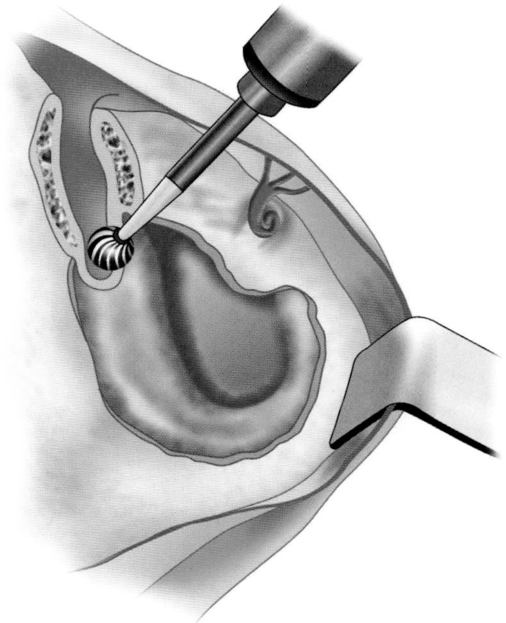

Fig. 4: Removal of the anterior bony nasolacrimal canal. Use of the mastoid drill facilitates exposure of the nasolacrimal duct approximately 1.5 cm inferior to the orbital rim

portion, an 8–12 mm bipedicled flap of inner nasal vestibular skin is created. This is achieved by creating an incision caudal to the upper lateral cartilages and nasal bones and extending toward the pyriform aperture and onto the nasal floor (Fig. 3). This flap is reapproximated to the free edge of the circumvestibular incision at the completion of the procedure, thus preventing postoperative nasal vestibule stenosis and retraction.

As mentioned previously, this approach facilitates excellent exposure for blunt and penetrating midface trauma. Access to bilateral medial and lateral buttresses, as well as horizontal buttresses is achieved readily. Open reduction and rigid fixation of Le Fort, medial and lateral orbital rim, orbital floor and zygomatic fractures can subsequently be attained.

Commonly, this approach is utilized for medial maxillectomy for benign and malignant neoplastic processes or for exposure to deeper spaces, such as the pterygopalatine fossa, sphenoid sinus, nasopharynx and middle skull base. The classic description of the medial maxillectomy involves en bloc resection of the lateral nasal wall, the medial 25–35% of the orbital floor and rim, lamina papyracea along with lacrimal fossa. Modifications include preservation of a bony framework of the inferior orbital rim and lateral pyriform aperture or removal of this frame with replacement and

rigid fixation with microplates at the end of the procedure. These modifications were developed to improve bony facial contour, though the authors have found similar cosmetic results by preserving the nasal bones, alveolus and 65–75% of the orbital rim.

As a common procedure, the authors will describe the medial maxillectomy in detail in this section. Medial maxillectomy begins with removal of the anterior wall of the maxillary sinus. This is best achieved with Kerrison Rongeurs with bone removal starting inferomedially and continuing superomedially toward the ethmoid air cells and superolaterally toward the zygomatic arch. Care must be taken to protect and preserve the infraorbital nerve. This is best done by leaving a narrow bony ledge around the infraorbital foramen. Once this is performed, the nasolacrimal sac and duct are addressed. This can be managed by simple transection at the level of the orbital rim, with or without stenting. However, the author's preferred technique is to remove the anterior bone of the nasolacrimal bony canal with a mastoid drill or fine Kerrison Rongeur, starting at the orbital rim and proceeding 10–15 mm inferiorly. The authors then mobilize the nasolacrimal duct and transect it distally (Fig. 4). The nasolacrimal duct is subsequently removed from the canal. The duct is then splayed with two opposing longitudinal cuts

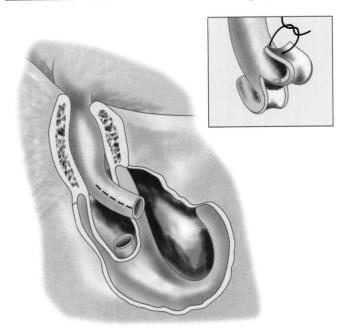

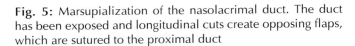

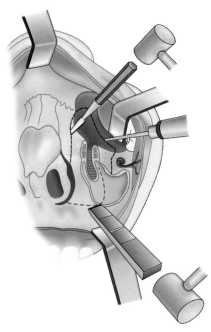

Fig. 5: Marsupialization of the nasolacrimal duct. The duct has been exposed and longitudinal cuts create opposing flaps, which are sutured to the proximal duct

Fig. 6: Creation of medial maxillectomy osteotomies. Note the anterior maxillary wall has been removed. Osteotomies proceed from a superomedial cut and then connect with oblique (orbital floor), inferior (nasal/maxillary floor) and posterior cuts

and the distal ends everted and sutured with 5-0 absorbable sutures to the remainder of the duct (Fig. 5). This prevents postoperative stenosis. Prior to bony cuts, the authors create a bipedicled flap of vestibular skin as previously described. Following this, conventional osteotomies are performed (Fig. 6). A cut is made along the nasal bone from the pyriform aperture to the glabella and connected to a posteriorly directed cut along or below and parallel to the frontoethmoidal suture line. The posterior extent of this frontoethmoidal cut is then connected to an oblique cut ending at the orbital rim, medial to the infraorbital foramen.

Medial osteotomies are made along the floor of the nasal cavity, separating the lateral nasal wall. Soft tissue cuts follow each bony osteotomy, freeing the specimen stepwise. The final cut is made with curved osteotomies or heavy curved scissors, freeing the specimen from the posterolateral nasal wall and ascending process of the palatine bone. This invariably exposes a bleeding sphenopalatine artery, which can be ligated directly. Alternatively, this can be addressed by ligating the internal maxillary artery in the pterygopalatine fossa after removing the ascending process of the palatine bone.

Special consideration can be given to other anatomical areas once the medial maxillectomy is complete. Orbital contents are exposed and the optic nerve may be exposed through systematic drill out toward the optic foramen.

The pterygopalatine fossa, infratemporal fossa and middle cranial fossa skull base can similarly be exposed by removing the posterior and lateral maxilla. Anterior sphenoidotomy can give wide access to the sella turcica and carotid artery. The anterior cranial base can be exposed through middle turbinate excision, though conventional literature supports need for frontal craniotomy or subfrontal approach for en bloc removal of neoplasms encroaching or involving the anterior cranial base. Traditional limitations for the MFD in accessing the frontal sinus can be overcome by performing ethmoidectomy first and then by detaching the medial canthal tendon to provide additional superiorly based soft tissue retraction. This maneuver allows complete exposure of the frontal sinus by removing its floor in a posterior-to-anterior direction, starting at the frontal outflow tract. Though rarely needed, an additional exposure can be obtained by removing the anterior frontal sinus wall in an inferomedial-to-superolateral direction.

At the conclusion of the extirpative procedure, the maxillectomy cavity is packed with antibiotic impregnated packing strips. Meticulous attention is paid to the previously mentioned intranasal and sublabial incisions. The intranasal incisions are closed with fine absorbable sutures with attention to proper alignment, projection and rotation. The sublabial incisions can be closed with 3-0 absorbable sutures. A nasal dorsal splint helps to reduce the postoperative edema.

POSTOPERATIVE TREATMENT

Postoperative considerations are similar to that of traditional approaches to the midfacial skeleton. Packing is removed in 1–3 days or may be left longer if formal craniotomy is combined with the MFD approach. Antibiotics are used while nasal packing is in place. Nasolacrimal stents, if placed, may be removed within 4–6 weeks. Aggressive nasal irrigation is begun immediately after packing is removed to facilitate debridement and prevent nasal crusting. In-office endoscopic-assisted debridement, akin to routine postoperative endoscopic sinus surgery debridement, may be helpful in reducing crusting.

HIGHLIGHTS

I. Indications
- Benign nasal cavity and paranasal sinus lesions (inverted papilloma, juvenile angiofibroma, and odontogenic and vascular lesions)
- Selected malignant nasal cavity and paranasal sinus lesions
- Facial trauma (midface fractures, NOE fractures, orbital floor reconstruction).

II. Contraindications
- None.

III. Special Preoperative Considerations
- Computed tomography (CT) scanning for evaluation of bony involvement (with special consideration to cranial base)
- Magnetic resonance imaging scanning to delineate soft tissue extent, periorbital invasion, dural involvement and to differentiate tumor from postobstructive inflammatory changes.

IV. Special Intraoperative Considerations
- Creation of bipedicled vestibular skin flap reduces risk of vestibular stenosis
- Marsupialization of the nasolacrimal duct prevents postoperative epiphora and obviates the need for stenting
- Detachment of medial canthal tendon facilitates superior exposure (reapproximation prevents postoperative telecanthus).

V. Special Postoperative Considerations
- Nasal packing for 1–3 days is generally sufficient
- Postoperative crusting and nasal congestion is common and should be expected
- Aggressive nasal irrigation and in-office debridement may alleviate symptoms.

VI. Complications
- Nasal crusting and congestion (reduced with irrigation)
- Facial hypesthesia or anesthesia (prolonged in less than 1% of cases)
- Oroantral fistula
- Epiphora from nasolacrimal stenosis
- Vestibular stenosis (reduced to 0.5% with bipedicled vestibular flap)
- Cranial nerve injury, dural injury, cerebral injury, CSF leak, pneumocephalus
- Esthetic changes to the nose.

REFERENCES

1. Portmann G, Retrouvey H. Le Cancer Du Nez, Gaston Doin et Cie, Paris. 1927.
2. Converse JM. Restoration of facial contour by bone grafts introduced through oral cavity. Plast Reconstr Surg. 1950;6(4):295-300.
3. Casson PR, Bonnano PC, Converse JM. The midfacial degloving procedure. Plast Reconstr Surg. 1974;53(1):102-3.
4. Conley JJ, Price JC. Sublabial approach to the nasal and nasopharyngeal cavities. Am J Surg. 1979;138(4):615-8.
5. Price JC. The midfacial degloving approach to the central skull base. Ear Nose Throat J. 1986;65(4):174-80.
6. Price JC, Holliday MJ, Johns ME, et al. The versatile midfacial degloving approach. Laryngoscope. 1988;98(3):291-5.
7. Maniglia AJ, Phillips DA. Midfacial degloving for the management of nasal, sinus and skull-base neoplasms. Otolaryngol Clin North Am. 1995;28(6):1127-43.
8. Har-El G, Lucente FE. Midfacial degloving approach to the nose, sinuses and skull base. Am J Rhinol. 1996;10:17-22.
9. Har-El G. Medial maxillectomy via midfacial degloving approach. Op Tech Otolaryngol Head Neck Surg. 1999;10:82-6.
10. Har-El G. Management of juvenile angiofibroma via midfacial degloving with medial maxillectomy. Op Tech Otolaryngol Head Neck Surg. 1999;10:107-8.
11. Har-El G. Anterior craniofacial resection without facial skin incisions—a review. Otolarygnol Head Neck Surg. 2004;130(6):780-7.
12. Buchwald C, Franzmann MB, Tos M. Sinonasal papillomas: a report of 82 cases in Copenhagen County, including a longitudinal epidemiological and clinical study. Laryngoscope. 1995;105(1):72-9.
13. Lawson W, Kaufman MR, Biller HF. Treatment outcomes in the management of inverted papilloma: an analysis of 160 cases. Laryngoscope. 2003;113(9):1548-56.
14. Howard DJ, Lund VJ. The midfacial degloving approach to sinonasal disease. J Laryngol Otol. 1992;106(12):1059-62.
15. Howard DJ, Lund VJ. The role of midfacial degloving in modern rhinological practice. J Laryngol Otol. 1999;113(10):885-7.

16. Maniglia AJ. Indications and techniques of midfacial degloving. A 15-year experience. Arch Otolaryngol Head Neck Surg. 1986;112(7):750-2.

17. Maniglia AJ, Phillips DA. Midfacial degloving for the management of nasal, sinus, and skull-base neoplasms. Otolaryngol Clin North Am. 1995;28(6):1127-43.

18. Baumann A, Ewers R. Midfacial degloving: an alternative approach for traumatic corrections in the midface. Int J Oral Maxillofac Surg. 2001;30(4):272-7.

19. Browne JD. Skull base tumor surgery: The midfacial degloving procedure for nasal, sinus, and nasopharyngeal tumors. Otolaryngol Clin North Am. 2001;34(6):1095-10 1201.

20. Cultrara A, Turk JB, Har-El G. Midfacial degloving approach for repair of naso-orbitoethmoid and midfacial fractures. Arch Facial Plast Surg. 2004;6(2):133-5.

ADDITIONAL READING

1. Browne JD. Skull base tumor surgery: The midfacial degloving procedure for nasal, sinus, and nasopharyngeal tumors. Otolaryngol Clin North Am. 2001;34(6):1095-104,viii.

2. Cultrara A, Turk JB, Har-El G. Midfacial degloving approach for repair of naso-orbitoethmoid and midfacial fractures. Arch Facial Plast Surg. 2004;6(2):133-5.

3. Har-El G. Anterior craniofacial resection without facial skin incisions—a review. Otolarygnol Head Neck Surg. 2004;130(6):780-7.

4. Har-El G, Lucente FE. Midfacial degloving approach to the nose, sinuses and skull base. Am J Rhinol. 1996;10:17-22.

5. Har-El G. Medial maxillectomy via midfacial degloving approach. Op Tech Otolaryngol Head Neck Surg. 1999;10:82-6.

Chapter 2

Maxillary Swing Approach to Central Skull Base

William Ignace Wei

INTRODUCTION

The central skull base includes the nasopharynx, the sphenoid sinus, paranasopharyngeal space, pterygoid plates and laterally it extends to the medial aspect of the condyle of mandible. The region is located in the center of the head and is over 10 cm deep from the skin surface in all directions. It is difficult to expose this region adequately for surgical resection of pathologies; this is particularly so when the lesion is malignant and has infiltrated nearby structures.

The concept of maxillary swing approach to the central skull base originated from the observation that during maxillectomy for carcinoma of the maxillary antrum, the central skull base was widely exposed when the maxilla bone was removed. Then this anterolateral approach was developed; the maxillary antrum, including the lateral wall and floor attached to the anterior cheek flap could be swung laterally as an osteocutaneous flap to expose the central skull base. After resection of the pathology in the region, the maxillary antrum could be returned to its original position and fixed to the facial skeleton.

The surgical approach involves a Weber-Ferguson facial incision as for maxillectomy, incision on the palate, osteotomies of the anterior wall, medial wall of the maxillary antrum and lower part of the zygomatic arch. The pterygoid plates are also separated from the maxillary tuberosity. This anterolateral approach exposes the central skull base on the side of the swing and with removal of the posterior part of the nasal septum; the exposure extends to the contralateral aspect. Theoretically, with a bilateral maxillary swing, the entire central skull base can be exposed adequately.

The maxillary swing approach to the central skull base is applicable for the resection of pathologies in the region, such as recurrent or residual nasopharyngeal carcinoma after chemoradiation and other tumors in the region, such as chordoma, sarcoma, melanoma and minor salivary gland tumor. Extensive benign pathologies in the central skull base can also be comfortably removed with this approach and this includes schwannoma, recurrent deep lobe parotid gland tumor. Patients with osteoradionecrosis of the central skull base may present with headache, bleeding or sepsis, with this approach; the necrotic bone can be removed and the defect could be covered with a microvascular free flap, which facilitates healing.

With the wide exposure of the region following the swing of the maxilla, the internal carotid artery lying in the paranasopharyngeal space can be identified visually or with palpation, thus avoiding its injury during tumor extirpation, especially during the dissection of the paranasopharyngeal lymph node. A microvascular free flap can also be employed to cover the exposed vessel and the raw area following removal of tumor. With this additional new vascular supply, further adjuvant therapy can be considered.

The morbidity associated with the operation was in general acceptable. The facial scar usually heals well and becomes less obvious with time. The development of significant trismus in patients who underwent previous radiation can be managed with passive stretching and this usually, is not a serious problem. With the resection of the eustachian tube, the patient frequently develops serous otitis media on the side of the swing and this will result in some hearing deterioration.

PREOPERATIVE EVALUATION AND ANESTHESIA

Patients undergoing the maxillary swing procedure need a full cardiopulmonary assessment to determine whether the patient can stand the procedure, as occasionally the blood loss may be significant. The interalveolar distance should be at least 3 cm; otherwise, it is difficult to raise the palatal flap and to insert the curved osteotome transorally to separate the pterygoid plates from maxillary tuberosity. The interalveolar distance also prompts an anesthetist to consider the appropriate route to insert the endotracheal tube. An upper alveolar dental plate (Fig. 1) is fabricated before the operation; this is used to clip onto the teeth on the upper alveolus with the return of the swung maxilla, thus ensuring the correct dental alignment.

The extent of preoperative evaluation of patient depends on the pathology. For benign lesions, in addition to a full clinical examination, an endoscopic examination of the nasal cavities, nasopharynx, oropharynx together with a cross sectional imaging study, such as computed tomography (CT) or magnetic resonance imaging (MRI) to determine the extent of the pathology, are essential. For malignant lesions, MRI with contrast is carried out to see the proximity of tumor to the internal carotid artery and involvement of other soft tissue in the regions, such as paranasopharyngeal lymph nodes. Computed tomography with bone window should be carried out to see whether the clivus or skull base bone is affected. For large primary tumor or tumor with high metastatic potential, positron emission tomography (PET) is indicated to rule out distant metastasis.

The operation is done under general anesthesia with the patient in supine position. The head lies on a head ring to allow turning and there is no need for support behind the shoulder to extend the neck, unless a neck dissection or neck exploration is also planned. Endotracheal intubation is carried out through the mouth, if possible, as this avoids disturbance of the nasopharynx pathology. Then a temporary tracheostomy is carried out and the endotracheal tube is withdrawn. The tracheostomy is optional, as the procedure can be carried out with the transoral endotracheal tube in position. The tube, however, interferes to a certain extent with raising of the palatal flap and osteotomy of the hard palate.

As the nose and nasopharynx is usually packed at the completion of the procedure and discharge from raw surface in the nasopharynx and oropharynx may lead to partial airway obstruction, a temporary tracheostomy aids to maintain the airway and if it is not done following endotracheal intubation, it is usually carried out at completion of the operation.

Eye ointment is placed in the contralateral eye, which is drafted off the operative field. The oral cavity and the nasal cavities are irrigated with copious amount of antiseptic solution, such as chlorohexidine. Preoperative intravenous antibiotics are given, which usually includes a metronidazole for anaerobic bacteria and a cephalosporin for aerobic organisms.

SURGICAL TECHNIQUES

Endoscopic examination to confirm the extent of the recurrent tumor in the nasopharynx is carried out before the incision (Fig. 2). The CT (Fig. 3) images are reviewed again to confirm that there is no involvement of skull base bone or the clivus. Detailed tumor extent is further ascertained with contrast MRI as in Figures 4 and 5.

The Weber-Ferguson facial incision (Fig. 6) is used. The horizontal limb is placed about 5 mm below and parallel to the edge of the lower eyelid. The incision over the lip is designed to be zigzag to prevent postoperative contracture. The horizontal limb curves down laterally along the skin crease to stop at about 0.5 cm above the lower edge of the zygomatic arch. Tarsorrhaphy is done for the eye on the side of swing to protect the cornea.

The lip incision on the lingual surface continues to extend posteriorly to stop between the two central incisors. The palatal wound is a curved incision placed at a distance of 0.5 mm from the teeth margin, continued posteriorly until the last molar tooth and then turned laterally behind it to stop just before reaching the buccal mucosa (Fig. 7). This allows an elevation of soft tissue and mucoperiosteum over the hard palate as a flap.

The skin incision over the face goes through skin, subcutaneous tissue and also the orbicularis oculi muscle (Fig. 8). The thin muscle is lifted together with the facial skin

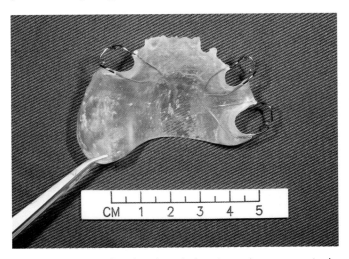

Fig. 1: An upper alveolus dental plate is made preoperatively, this will ensure accurate dental alignment when the maxilla is returned to its original position

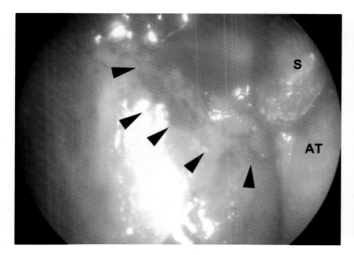

Fig. 2: Endoscopic view of left side recurrent nasopharyngeal carcinoma (arrowheads). The main tumor was partly covered by the medial crura of the auditory tube (AT), which is retracted by the tip of the metal sucker (S)

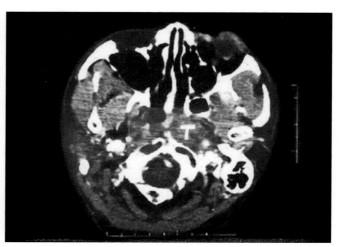

Fig. 3: Computed tomography showing the tumor (T), there was no bone erosion

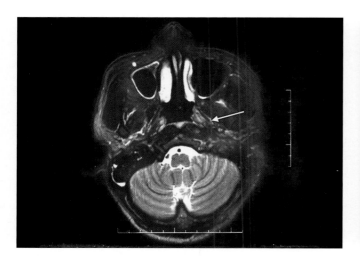

Fig. 4: Magnetic resonance imaging showing the extent of the abnormal soft tissue (arrow), it is clearer than the image of computed tomography in Figure 3

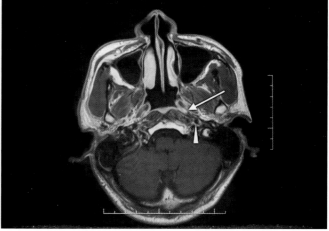

Fig. 5: Contrast magnetic resonance imaging, showing clearly the deep infiltrative extent of the tumor (arrow), which is not affecting the internal carotid artery (arrowhead)

until the orbital rim is reached. Lifting the muscle with the skin maintains the blood supply of the overlying skin and this is particularly important, if the patient has previous radiation treatment. Care is taken to avoid cutting the orbital septum or else the periorbital fat will herniate into the wound. If it happens, it is not harmful; but becomes a nuisance during the elevation of the facial flap. The skin incision over the lip is continued and the orbicularis oculi muscle is divided in the line of skin incision. The labial vessels encountered during the dissection are divided and tied as in Figure 9.

The incision on the anterior cheek goes down to the anterior wall of the maxilla. Limited amount of soft tissue

over the anterior wall of the maxilla is elevated to expose just the strip of bone for osteotomy (Fig 10). The osteotomy site is 0.5 cm below the inferior orbital rim, it sometimes goes through the infraorbital foramen. The infraorbital nerve is identified and divided between clamps. This reduces blood loss when the oscillating saw cuts through the infraorbital foramen.

The osteotomy over the anterior wall of maxilla extends horizontally, laterally to middle part of the zygomatic arch and then turns downwards through the lower edge of the arch. Only the lower part of the zygomatic arch is divided and after the completion of the osteotomy, the inferior

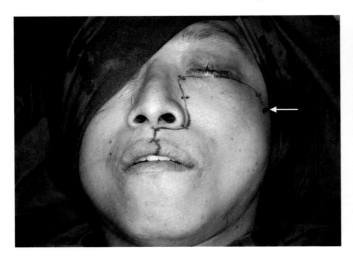

Fig. 6: Weber-Ferguson incision on the face is marked and tattoo points are made along the incision at the critical points to facilitate precise skin apposition on closure of the facial wound. The lower edge of the zygoma is also marked (arrow)

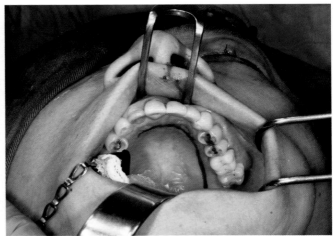

Fig. 7: The incision on the palate is shown, posteriorly it curves laterally behind the last molar tooth

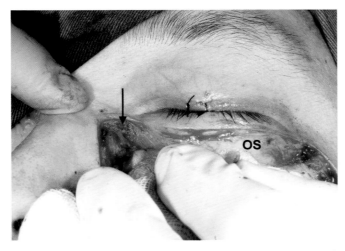

Fig. 8: The facial skin incision includes the orbicularis oculi muscle (arrow), which is elevated with the flap. The orbital septum (OS) is not disturbed

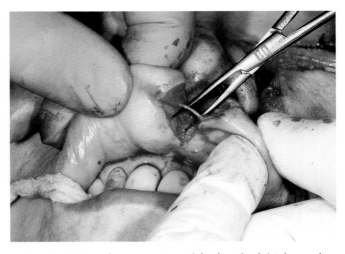

Fig. 9: During the separation of the lip, the labial vessel is identified and divided

orbital rim remains attached to the facial skeleton through the zygoma as in Figure 11.

Before the osteotomy, a four-hole titanium plate is placed across the osteotomy line, holes are drilled, screws are inserted and then removed. These drilled holes before osteotomy will ensure accurate position of the maxilla bone when it will be returned to its original position, after tumor resection. After removal of the screws, the holes are marked with gentian violet to facilitate their identification (Fig. 12). The soft tissue over the midline is elevated to expose the underlying bone, during planning for a midline osteotomy.

Sometimes the patient may have a high nasal spine (Fig. 13), this can be removed with a burr or a rongeur (Fig. 14), creating a flat bony surface where the second titanium plate can be placed. Holes are drilled and screws are inserted and removed. This procedure is similar to the plate over the zygomatic arch. Sometimes with a high nasal spine, a five-hole titanium plate may be used, as the elevated bone will take up some length of the plate.

Before osteotomies are carried out, soft tissue and mucoperiosteum over the hard palate have to be lifted off the bony hard palate (Fig. 15). The palatal wound is incised down

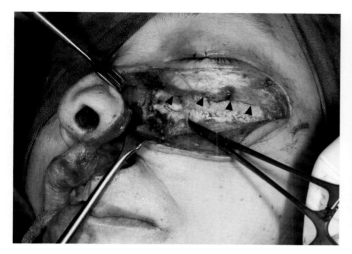

Fig. 10: Limited amount of soft tissue is lifted over the anterior wall of the maxilla to expose a narrow strip of anterior wall of the maxilla for osteotomy, which is about 0.5 cm below the inferior orbital margin (arrowheads). The infraorbital nerve is identified and divided before the osteotomy

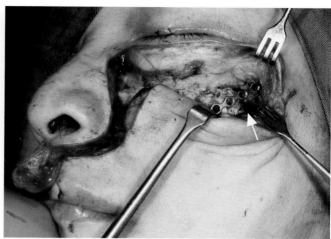

Fig. 11: The lower border of the zygomatic arch is identified (arrow). The planned osteotomy on the anterior wall of the maxilla extends laterally towards the middle of the zygomatic arch and then turned down to divide the lower part of the zygomatic arch. A four-hole titanium plate is placed across the planned osteotomy line

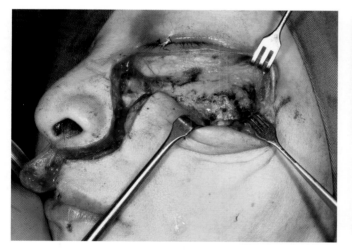

Fig. 12: The holes were drilled before osteotomy screws were inserted and removed, the screw holes are marked with gentian violet

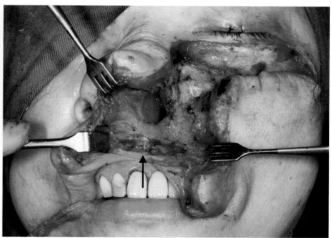

Fig. 13: The patient has a high nasal spine (arrow)

to bone and the soft tissue together with the mucoperiosteum is lifted with a sharp periosteal elevator. This elevation is done with the elevator scrapping on the bony hard palate. As long as the dissection is close to bone, the flap can be lifted intact, thereby showing the greater palatine vessels coming through the palatine foramen (Fig. 16). This is divided and then the palatal flap can be raised further, going medially across the midline and posteriorly to reach the posterior edge of the hard palate. The attachment of the soft palate on the

hard palate is divided with diathermy and the nasal cavity is entered (Fig. 17). A curved osteotome (Figs 18A and B) is inserted into the groove between the maxillary tuberosity and the pterygoid plates. The groove lies posterolaterally behind the hamulus, which can be palpated with finger. The osteotome has to be curved so that when it is placed in the groove and driven by the mallet, it goes vertically upwards separating the posterior wall of the maxillary antrum from the pterygoid plates as in Figure 19.

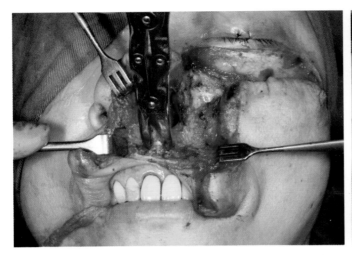

Fig. 14: The high nasal spine is removed and creates a flat surface to apply the titanium plate for a midline osteotomy

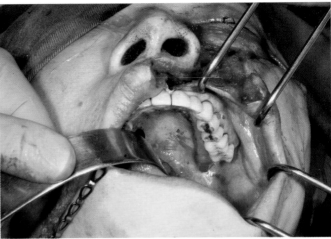

Fig. 15: The incision on the palate is curved laterally behind the last molar tooth

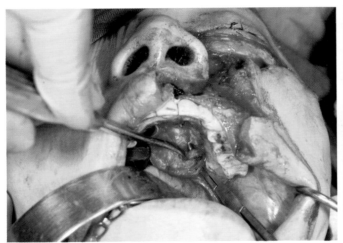

Fig. 16: After lifting the soft tissue and mucoperiosteum over the hard palate, the greater palatine vessels are identified and isolated

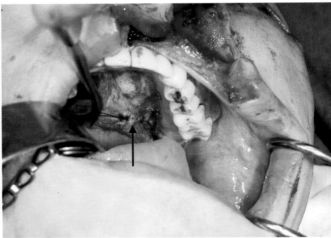

Fig. 17: The greater palatine vessel is divided (arrow)

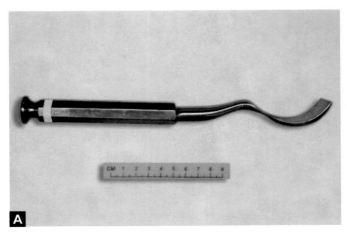

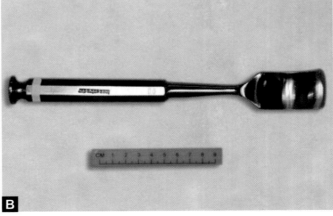

Figs 18A and B: The curved osteotome, side and front view

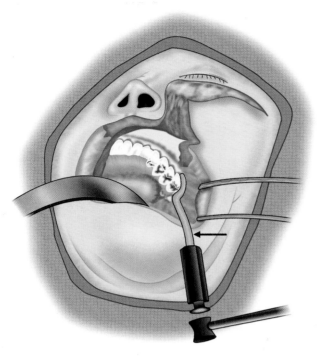

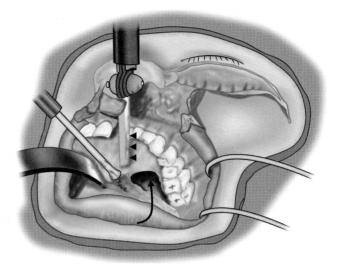

Fig. 20: The oscillating saw blade can be seen cutting through the hard palate in the midline, soft palate (arrowheads) is detached from the curved posterior edge of the hard palate and the nasal cavity can be seen (curved arrow)

Fig. 19: The curved osteotome (arrow) is inserted in the groove between the maxillary tuberosity and the pterygoid plates. By hitting on the head of the handle, the blade of the osteotome cuts vertically upwards to separate the maxillary tuberosity from the pterygoid plates

An oscillating saw with a long and thin blade divides the hard palate from anterior to posterior and from superior to inferior. The lifted mucoperiosteal palatal flap is retracted from the path of the osteotomy and protected. This oscillating saw, cuts through the entire hard palate and lower part of the nasal septum, if there is a septal deviation. Blood loss is minimal with this osteotomy, so it is carried out as the first osteotomy (Fig. 20). Then the osteotomy of the anterior wall of the maxilla is carried out also with long thin blade. The blade goes through the antrum and divides the lateral wall on its way until it reaches and cuts the post wall. The last osteotomy goes through the medial wall of the antrum or the lateral wall of the nose and this is placed above the inferior turbinate and below the middle turbinate.

After completion of the osteotomies, the maxilla bone drops down, but remains attached to the anterior cheek flap (Fig. 21). Then the whole osteocutaneous complex is retracted laterally to expose the nasopharynx and paranasopharyngeal space. Pathologies in the region can be removed under direct vision with this exposure (Figs 22 and 23). The posterior part of the nasal septum is removed to increase the exposure of the contralateral nasopharynx as in Figure 24.

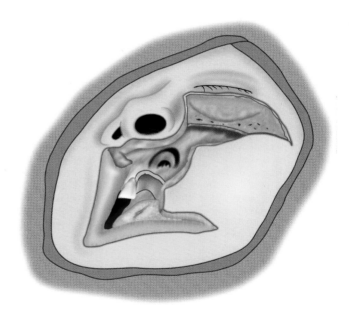

Fig. 21: After completion of all the osteotomies, the maxilla bone (MB) is dropped down but remained attached to the anterior cheek flap

With the maxilla swung laterally, the tumor with its surrounding tissue is adequately exposed and can be removed with conventional instruments (Fig. 25). The paranasopharyngeal space is also exposed (Fig. 26) and pathologies if present in the region can also be adequately

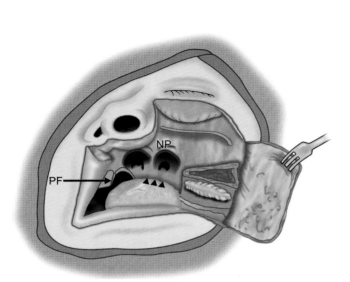

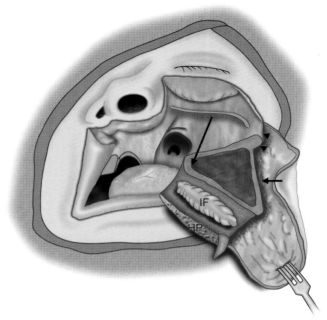

Fig. 22: The maxillary antrum is retracted laterally to expose the nasopharynx (NP), the palatal flap (PF) and the anterior part of the soft palate (arrowheads) are shown

Fig. 23: The maxillary antrum with intact walls, attached to the anterior cheek flap is retracted laterally. Medial wall with the inferior turbinate (IF) and the hard palate (HP), posterior wall (arrow), anterior wall with the infraorbital foramen (half arrow) encloses the triangular maxillary antrum. A short segment of zygomatic arch is also shown (arrowheads)

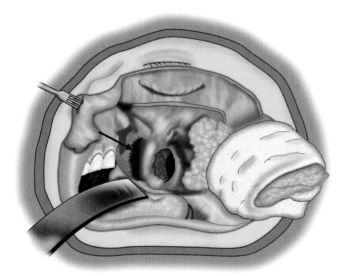

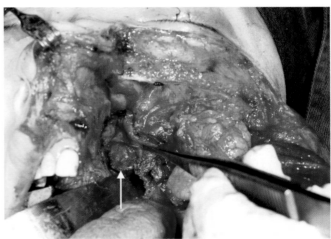

Fig. 24: The entire maxillary antrum is retracted laterally with gauze, exposing the nasopharynx and paranasopharyngeal space. The tissue to be removed is marked with gentian violet. The posterior part of the nasal septum is included in the resection to increase the exposure of the opposite nasopharynx. Arrow showing the resection line on posterior part of nasal septum

Fig. 25: With the nasopharynx adequately exposed, the recurrent tumor with surrounding tissue (arrow) is removed under direct vision

removed (Fig. 27). With the removal of the posterior part of nasal septum, the resection can be extended to the opposite nasopharyngeal wall (Fig. 28). Following this wide exposure,

en bloc resection of the nasopharyngeal carcinoma can be carried out and the resection includes the eustachian tube crura (Fig. 29). The inferior turbinate on the side of the swing is resected (Fig. 30). The mucosa over the turbinate is taken off and the submucosal tissue is trimmed to become a

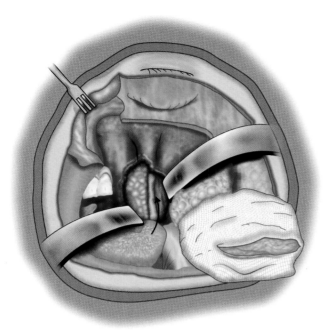

Fig. 26: The dissection could include some of the paranasopharyngeal tissues (arrow)

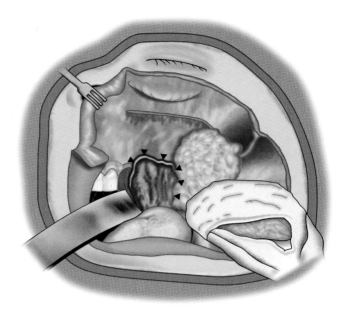

Fig. 27: The defect (arrowheads) in the nasopharynx after completion of nasopharyngectomy

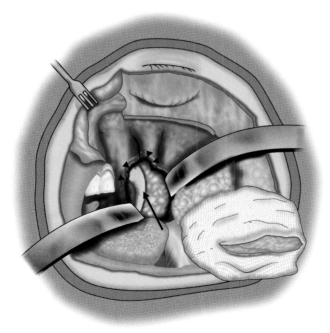

Fig. 28: After nasopharyngectomy and removing posterior part of the nasal septum (arrowheads), the lateral wall of the contralateral nasopharynx can be seen (arrow)

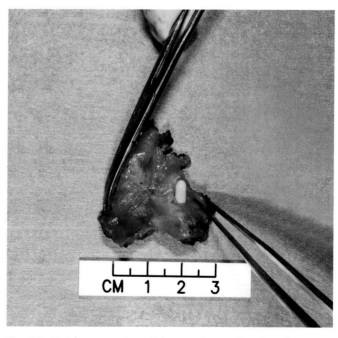

Fig. 29: En bloc resection of the specimen, showing the tumor (T) lying close to the medial crura of the Eustachian tube opening (marked with a yellow tube)

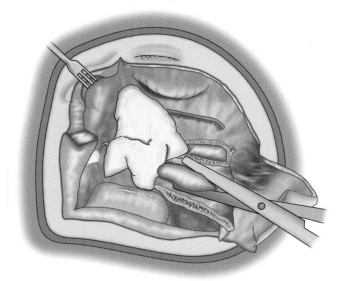

Fig. 30: The inferior turbinate (IF) on the side of the swing was removed by scissors

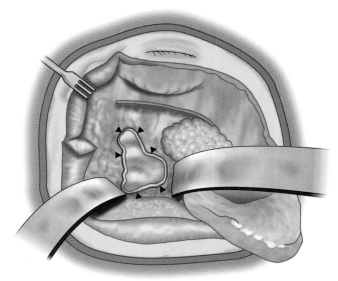

Fig. 31: Inferior turbinate mucosa (arrowheads) is laid over the raw area in the nasopharynx as a free mucosal graft

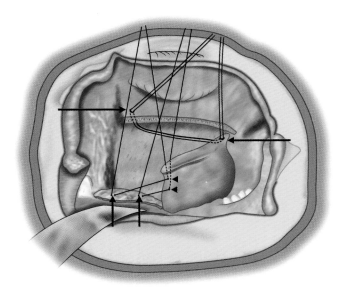

Fig. 32: Holes are drilled on the posterior edge of the hard palate (arrowheads) and stitches passing through the anterior border of the soft palate (half arrows) also passes through these holes. On tying these sutures, the soft palate is reattached to the posterior edge of the hard palate. Holes are drilled on the nasal spine and superior medial corner of the anterior wall of the maxilla (arrows). A wire is passed through the holes and when tightens, act as a fixing point for the maxilla

thin and nearly transparent mucosa. This is laid onto the raw area in the nasopharynx as a free graft (Fig. 31). Frequently, this mucosal graft survives and even if it does not, it serves as a temporary dressing.

On the posterior edge of the hard palate, 2–3 holes are drilled. Separate sutures passing through the anterior cut edge of the soft palate also pass through these holes. These sutures attach the soft palate back to the hard palate. A hole is drilled on the base of the nasal bone and a corresponding hole is drilled on the superomedial part of the anterior wall of the maxilla, a size 26 wire is passed through these holes. When the maxilla returns to its original position, it can be tightened to give addition fixation as in Figure 32.

The maxilla is then returned to its original position. The sutures that attach the soft palate to the hard palate are tied and the intraoral placement of the prefabricated dental plate ensures accurate repositioning of the maxilla as in Figure 33.

While the maxilla is returned to its original position, it is held with the hand, the two titanium plates are placed onto the predrilled screw holes and the screws are inserted. The wire on the superomedial angle of the anterior wall of the maxilla is also tightened to give additional support as Figure 34.

The dental plate is then removed and the palatal flap returned. To fix the posterior part of the flap to the alveolar

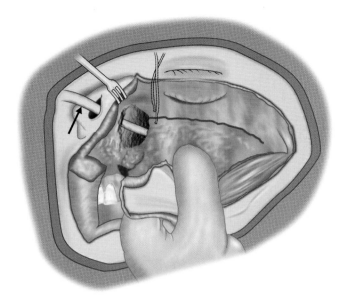

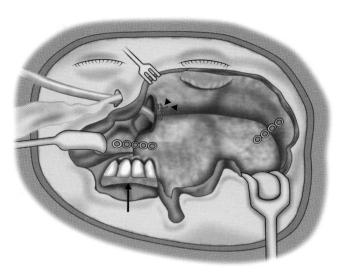

Fig. 33: The osteocutaneous complex is returned, the prefabricated dental plate can be inserted to help in the accurate repositioning of the swung maxilla. The wire over the medial superior angle can be tightened after the maxilla has returned to its original position. A nasogastric tube (arrow) is inserted in the opposite nose for postoperative feeding. A Foley's catheter is inserted and balloon inflated to hold the mucosal graft in position

Fig. 34: With the insertion of the dental plate with wire hooking onto the teeth (arrow), precise return of the maxilla to its original position can be achieved. The titanium plates and screws are inserted. The tightening of the wire at the superomedial angle (arrowhead) of the anterior wall of the maxilla gives additional stability

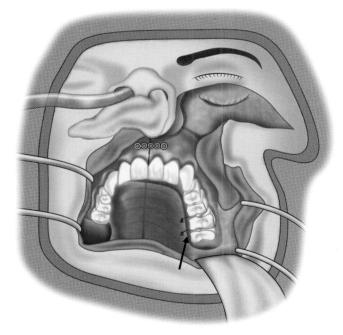

Fig. 35: The dental palate is removed and the palatal flap is sutured by two stitches (arrow) to the alveolar margin. The rest of the palatal flap is returned and held in position with the reinsertion of the dental plate. The nasal cavity is packed with an antiseptic gauze

margin, 2–3 sutures are used (Fig. 35). The dental plate is re-inserted to keep the palatal flap in position and this plate was left in position into the postoperative period. Nasal cavity is packed with antiseptic ribbon gauze and the facial wound is closed in layers as in Figure 36.

POSTOPERATIVE TREATMENT

Patient returns to ward after the anesthetic effect is over and there is no need for ventilator support. The tracheostomy allows frequent suction of secretions from the trachea as in the early postoperative period, patient tends to aspirate. The tracheostomy tube is removed when patient can cough adequately, to keep the airway patent and this may range between 2 days and 4 days. The dental plate is removed on the third day after operation and nasogastric tube feeding starts from the second day, after operation. The Foley's catheter and nasal packings are removed within 1 week of operation. The nasogastric tube sometimes is still in situ for feeding as although the patient is allowed to take fluid diet orally, the amount is usually not enough during the early postoperative period (Figs 37 and 38).

At 2 weeks after operation, the facial wound has healed (Fig. 39) and the patient can take full oral diet. Facial function has returned (Fig. 40). The patient has trismus (Fig. 41) and

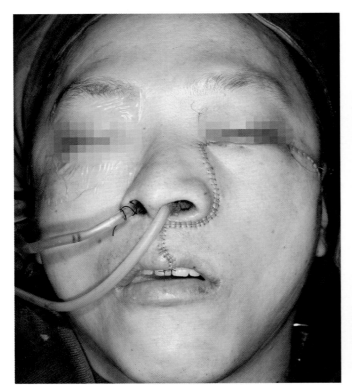

Fig. 36: The soft tissue and the
skin are closed in layers

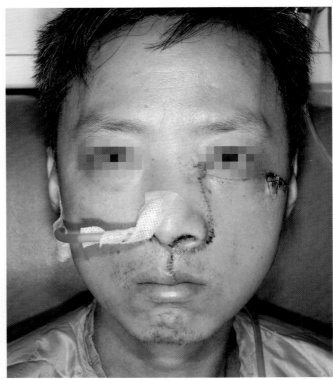

Fig. 37: Patient on the seventh day after the operation,
the nasogastric tube is in place

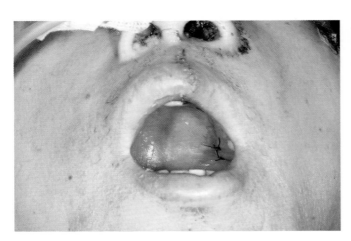

Fig. 38: Patient on the 7th day after operation,
the palatal flap appeared healthy

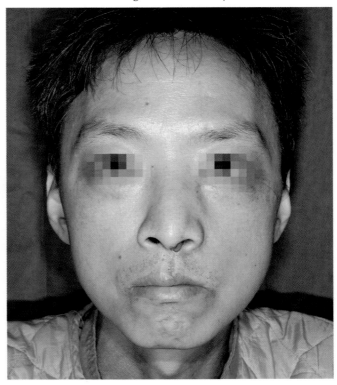

Fig. 39: Patient two weeks after the operation,
all tubes are removed, the wound has healed

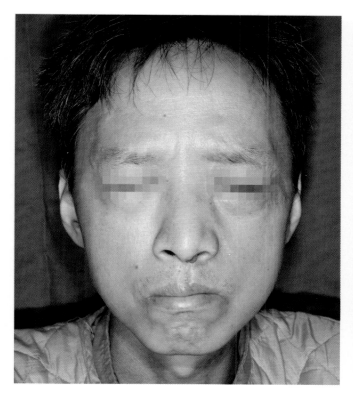

Fig. 40: Patient two weeks after operation, the facial function has returned to normal

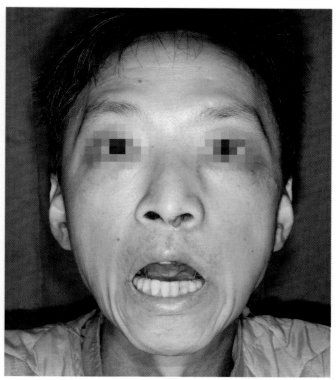

Fig. 41: Patient two weeks after the operation, he has trismus which will respond to conservative management

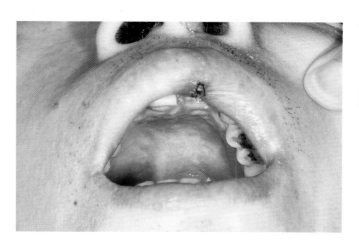

Fig. 42: Patient at two weeks after operation, the palatal wound has healed and the palatal flap has survived

this usually responds to conservative management, such as passive stretching. The palatal wound has completely healed (Fig. 42).

Endoscopic examination of the nasal cavity starts at about 2 weeks after the operation, debris and secretions are removed and this procedure is repeated at 1–2 weeks intervals, depending on the amount of debris and secretion.

The patient is then followed up at regular intervals to monitor the status of the pathology in the nasopharynx.

HIGHLIGHTS

I. Indications
  • Localized lesion in the central skull base, such as recurrent nasopharyngeal carcinoma after chemoradiation, chordoma, schwannoma, angiofibroma and other tumors in the nasopharynx, large benign salivary gland tumors, sarcoma, etc.

II. Contraindications
  • When the tumor has invaded the skull base bone and curative resection is not likely
  • When the internal carotid artery is encased by the malignant disease
  • When the blood supply to the maxillary antrum has been disturbed, such as a previous midfacial deglove procedure.

III. Special Preoperative Considerations
Evaluation of the exact extent of the pathology, their extension and possible infiltration of surrounding structures.

IV. Special Intraoperative Considerations

Precise osteotomy is essential to avoid fracture of the facial bone and to reduce blood loss during the operation.

V. Special Postoperative Considerations

Early rehabilitation to relieve the trismus.

VI. Complications

- Injury of the internal carotid artery and dura at the skull base during operation
- Osteoradionecrosis of part of the maxilla bone is a possibility, although this is unusual.

ADDITIONAL READING

1. Chan JY, Chow VL, Tsang R, Wei WI. Nasopharyngectomy for locally advanced recurrent nasopharyngeal carcinoma: exploring the limits. Head Neck. 2012;34(7):923-8.

2. NG RW, Wei WI. Elimination of palatal fistula after the maxillary swing procedure. Head Neck. 2005;27(7): 608-12.

3. Wei WI, Chan JY, Ng RW, Ho WK. Surgical salvage of persistent or recurrent nasopharyngeal carcinoma with maxillary swing approach—Critical appraisal after 2 decades. Head Neck. 2011;33(7):969-75.

4. Wei WI, Ho CM, Yuen PW, et al. Maxillary swing approach for resection of tumors in and around the nasopharynx. Arch of Otolaryngol Head and Neck Surgery. 1995;121(6): 638-42.

5. Wei WI, Lam KH, Sham JS. New approach to the nasopharynx: the maxillary swing approach. Head Neck. 1991;13(3):200-7.

6. Wei WI, Sham JS. Nasopharyngeal Carcinoma. Lancet. 2005;365(9476):2041-54.

7. Wei WI. Nasopharyngeal cancer: Current status of Management: a New York Head and Neck Society Lecture. Arch Otolaryngol Head Neck Surg. 2001;127(7):766-9.

Chapter **3**

Minimally Invasive Endoscopic Staple Diverticulotomy for Zenker's Diverticulum

Daniel Zikk, Amir Szold

INTRODUCTION

Zenker's diverticulum is a mucosal outpouching through fibers of the inferior constrictor and the cricopharyngeal muscles (Fig. 1).[1] A clear understanding of the pathogenesis of this diverticulum is lacking, but most theories have focused on esophageal dysfunction and on anatomic defects of the cricopharyngeal muscle.[2] Zenker's diverticulum typically affects elderly patients, especially males. A Zenker diverticulum carries with it a high frequency of retention of food elements within its pouch. These food elements and secretions frequently lead to complaints of upper esophageal dysphagia, regurgitation of undigested food, aspiration, noisy deglutition, halitosis and changes in voice. Mild-to-moderate weight loss is frequent. Aspiration and pneumonia are potentially serious complications,[3] while squamous cell carcinoma in a Zenker's diverticulum is a very rare condition.[4]

The diagnosis of Zenker's diverticulum is usually confirmed by a barium swallow or as an accidental finding during esophagogastroscopy.

The minimally invasive endoscopic approach to Zenker's diverticulum was first described by Mosher[5] in 1913 and by Dohlman and Mattsson[6] in 1960. Since then, several series using this technique with either electrocoagulation, laser or harmonic scalpel has been reported.[7-10] However, even with refinement of the surgical technique, surgeons have continued to be reluctant to use endoscopic treatment because of concern about the sutureless division of the common wall, which could lead to bleeding, perforation, cervical soft tissue infection and mediastinitis. In order to address this concern, Collard et al.[11] introduced in 1993, the endoscopic stapling technique using an endosurgical stapler that simultaneously divides the common wall between the esophagus and the diverticulum, and then stapling the wound edges to close them. In recent studies, the endoscopic approach by means of the stapling technique turned out to be minimally invasive, effective, safe, fast and associated with short hospital stay, short interval from surgery to oral intake, rapid convalescence and a very low complication rate.[12-14] In the following article, the management and surgical technique of the endoscopic stapled diverticulotomy for Zenker's diverticulum will be discussed.

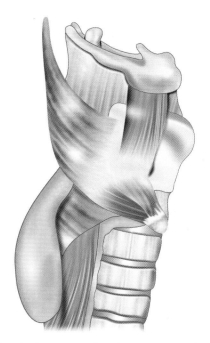

Fig. 1: Anatomy of Zenker's diverticulum

PREOPERATIVE EVALUATION AND ANESTHESIA

The preoperative work-up includes history, physical examination and imaging of the upper digestive tract with contrast media. The most common presenting symptoms of Zenker's diverticulum are dysphagia, nocturnal regurgitation of undigested food, aspiration, noisy deglutition, halitosis and complaints of changes in voice quality. Preoperative laryngoscopy to assess pharyngeal and vocal cord integrity, and mobility is required.

Imaging of the upper esophageal tract preoperatively is essential. These include barium swallow study (Figs 2A to C) of the upper gastrointestinal tract and in certain cases computerized tomography of the neck and upper mediastinum (Fig. 3). Computerized tomography is advocated especially in cases where the pouch is very large and extends toward the lower neck and mediastinum.

Endoscopic staple diverticulotomy for Zenker's diverticulum is carried out under general anesthesia with oral endotracheal intubation. To allow extension of the neck and low tension of the tongue and lower jaw, muscle relaxants are used throughout the procedure.

Before 1 hour of operation, the patient is given intravenous second-generation cephalosporin.

SURGICAL TECHNIQUE

The patient is placed supine on the operating table with the neck extended and the surgeon sitting behind the patient's head. A dental protection is placed on the upper and lower dentition. The patient is intubated with an endotracheal tube smaller than the standard tubing (i.e. 6 mm outside diameter tube for 70 kg patient). The endotracheal tube should be positioned to the left side of the mouth away from the operative field. A double-lipped Weerda diverticuloscope (Karl Storz, Tuttlingen, Germany) is then lubricated with 2% lidocaine gel and is placed under direct vision, into the oral cavity and pharynx (Fig. 4). The two lips of the Weerda diverticuloscope can be approximated and angulated according to the patient's anatomy. The upper blade of the diverticuloscope is inserted into the esophageal lumen and the lower blade into the diverticulum (Figs 5A and B). After clear visualization of the esophageal lumen, the diverticular pouch and the interposed bridge, the diverticuloscope is fixed and held in place by means of laryngoscope holder and chest support. The diverticular pouch is washed by normal saline, cleaned from undigested food along with secretions and is inspected. A 5.0 mm 0° rigid endoscope is inserted alongside to an Endo-GIA 35 mm (Figs 6A and B) endoscopic stapler (Ethicon Inc., Somerville, NJ, USA). The stapler is applied under endoscopic vision through the scope; one arm is placed into the diverticular pouch and the other one in the esophageal lumen. After midline approximation of the two arms, the stapler is fired dividing the common wall between the esophagus and the diverticulum and at same time, stapling together the esophageal and the diverticular wall. One to three applications of the stapler are used until the common wall is completely divided. After the removal of the stapler, the edges retract laterally on the action of the cricopharyngeal

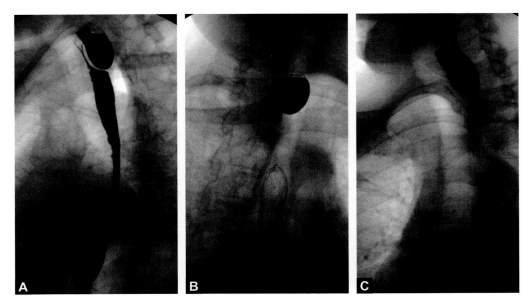

Figs 2A to C: Barium swallow study images of a patient with medium size Zenker's diverticulum. (A and C) Lateral images; (B) Anteroposterior (AP) image

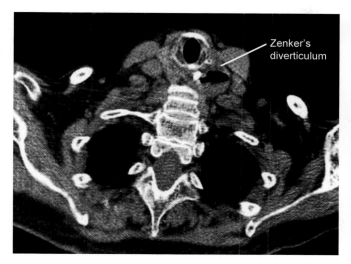

Fig. 3: Computed tomographic image of a patient with large Zenker's diverticulum

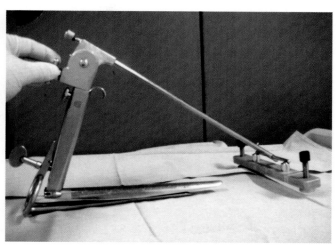

Fig. 4: A double-lipped Weerda diverticuloscope (Karl Storz, Tuttlingen, Germany)

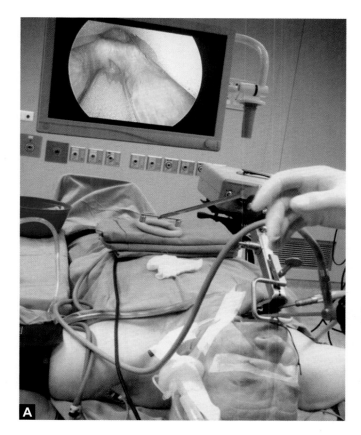

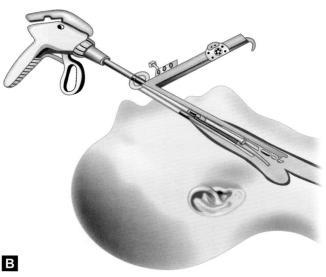

Figs 5A and B: (A) Weerda diverticuloscope in place. Endoscopic view; the upper blade of the diverticuloscope is in the esophageal lumen and the lower blade in the diverticulum. A clear visualization of the esophageal lumen, the diverticular pouch and the interposed bridge is seen; (B) Schematic drawing of surgical instruments in place

muscle that had just been divided, resulting in a common cavity (Figs 7A to C). The operative field is inspected for bleeding and the Weerda diverticuloscope is removed. The use of electrocautery is rarely needed. The use of low voltage and fully insulated instruments are mandatory. Nasogastric tube is not applied.

POSTOPERATIVE EVALUATION

Routine perioperative plain lateral neck and anteroposterior (AP) chest X-rays are done a day after the operation. Intravenous second-generation cephalosporin is adminis-

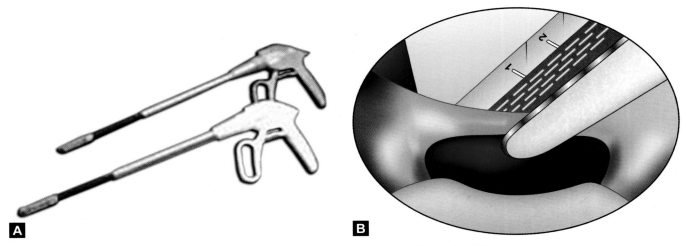

Figs 6A and B: (A) An Endo-GIA 35-mm endoscopic stapler (Ethicon Inc., Somerville, NJ, USA);(B) Stapler over the common wall before incision

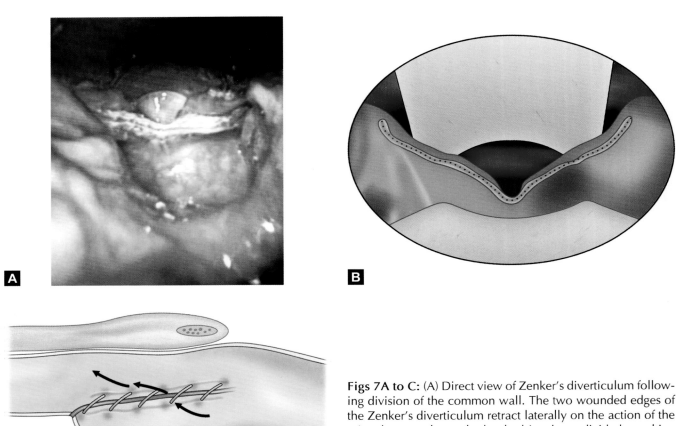

Figs 7A to C: (A) Direct view of Zenker's diverticulum following division of the common wall. The two wounded edges of the Zenker's diverticulum retract laterally on the action of the cricopharyngeal muscle that had just been divided, resulting in a common cavity; (B) Schematic representation of direct view of Zenker's diverticulum following division of the common wall; (C) A schematic representation of the lateral view of Zenker's diverticulum following division of the common wall

tered for additional 2 days. The patient stays in the hospital for two nights. The patient is allowed to have liquid food after 24 hours and is maintained on soft diet for additional 10 days. Patients are assessed for 1 week after surgery for postoperative results. Follow-up evaluation continues in the outpatient clinic at variable intervals, according to the clinical course and the relief of symptoms. Postoperative radiologic assessment of the surgical site with barium swallow video fluoroscopy is usually taken; one or two months after the operation whenever needed and must be interpreted with understanding of the surgical intent. Findings that indicate a successful result include: reduced height of the partition wall, easy passage of barium into the esophagus and reduced height of barium in the residual sac.

COMMENTS

The goal of surgical treatment of Zenker's diverticulum is to eliminate the accumulation of undigested food in the pouch and to release the increased pressure of the upper esophageal sphincter, which is believed to be one of the causes in the development of Zenker's diverticulum. These goals can be achieved by either open neck surgery or via minimally invasive endoscopic techniques. A typical patient with Zenker's diverticulum is elderly and suffers with multiple medical problems. Ideal management is in achieving these goals and reducing the operative risk, operative time and hospitalization. For many years, patients with symptomatic Zenker's diverticulum were treated by an open cervical excision of the diverticular sac with or without cricopharyngeal myotomy. Despite of relatively high success rates, this technique was characterized by unacceptable mortality rates (2%), high complication rate (10–30%) and protracted convalescence period. The minimally invasive endoscopic staple diverticulotomy for Zenker's diverticulum is an elegant solution that offers brief operative exposure, short anesthesia with hospital stay and rapid convalescence and resolution of the symptoms caused by the diverticulum. With this technique, not only the neck incision is avoided, but the patient is allowed to resume oral intake rapidly. Further advantages are the high success rates and decreased morbidity associated with this technique. Series published since 1993 prove that minimally invasive endoscopic staple diverticulotomy for Zenker's diverticulum, to be superior to all other techniques, both external and endoscopic.[12-14]

HIGHLIGHTS

I. Indications
- Symptoms

  - Upper esophageal dysphagia, regurgitation of undigested food, aspiration, recurrent aspiration pneumonia, weight loss, chronic laryngitis and hoarseness
- Findings
  - Stasis of saliva and undigested food at the hypopharynx
- Suspicious malignancy.

II. Contraindications
- Trismus
- Stiffness and immobility of the neck
- Medically unfit for surgery
- Coexistent oral and/or pharyngeal pathologies preventing introduction of the endoscopic surgical instruments.

III. Special Preoperative Considerations
- Barium swallow study or CT of the neck
- Laryngoscopy to evaluate the integrity of the pharynx and larynx
- Intravenous second-generation cephalosporin, 1 hour prior to surgery.

IV. Special Intraoperative Considerations
- Dental protection of the upper and lower dentition
- Lubrification of the Weerda diverticuloscope by 2% lidocaine gel
- Careful introduction of the Weerda diverticuloscope, always under direct vision.

V. Special Postoperative Considerations
- Check for the presence of air in the neck by palpation or imaging if needed
- Assess integrity of the upper esophageal tract before allowing the patients to resume liquid food after operation.

VI. Complications
- Dental injury
- Bleeding
- Mediastinitis
- Esophageal or pharyngeal perforation
- Diverticulum perforation
- Cervical emphysema.

REFERENCES

1. Ludlow A. A case of obstructed deglutition from a preternatural dilatation of and bag formed in the pharynx. Medical Observations and Enquiries. Society of Physicians, 2nd edition. London. 1769;3:85-101.
2. Zenker FA, von Ziemssen H. Krankenheiten des oesopahgus. In: von Ziemssen H (Ed). Heandbuch der Speciellen Pathologie and Therapie. Volume 7 (Suppl.). Leipzig: FCW Vogel; 1877. pp. 1-87.

3. Siddiq MA, Sood S, Strachan D. Pharyngeal pouch (Zenker's diverticulum). Postgrad Med J. 2001;77(910):506-11.

4. Brücher BL, Sarbia M, Oestreicher E, et al. Squamous cell carcinoma and Zenker diverticulum. Dis Esophagus. 2007;20(1):75-8.

5. Mosher HP. Webs and pouches of the esophagus: their diagnosis and treatment. Surg Gynecol Obstet. 1917;25: 175-87.

6. Dohlman G, Mattsson O. The endoscopic operation for hypopharyngeal diverticula: a roentgencinematographic study. AMA Arch Otolaryngol. 1960;71:744-52.

7. Kos MP, David EF, Mahieu HF. Endoscopic carbon dioxide laser Zenker's diverticulotomy revisited. Ann Otol Rhinol Laryngol. 2009;118(7):512-8.

8. Ferreira LE, Simmons DT, Baron TH. Zenker's diverticula: pathophysiology, clinical presentation, and flexible endoscopic management. Dis Esophagus. 2008;21(1): 1-8.

9. Bonavina L, Bona D, Abraham M, et al. Long-term results of endosurgical and open surgical approach for Zenker diverticulum. World J Gastroenterol. 2007;13(18):2586-9.

10. Sharp DB, Newman JR, Magnuson JS. Endoscopic management of Zenker's diverticulum: stapler assisted versus Harmonic Ace. Laryngoscope. 2009;119(10):1906-12.

11. Collard JM, Otte JB, Kestens PJ. Endoscopic stapling technique of esophagodiverticulostomy for Zenker's diverticulum. Ann Thorac Surg. 1993;56(3):573-6.

12. Wasserzug O, Zikk D, Raziel A, et al. Endoscopically stapled diverticulostomy for Zenker's diverticulum: results of a multidisciplinary team approach. Surg Endosc. 2009;17(3):168-71.

13. Roth JA, Sigston E, Vallance N. Endoscopic stapling of pharyngeal pouch: a 10-year review of single versus multiple staple rows. Otolaryngol Head Neck Surg. 2009;140(2):245-9.

14. Manni JJ, Kremer B, Rinkel RN. The endoscopic stapler diverticulotomy for Zenker's diverticulum. Eur Arch Otorhinolaryngol. 2004;261(2):68-70.

Chapter **4**

Radical Neck Dissection

Claudio R Cernea, Lenine G Brandão

INTRODUCTION

The radical neck dissection is the most characteristic surgical procedure of the specialty of head and neck surgery. It was originally described by Crile in 1906[1] and its technique remained virtually unchanged to the present day. It is noteworthy that a very similar procedure was reported by F Jawdynski[2] 18 years earlier, but as it was published only in Polish, very few surgeons acknowledged it. With almost no modification[3] this operation was popularized by Martin,[4] during the decades of 1940s and 1950s.

In fact, squamous cell carcinomas of the upper aerodigestive tract form a perfect model for this operation, for several reasons. The initial spread of these cancers involves the regional cervical lymph nodes, usually in a relatively predictable sequence. Hematogenic metastases appear later. Therefore, comprehensive locoregional treatment actually reduces the recurrence rate and enhances tumor-related survival. In addition, the most commonly involved cervical lymphatic chains are readily accessible to excision using a fairly standard technique, in contrast with other anatomic locations within the human body. Finally, important anatomic structures like the carotid artery and brachial plexus are spared, whereas others like the internal jugular vein and the accessory nerve are unfortunately sacrificed.

By definition, a radical neck dissection encompasses all five major lymph node levels of the neck: (i) level I (submandibular and submental); (ii) level II (superior third of jugular vein); (iii) level III (middle third of jugular vein); (iv) level IV (inferior third of jugular vein) and; (v) level V (posterior triangle). As already mentioned, the internal jugular vein, the accessory nerve and the sternocleidomastoid muscle are included in the specimen as well.

During the decade of 1960s[5,6] and later, in the decade of 1980s,[7] several modifications of the radical neck dissection were described and are discussed in other chapters of this book.

PREOPERATIVE EVALUATION AND ANESTHESIA

In approximately 90% of patients with clinically evident neck metastases, a primary cancer can be identified, usually within the head and neck area. Therefore, a thorough preoperative evaluation must be performed, including a triple endoscopy. In addition to this, imaging methods are required. The radical neck dissection is indicated for advanced neck disease, often a N3 neck, in which there is capsular rupture and potential invasion of surrounding structures, either microscopically or macroscopically. In these instances, it is mandatory to fully evaluate the limits of the metastatic mass to properly plan the surgical strategy or eventually, to contraindicate the surgical procedure (refer to highlights). In other words, it is advisable to plan a radical neck dissection instead of a modified neck dissection in a patient with clinical and radiological findings, suggestive of gross extracapsular spread in the neck as in Figure 1.

Evidently, it is important to evaluate the clinical status of the patient, paying attention to any possible clinical comorbidity. The operation is performed under general anesthesia, and the indication of tracheostomy depends upon the surgical treatment of the primary tumor, at the time of the neck dissection.

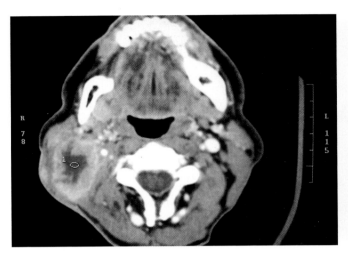

Fig. 1: Neck metastases on level II with radiological signs of gross extracapsular spread

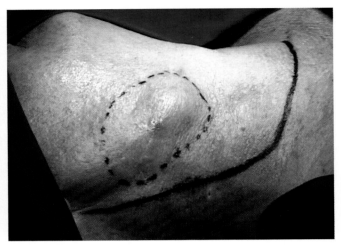

Fig. 2: A 42-year-old male with a squamous cell carcinoma metastatic to the neck with unknown primary staged T0N3M0; the L-shaped incision on the right neck is demonstrated

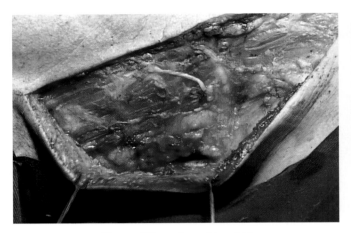

Fig. 3: Dissection of level V

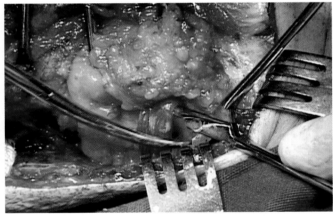

Fig. 4: Section of the omohyoid muscle in level V

SURGICAL TECHNIQUE

The choice of the incision also depends on the concomitant resection of the primary cancer, if indicated. In the original technique published by Crile and popularized by Martin, a "glass of wine" shape was usually recommended. The disadvantage of this design is to create a critical point exactly at the trifurcation, which can potentially expose the carotid artery; should a flap dehiscence occur. Hence, the authors only perform this incision when a paramedian mandibulotomy is planned in order to offer wide exposure of posteriorly located oropharyngeal or skull base tumors. The authors' favorite approach is an L-shaped incision, which enables safe access to all five lymphatic levels encompassed by the radical neck dissection with a more reliable flap design as in Figure 2.

The flaps are raised in a subplatysmal plane, except if there is invasion of the platysma muscle. In this circumstance, the skin is also involved and a conventional or free flap is indicated for reconstruction.

The dissection is started by exposing the anterior border of the trapezius muscle, which is the posterior boundary of the radical neck dissection. Therefore, the whole contents of level V and the posterior aspect of levels III and IV are dissected and pushed anteriorly (Fig. 3). The omohyoid muscle is cut and its anterior stump helps to pull the specimen anteriorly (Fig. 4). As this is a classical radical neck dissection, the accessory nerve is transected. However, the motor branches of the cervical plexus are preserved if oncologically safe, in order to preserve some motor supply to the trapezius muscle as well as to the elevator of the scapula.

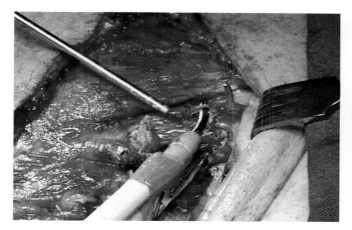

Fig. 5: Section of the clavicular head of the
sternocleidomastoid muscle

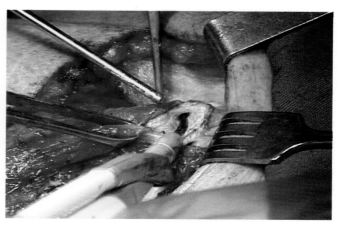

Fig. 6: Section of the sternal head of the
sternocleidomastoid muscle

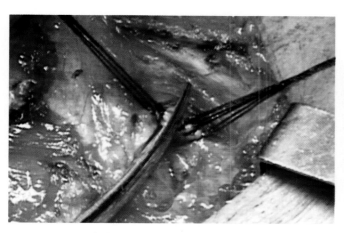

Fig. 7: Triple ligature and section of the inferior part
of the internal jugular vein

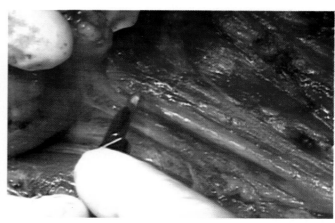

Fig. 8: Dissection of the vagus nerve and of the
common carotid artery

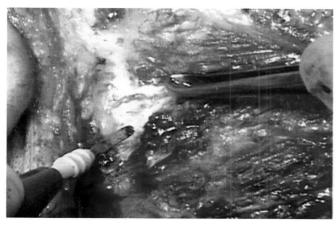

Fig. 9: Section of the mastoid origin of the
sternocleidomastoid muscle

The clavicular and sternal heads of the sternocleidomastoid muscles are cut (Figs 5 and 6) and the internal jugular vein is triple tied and transected, close to the junction with the subclavian vein (Fig. 7). On the left side, extra caution must be exerted to avoid injury to the thoracic duct. If any chyle leak is detected at this point, its origin should be identified and carefully tied. The authors have developed a yet unpublished maneuver; after disconnecting the ventilator, an abdominal compression exerted by one member of the surgical team can help to increase the lymphatic flow in the thoracic duct and to better demonstrate the fistula.

The surgeon must identify the vagus nerve, the common carotid artery and the phrenic nerve, avoiding any unexpected injury (Fig. 8). The whole specimen is then mobilized cranially.

The next step is the section of the mastoid insertions of the sternocleidomastoid muscle (Fig. 9), with identification of the posterior belly of the digastric muscle. Medially and cranially, the upper portion of the internal jugular vein is identified and again, it is triple ligated and cut (Fig. 10). The accessory nerve is also cut at this point. Care is taken to avoid injury to the internal carotid artery and the hypoglossal nerve.

The dissection continues from lateral to medial, toward level I (Fig. 11), with the identification and preservation of the following structures: the marginal mandibular nerve, the lingual nerve and the hypoglossal nerve. All contents of the submandibular and submental regions are then removed in continuity with the rest of the specimen (Fig. 12).

The final view of the operative field shows the extension of this operation as in Figure 13.

Very meticulous check of any residual bleeding is performed under pulmonary hyperpressure. A suction drain is placed and the wound is closed in layers as in Figure 14.

POSTOPERATIVE TREATMENT

Immediate postoperative care is usually not complex, except if there is a dehiscence of the incision, with exposure of the carotid artery. This serious complication may lead to arterial blow out, which is obviously associated with significant morbidity and mortality. Thus, this dehiscence should be

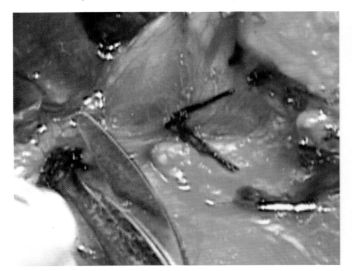

Fig. 10: Triple ligature and section of the superior part of the internal jugular vein at the jugular foramen

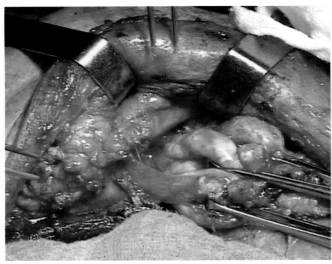

Fig. 11: Dissection of the contents of level I

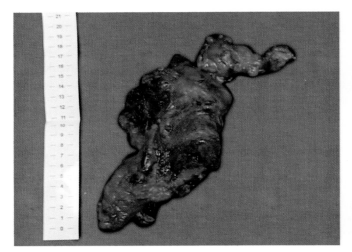

Fig. 12: The surgical specimen, including the five nodal levels, the sternocleidomastoid muscle, the internal jugular vein and the XI nerve

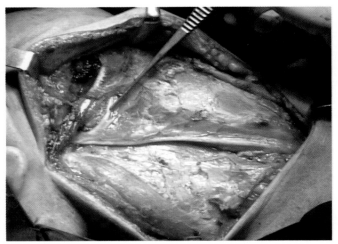

Fig. 13: The final operative field with the forceps pointing at the XII nerve

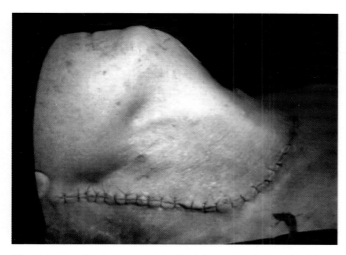

Fig. 14: The final aspect of the incision with the suction drain

corrected by resuturing the wound or eventually, with the use of a well-vascularized flap to cover the exposed artery.

After neck dissections, usually there is a reasonable amount of fluid that is produced. However, if the volume of drainage exceeds hundreds of milliliter, particularly after a left radical neck dissection, a chyle fistula should be considered. Most fistulas are managed conservatively but in few instances a surgical revision is necessary.

The most important long-term complication is disability of the shoulder, secondary to definitive paralysis of the accessory nerve. To minimize the effect of this nerve injury, every effort must be made to preserve the motor roots of the cervical plexus to the other cervical agonist muscles, especially the elevator of the scapula. Also, it is important to begin physical therapy rehabilitation of the corresponding upper limb as soon as possible.

If a radical neck dissection is performed, probably the patient has a rather extensive nodal disease. The best oncological results are achieved with the postoperative adjuvant radiotherapy or chemoradiotherapy, which ideally should start as soon as the wound is healed and preferably, not after six weeks.

HIGHLIGHTS

I. Indications
- Advanced metastatic disease in the neck, with clear extracapsular spread and potential or proven invasion of some surrounding structures.

II. Contraindications
- Relative
  - Circumferential invasion of the carotid artery, invasion of deep neck muscles
- Absolute
  - Invasion of skull base, vertebrae and major vessels at the thoracic inlet. Impossible to control the primary tumor and the extensive distant metastases.

III. Special Preoperative Considerations
- Be sure that the primary tumor can be controlled and that there is no extensive distant disease
- Plan adequately the design of your incision to contemplate the resection of the primary tumor
- Be prepared to reconstruct the carotid artery, if an invasion is suspected
- Be prepared to use a distant or free flap, when dealing with very extensive extracapsular spread.

IV. Special Intraoperative Considerations
- Perform very meticulous hemostasis at all times
- When doing a bilateral neck dissection, always start in the less involved side; should an internal jugular vein be needed on this side, it is advisable to postpone the contralateral radical neck dissection for at least 2 weeks, to enable the development of collateral venous circulation, to avoid intracranial venous hypertension
- Be sure to properly ligate the two remaining stumps of the internal jugular vein; any hemorrhage at these levels could be extremely difficult to control.

V. Special Postoperative Considerations
- Leave a very light dressing on the incision, enabling early detection of wound dehiscence or flap necrosis
- Monitor the drainage volume, especially after left radical neck dissections, to detect chyle fistulas
- Pay attention to excessively high urinary volume and/or disorientation, which can be early signs of the syndrome of inappropriate secretion of antidiuretic hormone (ADH)
- Start physical rehabilitation of the ipsilateral shoulder as soon as possible.

VI. Complications
- Hematomas
- Hemorrhages
- Flap necrosis
- Wound dehiscence
- Chyle fistula
- Unexpected nerve injuries
- Cerebrovascular accident
- Syndrome of inappropriate secretion of ADH
- Cervical edema, brain edema (bilateral dissections).

REFERENCES

1. Crile G. Landmark article, 1906: Excision of cancer of the head and neck. With special reference to the plan of dissection based on one hundred and thirty-two patients. JAMA. 1987;258(22):1780-4.

2. Jawdynski FI. Przypadek raka pierwotnego syzi. T.z. raka skrzelowego volkmann'a. Wyciecie nowotworu wraz z rezekcyja tetnicy szjowej wspolnej i zyly szyjowej wewnetrznej. Wyzdrowieneie Gaz Lek. 1888;28:530-5.

3. Subramanian S, Chiesa C, LyubaevV, et al. The evolution of surgery in the management of neck metastases. Acta Otorhinolaryngol Ital. 2006;26(6):309-16.

4. Martin H, Del Valle B, Ehrlich H, et al. Neck dissection. Cancer. 1951;4:441-99.

5. Suárez O. El problema de las metastasis linfaticas y alejadas del cancer de laringe e hipofaringe. Rev Otorrinolaryngol. 1963;23:83-99.

6. Bocca E, Pignataro O. A conservation technique in radical neck dissection. Ann Otol Rhinol Laryngol. 1967;76(5):975-87.

7. Bocca E, Pignataro O, Sasaki CT. Functional neck dissection. A description of operative technique. Arch Otolaryngol. 1980;106(9):524-7.

Chapter **5**

Total Parotidectomy

Eugene N Myers, Robert L Ferris, Joshua Dunklebarger

INTRODUCTION

Total parotidectomy reflects a spectrum of operations to treat a wide variety of pathological disorders of the parotid gland. These disorders range from chronic sialadenitis to highly malignant tumors, which may involve the entire parotid gland, the facial nerve and adjacent structures. A variety of modifications of total parotidectomy must be adapted to these pathologies, considering the disease pathogenesis and progression.

Carwardine (1907) is said to have been the first to remove the parotid gland with the identification and preservation of the facial nerve. Sistrunk in 1921 reported 112 cases of parotidectomy in which he identified the cervical branch of the facial nerve adjacent to the submandibular gland; which he dissected retrograde to the main trunk, preserved the facial nerve and dissected out the tumor with a remarkably low incidence of facial nerve injury or tumor recurrence.

It was not until 1958 that Beahrs and Adson in their milestone work at the Mayo Clinic described the surgical anatomy of the facial nerve and a technique of parotidectomy, which included initial identification of the main trunk of the facial nerve as it exits the stylomastoid foramen and then, dissecting the individual branches anteriorly. This set the stage for their later milestone publication.

Experience with 1360 primary parotid tumors examined the results of the surgical treatment of parotid tumors during the two consecutive 15-year periods: (i) 1940 to 1954 and (ii) 1955 to 1969. Local excision was used in the early series while in the later one, a superficial or total parotidectomy with the identification and preservation of the facial nerve was done. This procedure later became the treatment of choice due to the decreased incidence of tumor recurrence and facial nerve paralysis. Since that report, superficial parotidectomy with facial nerve dissection has become the most frequently performed operations in the United States for tumors involving the superficial lobe of the parotid gland.

HA Kidd (1950) was the first to describe a total parotidectomy with preservation of the facial nerve. Kerry Olsen of the Mayo Clinic posed the question: "What constitutes a total parotidectomy?" His answer: "In general, total parotidectomy consists of removing both the superficial portion of the gland and the entire deep lobe beneath the facial nerve. In extreme cases, the operation may also include removal of the peripheral facial nerve and even the surrounding muscle, bone and skin. The practice of a more extensive version of the operation is seldom indicated in cases of advanced malignancy."

Olsen posed a second question: "When does the surgeon need to contemplate total parotidectomy?" Multifocal tumors such as Warthin's tumor, despite its benign behavior, may require total parotidectomy in order to ensure its complete removal. Benign tumors arising in the deep lobe often requires initial elevation or removal of the superficial lobe followed by mobilization of the facial nerve before removal of the deep portion of the gland. Tumors arising in the deep lobe of the parotid gland with an extension to the parapharyngeal space will require removal of the deep lobe together with the dissection of the parapharyngeal space. Malignant tumors of the parotid gland, except for low-grade tumors, usually require total removal of the gland. All high-grade tumors arising in the superficial lobe of the parotid gland require total parotidectomy with an attention to the intra- and periparotid lymph nodes. Tumors that spread outside the parotid gland or involve the facial nerve, usually require total parotidectomy and neck dissection, malignant tumors which originate in the facial skin and invade the parotid gland, usually require total parotidectomy. Squamous cell carcinoma and malignant melanoma of the facial skin may metastasize to the lymph nodes of the parotid gland and requires a total parotidectomy to remove the intra- and extraparotid lymph nodes as well as a neck dissection.

In all of the above mentioned variations on the theme of total parotidectomy, every effort should be made to preserve the facial nerve in patients whose facial nerve is not affected by tumor. While this may sound risky from the oncologic point of view, the close margins on the nerve can be neutralized with the use of postoperative radiotherapy.

PREOPERATIVE EVALUATION AND ANESTHESIA

The evaluation of the patient for parotid surgery should always start with a thorough and concise history including any prior radiation exposure. Emphasis should be given to tumor presentation. A history of slow or rapid growth, pain, facial paresis or paralysis, and overlying skin changes or an associated mass in the neck is very helpful in differentiating between benign and malignant tumors. The triad of recent onset of pain, facial paralysis and a mass in the parotid gland (Fig. 1) are pathognomonic for a malignant tumor of the parotid gland, so the presence or absence of these symptoms must be elicited directly. Information should also be sought about the presence of skin cancers or lesions, which may have been excised or biopsied recently in the facial, temporal,

auricular and postauricular areas. Cigarette smoking may be a valuable clue, since patients with Warthin's tumor often have a history of substantial tobacco use. A history of Sjögren's syndrome, chronic or recurrent sialadenitis with swelling particularly associated with calculi is very valuable clue in making a diagnosis.

Naturally, a history of the patient's general medical condition is important in order to be able to determine whether they require a preoperative medical evaluation. Patients with multisystem disease or poorly controlled medical problems will need to be stabilized prior to surgery. This is particularly important in older patients who are often those having more advanced disease and will have to undergo lengthy extirpative and reconstructive procedures. Inquiry must be made into the use of any type of coagulation disorder or the use of medications, which have anticoagulant properties, such as aspirin, ibuprofen and warfarin.

A complete examination of the head and neck must be carried out. Note should be made of the size and degree of mobility of the mass(es) in the parotid gland. Infiltration or ulceration of the skin by cancer or fixation of the skin to underlying structures should be recorded. The skin in the lymphatic drainage basin of the parotid gland should be inspected for the presence of squamous cell carcinoma or melanoma. Facial nerve function should be evaluated and graded according to the House-Brackmann grading system for postoperative comparison. The presence or absence of a mass in the area of the soft palate and lateral pharyngeal wall suggests parapharyngeal space extension of a deep lobe parotid tumor (Fig. 2A). This should be confirmed by imaging studies (Fig. 2B). The neck must be palpated to detect enlarged lymph nodes and the size and mobility of the nodes should be measured and recorded.

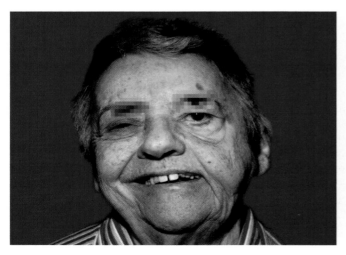

Fig. 1: Patient with recent onset of pain, a mass in the left parotid gland and facial nerve paralysis

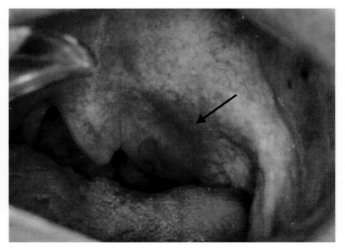

Fig. 2A: Patient with mass in the parapharyngeal space (arrow)

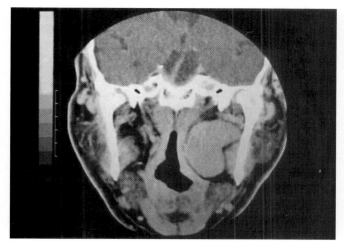

Fig. 2B: CT scan demonstrating a deep lobe parotid tumor with extension into the parapharyngeal space

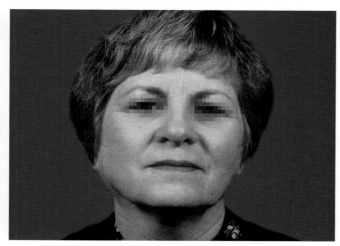

Fig. 3A: Patient with a mass in the right parotid gland which was not mobile on palpation

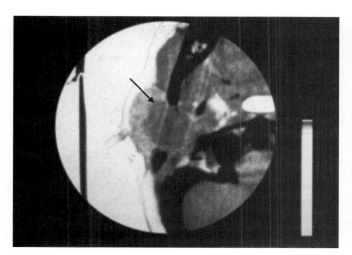

Fig. 3B: MRI demonstrating tumor of the deep lobe (arrow)

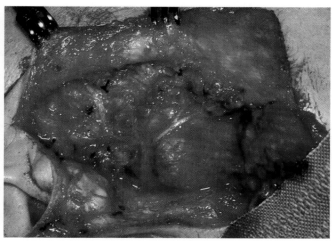

Fig. 3C: Facial nerve adherent to the capsule of a tumor of the deep lobe of the parotid gland

The role of imaging studies prior to parotidectomy is somewhat controversial, but it is usually agreed that imaging is not necessary for a mobile mass in the superficial lobe of the parotid gland with benign characteristics on history and physical examination. Most tumors of the parotid gland occur in the "tail of the parotid" (inferior aspect of the parotid gland) and up to 90% of these are benign. When confronted with a mass which is either partially or completely immobile (Fig. 3A) the possibility of a deep lobe parotid tumor with or without extension into the parapharyngeal space should be considered. In such cases, imaging studies (Fig. 3B) will provide information which will be valuable in organizing a comprehensive plan of management. Tumors, which are relatively immobile, and are either fixed or very close to

the external auditory meatus, suggests the possibility that the main trunk of the facial nerve will not be identifiable at the stylomastoid foramen (Fig. 3C). Imaging should be carried out to corroborate this impression. The temporal bone, mastoid air cell system and the skull base should be included in order to rule out the involvement of these areas and to provide a "road map" for the otologist, if opening the mastoid and mobilizing the facial nerve out of the Fallopian canal becomes necessary.

Magnetic resonance imaging (MRI) with gadolinium provides important information regarding the consistency and the extent of the tumor and its relationship to the surrounding structures. CT scanning with contrast may also be helpful in obtaining information regarding the relationship of the tumor to the adjacent bone or vascular structures. Co-registered positron emission tomography-computed tomography (PET-CT) scanning has come into recent popularity and has proved to be useful in the preliminary staging of malignant tumors in order to rule out distant metastasis. This study establishes a baseline against which post-treatment scans could be compared.

Fine needle aspiration biopsy (FNAB) in the evaluation of parotid masses is also somewhat controversial. The test result largely depends up on the operator and the interpreter; a negative biopsy for malignancy does not necessarily rule out malignancy or the vice-versa. The use of FNAB may be useful in ruling out cancer in patients with bilateral parotid tumors, especially to those patients who are in poor general health or who are reluctant to undergo removal of the mass. In patients with an obvious malignancy, presenting with pain and facial nerve paralysis, FNAB may be helpful in characterizing the type of malignancy, which is useful in pretreatment planning.

Surgery remains the mainstay of initial treatment in most of the patients with a tumor in the parotid gland. After the patient has been thoroughly evaluated, the surgeon will devise a plan of action for effective management. An elaborate discussion with the patient and his family members will help them in understanding the treatment plan thoroughly. The most important goal in effecting a cure is complete tumor removal, appropriate management of cervical lymphatics, facial nerve preservation when oncologically safe and rehabilitation procedures, when the nerve is resected.

Surgery of the parotid gland is really the surgery of the facial nerve. The entire operation, including placement of the incisions, any unavoidable cosmetic defect, the ever present possibility of facial nerve paralysis or paresis, and the need for reconstruction of the nerve or any adjacent skin, must be thoroughly discussed with the patient. It is important that the patient and his family understand the risks and benefits of the procedure as well as the potential consequences and complications prior to proceeding.

The operation of total parotidectomy is always performed with the patient under general endotracheal anesthesia. Adjustments in the anesthesia plan must be made in accordance with the patient's medical comorbidities and the estimated length of the operation. Once general anesthesia is induced, the endotracheal tube is placed toward the side opposite of the operative field and taped to the area of the oral commissure in order to stabilize it. The patient's head is then turned toward the side opposite to the tumor. A folded sheet is placed under the shoulders to extend the neck. If an electrophysiological monitoring is to be used, electrodes are inserted in the appropriate areas of the face prior to the prepping and draping. The face and neck are painted with Betadine solution. If a graft from a distant site

is contemplated, that site should also receive a sterile prep. Drapes should be applied in such a way that the face and neck are exposed and the drape is fixed to the skin with staples. Draping of distant donor sites is also carried out at this time.

Paralytic agents should not be used after inducing anesthesia in order to be able to properly identify the main trunk of the facial nerve. The dissection is performed under direct vision using landmarks such as the cartilaginous tragal pointer and the styloid process. The nerve is often identified by movement of the face caused by stimulation when the nerve is touched by the instrument during dissection. After the main trunk is identified, further dissection is carried along the branches of the nerve. When the nerve is touched by the instrument, facial twitching alerts the surgeon to the presence of the nerve branches. The use of paralytic agents would eliminate this safety feature.

Intraoperative electrophysiological facial monitoring is routinely used by some surgeons and never used by others. The indications for such monitoring includes patients with recurrent sialadenitis, patients who have recurrent tumors (benign or malignant), a patient reoperated for other indications unless the facial nerve was never previously identified and dissected. The operative field in such patients is usually very fibrotic and the landmarks may be obscured by the disease process or by multiple masses of recurrent tumor. In such cases, monitoring is useful in helping to prevent injury to the facial nerve.

In most cases of total parotidectomy, blood replacement is not necessary although there are occasions when it may be required. Therefore, blood should be ordered preoperatively and the blood bank should be alerted to the potential need for transfusion. Patients undergoing lengthy procedures, such as those requiring microvascular free flap transfer with or without facial nerve reconstruction, will require careful attention to fluid and electrolyte replacement during the operative period. The body of the patient should be kept warm with blankets to prevent hypothermia, particularly in patients undergoing microvascular free flap transfer in order to prevent thrombosis of the blood vessels in the graft.

SURGICAL TECHNIQUE

After the patient is prepped and draped as described earlier, the incision is outlined with a marking pen (Fig. 4A) and made with a scalpel or by use of electrocautery with a very fine needle tip or using a Shaw scalpel. This does not cause excessive scarring and saves a good bit of time in not having to go back and identify and coagulate the individual bleeders. Incision is made in the natural skin fold in the preauricular area and is carried posterior to the earlobe in a curvilinear fashion

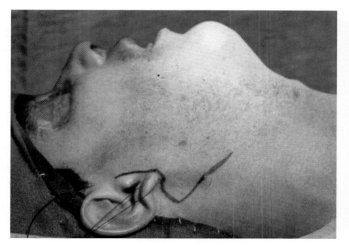

Fig. 4A: Incision for parotidectomy

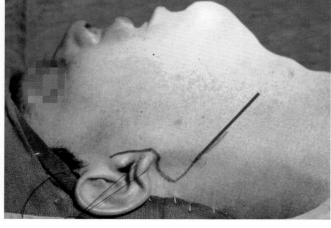

Fig. 4B: Extension of incision for submandibular gland dissection

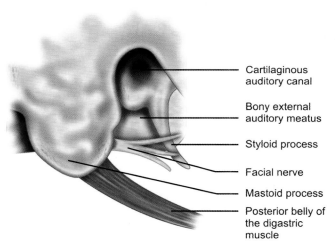

Cartilaginous auditory canal

Bony external auditory meatus

Styloid process

Facial nerve

Mastoid process

Posterior belly of the digastric muscle

Fig. 5: Landmarks used in identification of the main trunk of the facial nerve

and carried down to the natural skin fold in the neck. If the patient has a deep lobe parotid tumor with parapharyngeal space extension, the incision should be extended anteriorly in order to be able to mobilize the submandibular gland (Fig. 4B). In patients who will have a neck dissection associated with a total parotidectomy, the incision is carried down just posterior to the sternocleidomastoid muscle and continued in a transverse fashion just above the clavicle. The flaps are then undermined in the subcutaneous plane and sewn to the drapes with 0 silk suture. The posterior skin flap is then elevated in order to identify the sternocleidomastoid muscle. The parotid gland is elevated off the sternocleidomastoid muscle. The greater auricular nerve is isolated and usually divided. A small posterior nerve branch may be preserved if anatomically and oncologically possible.

The following landmarks are identified using sharp and blunt dissection: the mastoid tip, the cartilaginous and bony external auditory meatus (Fig. 5). The posterior belly of the digastric muscle is at the same depth as the facial nerve. This dissection allows the gland to be separated from the muscle. The stylomastoid foramen where the facial nerve exits the temporal bone, is located between the bony external auditory meatus and the mastoid tip. The soft tissues are elevated off the cartilaginous pointer, which is helpful since this structure points to the area approximately 1 cm from the main trunk of the facial nerve. The parotid masseteric fascia is undermined and incised. This allows anterior displacement of the gland with small right angle retractors. Dissection is then carried along with a blunt tip scissors or a curved hemostat, using a small forcep to grasp bits of tissue until the main trunk of the facial nerve is identified. Dissecting in a plane parallel and just lateral to the nerve, a tunnel can be formed over the nerve and with the facial nerve in full vision, the tissue overlying the nerve is incised (Fig. 6). The blunt retractors are then moved anteriorly and this maneuver is repeated until the bifurcation of the facial nerve is identified. When the tunnel is developed the clamp is spread and the parotid tissue is divided by the surgeon or an assistant using scissors, scalpel or Shaw knife. When a deep lobe tumor is present, the main trunk of the facial nerve may be displaced laterally and may be encountered sooner than expected. In children, the main trunk may not be as deep as in adults. Dissection is then carried along the small branches of the facial nerve anteriorly until the anterior border of the masseter muscle, which is the anterior extent of the parotid gland, is reached. This completely mobilizes the superficial lobe of the parotid gland. As the gland is dissected anteriorly, it becomes pedicled on the most anterior portion of the gland and Stensen's duct.

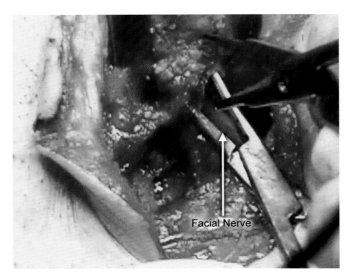

Fig. 6: Dissection of the parotid tissue in order to expose the main trunk of facial nerve. A tunnel is created over the nerve and the parotid tissue is incised

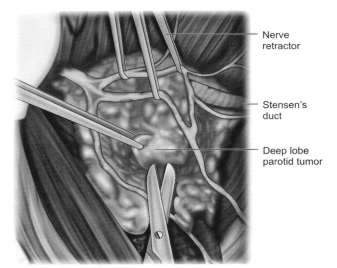

Fig. 7: Diagram of retraction of facial nerve and removal of deep lobe parotid tumor

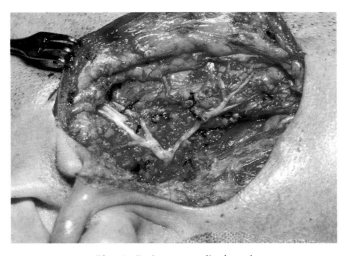

Fig. 8: Entire nerve displayed

At this point, some surgeons will incise the pedicle and excise the superficial lobe. However, since the superficial lobe is rarely involved by a deep lobe tumor, it is oncologically sound to preserve it, which is cosmetically beneficial to the patient since, it restores the normal anatomy.

Since the total parotidectomy is modified to accommodate a variety of pathologies, several different techniques will be described.

Benign Tumors of the Deep Lobe Parotid Gland

After the dissection described above, the entire deep lobe parotid tumor should be exposed. All or some of the branches of the facial nerve will be splayed out over the tumor and adhere to its capsule. Using blunt tip scissors or a curved hemostat the branches of the nerve in contact with the tumor are undermined and gently separated from the capsule of the tumor. Nerve retractors are used to retract the nerve as it is mobilized off the gland. Once the branches of the nerve have been mobilized and retracted, the tumor is removed by sharp and blunt dissections (Fig. 7). The tumor is then sent to pathology and the wound is irrigated. Hemostasis is obtained, entire nerve is displayed (Fig. 8) and hemovac drains are placed. Using the electrical stimulator, the facial nerve is tested from the main trunk to the most peripheral branches. If the nerve stimulates normally, normal facial function is expected. If the nerve is anatomically intact but does not stimulate, it is likely that all or some of the facial muscles will not function postoperatively. Facial function should begin within three months and the patient should be so advised. Antibiotics are not used during or after this procedure. If the superficial lobe has been preserved, it is sewn back into place using chromic catgut sutures. The skin is closed with sutures and steri-strips are placed on the incision.

Malignant Tumors of the Parotid Gland

Patients with a high-grade malignant tumor of the parotid gland should have a total parotidectomy carried out as described above. Patients who present facial nerve without paralysis, requires meticulous dissection of the facial nerve which should be carried out in making every effort to preserve it. Sometimes, despite the fact that the patient has good facial function, there may be encasement or invasion of the entire facial nerve or more likely branches of the facial nerve, such as the ramus mandibularis. In locally advanced cancer, it may not be possible to identify the main trunk of the facial nerve as described above. In such cases, a mastoidectomy is done; the Fallopian canal is opened and the facial nerve is mobilized. After transecting the nerve, frozen sections are obtained to ensure clear margins. In those cases, branches of the facial nerve may be removed and as many branches as possible are preserved. When the nerve is transected, samples of the nerve from the proximal and distal ends are sent for frozen section analysis to ensure clear margins.

When the patient has invasion of the facial nerve, the nerve is transected near the stylomastoid foramen and frozen section margins are obtained from the proximal portion of the nerve. Prior to proceeding with excision of the gland, the peripheral branches of the facial nerve are identified, marked appropriately with vessel loops and if not involved by tumor, preserved for reconstruction. Dissection is then carried out as described above, removing the masseter muscle with a deep margin of resection; together with the entire parotid gland. Aggressive tumors may involve the mandible or the temporal bone, making it necessary to remove all or some of these structures to ensure clear margins. Frozen sections are obtained to assure tumor clearance. If frozen sections are positive; more tissue must be resected since leaving a positive margin places the patient on a "death trajectory." Neck dissection usually follows after the parotidectomy. Facial nerve reconstruction procedures are then carried out. If replacement of the overlying skin is necessary, either a regional pedicle flap or microvascular free tissue transfer technique may be used.

Cancer of the Skin Invading the Parotid Gland

A total parotidectomy should be carried out in continuity with the cancer and the surrounding skin. Neck dissection should be carried out after the removal of parotidectomy specimen. Reconstruction of the defect may include facial nerve grafting, if the nerve is taken and resurfaced, where the skin has been excised (Figs 9A to F). This is usually done at the time of parotidectomy and may include a regional pedicle flap such as a cervical-pectoral rotation flap, often with a pectoralis major flap to provide bulk under the rotation flap, latissimus dorsi flap or a microvascular free tissue transfer (Fig. 10). Some surgeons prefer to delay the reconstruction until the status of all the margins are assured by permanent sections.

Metastatic Cancer to the Parotid Lymph Nodes

Squamous cell carcinoma, malignant melanoma or Merkel cell carcinoma arising in the skin of the auricle, temple, facial skin or brow may metastasize to the intra- or periparotid lymph nodes. A total parotidectomy, as described above should be carried out attempting to preserve the facial nerve (Figs 11A to F). Any documented or suspicious lesions in the above mentioned areas of the skin should also be excised. Patients with a primary cancer of the auricle may require auriculectomy. A neck dissection should be carried out after the specimen is removed since patients with cancer metastatic to the parotid nodes often have metastases in the neck.

Deep Lobe Parotid Tumor with Parapharyngeal Space Extension

Patients undergoing surgery for a deep lobe tumor with an extension into the parapharyngeal space (Figs 12A to H) should first undergo complete mobilization of the submandibular gland, which is facilitated by ligation of the facial artery, when it emerges deep to the digastric muscle.

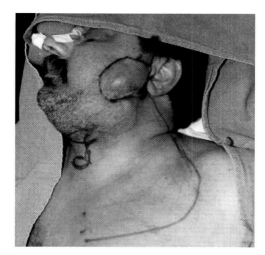

Fig. 9A: Patient with cancer of the parotid gland with invasion of skin. Expected excision of skin and design of cervical pectoral rotation flap

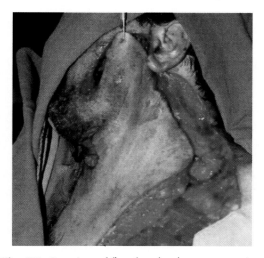

Fig. 9B: Rotation of flap for cheek reconstruction

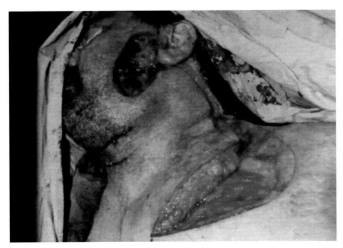

Fig. 9C: Design of pectoral muscle flap to be placed under the rotation skin flap to provide bulk for contour

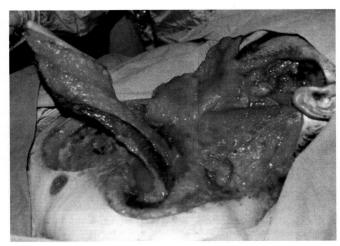

Fig. 9D: Pectoralis muscle flap elevated

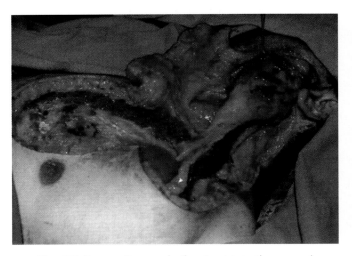

Fig. 9E: Pectoralis muscle flap inset into the wound

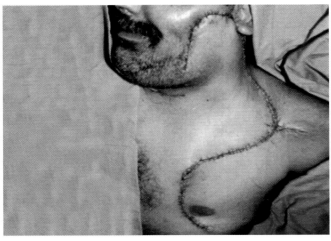

Fig. 9F: Inset of rotation flap. Closure of donor sites

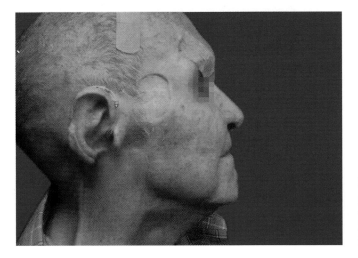

Fig. 10: Patient with cancer of the skin invading parotid. Total parotidectomy with facial nerve preservation and excision of overlying skin and neck dissection. Defect resurfaced with latissimus dorsi flap. Patient previously had cancers removed from the auricle and temporal area

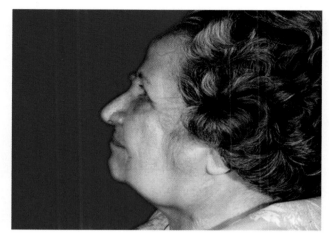

Fig. 11A: Patient with squamous cell carcinoma metastatic to the lymph nodes in the parotid gland and left side of the neck

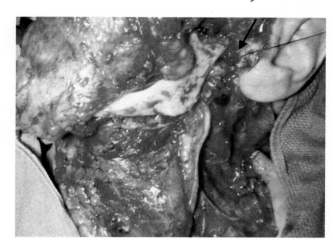

Fig. 11B: Entire facial nerve and parotid gland excised with neck dissection. Facial nerve resected and marked with a black silk suture

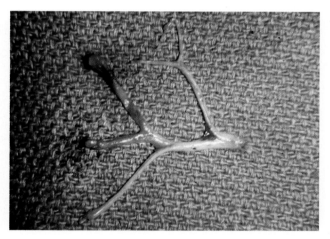

Fig. 11C: Branch of fourth cervical nerve (cervical plexus) prepared for grafting

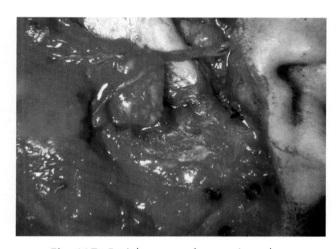

Fig. 11D: Facial nerve grafts sewn into place

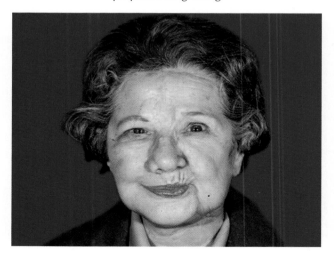

Fig. 11E: Patient smiling

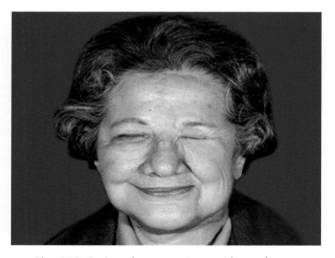

Fig. 11F: Patient demonstrating good eye closure

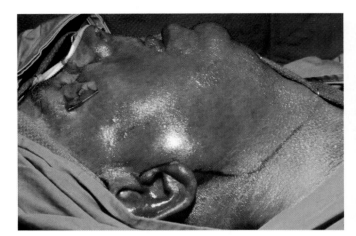

Fig. 12A: Man with a large tumor of the deep lobe of the parotid gland with massive extension into the parapharyngeal space. Incision extended anteriorly on the neck to allow dissection of the submandibular triangle

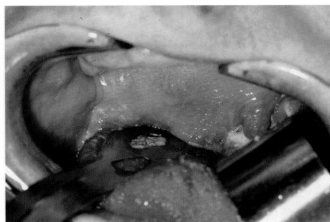

Fig. 12B: Same patient with parapharyngeal space involvement displacing uvula into contact with the left tonsil

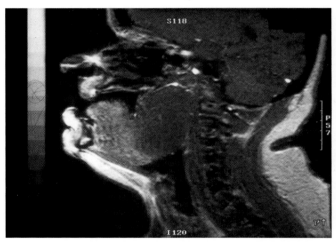

Fig. 12C: MRI identifying large mass occluding the pharyngeal airway

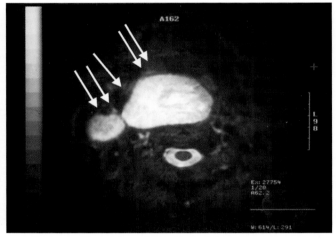

Fig. 12D: MRI of deep lobe parotid tumor demonstrating extension into parapharyngeal space. Note: Groove made by stylomandibular ligament (arrows)

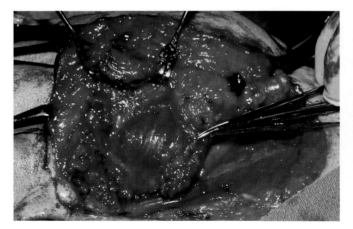

Fig. 12E: Large deep lobe parotid tumor with nerve splayed out and attached to the tumor

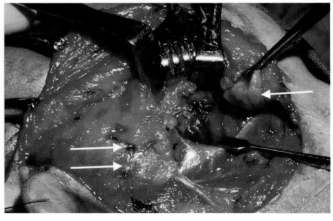

Fig. 12F: Submandibular gland mobilized anteriorly (arrow) to disclose the mass in the parapharyngeal space (2 arrows)

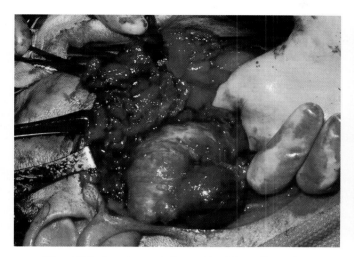

Fig. 12G: Specimen delivered by blunt dissection

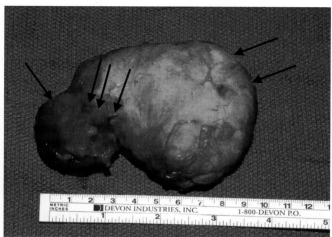

Fig. 12H: Specimen demonstrates deep lobe parotid tumor (arrow) with large parapharyngeal space extension (2 arrows). Note: Groove made by stylomandibular ligament (3 arrows)

The apex of the parapharyngeal space is in the submandibular triangle and mobilizing the gland facilitates dissection into the parapharyngeal space. After approaching the deep lobe as described above and mobilizing and gently retracting the facial nerve, the tumor and its parapharyngeal space extensions are mobilized by sharp and blunt dissection. The parapharyngeal extension lies invariably into the prestyloid parapharyngeal space which has no neurovascular structures of concern. After hemostasis has been obtained, the wound is irrigated. Hemovac drains are placed in the parapharyngeal space and the parotid bed and the wounds are closed in layers. A pressure dressing is applied. It is rarely necessary to split the mandible for added exposure.

Chronic Sialadenitis

Hayes Martin in 1964, stated that, "complete excision of the parotid gland is difficult because the gland has an indistinct capsule and the borders of the gland are somewhat difficult to distinguish from subcutaneous fat. The attempt to remove every particle of the parotid tissue is probably seldom necessary or advisable. On the other hand, given sufficient time and patience practically all of the gland can be removed with preservation of the facial nerve."

The facial nerve can usually be identified as described above since the main trunk of the facial nerve is not usually subjected to changes from infection. After the nerve is identified, dissection is carried anteriorly. Once the dissection is in the parenchyma of the gland, chronic infection and scarring may make identification and dissection of the facial nerve challenging. We suggest the use of electrophysiological facial monitoring in these cases to help in identifying the

peripheral branches of the nerve. If scarring prevents identification of the more proximal branches, an effort should be made to identify a peripheral branch, such as the ramus mandibularis or buccal branch and carry out a retrograde dissection along the nerve until the main trunk is identified and then dissection may be resumed anteriorly.

A total parotidectomy is carried out and is pedicled on Stensen's duct. The duct is skeletonized into the buccal mucosa (Fig. 13A). Attention is paid to making certain that there are no stones in the distal end of the duct. The duct is then excised including the punctum in the buccal mucosa (Fig. 13B). The mucosal defect is sutured or closed. Any remnants of the parotid gland are removed in a piecemeal, which usually involves mobilization of branches of the facial nerve. The procedure is completed as described above. Perioperative intravenous antibiotics are given.

Recurrent Tumors

Patients with recurrent tumors, either benign or malignant, should undergo identification of the main trunk of the facial nerve and then dissection is performed through total parotidectomy as described above for chronic sialadenitis. Electrophysiological facial nerve monitoring is used as in chronic sialadenitis cases. This is usually not a problem since the most common cause of recurrence is that, a formal parotidectomy with facial nerve dissection was not done at the initial operation. This leaves the area of the main trunk without scarring. The most common recurrent tumor is pleomorphic adenoma (Fig. 14A). These are usually not single, but rather occur as multiple small nodules and frequently there will be parotid tissue remaining because the

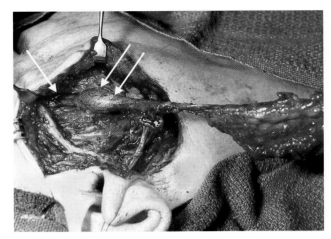

Fig. 13A: Dissection of Stensen's duct into the buccal mucosa (arrow). Large calculus in distal duct (2 arrows)

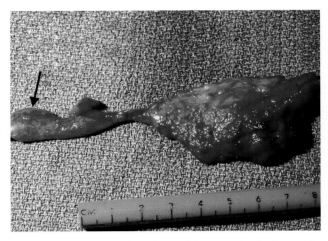

Fig. 13B: Specimen of total parotidectomy including entire Stensen's duct and calculus (arrow)

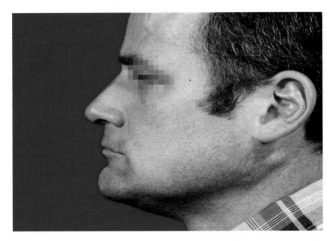

Fig. 14A: Patient with recurrent pleomorphic adenoma. The tumor has been enucleated and parotidectomy was not done originally

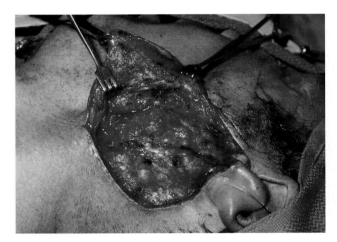

Fig. 14B: Exposure of gland reveals multiple recurrences

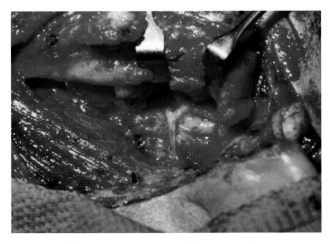

Fig. 14C: Facial nerve exposed. Total parotidectomy was then carried out with facial nerve dissection

recurrence is usually related to incomplete removal for the first time when the surgery was done. In this form of total parotidectomy, every effort should be made to preserve all branches of the facial nerve, but it may not be possible in some cases as in Figures 14B and C.

POSTOPERATIVE TREATMENT

The patient is extubated and transferred to the recovery room for observation. Drains are maintained on suction and if only the parotid gland is involved, the drain is usually removed within the first 24 hours. If a neck dissection is included the drains may remain longer. The compression dressing is removed after the drains are removed. The wound is closed with absorbable sutures, which are left in place

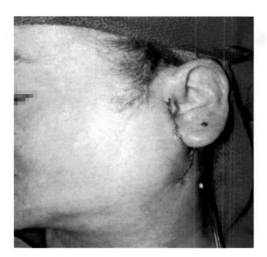

Fig. 15A: Patient with hematoma in wound. History of chronic aspirin ingestion despite urging to stop

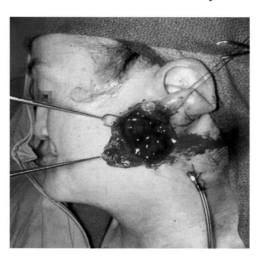

Fig. 15B: Blood clot exposed—bleeding is stopped—the wound is irrigated and the hemovac drain is replaced with a new one

until the patient is seen in the office approximately 1 week postoperative. If the wound appears to be healing well, the steri-strips and sutures are removed.

Since the greater auricular nerve is routinely sacrificed, the patients have to undergo an anesthesia of the earlobe. This may be somewhat annoying at first, but after approximately 1 year, most patients have no complaints.

It is important to be compulsive about intraoperative hemostasis in order to prevent hematoma, which occurs in a very small percentage of patients. The authors' experience indicates that hematoma is more likely to occur in patients who are taking aspirin or nonsteroidal anti-inflammatory drugs and we always counsel patients against the use of such medications for 7 to 10 days prior to surgery. When a hematoma is detected (Fig. 15A), the patient should be returned to the operation room and under general anesthesia, the wound is opened, the hematoma is evacuated and the wound is explored. Ordinarily, there are no large bleeding vessels, but rather a general oozing is found. The facial nerve, of course, must be in full view in the operative field always in order to protect it, which is safe to take care of the bleeding areas with clamps and sutures, but with diffuse oozing it may be necessary to use bipolar cautery in the areas away from the nerve. The wound is copiously irrigated. New hemovac drains are placed because of clot formation in the original drains (Fig. 15B).

Postoperative wound infections are very rare. Arriaga and Myers reported a series of 175 parotidectomies performed without antibiotics; infection occurred in less than 5% of patients. Therefore, routine administration of antibiotics is not justified. If the wound becomes infected, antibiotics should be given. Patients operated for chronic sialadenitis

should be given perioperative antibiotics. Oral antibiotics are routinely prescribed for 2 weeks to prevent postoperative infection and to ensure complete healing.

Postoperative sialocele usually occurs in patients with superficial lobe parotidectomy and is not seen in patients with total parotidectomy, since theoretically all of the functioning parotid tissue has been removed.

Patients who have had the microvascular free tissue transfer will require intensive nursing care and monitoring. Surgery which includes microvascular flaps is usually performed in older patients and due to the length of the operation and the administration of large quantities of fluids, these patients are usually admitted directly to the intensive care unit (ICU) and diuresed over the next several days. It is important for the surgical team to monitor the drains, remove them and remove the dressings as appropriate. The use of Doppler monitors is helpful in determining whether the pulse is present at the anastomotic site indicating that the vessel is patent. If not, a thrombosis of the artery or vein should be suspected and the patient is taken back to the operation room as quickly as possible for thrombectomy and reanastomosis.

Inadvertent injury to the facial nerve occurs in 3–5% of the cases. This may be due to excessive stimulation of the nerve intraoperatively or stretching the nerve during retraction. At the completion of the surgery, if the facial nerve is anatomically intact and the nerve is functional, as demonstrated by the use of the nerve stimulator, the full return of function is expected. At times, when the nerve is anatomically intact but the face does not move with the use of nerve stimulator, probably due to the weakness of all or some of the nerve branches for up to three months when a full recovery is expected. The etiology is thought to be due to the pressure or traction on the nerves during the surgery. When the nerve has been resected, a gold weight should be placed on the upper eyelid in the postoperative period. The ability to close the eye can be determined by taping various weights to the eyelid and the one which produces total closure of the eyelid is chosen for insertion into the upper eyelid. This is done under local anesthesia by making an incision in the skin crease, above the tarsal plate of the upper eyelid. The skin is undermined to form a subcutaneous pocket and a gold weight is inserted to ensure complete eye closure. Patients with partial functional recovery following the facial nerve reconstruction surgery often will have an ectropion of the lower eyelid, which could be repaired by V excision and partial tarsorrhaphy.

Patients who have had total parotidectomy have a much higher incidence of Frey's syndrome (gustatory sweating) than those who have superficial or partial lobectomy, based on the removal of the auriculotemporal nerve in the superior deep portion of the gland, as it leaves the infratemporal fossa. The gustatory sweating can be abolished by injection of Botox into the skin in the area, in which sweating occurs guided by the use of Minor's starch-iodine test (Fig. 16). The injections usually abolish the sweating for up to 1 year or in some patients permanently and do not cause facial paralysis.

First bite syndrome is characterized by pain in the area of the resected parotid gland, when the patient takes the first bite into the meal. The more the patients chew and eat, the quicker the symptoms disappear. It is unlikely that the first bite syndrome would occur when total parotidectomy is carried out.

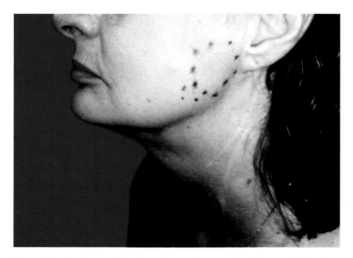

Fig. 16: Patient with Frey's syndrome for Botox injection. Circle drawn on skin is the area of sweating identified by Minor's starch-iodine test

Patients who have had undergone reconstruction of the facial nerve with free nerve grafting, usually, have no facial function until at the early 6 months or more likely by 9 months, with the complete return of function within 1 year. It is helpful to have the patients undergo physical therapy with an individual, experienced in facial nerve rehabilitation. The first sign of return of function is usually the straight horizontal oral commissure rather than the sagging oral commissure seen in complete facial nerve paralysis. The midface always does better than the ramus mandibularis or the frontalis muscle, which rarely regains function despite meticulous surgical techniques when compared in approximation over the other nerves.

HIGHLIGHTS

I. Indications
- Deep lobe parotid tumors (benign/malignant)
- Malignant tumors of the superficial lobe
- Recurrent tumors (benign/malignant)
- Metastatic cancer to the parotid gland
- Cancer of the skin invading the parotid gland
- Chronic or recurrent sialadenitis.

II. Contraindications
- Lymphoma
- Skull base invasion
- Metastatic cancer involving distant sites
- Patient medically unfit for surgery
- Patient refuses surgery.

III. Special Preoperative Considerations
- Thorough patient evaluation
- Appropriate imaging studies
- Biopsy as necessary
- Evaluation by other members of the surgical team, e.g. otologist, plastic surgeon when necessary
- Thorough patient counseling and informed consent.

IV. Special Intraoperative Considerations
- Facial nerve monitoring, especially for patients with recurrent tumor or chronic sialadenitis
- Availability of pathologist for frozen section review of tissues to assure complete tumor removal
- Antibiotics necessary only for patients with chronic sialadenitis
- A mastoid approach may be necessary if the facial nerve cannot be identified in the area of the stylomastoid foramen
- Immediate reconstruction of the facial nerve is more successful than delayed reconstruction
- Peripheral branches of the facial nerve should be identified and preserved for reconstruction in cases, when the main trunk of the nerve is removed

- Ligation of branches of the external carotid artery and retromandibular vein can prevent excessive blood loss
- Total parotidectomy may be extended to include resection of the facial nerve, temporal bone resection, partial mandibulectomy, resection of the overlying skin and adjacent musculature
- Neck dissection should be included in resection of high-grade malignant tumors and skin cancer metastatic to the parotid lymph nodes
- Removal of the parapharyngeal space extension of a deep lobe parotid tumor is facilitated by the mobilization of the submandibular gland
- A reconstructive surgeon should be available if the facial nerve is removed or skin is excised.

V. Special Postoperative Considerations

- Gold weight should be inserted into upper eyelid for patients with facial nerve paralysis
- Frey's syndrome may be treated with injections of Botox
- Patients with high-grade parotid cancer should receive adjunctive radiation therapy.

VI. Complications

- Facial nerve paralysis
- Frey's syndrome (syndrome of gustatory sweating)
- Hematoma
- Recurrent tumor.

ADDITIONAL READING

1. An Atlas of Head and Neck Surgery. Lore JM and Medina J (Eds). 4th edition. Philadelphia:Elsevier/Saunders; 2004.
2. Arriaga MA, Myers EN. The surgical management of chronic parotitis. Laryngoscope. 1990;100(12):1270-5.
3. Johns ME. Total parotidectomy. In: Johns ME, Price JC, Mattox DE (Eds). Atlas of Head and Neck Surgery, Volume 1. Philadelphia: BC Decker; 1990.
4. Johnson JT. Parotidectomy. In: Myers EN (Ed). Operative Oto-laryngology – Head and Neck Surgery, 2nd Edition. Saunders/Elsevier; 2008.
5. McCammin SD, Patel SG. Management of salivary gland neoplasms. In: deSouza C (Ed). Head and Neck Surgery. New Delhi: Jaypee Brothers Medical Publishers; 2009.
6. Moore EJ, KerryD Olsen. Total parotidectomy. In: Salivary Gland Disorders, Myers EN, Ferris RL (Eds). Heidelberg, Germany: Springer Co; 2007.
7. Myers EN, Johnson JT. Management of tumors of the parapharyngeal space. In: Myers EN (Ed). Operative Otolar-yngology – Head and Neck Surgery, 2nd edition. Saunders/Elsevier; 2008.
8. Simental A, Carrau RL. Malignant neoplasms of the salivary glands. In: Cummings CW, et al (Eds). Cummings Otolaryn-gology–Head and Neck Surgery, 4th edition. Philadelphia: Elsevier/Mosby; 2005.
9. Surgery of Head and Neck Tumors. Martin Hayes B (Ed). New York: Hoeber-Harper; 1964.

Chapter **6**

Resection of Lymphangiomas and Hemangiomas of the Neck and Face in Pediatric Patients

Jochen A Werner, Behfar Eivazi

INTRODUCTION

The successful treatment of vascular anomalies depends on profound knowledge of the biologic behavior of vascular lesions and their correct classification. On the basis of the clinical course and biologic properties, Mulliken and Glowacki developed a classification that was included in the official classification by the International Society for the Study of Vascular Anomalies (ISSVA) and has remained still valid. The main differentiation has to be made between hemangiomas and vascular malformations. Hemangiomas represent an entire different entity than vascular malformations since their biologic behavior is based on proliferation and cell division. They are real "tumors". Vascular malformations, on the other hand, are the result of abnormalities in the development of vascular components during embryogenesis. The differentiation between these two entities is the first step toward determining an accurate diagnosis and the first-line therapy regimen.

INFANTILE HEMANGIOMAS

Infantile hemangiomas are proliferating embryonal tumors and have to be classified according to the stage, growth pattern, appearance and the organ specificity. In the early or initial phase, they may partially appear for a few days. Depending on the type of growth, they are diffuse, infiltrating the surrounding tissue or in case of limited growth, are sharply demarcated. During the proliferation phase, a cutaneously located infantile hemangioma proliferates at a different pace, while spreading in size by exophytic or endophytic

subcutaneous growth. The maturation phase follows in which proliferation comes to a halt. The regression phase occurs, which is followed by the phase of the fibrolipomatous transformation. This is usually completed by the sixth birthday in cutaneous localized hemangiomas. Regression proceeds usually faster in localized, than in diffused infiltrating cutaneous or subcutaneous hemangiomas.

Hemangiomas can show a more plane, but segmental growth pattern which can follow developmental segments of the face. These so-called "segmental hemangiomas" are rare, but when located in the head and face area, they are often more problematic than localized hemangiomas. Complications are mostly ulcerations or functional compromises. Segmental hemangioma in the so-called "beard" area or the upper frontal part of the chest are often associated with involvement of the upper respiratory tract and might lead to life-threatening breathing problems. The so-called PHACE(S) syndrome (P, posterior fossa malformation; H, segmental hemangioma; A, arterial anomalies; C, coarctation of aorta; E, eye malformations; S, cleft sternum) is a syndromal form of manifestation of segmental hemangiomas in the head area combined with cerebral, ophthalmological and/or cardiac malformations.

VASCULAR MALFORMATIONS

Vascular malformations are classified according to the predominantly involved portions of the vascular system and subdivided into capillary, venous, arteriovenous, lymphatic and hemolymphatic malformations. Another clinically relevant property is their flow behavior. There is a differentiation between low-flow lesions (so called low or no-flow malformations), such as lymphatic, capillary and venous malformations and high-flow lesions such as arteriovenous malformations and arteriovenous fistulas. Vascular malformations of the head and neck area reveal an inhomogeneous pattern of onset and symptoms, depending on their size, location, morphology and also on their flow behavior. A common feature of all vascular malformations is that they can encounter in all organs and regions of the body. They can appear in singular, multiple or disseminated forms and may vary in their growth pattern, from well-demarcated to diffuse infiltrating shapes. Their appearance can be an isolated, multiple or complex form, e.g. as a part of a syndromal disease. Their growth pace usually behaves proportional to the growth of the body. Acute volume increase and associated clinical symptoms are observed during hormonal fluctuations (e.g. puberty), by infections because of thrombosis, hemorrhage or by trauma. The main difference to hemangiomas is the fact that a spontaneous regression of vascular malformations generally never occurs. In the head and neck high-flow malformations are less frequently observed than low-flow lesions. Both kinds may cause significant clinical symptoms due to space occupation, bleeding or ulcerations. When any of the following organs, i.e. the upper aerodigestive tract, the visual or auditory system, the skin or the facial skeleton are affected, it can result in various and inhomogenous pattern of clinical symptoms and esthetic compromises.

High-Flow/Arteriovenous Malformations

Arteriovenous malformations (AVMs) present often an unpredictable clinical course. They might appear as an asymptomatic lesion like a limited birth mark or as a palpable or pulsatile mass. Clinical symptoms can be secondary to compression of the adjacent normal structure or because of hemorrhage. Extended AVMs might cause further cardiac symptoms due to high output, heart failure or ischemic tissue necrosis due to a "steal" phenomenon. The AVM may initially remain undetected. However, throughout the patient's life, it may show a gradual enlargement proportional to the growth of the individual or it may develop in an expanding pattern as a result of many, still unexplained factors, like hormonal changes or trauma. This might explain the fact that these lesions are rarely diagnosed and treated in pediatric patients.

Low-Flow Malformations

Capillary Malformations

The port wine stain is a classic example for capillary malformations. If untreated, they may become more nodular during the course of time and increasingly involve the subcutaneous and soft tissue. They occur in approximately 0.3% of all newborns and often expand along the branches of the trigeminal nerve. These cases, on the other hand, are sometimes associated with syndromes, such as the Sturge-Weber syndrome and require an ophthalmological and neurological examination. Treatment with pulsed dye laser is standard for port wine stains.

Venous Malformations

Venous malformations are developmental errors comprised of dysplastic venous vessels. They manifest as a compressible, livid, bluish vascular mass or as a patch. If the upper aerodigestive tract is affected, these lesions may cause clinical symptoms like dysphagia, dyspnea, dysphonia, pain or bleeding. Additionally, the involvement of the lips, the visual parts of the oral cavity or the oropharynx may further cause psychical strain, anxiety reactions, limitations of oral and dental hygiene and restrictions of intimate activities. Further symptoms such as pain or stasis are caused by thombosis and phleboliths.

Lymphatic Malformations

The head and neck region is the most common site of lymphatic malformations (syn. lymphangiomas). About 40% of lymphangiomas are identifiable as such in the neonatal period, 75% by the end of the second year of life. Extended lymphangiomas are increasingly diagnosed prenatally by ultrasound screening. Typically, they show an abrupt volume increase in context with infections, often accompanied with intralesional hemorrhage, responsible for symptom exacerbation. In addition to their primary space occupying character, lymphangiomas can infiltrate the affected organs like the parotid gland, the tongue or the larynx. Lymphangiomas are classified according to their morphological aspects as "microcystic", "macrocystic" or "combined". A major reason for functional impairment in the head-neck area is the infestation of the tongue. For an appropriate care and therapy planning lymphatic malformations involving the tongue are graded according to their extent into four stages as follows:

Stage I: Isolated superficial microcystic lymphatic malformations of the tongue.

Stage II: Isolated lymphatic malformations of the tongue with muscle involvement:
   a. involving a part of the tongue
   b. involving the whole tongue.

Stage III: Microcystic lymphatic malformations of the tongue and the floor of mouth.

Stage IV: Extensive microcystic lymphatic malformations involving the tongue, the floor of mouth and further cervical structures.

PREOPERATIVE AND INTRAOPERATIVE DIAGNOSTIC AND PREVENTIVE MEASURES

Preoperative Imaging

B-mode ultrasound combined with color coded duplex sonography is performed for all accessible lesions. This is usually sufficient for circumscribed and superficial lesions. In all other cases, further radiological evaluation is necessary including magnetic resonance imaging (MRI) of the head and neck. In cases, of involvement of the facial skeleton, axial and coronal computed tomography (CT) is required. A diagnostic angiography is performed on all extended high-flow lesions and for extended cases without a determinate flow behavior. The CT angiography, which is an imaging technique to visualize blood vessels with the help of computer tomography, is gaining an increasing value especially for extended arteriovenous malformations of the head and neck. Based on a multislice CT, the vascular regions of interest are scanned during which a rapid intravenous injection of iodinated contrast medium is administered. This results in a representation of the vascular structure in layers, which can be obtained using a computerized 3D representation.

Preoperative Laboratory Tests and Preparations of Blood Products

All invasive interventions on extended vascular anomalies bear the risk of significant bleeding. This fact has to be considered during planning and scheduling of a surgery. Prior to surgery, beside routine laboratory parameters like electrolytes, blood count, TSH levels, urea and creatinine, determination of blood group and preparation of erythrocyte concentrate is routinely performed. The amount of erythrocyte concentrate required depends on the estimated extent of surgery. Further, the patients have to be advised about the possibility of donation of own blood for a planned surgery. If multiple donations are necessary, they should be performed in weekly intervals. The last session for donation of own blood has to be performed at least 10 days before surgery.

A detailed coagulation analysis is needed in order to identify the patients at increased risk of bleeding. This proceeding is supported by the fact that a relevant proportion of the patients with congenital vascular malformations of the head and neck show an impaired primary hemostasis. A thorough analysis of the hemostasis might be necessary since intraoperative or postoperative bleeding in patients with congenital vascular malformation may increase morbidity and can potentially be life-threatening to the patient, if an unrecognized hemostatic defect exists. Generalized hemostatic tests in patients with extensive congenital vascular malformations are recommended, especially in cases where even a minimal blood loss can raise a problem like in small children. The preoperative hemostatic tests should include blood cell count, platelet count, prothrombin time, activated partial thromboplastin time, fibrinogen levels and PFA-Epi. In case of prolonged PFA-Epi, additional tests such as levels of PFA-ADP, Von Willebrand factor and D-dimers may also be required. Furthermore, in selected cases factor analysis can also be done. Advanced venous malformation can be asscoiated with a so-called "localized intravascular coagulopathy", indicating the risk of a disseminated intravascular coagulopathy. Localized intravascular coagulopathy is associated with elevated D-dimer levels and decreased fibrinogen levels. In these cases a preventive stabilization of the hemostasis can be achieved by administration of low-molecular weight heparin medication prior to surgery.

Preoperative Embolization for High-Flow Vascular Malformations

High-flow vascular malformations represent a considerable treatment challenge because of the complex anatomic and hemorrhagic characteristics of the lesion. Therapy of choice for most extended high-flow malformations is a combination of endovascular and surgical treatment, which allows otherwise inoperable lesions to be successfully treated. Embolization, as preoperative adjuvant therapy may lead to a significant devascularization and reduces the bleeding intensity. The choice of the interventional approach (transarterial, direct puncture or combined mode) and the appropriate embolic agent is made individually for each case. Beside microparticles and coils, liquid embolic agents like Onyx® or Histoacryl® (N-butyl cyanoacrylate) are increasingly preferred for use in the treatment of craniofacial AV malformations.

Special Intraoperative Preventive Measures

Surgery of extended vascular malformations, especially venous malformations is associated with a non-negligible risk of air embolism. Both volume and rate of air accumulation are dependent on the size of the vascular lumen as well as the pressure gradient. Transesophageal echocardiography is a very sensitive method, which is routinely used as a monitoring device for detection of air embolisms during surgery. The sensitivity is further improved in combination with a precordial Doppler. Further, the placement of a central venous catheter in the right atrium is necessary to aspirate air in case of embolism.

To further decrease the homologous transfusion requirements, the operation theater is equipped with an autologous transfusion device (e.g. Cell-Saver®), which is nowadays a mandatory tool for the operative management of advanced vascular malformations. The above performances demonstrate that a close interdisciplinary cooperation in a highly specialized center is an essential prerequisite for successful treatment of extensive vascular malformations.

TREATMENT OF HEMANGIOMAS

Infantile hemangiomas are self limiting, proliferative lesions with a tendency to spontaneous regression. The crucial factor for an indication to treat a hemangioma is the growth behavior and the expected esthetic or functional impairments. An "active observation" on hemangiomas without excessive growth tendency and without esthetic or functional compromise is almost always justified.

Traditionally, established treatment concepts include systemic steroid therapy, conventional surgery and laser therapy. The cryotherapy is suitable for localized and superficial findings only. Interferon therapy is performed for extensive, life-threatening and otherwise uncontrollable cases.

Atrophic skin changes and hypopigmentation are frequently observed after laser treatments and cryotherapy. The improper use of lasers leads to massive wound healing disturbances, ulcerations, tissue necrosis and excessive scarring (Fig. 1). Revision surgery is mandatory in these failed cases.

The surprising observation of the inhibitory effect of the beta blocker propranolol on proliferating hemangiomas of the infancy overwhelmed the physicians who deal daily with the management of hemangiomas. Propranolol is a nonselective β2-blocker. Possible explanations for the effect of propranolol on hemangiomas are a decrease in blood flow and accelerated endovasal coagulation by narrowing of the hemangioma supplying capillary vessels. Further reduced expression of vascular endothelial growth factor (VEGF) and basic fibroblast growth factor (bFGF), which in turn can represent markers of proliferative hemangiomas, are discussed as responsible mechanisms. The dose of propranolol used for hemangiomas is 2 mg/kg bw per day, divided into three doses. This is usually continued for a period of up to 6 months. Recent observations in pediatric patients with infantile hemangiomas of the head and neck are promising and suggest a paradigm shift in the treatment of hemangiomas. In particular, the adverse effects in strict compliance with pediatric and cardiologic controls are considered as negligible. The surgery for infantile hemangiomas is reserved for nonresponders to the beta blocker therapy, revision cases and for correction of remnants or the residual fibrous fatty tissue.

SURGERY OF VENOUS MALFORMATIONS

Treatment of venous malformations of the head and neck is challenging. In cases of diffuse facial or cervicofacial spread, a complete conventional surgical treatment is often not possible. The choice of the optimal therapy for mucosal venous malformations of the upper aerodigestive tract depends on the location, size and extension of the lesion. The Nd:YAG laser is a suitable tool for most venous malformations of the mucosa and delivers good results with a very low incidence of complications. The CO_2 laser is suitable for lesions, which are well defined, circumscribed and accessible to a complete excision. Open surgical approaches are necessary for otherwise not sufficiently treatable findings like extensive lesions, to achieve optimal esthetic result by involvement of further parts of the facial or cervical soft tissue and to remove phleboliths, if they cause pain and stasis.

Technique of Nd:YAG Laser Therapy

In general, every therapeutical intervention with laser should be performed only by trained personnel. Depending on local regulations, the interventions have to be supervised by the officials for laser safety and comply with the laser safety regulations.

Nd:YAG laser therapy (interstitial or noncontact technique) is usually performed under general anesthesia. Treatment is carried out under ultrasound or endoscopic control. Power density normally ranges from 500 W/cm² to 3000 W/cm². The chosen power density depends on the tissue effect of the laser radiation. To protect the tissue from serious

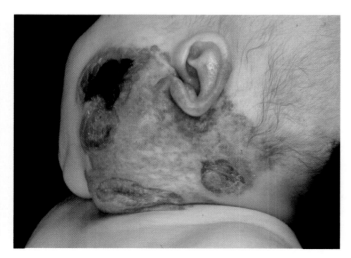

Fig. 1: Necrosis and ulcerations after excessive interstitial laser therapy of a parotideal hemangioma, performed in a peripheric department

heat damage, the Nd:YAG laser radiation should be applied exclusively with simultaneous tissue cooling. This is carried out with ice cubes (not containing air bubbles) or with an ice cold Ringer's solution for "enoral" or "endopharyngeal" treatment. The depth of penetration of the laser radiation can be increased by tissue compression with a piece of ice. For interstitial Nd:YAG laser therapy the laser light is applied via a bare fiber directly onto the vascular tissue. For non-contact therapy, laser is applied on the lesion's surface in multiple single spots or under a continuous movement of the laser beam starting from the peripheral border of the lesion to its center. This is continued, until shrinkage and pallor of the lesion is visualized. Treatment is repeated in multiple sessions, depending on the extent and infestation of diverse regions.

Nd:YAG Laser Therapy of Venous Malformations (Laryngeal and Pharyngeal Regions)

First the inspection of the upper aerodigestive tract by endoscopy and photo documentations of findings are performed (Figs 2A and B). As a first therapeutic step, the Nd:YAG laser therapy is performed in the area of the oral cavity or oropharynx in noncontact form. The laser therapy is initiated with a power level of 8 watts, which can be gradually increased up to 25 watts, depending on the response of the tissue. Cooling is performed by dumping of ice cold Ringer's solution into the oral cavity. Multiple laser spots are set or the beam is continuously applied from the periphery of the lesion (Figs 2C and D). After an interval of 2–3 months

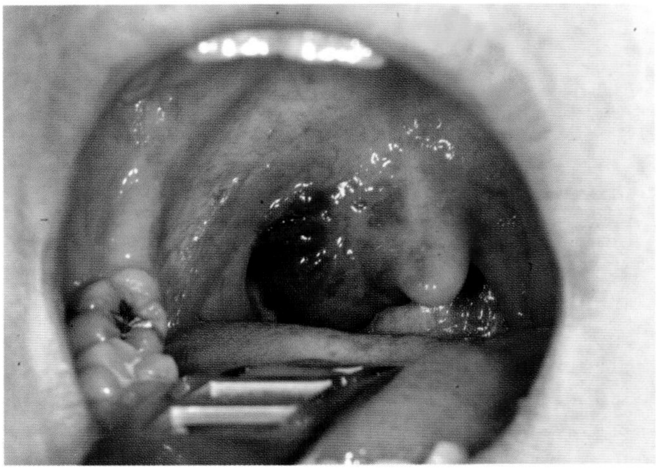

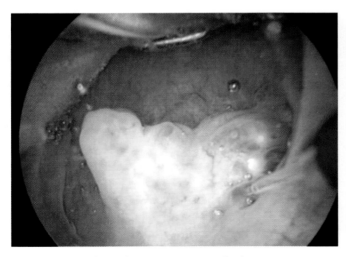

Fig. 2A: Venous malformation of oropharynx accessible to Nd:YAG laser therapy

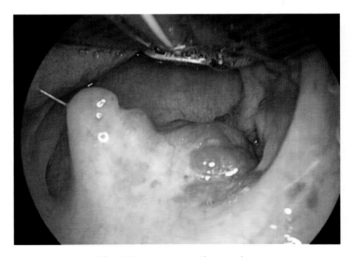

Fig. 2B: Intraoperative setting of the lesion

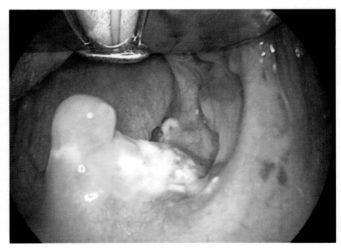

Fig. 2C: Multiple laser spots are applied in noncontact technique, cooling is performed by cold Ringer's solution

Fig. 2D: Status after completed session of Nd:YAG laser application

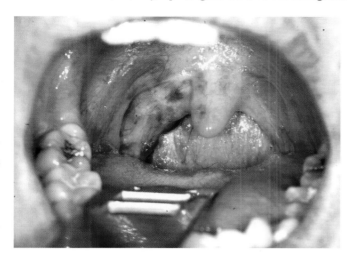

Fig. 2E: Status three months after Nd:YAG laser therapy

(Fig. 2E), the laser therapy of the lower areas like hypopharynx or larynx is carried out by the same technique. In extended cases with risk of obstruction of the upper airways by edema, the procedure should be performed on at least two settings.

CO$_2$ Laser Resection

Marginal and circumscribed lesions, for example if located on the lingual edge or medial wall of oropharynx, are well suited for excision by CO$_2$ laser. Technical details of tissue excision by CO$_2$ laser are identical to those described for treatment of benign and malignant tissue changes in the upper aerodigestive tract and are not further explained in detail in this chapter.

Selective Removal of Phleboliths

Depending on the anatomic site, phleboliths are removed under ultrasound guidance, microscopic or manual control. Phleboliths in facial regions are removed additionally under neuromonitoring of the facial nerve with microscopic approach.

Technique for Removal of Phleboliths in Parotideal Region

After drawing the planned incision line and marking the phlebolith, the skin is cut with a number 15 blade in an S-shape, according to an incision for lateral parotidectomy. After incision of the skin and platysma, the frontal edge of the sternocleidomastoid and anterior part of the digastric muscle are identified. The mandibular arch of the facial nerve is identified and followed to its peripheral extension. The nerve is maintained to the periphery under microscopic vision and neuromonitoring. The phlebolith is now prepared and dissected gently from the neural branches. It is then dissolved

from the vascular malformation by meticulous preparation and hemostasis. Wound closure is then performed after insertion of a number 8 suction drainage in two layers as in Figures 3A to E.

TREATMENT OF LYMPHATIC MALFORMATIONS

Sclerotherapy with OK-432 (Picibanil®)

A popular substance for sclerosing therapy of lymphangiomas is Picibanil® (OK-432). This agent is a lyophilized mixture of *Streptococcus pyogenes* (serology group A) and causes an inflammation in the treated tissue, which leads to a not yet fully understood immunological cascade. The immunological reaction leads to fibrosis and volume reduction. Picibanil® has proven particularly useful for the treatment of singular, macrocystic lymphangiomas. Microcystic lymphangiomas with cyst diameter less than 1 cm and infiltrative lymphangiomas in the parotid gland and the tongue are not suitable for treatment with OK-432.

First, the cyst is punctured and 50–90% of the fluid content is drained. In larger cysts 10–20 ml solution of Picibanil® at a total dose of 0.1–0.2 mg is then introduced into the punctured cyst. The maximum dose per session should not exceed 0.3 mg. The time interval between two treatment sessions should be at least 6 weeks. The procedure is performed routinely under ultrasound guidance.

Sclerotherapy with Doxycycline

Doxycycline is a broad-spectrum antibiotic in routine clinical use. Further it is also a nonspecific matrix metalloproteinase inhibitor, which is important in angiogenesis. This sclerosant seems to be safe and effective also for macrocystic lymphatic malformations. The cysts are punctured and the fluid contents are aspirated as much as possible. After a solution with a concentration of 10 mg/ml doxycycline is made, the sclerosant is injected in smaller cysts under ultrasound control. For larger cervical lesion, doxycycline is injected, retained in the lesion for 4–8 hours and re-aspirated again. The aspiration is performed through a previously inserted draining catheter. Further injections are made every other day until the drainage of the cystic fluid ceases. Maximum dose of 20 mg/kg or total of 1000 mg of doxycycline should not be exceeded per therapy session.

Laser Treatment of Microcystic Lymphatic Malformations

Because of the diffuse nature of microcystic lymphatic malformations it is often difficult to distinguish between involved and healthy tissue. A complete extirpation is

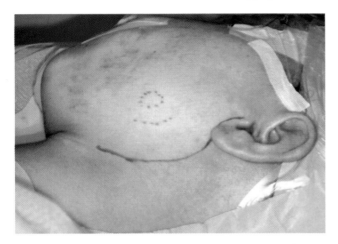

Fig. 3A: Drawing of the planned incision and marking of the phlebolith in facial venous malformation

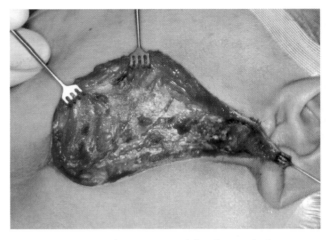

Fig. 3B: Status after incision of the skin and platysma

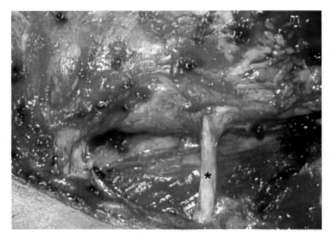

Fig. 3C: Identification of the frontal edge of the sternocleido-mastoid, the anterior part of the digastric muscle and the mandibular arch of the facial nerve (*)

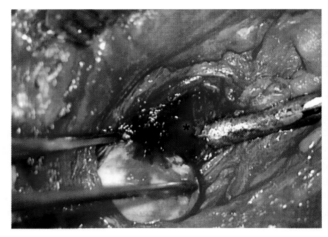

Fig. 3D: Dissection of the phlebolith from the vascular malformation (*) by meticulous preparation and hemostasis

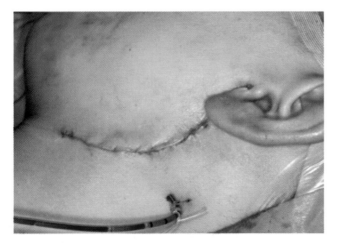

Fig. 3E: Wound closure after insertion of a number 8 suction drainage

rarely possible. The use of CO_2 laser is effective in the treatment of lymphatic malformation of the mucosa for debulking, excision or vaporization. The advantages of CO_2 laser therapy in comparison to conventional surgery include less postoperative edema, less tissue trauma and less blood loss. The laser ablation of lymphatic malformation vesicles prevents repetitive bleeding and painful swelling. Vaporization of bleeding areas is performed with the CO_2 laser in a defocused mode with a laser power of 8–15 watts. Superficial lymph cysts are often connected with deeper cysts in the underlying muscle. CO_2 ablation of the deeper parts of the tissue (e.g. tongue) is combined with interstitial application of Nd:YAG laser light. Moderately deep components, which do not infiltrate the tongue muscles can be dissected as thin slices in ablative technique as in Figures 4A to C.

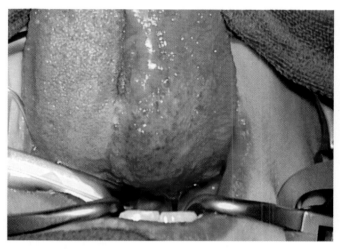

Fig. 4A: Previously treated microcystic lymphatic malformation of the tongue with residual vesicles in the dorsal part

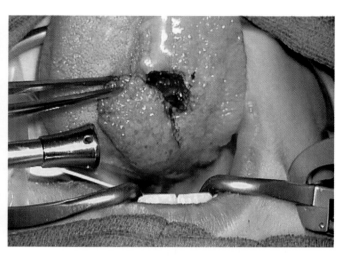

Fig. 4B: Dissection of a slice of the surface from the muscle layer

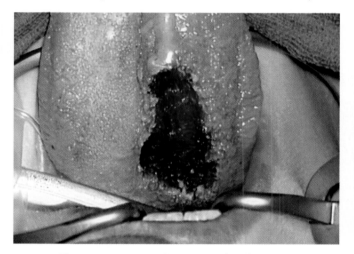

Fig. 4C: Intraoperative status after dissection

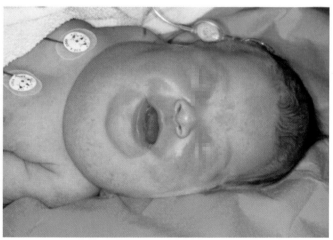

Fig. 5A: Three days old female with extended bilateral lymphatic malformation of the neck

Re-epithelialization after CO_2 laser ablation is usually complete after 1–2 weeks. The scarring is limited and usually a desired side effect is reduced recurrence of the vesicles.

Surgery of Extended Bilateral Lymphatic Malformations

Advanced lymphatic malformations of the head and neck are neither suitable to laser therapy nor to sclerotherapy. Therapy of choice, especially if accompanied with functional impairment like dyspnea or severe dysphagia is an extended conventional surgical resection within few days after the birth. An exemplary operation for extensive cervical lesion is described below as in Figures 5A and B.

First, a horizontal skin incision in a preformed skin fold of the neck is made using a number 15 blade. Beginning craniolaterally and starting from the (more) affected side,

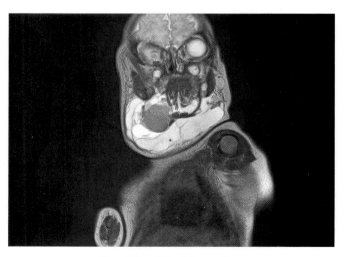

Fig. 5B: MRI of the patient

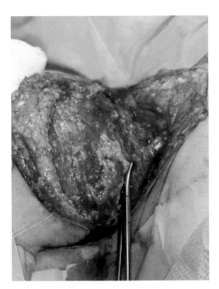

Fig. 5C: Intraoperative situs, the incision is extended to the contralateral side, the multicystic mass is already visualized

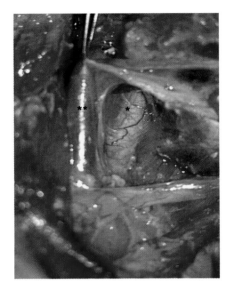

Fig. 5D: Identification of common carotid artery (*) and internal jugular vein (**)

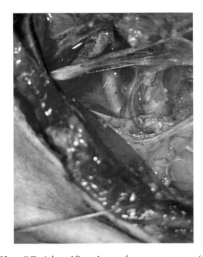

Fig. 5E: Identification of vagus nerve (*)

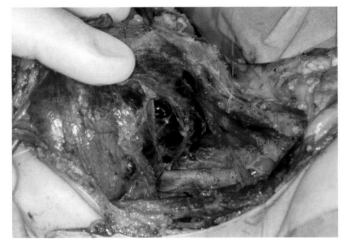

Fig. 5F: The lymphangioma is elevated and rolled over the median part of the neck

the incision is extended through the median slightly to the contralateral side. After dissection of the entire skin flap, the multicystic mass is usually already visualized (Fig. 5C). The common carotid artery, the internal jugular vein, the accessory, the vagus and hypoglossal nerves are then identified and prepared beside the digastric, the sternocleidomastoid and the stylohyoid muscles. The lymphangioma, which is almost always directly adjacent to the vascular and neural structures (Figs 5D and E) is elevated, gently dissected, from every single structure and rolled over the median to the contralateral side (Fig. 5F). The preparation is performed meticulously to keep the wall of the cysts intact. Any accidental opening

of the lymphangioma cysts immensely complicates further dissection. Once the median is reached, the anterior part of digastric muscle, the submandibular gland, the marginal arch of the facial nerve and the lingual nerve are identified and the lymphangioma is dissected also from the floor of the mouth (Fig. 5G). A protective tracheostomy is performed in cases of massive bilateral and pre-existing respiratory problems. An additional caudally located skin incision is performed to place the stoma in a separated cavity. After intubation through the stoma a suction drainage is inserted on each side. A two-layer closure of the wound cavity follows and the wound is dressed with a compression bandage. The

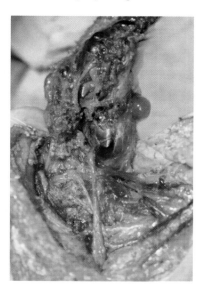

Fig. 5G: Elevation of the lymphangioma and dissection from the submandibular region and floor of the mouth

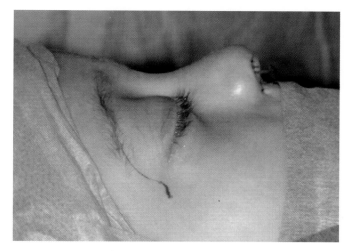

Fig. 6A: Drawn line for skin incision of lateral orbitotomy

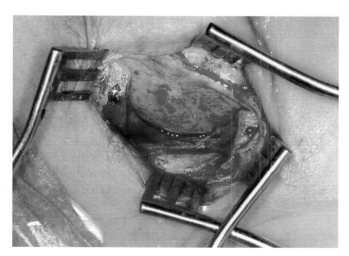

Fig. 6B: Exposure of the periorbit after resection of bony fragment and placement of drill holes

and also for lymphatic or other vascular malformations. A complete resection of lymphatic malformations of the orbit is only possible in rare cases. Access to the lateral orbit begins at the outer orbital rim. The lateral bony margin of the orbit is exposed after skin incision, which preferably begins from the lateral portion of the eyebrow (Fig. 6A). The resection borders of the bone are then marked. Four drill holes are made on each side for the subsequent fixation of the fragment. Using the Feldman saw and a chisel, the bony fragment is removed in the lateral area to expose the periorbit (Fig. 6B). This is then incised in a T-shape. The intraconal content is then visualized after preparation of the lacrimal gland and the lateral rectus muscle, under microscopic view (Fig. 6C). The lymphangioma is then followed up to peri- and retrobulbar areas and then excised. A drain is inserted before wound closure. The periorbit is readapted by a loose suture; the bony fragment of the lateral orbit is reinserted and fixed by suture of the previously created drill holes. The wound is then closed in two layers as in Figure 6D.

Intralesional Endoscopic Approach to Advanced Lymphatic Malformations of the Head and Neck

Endoscopic techniques have evolved to become an integral part of the surgical approach in different specialties and also in the head and neck area. Further, there are increasing efforts to establish endoscopic methods in the soft tissue surgery. Another innovative method is the endoscopic approach to advanced lymphatic malformations of the head and neck. This technique, which is still at a very early level, may improve the knowledge about the nature of these lesions and

contralateral (less affected) side is not radically operated at the first step. This is to safely exclude bilateral nerve damage. The decision on the further form of treatment and the appropriate timing for the residual lesion is made upon the further course and based on residual symptoms.

Surgery for Advanced Orbital Lymphatic Malformations by Lateral Orbitotomy

Orbital surgery is very strongly indicated, if the visual function is endangered by space occupying intraorbital lymphatic malformations. Lateral orbitotomy allows an appropriate approach to laterally accessible larger intraconal masses

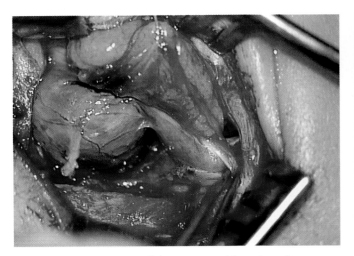

Fig. 6C: Exposure of the intraconal lymphangioma

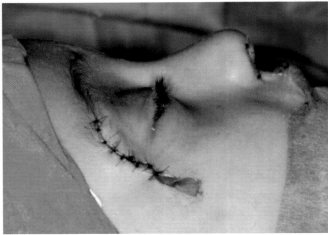

Fig. 6D: Wound closure after placement of a drain, loose re-adaption of the periorbit and reinsertion of the bony fragment

contribute to achieve better therapeutic results and reduce surgical complications.

The interventions are performed under general anesthesia in the operating theater. A rigid endoscope is used to perform the inspection of the lymphatic malformation by intralesional view. An endoscope with working channels for drainage and instillation of fluids and for insertion of surgical instruments (e.g. microscissors, biopsy clamp and coagulation electrode) may be used to carry out therapeutic interventions during the intralesional endoscopy. The transcutaneous approach can be performed according to a conventional access for open surgery or by a small skin incision with a length of 1–2 cm.

This method provides an internal view of the lymphatic malformation and enables the surgeon to gain further impression about the morphologic properties and serve as an additional diagnostic tool besides imaging studies like ultrasound, CT or MRI. Further, intralesional endoscopy reveals more detailed morphologic aspects like intralesional septation and vascularization, as well as intercystic correspondence and channel networks. These observations contribute to a more detailed analysis of the disease and a better explanation of the clinical findings.

The results of the sclerotherapy for advanced cases, even when performed on multiple settings, are often unsatisfactory. The evidence of intercystic connection and multiple septations may explain why the sclerosing agents may not reach a sufficient concentration to be effective in some regions. The creation of new cavities within a mixed lesion might make advanced lymphatic malformations more accessible for therapy with sclerosing agents. Other endoscopic procedures, which are commonly practiced in diverse specialties like gastroenterology and laparoscopic

surgery like coagulation of intralesional vessels, ligature of vessels by clips and dissection of membranes can also be performed for treatment of lymphatic malformations of the head and neck.

PERSPECTIVES IN ANTIANGIOGENIC TREATMENT

The interface of angioma therapy and tumor therapy seems to be very close, especially for the aspect of angiogenesis and of course the inhibited proliferation as promising therapeutic approach of advanced vascular malformations. During the past decade several new antiangiogenic drugs entered the market. These drugs included monoclonal antibodies such as bevacizumab (Avastin®, Roche/Genentech) that are directed against VEGF-A, a major key player in angiogenesis. Also small molecule kinase inhibitors such as Semaxanib and Sunitinib (SU5416 and SU011248, Pharmacia/Sugen) were developed that are directed against the tyrosine kinase domain of VEGFR-2. Another relatively new compound, Aflibercept (VEGF-trap, AVE0005, Sanofi-Aventis), was designed as a fusion protein of ligand-binding domains from VEGFR-1 and VEGFR-2 with the IgG1 Fc fragment. All of these drugs were primarily intended for use in cancer treatment. Naturally, they are also attractive candidates for the treatment of nonmalignant hypervascular diseases such as proliferative vascular malformations. Such studies are still very limited and only found in anecdotal reports. For example, bevacizumab, the most established antiangiogenic drug, exhibited therapeutic efficacy in the treatment of retinal capillary hemangiomas as a manifestation of von Hippel-Lindau disease. It is interesting, that well known compounds that are used for decades in the treatment of unrelated diseases appear to influence the proliferation of vascular tumors. As mentioned above, it was recently discovered that the β-blocker propranolol exhibits a dramatic antiangiogenic effect on proliferative hemangiomas and drugs that were discredited in the past such as thalidomide became significant again for antiangiogenic treatment of selected clinical cases. Lastly, highly proliferative vascular tumors can behave in its growth pattern like a true malignancy and threaten life functions. In these cases chemotherapy with vincristine could successfully control growth of the vascular tumor. Still little is known about the complex mechanisms that are underlying angioproliferative vascular diseases such as lymphangiomas, hemangiomas and arteriovenous malformations. A large amount of interdisciplinary work will be necessary to elucidate these basic mechanisms, as it is a prerequirement for the development of more potent and suitable drugs that effectively can be used in the treatment of these stigmatizing vascular tumors.

HIGHLIGHTS

I. Classification and Diagnosis
- Distinguish between infantile hemangiomas and vascular malformations
- Distinguish between high- and low-flow lesions.

II. Imaging
- B mode ultrasound and color Doppler are suitable for routine diagnostics
- MRI has to be performed in all extended cases
- CT is necessary for bony structures, consider CT angiography
- Conventional angiography indicated only for selected cases.

III. Blood Products and Coagulation Tests
- Offer opportunity of self donation
- Thorough coagulation analysis for advanced vascular malformation.

IV. Operation Safety
- Preoperative embolization for high-flow malformations
- Transesophageal echocardiography and Doppler to detect air embolism
- Autologous transfusion systems to reduce need of transfusions.

V. Therapeutic and Surgical Approach
- Propranolol is first line therapy for infantile hemangiomas
- Do not perform excessive laser coagulation for hemangiomas
- Nd:YAG laser is preferred for mucosal venous malformations

- CO_2 laser is suitable for excision of limited lesions
- Phleboliths in the facial region are removed under monitoring of N.VII
- OK-432 and doxycycline are suitable sclerosants for macrocystic lymphatic malformations
- Radical surgery is indicated for advanced obstructive lymphatic malformations.

VI. Innovations and Future Concepts
- Intralesional endoscopy is gaining importance for advanced lymphatic malformations
- Consider antiangiogenic therapy for otherwise uncontrollable cases.

ADDITIONAL READING

1. Ach T, Thiemeyer D, Hoeh AE, et al. Intravitreal bevacizumab for retinal capillary haemangioma: long-term results. Acta Ophthalmol. 2010;88(4):e137-8.
2. Chow LQ, Eckhardt SG. Sunitinib: from rational design to clinical efficacy. J Clin Oncol. 2007;25(7):884-96.
3. Chu QS. Aflibercept (AVE0005): an alternative strategy for inhibiting tumour angiogenesis by vascular endothelial growth factors. Expert Opin Biol Ther. 2009;9(2):263-71.
4. Eivazi B, Ardelean M, Bäumler W, et al. Update on hemangiomas and vascular malformations of the head and neck. Eur Arch Otorhinolaryngol. 2009;266(2):187-97.
5. Eivazi B, Sierra-Zuleta F, Ermisch S, et al. Therapy for prenatally diagnosed lymphangioma—multimodal procedure and interdisciplinary challenge. Z Geburtshilfe Neonatol. 2009;213:155-60.
6. Eivazi B, Teymoortash A, Stiller S, et al. Betablockers—new perspektives for infantile hemangiomas of the head and neck. Laryngorhinootologie. 2010;89(4):230-1.
7. Eivazi B, Wiegand S, Pfützner W, et al. Differential diagnosis of venous malformations of the upper aerodigestive tract. Laryngorhinootologie. 2009;88(11):700-8.
8. Fawcett SL, Grant I, Hall PN, et al. Vincristine as a treatment for a large hemangioma threatening vital functions. Br J Plast Surg. 2004;57(2):168-71.
9. Ferrara N, Hillan KJ, Gerber HP, et al. Discovery and development of bevacizumab, an anti-VEGF antibody for treating cancer. Nat Rev Drug Discov. 2004;3(5):391-400.
10. Léauté-Labrèze C, Dumas de la Roque E, Hubiche T, et al. Propranolol for severe hemangiomas of infancy. N Engl J Med. 2008;358(24):2649-51.
11. Piribauer M, Czech T, Dieckmann K, et al. Stabilization of a progressive hemangioblastoma under treatment with thalidomide. J Neurooncol. 2004;66(3):295-9.
12. Werner JA, Eivazi B, Folz BJ, et al. State of the art of classification, diagnostics and therapy for cervicofacial hemangiomas and vascular malformations. Laryngorhinootologie. 2006;85(12):883-91.

13. Werner JA, Lippert BM, Gottschlich S, et al. Ultrasound-guided interstitial Nd: YAG laser treatment of voluminous hemangiomas and vascular malformations in 92 patients. Laryngoscope. 1998;108(4 Pt 1):463-70.

14. Wiegand S, Eivazi B, Barth PJ, et al. Pathogenesis of lymphangiomas. Virchows Arch. 2008;453(1):1-8.

15. Wiegand S, Eivazi B, Karger R, et al. Surgery in patients with vascular malformations of the head and neck: Value of coagulation disorders. Phlebology. 2009;24:38-42.

16. Wiegand S, Eivazi B, Sel S, et al. Analysis of cytokine levels in human lymphangiomas. In Vivo. 2008;22(2):253-6.

17. Wiegand S, Eivazi B, Zimmermann A, et al. Microcystic lymphatic malformation of the tongue—diagnosis, classification and treatment. Arch Otolaryngol Head Neck Surgery. 2009;135(10):976-83.

18. Wiegand S, Eivazi B, Zimmermann AP, et al. Evaluation of children with lymphatic malformations of the head and neck using the Cologne Disease Score. Int J Pediatr Otorhinolaryngol. 2009;73(7):955-8.

19. Zimmermann AP, Eivazi B, Wiegand S, et al. Orbital lymphatic malformation showing the symptoms of orbital complications of acute rhinosinusitis in children: a report of 2 cases. Int J Pediatr Otorhinolaryngol. 2010;74(4): 338-42.

Chapter 7

Maxillofacial Prosthetics and Rehabilitation

Mordechai Sela, Anat Buller Sharon

INTRODUCTION

This chapter deals with the intraoral as well as the extraoral maxillofacial prosthetic rehabilitation. The field of maxillofacial rehabilitation is dedicated to the prosthetic correction and management of maxillofacial defects acquired from surgical ablation and cancer, traumatic injuries or congenital alterations in growth and development (AAMP, 2008).

Large defects in the head and neck region, i.e. missing anatomical organs in patients whose maxillary sinus, hard and/or soft palate have been removed by radical surgery, is one of the greatest challenges in the field of maxillofacial rehabilitation.

The main objective of the treatment is to establish a comfortable prosthesis that restores speech, deglutition and mastication. The maxillary defect created by cancer surgery is best closed by obturation.

Obturator treatment consists of three stages:
1. The surgical obturator is inserted in the operation room immediately after surgery. It provides tissue and surgical dressing support, enables swallowing, speech and communication. The surgical obturator is planned in co-operation with the surgeon before the operation, prefabricated in advance and adapted to the defect in the course of the operation. After 1 week of surgery, the surgical obturator is removed, relined and adjusted to the healing process at the site of the surgery.
2. The interim obturator is usually fitted 6 weeks post surgery, after initial healing. The interim obturator allows the patient to function better and with greater comfort.
3. The definitive obturator is provided once the tissue has stabilized and no further changes are expected, usually six months following surgery and chemoradiation.

Prosthetic obturation is influenced by the size and location of the defect of remaining structures. Co-operation between a surgeon and a prosthodontist would result in sorting out the defect, making it easier to obturate and would lead to an efficient functional prosthesis.

The design of the obturator is based on the basics of prosthodontic principles: support, retention and stability. Routine maintenance is necessary to provide comfort, good function and esthetic importance.

EXTRAORAL REHABILITATION

Extraoral rehabilitation is used to treat patients who have undergone mutilating surgery resulting in facial disfigurement such as loss of the nose, ear and other complex organs. The defects can be artificially restored with a silicone prosthesis, which is anchored to a soft tissue or bone by a medical adhesive or with the help of an osseointegrated implant.

Rehabilitation Post-Maxillectomy in Adults (A Case Report)

A 48-year-old Caucasian female was diagnosed with squamous cell carcinoma of the maxillary sinus. The tumor was manifested in the oral cavity by a substantial swelling of the left maxilla, gingival vestibule and maxillary sinus (Fig. 1). Clinically, the tumor reached the midline of the maxilla. Computed tomography (CT) scan revealed that the tumor occupied the maxillary left sinus and was expanding toward the orbital rim and temporomandibular fossa (Fig. 2). A surgical obturator was planned according to the clinical findings, in co-operation with the head and neck surgeon. Removal of the tumor created a large defect that included the left maxilla, maxillary sinus and orbital rim (Fig. 3). Without rehabilitation, the defect would not restore the normal oral functions such as swallowing, speech and breathing, and would cause significant esthetic damage. The large excised tumor (7 cm × 9 cm) included the teeth, maxillary sinus and the orbital rim (Fig. 4). A surgical obturator was fitted to the site of the excision. The surgical obturator helps to maintain hemostasis (Fig. 5), improves esthetics (Fig. 6) and enables speech and deglutition. The surgical obturator was removed a week post-maxillectomy and the patient was irradiated with 70 Gy (Fig. 7).

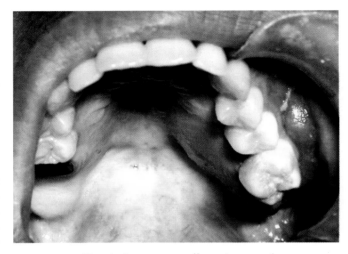

Fig. 1: Squamous cell carcinoma of left maxilla, intraoral view

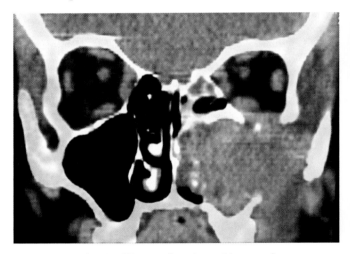

Fig. 2: CT scan showing widespread involvement of the maxillary sinus

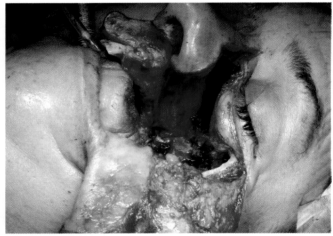

Fig. 3: Maxillectomy defect following surgery

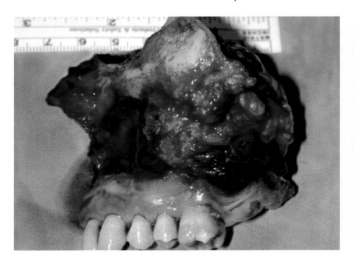

Fig. 4: Tumor specimen

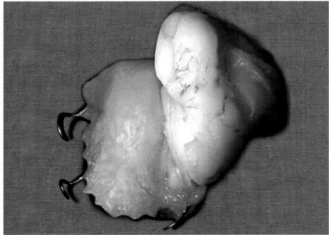

Fig. 5: The surgical obturator made out of acrylic and silicone

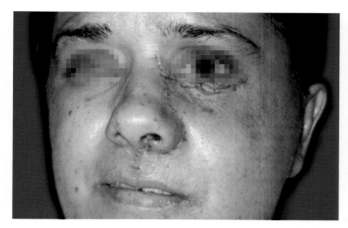

Fig. 6: One week post surgery, surgical obturator in place

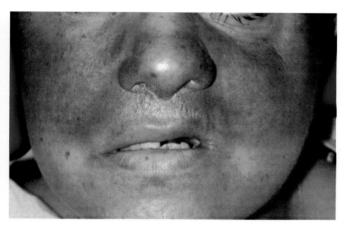

Fig. 7: Irradiated patient (70 Gy). Note mucositis in left nostril

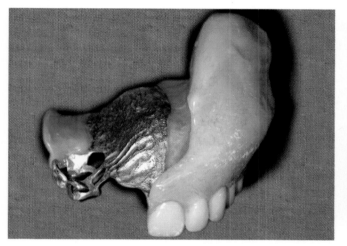

Fig. 8A: Definitive obturator

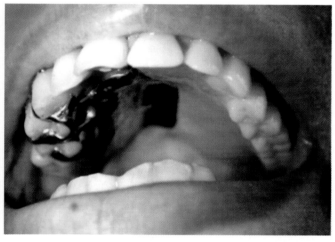

Fig. 8B: Definitive obturator in oral cavity

The most remarkable side effect of the radiation therapy was dermatitis. The difference in skin color well demonstrated the field of radiation. Palliative treatment was also provided during the period of radiation to ease and relieve other side effects of radiation, such as radiation mucositis as seen in the nasal mucosa in Figure 7, xerostomia and trismus. After 6 months, the final obturator was fabricated (Figs 8A and B). Teeth, alveolar bone and the hard and soft palate were restored.

Maxillofacial Rehabilitation in Children

The incidence of tumors in children differs to that in adults. Most of them are lymphomas, sarcomas and thyroid malignancies. The main prosthetic strategies are the same as those described above. Management of children during treatment and the relationship with their parents are main concerns. Changes and modulation of the obturator should

be made frequently in accordance with the patient's growth and development.

Rehabilitation of a Pediatric Patient (A Case Report)

A 10-year-old Caucasian boy was diagnosed with osteogenic sarcoma of the right maxilla (Fig. 9). The tumor was manifested as a hard swelling in the maxilla. A panoramic X-ray showed the difference between the right and the left sides of the maxilla. The tumor was seen as a radio-opaque area, which had displaced the teeth and destroyed the anatomical areas (Fig. 10). CT scan revealed that the tumor occupied the right maxillary sinus and had penetrated into the soft tissues of the face (Fig. 11). The clinical intraoral view (Fig. 12) showed the dimensions of the tumor. Since, the hard and soft palate were involved and there was erosion of the oral mucosa, the child was a candidate for subtotal

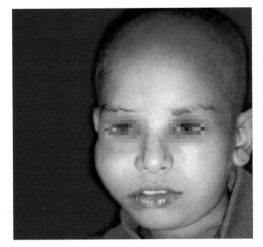

Fig. 9: Osteogenic sarcoma of right maxilla

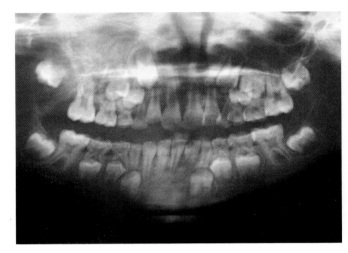

Fig. 10: Panoramic radiograph of the tumor

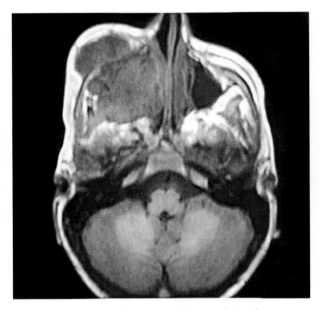

Fig. 11: CT scan showing widespread involvement of the maxillary sinus

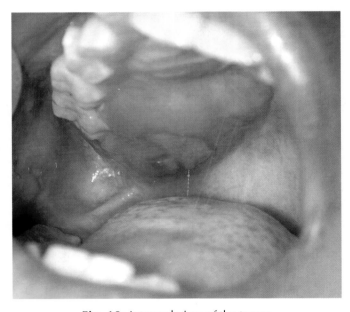

Fig. 12: Intraoral view of the tumor

maxillectomy. Rehabilitation was complicated because very little supporting tissues remained on the oral cavity for retention of the obturator. Upon surgery, exposure of the maxilla clearly revealed the tumor. On the left side, a palatal incision was made between the canine and the first premolar and on the posterior side, close to the base of the skull (Fig. 13). When possible, the transalveolar cut should be made through the socket of the tooth adjacent to the site of surgery. This will provide the remaining tooth with greater bony attachment and a more suitable abutment for the obturator.

The large excised tumor (11 cm × 7 cm) included most of the maxilla, teeth, maxillary sinus, orbital rim and soft palate (Fig. 14). It was clear that without rehabilitation of the missing organs, the oral functions would be heavily compromised. Most of the surgical obturator was fabricated in the operating room, according to the extent of the surgery and inserted into the oral cavity to replace the missing maxilla (Fig. 15). The flap was then sutured back in place (Fig. 16). A week post surgery, the surgical obturator was removed and the child and his parents were taught how to handle the obturator (Fig. 17). The oral hygiene of the obturator, adjacent tissues and the remaining teeth were strictly maintained in order not to delay the healing process. After three months, chemoradiation therapy

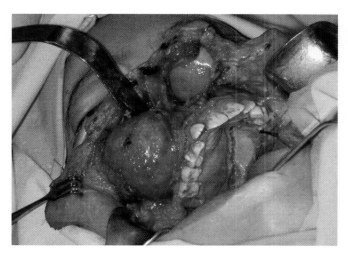

Fig. 13: The tumor as exposed during maxillectomy

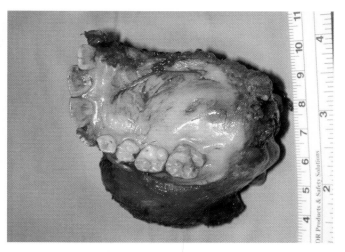

Fig. 14: Tumor specimen

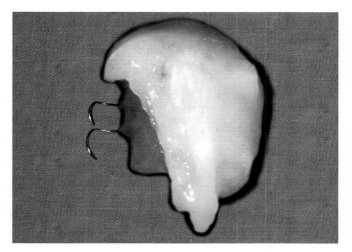

Fig. 15: Surgical obturator made out of acrylic and silicone

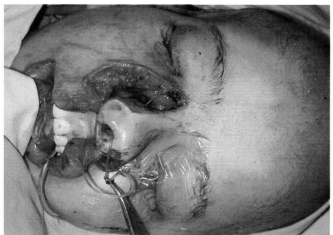

Fig. 16: Obturator replaced the resected region, flap sutured back in place

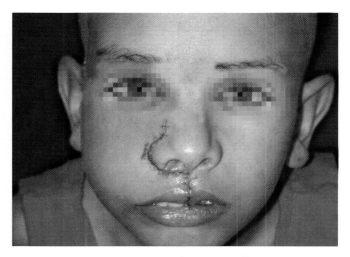

Fig. 17: Patient a week post maxillectomy; surgical obturator in oral cavity

was completed. The definitive obturator was constructed six months post surgery, when the tissues had stabilized (Fig. 18). The definitive obturator included the missing teeth, alveolar bone and maxillary sinus. Retention was provided by the residual teeth, the soft palate and the entrance to the pharynx, as well as the remaining concha. To facilitate insertion of the obturator and in order to avoid injury of the healthy tissue, the upper part of the obturator was made of silicone. Without the prosthesis, the soft tissues on the right side of the face would relapse (Fig. 19). The definitive obturator (Fig. 20) should be adjusted frequently according to the child's growth and development.

EXTRAORAL PROSTHETICS

After extensive surgery in the head and neck region, patients suffer from major deformations and mutilation. Missing

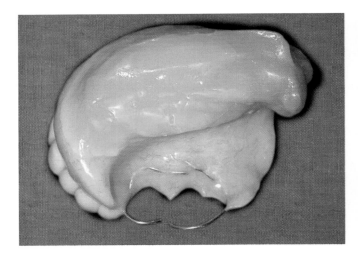

Fig. 18: Definitive obturator

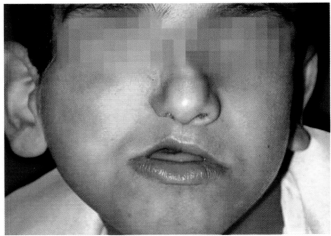

Fig. 19: Patient without the obturator.
Note relapse of lip and cheek

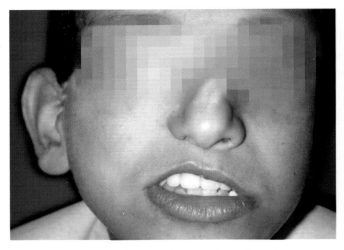

Fig. 20: Definitive obturator in oral cavity.
Note lip and cheek support

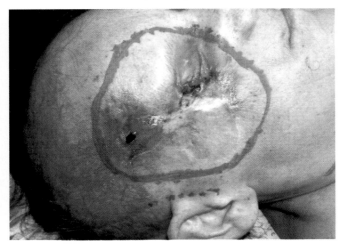

Fig. 21: Squamous cell carcinoma
of right orbital region

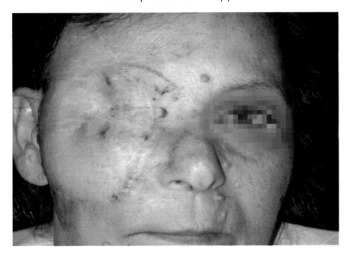

Fig. 22: Patient post exenteration of
right orbit and free abdominal flap

organs such as eyes, nose and ears cause a major esthetic deformation. To complete missing organs in such patients, silicon extraoral prostheses are used.

Oculofacial Prosthesis and Rehabilitation Post Exenteration (A Case Report)

A 63-year-old Caucasian female was diagnosed with squamous cell carcinoma of right orbit (Fig. 21). She underwent exenteration and was reconstructed with a free abdominal flap. After three months, she was referred to author's clinic for prosthetic rehabilitation (Fig. 22). A moulage of the defect and the adjacent tissue was made (Fig. 23) using irreversible hydrocolloid material reinforced with plaster of paris. A cast of the impression was made and a wax-up model of the missing area was carved out (Fig. 24). The wax model was tried on the patient's face and all the required changes to improve the esthetics were made at this

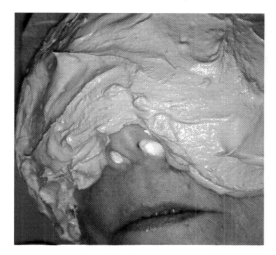

Fig. 23: Moulage of the face

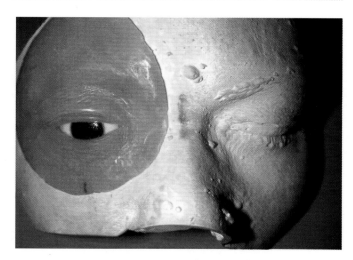

Fig. 24: Wax-up model of orbital region

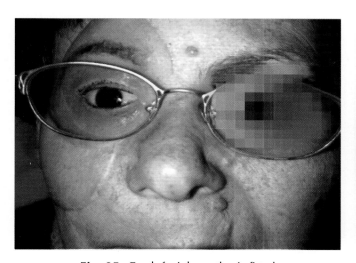

Fig. 25: Oculofacial prosthesis fitted

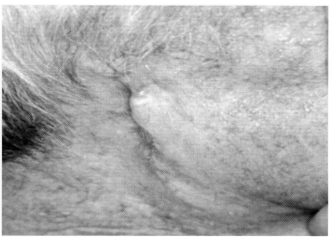

Fig. 26: Patient post removal of right ear due to basal cell carcinoma

stage. The wax model was converted into a silicon prosthesis that was attached to the skin with a medical adhesive (Fig. 25). The prosthesis resembles the soft tissue texture and is dyed with external pigments to match the facial skin. The prosthesis includes the missing eye as well as the missing surrounding orbital tissue.

Prosthesis Retention by Implants

Another means for retention of silicone prostheses, other than medical adhesives, is osseointegrated implants.

Ear Prosthesis (A Case Report)

An 88-year-old male underwent removal of the external right ear, due to basal cell carcinoma (Fig. 26). As can be seen in the Figure 26, the tragus was left in this region, as well as the entrance to the external acoustic canal. It was decided to use short implants that would be placed in the mastoid region in order to retain the prosthesis. The exact site for insertion of the implant was determined by the location of the future prosthesis. Two implants were inserted into the mastoid area (Fig. 27). After 4 weeks of surgery, the implants were loaded (Figs 28A and B) with the ear prosthesis. The working procedure for the silicone ear is very similar to those described for the orbital prosthesis. Gold attachments, which serve as retainers for the implants were embedded in the inner aspect of the ear (Fig. 29). The final product (Fig. 30) shows the similarity of the ear prosthesis to the anatomy of the original ear. The prosthesis was attached to the implants with good retention. Satisfactory esthetics, symmetry and even retention of the patient's glasses (necessary in this case) were achieved.

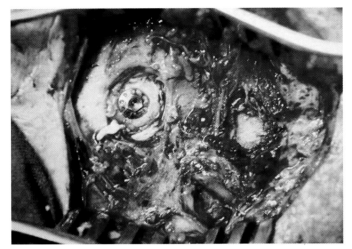

Fig. 27: Implant location in the mastoid region

Nose Prosthesis (A Case Report)

A 54-year-old Caucasian female was diagnosed with squamous cell carcinoma of the right nose (Fig. 31). The tumor displaced the nostril and the ala nasi. Surgical removal of the tumor created an extensive defect (Fig. 32). The first priority was to close the defect with a flap (rotational or forehead). Surgeons preferred a follow-up period of 1 year before final surgical closure. As a temporary solution, a silicone prosthesis was made. The technique for this procedure is the same as for the ear and orbital prosthesis described above. In this patient, the prosthesis was attached to the skin by medical adhesive (Fig. 33). The cosmetic results were extremely satisfactory. The prosthesis provided adequate breathing through the affected nostril and met the patient's esthetic requirements. Most patients delay the surgical closure at this stage.

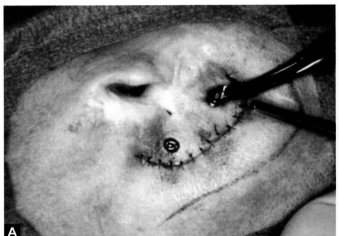
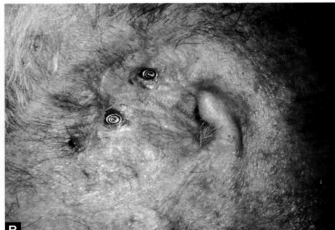

Figs 28A and B: (A) Final stage of implant insertion; (B) Implants ready to be loaded

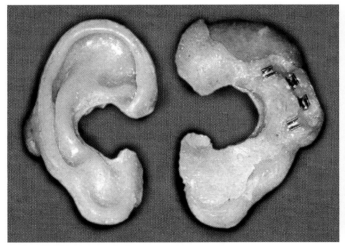

Fig. 29: Inner and outer aspects of the prosthesis. Note the gold attachments in the inner aspect

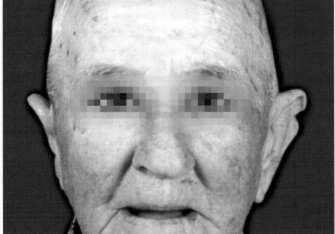

Fig. 30: Ear prosthesis attached to implants

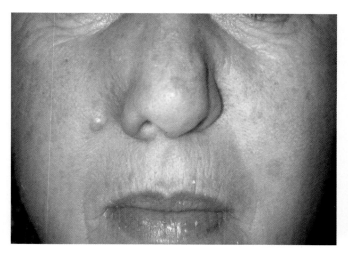

Fig. 31: Squamous cell carcinoma of the nose

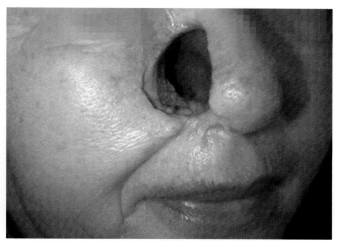

Fig. 32: Defect following tumor resection

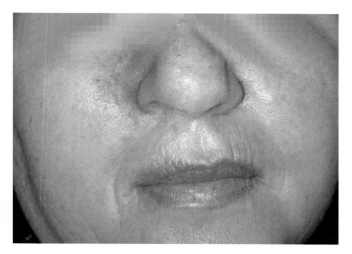

Fig. 33: Nose prosthesis fitted

The advantage of this kind of prosthesis is the predictability of the final result, because already in the try-in phase, a first impression is obtained regarding the future appearance of the final prosthesis. Another critical advantage is the conservative treatment applied for rehabilitation, which does not involve radical or invasive procedures.

SUMMARY

Maxillofacial rehabilitation is the art and science of anatomical, functional and esthetic reconstruction with the aid of prostheses, for defects in the head and neck region resulting from major surgery, trauma or congenital malformations.

The most important objectives of the maxillofacial rehabilitation include:
- Restoration of function and esthetics
- Protection of tissues
- Psychological influence.

The materials used in constructing the prostheses do not irritate the tissues; the prostheses are comfortable and readily handled by the patient.

This chapter deals with extraoral and intraoral prostheses, which are made after extensive surgical treatment and reconstruction of the affected function and esthetics.

Cooperation with the surgeon before and during the course of surgery is very important and leads to better prosthetic results and comfort for the patient. This field enables such patients to achieve prosthetic rehabilitation with a high degree of esthetics, giving them the possibility to "return to life," after mutilating surgery without any apprehensions.

In the near coming future, with the development of microvascular surgery, we hope that the use of obturators will decrease. Treatment will be performed at the time of resection and rehabilitation will be based on fixed prostheses. This future technique will provide good quality of life for head and neck cancer patients.

ADDITIONAL READING

1. Black WB. Surgical obturation using a gated prosthesis. J Prosthet Dent. 1992;68(2):339-42.
2. Chalian VA, Drane JB, Standish SM. Maxillofacial prosthetics: multidisciplinary practice. Baltimore: The Williams and Wilkins Company; 1972.
3. Driscoll CF, Hughes B, Ostrowski JS. Naturally occurring undercuts in the retention of an interim oculofacial prosthesis. J Prosthet Dent. 1992;68(4):652-4.

4. Hecker DM. Maxillofacial rehabilitation of a large facial defect resulting from an arteriovenous malformation utilizing a two-piece prosthesis. J Prosthet Dent. 2003;89(2):109-13.

5. Marunick MT, Mahmassani O, Klein B, et al. The effect of surgical intervention for head and neck cancer on whole salivary flow: a pilot study. J Prosthet Dent. 1993;70(2):154-7.

6. Ma T, Johnson M. A technique for fabrication of interim midface prostheses. J Prosthet Dent. 1992;68(6):940-2.

7. Ord RA, Blanchaert RH. Oral cancer: the dentist's role in diagnosis, management, rehabilitation and prevention. Quintessence Publishing Co Inc; 2000.

8. Rautava J, Luukkaa M, Heikinheimo K, et al. Squamous cell carcinomas arising from different types of oral epithelia differ in their tumor and patient characteristics and survival. Oral Oncology. 2007;43:911-9.

9. Taylor TD. Clinical Maxillofacial Prosthetics. Quintessence Publishing Co Inc; 2000.

10. Thomaidis V, Seretis K, Fiska A, et al. The scalping forehead flap in nasal reconstruction: report of 2 cases. J Oral Maxillofac Surg. 2007;65(3):532-40.

11. Thomas KF. The Art of Clinical Anaplastology. S Thomas Publishing; 2006.

Chapter 8

Sentinel Node Biopsy

Francisco J Civantos

INTRODUCTION

Sentinel lymph node biopsy (SLNB) offers a less invasive technique, as an alternative to formal neck dissection, which allows the surgeon to excise and meticulously examine the primary draining lymph nodes in the clinically N0 neck. Morton et al. reintroduced this concept to surgical practice in a landmark publication describing the technique and their early prospective clinical experience with SLNB using blue dye in patients with clinically node negative cutaneous malignant melanoma.[1,2] Using injection of blue dye at the primary site, 259 sentinel nodes were identified in 194 out of 237 lymphatic nodal basins and the incidence of false-negative sentinel nodes (i.e. the identified sentinel node is found to be disease-free when metastatic disease is present in the regional lymphatic vessels) was less than 1%.[2] Their model of initial sentinel node biopsy, followed by complete lymphadenectomy, detailed pathological analysis and correlation of findings has been used to validate this technique at multiple anatomical sites in subsequent trials.

SLNB has been validated as an accurate means of staging the lymphatics relative to formal lymphadenectomy in cutaneous melanoma.[3]

Alex and Krag subsequently developed the use of radionuclides, nuclear imaging and a hand-held gamma probe to identify sentinel lymph nodes in the clinically N0 neck.[4,5] Based on their work, sentinel node biopsy has more recently been performed using peritumoral intradermal injections of unfiltered ^{99m}Tc sulphur colloid or other radiotracer and intraoperative gamma detection probes. The use of ^{99m}Tc sulphur colloid and the gamma probe allows direct placement of the biopsy incision over the radiolabeled sentinel node(s) and the probe directs dissection straight to the node without disturbing the surrounding tissues. Sentinel node biopsy in melanoma using the gamma probe resulted in retrieval of sentinel nodes in 82–100% of cases, with a very low incidence of false-negatives confirmed by early follow-up.[6-10] Additionally, a higher than expected incidence of bilateral drainage, "skip" drainage to a more distant node in a group than might be anticipated from the location of the primary melanoma, drainage to multiple lymph node groups in the neck and unorthodox ipsilateral patterns of lymphatic drainage have been documented.[9-11]

Management of the N0 neck in patients with early invasive squamous cell carcinoma of the head and neck is controversial. This controversy is particularly well illustrated for early oral cancers that can be excised transorally. Simple close observation of the lymphatic basin has been traditionally used in order to avoid the morbidity of prophylactic neck dissection or irradiation in the majority of patients, in whom neck metastases will truly never develop.[12-15] On the contrary, the weight of opinion in the recent literature argues against a generalized "watchful waiting" approach [16-18] and favors treatment for patients at risk for cervical metastases. Patients at risk have been identified by characteristics of the primary lesion, such as thickness greater than 4 mm, size greater than 2 cm, anatomic location, microinvasion, perineural infiltration, etc.[19-24]

Computed tomography (CT), magnetic resonance imaging (MRI) and ultrasonography have been used to betterly identify grossly involved nonpalpable nodes and increase the safety of the "watchful waiting" approach. However, significant limitations exist in terms of specificity and sensitivity because imaging modalities are incapable of identifying very small and even microscopic, subclinical metastases.

The controversy surrounding the management of the N0 neck in mucosal squamous carcinoma of the head and neck is analogous to that of elective regional lymphadenectomy in patients with invasive, intermediate risk clinical node negative melanoma. Experience from multiple centers has demonstrated that the presence or absence of occult melanoma metastases to regional nodes can be determined with a high degree of accuracy using the less invasive sentinel node biopsy technique. Patients with negative sentinel nodes can thereby be spared with the expense and morbidity of surgery from which they could realize no benefit, whereas those with positive sentinel nodes proceed to lymphadenectomy for compelling therapeutic indications.

As has occurred in clinically negative node melanoma, sentinel node biopsy ultimately offers the exciting possibility of identifying those patients with clinically negative node carcinomas of the other head and neck sites and histologies which harbor occult metastases in the cervical lymphatics. It is important that a complete understanding of the technique including an established false-negative rate, be available for each tumor type, before incorporating it into routine clinical practice.

SENTINEL LYMPH NODE BIOPSY FOR HEAD AND NECK SQUAMOUS CELL CARCINOMA

Between 1996 and 2000, multiple sites initiated single institutional trials for studying sentinel node biopsy for oral cancer; the most accessible mucosal site.[25-32] More than 60 single institution trials, two international conference consensus documents and a meta-analysis have since been published regarding this topic.[33-35] In particular, the group in Canniesburn, Scotland has been a major advocate for this technique in Europe, where a considerable number of institutions and groups have published elegant validation series, comparing pathological results of sentinel node biopsies to that of immediate completion neck dissection; not only looking at overall results, but assessing issues, such as, learning curves, proper pathological analysis and various details of surgical technique. Ross et al.[31] were the first to publish preliminary results regarding sentinel node biopsy alone, without the completion of neck dissection, for oral cavity cancer. The American College of Surgeons Oncology Group completed a multi-institutional pathological valida-tion study of the sentinel node biopsy, which compared the novice surgeons to experienced surgeons and reported an overall 96% negative predictive value.[36]

Several smaller series have extended this technique to hypopharyngeal and supraglottic sites in conjunction with endoscopic resection.[37] There has also been series describing the experience with head and neck cutaneous lesions other than the melanomas, including selected high-risk squamous cell carcinomas of the skin, Merkel cell carcinomas and other lesions.[38-41] It has been demonstrated in the literature that predictive values of a negative sentinel lymph node may vary between 90% and 100%, and the significant upstaging of the lymphatic basin occurs with this technique, relative to standard formal lymphadenectomy. Unexpected patterns of lymphatic drainage can occur, including unanticipated contralateral drainage, which may be missed with standard lymphadenectomies. In addition, fine step sectioning and immunohistochemistry is essential in properly evaluating the sentinel lymph node and significantly improving the negative predictive value.

Although, sentinel node biopsy has become a standard approach to the lymphatic basins for head and neck melanoma, there has been reluctance to adopt this procedure for mucosal squamous cell carcinoma. Significant concerns exist regarding the possible need for a staged surgery in minority of patients, whose sentinel nodes are detected to be positive only on final pathology, as well as the risk of false-negatives in a highly curable setting. A false-negative sentinel node biopsy carries a great importance because in a selective neck dissection it does not always accurately diagnose metastases, but also provides therapy to the lymphatic field, while sentinel node biopsy leaves the highest risk lymphatic basins untreated. False-negatives can occur for technical reasons, such as, incomplete injection, inadequate radiological imaging, failure to remove all radioactive nodes due to background radioactivity or desire to avoid more complex anatomical areas and other multiple factors. However, even if technically perfect, there are theoretical limitations to the ability of sentinel node biopsy to pickup every lymphatic metastases, including the limitations of standard histopathological techniques to detect the minimal disease, the theoretical potential for metastases to lodge in distal nodes, while being eliminated in more proximal ones (termed "skip" metastases) and the potential for nonlymphatic gross disease that is below the threshold of imaging. Given the fairly moderate morbidity of selective neck dissection, these concerns are enough to keep many surgeons from offering patients this technique for mucosal cancers.[42]

Selective neck dissection remains attractive as an accu-rate, minimally invasive technique for staging the cervical lymphatics in spite of these issues. It is therefore, important that statistically significant, quality-controlled data should be generated before accepting the less invasive sentinel node biopsy approach. Excellent pathological validation data exists, but data regarding long term follow-up of patients with oral cancer, who receive sentinel node biopsy alone, is still being collected and other mucosal sites in the upper aerodigestive tract have only started to be evaluated. On the other hand, patients occasionally present with lesions that clinically appear relatively superficial (i.e. <4 mm depth of invasion suspected) and these represent a group where the "watchful waiting" approach remains the standard of care. In this group, the sentinel node biopsy approach might theoretically represent a more aggressive approach for patients that desire an evaluation of the lymphatics beyond the current standard. Furthermore, for selected lesions, which are at the borderline in terms of thickness and stage, sentinel node biopsy provides an intermediate approach between watchful waiting and selective neck dissection.

GAMMA PROBE GUIDED SELECTIVE NECK DISSECTION

The introduction of sentinel node biopsy for sites, such as, breast and oral cavity, where there is an established pattern of lymphatic drainage and a generally accepted procedure for selective lymphadenectomy with acceptable morbidity, has led to the concept of "gamma probe guided selective neck dissection." In this procedure, patients who are advised to consider lymphadenectomy are offered concurrent sentinel node mapping and biopsy along with the formal dissection. This procedure allows the performance validation studies, but is also offered in order to obtain the benefit of more accurate mapping and staging through fine sectioning and immunohistochemistry of the sentinel node. Many patients, who would have been staged as N0, are upstaged to N1 based on this technique. This allows for closer follow-up evaluation, consideration of radiological imaging and possible adjuvant radiation. In review of the literature for oral cancer, this could be anticipated to occur in 10–20% of the cases.[27,28,31,43,44] The technique also allows the identification of unusual patterns of lymphatic drainage and selective neck dissection by ensuring that all lymph nodes at risk are removed. For example, with oral cavity cancer one might detect contralateral nodes, perifacial nodes and very posterior nodes in the jugular region bordering on level V that might have been left out of a selective neck dissection, but proved to represent an important direct drainage patterns from the primary tumor. There is sufficient data on the use of this technique currently available and the potential benefits are sufficiently documented that an argument regarding the use of this approach as an adjunct to formal lymphadenectomy is justifiable, could potentially benefit the patient and is of low risk. The addition of a preoperative tumoral injection and prolongation of the surgery by less than an hour in most cases are unlikely to harm the patient and are outweighed by the benefits of more accurate staging and knowledge of drainage patterns as a guide to a better lymphadenectomy. Generally, this is the approach used to gain experience with sentinel node technology by surgeons experienced in selective neck dissection.

CONTROVERSIES REGARDING SURGICAL TECHNIQUE

The importance of understanding the true predictive value of a negative sentinel node biopsy is complicated by the variations in surgical technique in practice, which could in theory alter the accuracy of the results obtained. Some groups exclusively use either radiotracers transported by lymph fluid [37,45,46] or combined with blue dye®.[44,47-49] In this context, Ross et al.[44] mentioned that the false-negative rate is not significantly reduced by additional color lymphography. He affirmed that the radioactive marking of the sentinel nodes (SN) represent the basis of sentinel lymphadenectomy in head and neck.

In addition, application of blue dye® does entail some risk of complications. Accidental injury of the lymphatics leads to an extravasation of the dye with resulting staining of adjacent tissues and reduction in intraoperative visualization. Especially, in the area of the cervical soft tissues and the oral primary site with their numerous neural and vascular structures, assessing tissue color and texture is of great importance in oncologic surgery. Furthermore, in 1985 Longnecker et al.[50] reported a 2% incidence of anaphylaxis after subcutaneous injection of blue dye®.

Intraoperative or preoperative tracer injection[37,45,46,48,49,51,52] and intraoperative lymphatic mapping detecting several "hot" nodes within the lymphatic draining basin during the selective neck dissection are performed by some groups. Intraoperative lymphatic mapping is performed after elevation of the cutaneous flaps, following mobilization and dissection of the neck dissection specimen. This latter approach to gamma probe guided neck dissection have the disadvantage of neither developing the surgeon's ability to perform the minimally invasive sentinel node biopsy, nor can be considered adequate for comparative study of the two techniques.[52]

SURGICAL TECHNIQUE (CONTRAST BETWEEN ORAL AND CUTANEOUS LESIONS)

There are multiple steps involved in the sentinel node biopsy technique for mucosal lesions. They are as follows:

Step 1
Patient Selection

An appropriate patient is the one with a significant risk of lymphatic micrometastases, who is also unlikely to have distant metastases with a small, injectable lesion.[53] Since, early oral cavity cancer has less risk of distant metastases than melanoma, the manner in which these patients need to be approached is a bit different from the way we approach melanoma patients. It is very important not to miss potentially curable micrometastases and reasonable to consider using the technique for lesions that are larger and more invasive than what would be considered appropriate for a melanoma. Nonetheless, multiple series have confirmed that the technique is not appropriate for T3 and T4 primary tumors due to the significant volume of tissue that would need to be injected; the excessively large number of radioactive nodes generated, the greater risk that grossly positive nodes exist, the potential for false-negatives due to incomplete injection and the technical futility of removing a large number of nodes in piecemeal fashion. On the contrary, the technique is best applied to T1 and smaller T2 lesions. If a lesion is less than 4 cm in maximal diameter but has significant tongue fixation or other manifestation of deep invasion, then this is truly a T4 lesion and the results with sentinel node biopsy are unlikely to prove accurate and useful.

If the primary tumor meets the above criteria, the next issue is whether the neck is grossly involved. While the sentinel node technique is an excellent technique for detecting micrometastases, it is less useful for detecting nonpalpable but grossly involved lymph nodes. This appears to be particularly true with squamous cell carcinoma. It is postulated that when a large percentage of the lymph node is replaced by cancer, physiologic obstruction occurs and alternative patterns of lymphatic drainage develop. Extranodal squamous cell carcinoma in the neck tissues, by definition, cannot be detected by sentinel node biopsy. It is important to detect the presence of such gross disease on preoperative imaging and avoid applying this technique, to that group of patients, in order to avoid false-positives. Generally, contrast enhanced computerized tomography or magnetic resonance imaging (if iodine allergic) are the imaging modalities used. These should be strictly interpreted. The role of positron emission tomography remains to be delineated, but this may ultimately also prove useful in ruling out such gross disease. It should be kept in mind that the sentinel node technology represents an excellent technique for detection of micrometastases in patients felt to have a reasonably low-risk of metastases, but is not as accurate at detecting grossly involved nonfunctional nodes.

Step 2

Injection of the Primary Tumor

The injection is performed prior to the surgical procedure, generally on the morning of surgery, in the radiological suite. Injection is also sometimes performed late on a day before. Use 500 millicuries on the morning of surgery or a slightly higher dose the night before. While, awake injection and imaging in radiology, is the most commonly used technique; as we extend this procedure to endoscopically accessible oropharyngeal, supraglottic and hypopharyngeal lesions, it is likely that co-operative efforts with the nuclear radiologist and the use of portable cameras will allow for intraoperative endoscopic injection, with or without radiological imaging, and gamma probe guided sentinel node biopsy, without the need for uncomfortable injections on an awake patient. Theoretical advantages of injecting under general anesthesia, include better exposure of the primary tumor and avoidance of motion of the patient related to discomfort. This may eventually further increase the reliability of this method. Taking into account that the radiolocalization of the detected hot spot, does not represent the drainage of the primary tumor but the drainage of the tracer deposits, which are supposed to mimic the lymphatic drainage of the primary tumor, the impact of a thorough and representative tracer injection becomes evident. Due to density and direction of the head and neck lymphatics the primary tumor may drain into several alternative lymphatic pathways, all representing the first echelon of draining sentinel lymph nodes.

Nevertheless, due to regulatory issues related to the injection of radioactive substances and the lack of widely available portable nuclear imaging, awake injection remains the most commonly used technique at present. It is important to ensure that the patient is comfortable so that an adequate preoperative injection is obtained. The author uses topical anesthetic, mild oral sedation and lingual, inferior alveolar and/or sphenopalatine nerve blocks to ensure patient's comfort during manipulation and injection of the primary tumor. Direct injection of the tumor with local anesthesia should not be performed as it may affect uptake of the radionuclide and reportedly may even cause it to precipitate in the tissues. The injection technique involves narrow injection with a 25 gauge needle circumferentially encompassing the leading edge of the lesion and an additional injection in the center of the lesion (Fig. 1). Five tuberculin syringes with 1 ml aliquots of technetium 99 sulfur colloid, with a total radioactivity of 400 mCi (millicuries), would represent a standard dose to be given in the morning of the scheduled surgery. A slightly higher dose should be given the night before. These dosages are extrapolated from the practice for melanoma and have worked well for oral cavity cancer, but formal comparative evaluation of dosages and volumes for use in the oral cavity have yet to be performed.

In order to extend this technique to supraglottic and hypopharyngeal sites, arrangements must be made to handle radionuclide in the operating suite, generally involving participation of a nuclear medicine technician and endoscopic injection of the primary tumor must be performed. Subsequently, adequate time must be allowed for migration of radionuclide to the lymphatic basin and the gamma probe can be used to confirm this.

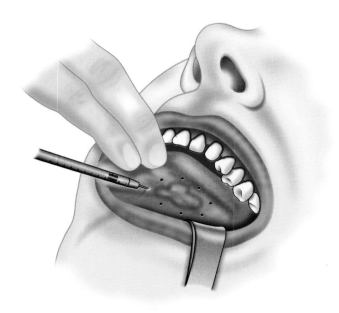

Fig. 1: A 1.5 inch needle and tuberculin syringe are used to inject gingerly, completely encompassing the lesion. Excess force should be avoided, so that nonphysiologic drainage patterns will not be opened. Sedation, topical anesthetics and nerve blocks can be used, but lidocaine should not be infiltrated into the bed of injection. Avoid injecting more widely or deeply than necessary, as the injected colloid will extravasate more widely than is apparent

For cutaneous lesions, it is well documented that a scar from a previous excisional biopsy can be injected to allow accurate sentinel node biopsy. Whether a previously excised oral lesion could undergo sentinel node excision by injection of an intraoral scar has yet to be determined. It is important to inject narrowly and not to inject into the deep tissues. The radionuclide will extravasate more widely in the oral cavity around the site of injection than in the skin and will usually go to the neck more quickly. There is no benefit in trying to inject a margin around the tumor, as this will lead to an unmanageable excess of radioactive nodes. However, injection must be just peripheral to the tumor in normal appearing tissue and not within the gross cancer, in order to allow migration into normal lymphatic channels. The author prefers to use unfiltered technetium 99 sulfur colloid. The presence of larger particles allows for retention of radioactivity in the proximal lymphatics. Retained particles at the site of primary injection are not a major issue as the author recommends removal of the primary tumor first. However, it is also possible to obtain good results using filtered technetium sulfur colloid and if there is a strong preference for addressing the lymphatics first, then this may

be preferable as there is a better clearance of background radioactivity from the primary site. More rapid migration of the filtered agent may also make it advantageous if injections of radionuclide are performed on the operation room table, at the start of the procedure rather than prior to the surgical procedure.

As discussed above, the use of blue dye concurrently with technetium sulfur colloid has become popular in sentinel node biopsy for melanoma. This is a reasonable technique for skin and certainly can help during the learning phase of the procedure, as the subtle blue dyed lymphatic vessels can be traced toward the sentinel node. Furthermore, reinjection of the blue dye is performed in the operating room under anesthesia and can provide a measure of security against inadequacy of preoperative injection due to patient discomfort. The most common approach, however, for the reasons previously mentioned, is to use the radionuclide alone for mucosal lesions. The author prefers to remove the primary tumor first to eliminate radioactive background at the primary site. When the technique is performed in this sequence, the blue dye has usually run through to the distal lymphatics by the time the oral resection is complete and margins are sent, making the dye less useful. The concept of injecting a second agent within the operating room for better accuracy is reasonable. However, there is currently a contrast agent, Sonazoid (GE Healthcare, Oslo, Norway) undergoing clinical trials that does not color the tissues, but can be identified by intraoperative ultrasound.[54] Sonazoid is a lipid stabilized suspension of 2 to 3.5 micron perfluorobutane microbubbles. This may some day provide an alternative to blue dye for those who desire a second tracer injection for increased accuracy.

Step 3

Nuclear Lymphatic Mapping

After injection, nuclear imaging of the lymphatics is obtained (Fig. 2). Single photon emission computed tomography (SPECT) technology, though not absolutely necessary, may eventually provide even better three dimensional localization of the sentinel node. The availability of both anteroposterior (AP) and lateral imaging will generally be adequate to guide the surgeon. A dynamic phase should be acquired with serial images for 1 hour following injection. These images should be acquired for one minute each. Transmission images should be acquired for 1–2 minutes in each new movement of the camera. While it is possible to perform sentinel node biopsy with the intraoperative gamma probe alone, the radiological image can be useful in providing a rough guide to the location of the sentinel node. It may provide for a more complete informed consent process by predicting unexpected drainage to the contralateral neck or other areas that were not expected to be involved.

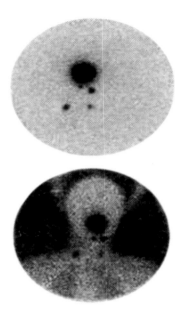

Fig. 2: Lymphoscintigram obtained after injection of a unilateral tongue cancer exhibiting significant bilateral lymphatic drainage

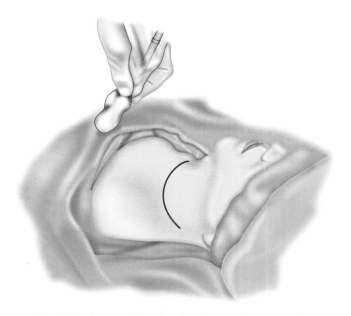

Fig. 3: Background reading is taken at the precordium

Step 4

Removal of the Primary Tumor

As mentioned above, the author prefers to resect the primary tumor transorally first. If the injection field is sufficiently narrow, this usually eliminates or greatly reduces background radioactivity at the primary site, or "shine through," that can confound the sentinel node identification. The usual, appropriate surgical margins with frozen section control should be obtained. In some situations, it may be necessary to perform the nodal biopsy prior to primary resection. Removal of the primary tumor first is less important, when the lymphatic basin is distant from the primary tumor and is often less of an issue for skin lesions (i.e. auricular scalp or nasal lesions). However, this can be important for lesions of the neck or preauricular skin where the lymphatics are immediately deep to the primary tumor. It is especially important for floor of mouth tumors due to the immediate proximity of the submandibular lymphatics.

Step 5

Gamma Probe Guided Sentinel Node Biopsy

The hand-held gamma probe is now used to confirm the location of the SLN(s), which was previously identified during lymphoscintigraphy. The skin is again marked with the location of the nodes. If the patient is to undergo sentinel node biopsy alone, with neck dissection planned only for positive findings intraoperatively or on permanent

histopathology, the incision can be drawn narrowly over the node. However, the incision must be consistent with the possibility of subsequent neck dissection and the planned incision for the formal lymphadenectomy should be considered. Alternatively, the incision can be drawn in the same line as that to be used for neck dissection; although shorter in length and flaps can be elevated. This latter approach is used when immediate gamma probe guided neck dissection is the plan. After the incision is made, subplatysmal flaps are elevated sufficiently to provide access to the hot area. The neck should first be carefully palpated in order to identify palpable gross lymphatic disease that may not be physiologically functional and hence may not take up radioactivity. The finding of gross cancer involvement would, of course, contraindicate sentinel node biopsy and mandate formal lymphadenectomy. If no gross disease is identified, the surgeon will now localize the sentinel node(s). Use of the probe to locate the nodes is not intuitive and it is best learned through instruction by a surgeon with experience in the technique. Initial readings are taken at the precordium and back table in order to assess the level of radioactivity (Fig. 3). Readings are also obtained from the resected tumor specimen and the bed of resection, in order to assess the level of anticipated background activity. The probe is slowly passed over the neck at a steady rate assessing the auditory input for radioactivity generated by the gamma probe. Care is taken to aim away from the primary resection bed. Since, the probe measures radioactivity over time, rapid or unsteady movement will lead to higher readings and louder auditory input and should be avoided. Using the steady constant motion, the probe is moved radially across each hot spot allowing the surgeon to determine the direction in which to proceed, in three dimensions, in order to locate the sentinel node. Using a fine hemostat or McCabe nerve dissector, the surgeon bluntly dissects toward the sentinel node (Fig. 4). Bipolar cautery can be used to divide the tissues to provide wider exposure. Use of paralytics and monopolar cautery should be avoided. After the dissection cavity is opened, the gamma probe is introduced into the space along the plane of dissection and angled in various directions in order to guide the surgeon to the sentinel node. The sentinel node is bluntly excised (Fig. 5). Probe readings (counts per minute) are recorded for initial readings taken while the node is in the patient, as well as for "ex vivo" readings of the extracted node, away from the patient (Fig. 6). Readings are taken repeatedly from the resection bed to ensure that there are no adjacent hot nodes, which are also to be removed (Fig. 7). Any lymph node exhibiting 10% or more of the radioactivity of the most radioactive node in the same anatomic area will be considered an additional SLN and will be harvested separately. If there are a large number of highly radioactive nodes (i.e. more than six), this essentially represents a failure of the technique and piecemeal removal of a large number of nodes is not recommended. The surgeon should proceed to selective neck dissection, if indicated. In the case, where there is a very hot sentinel node in a specific area, there may be a relatively hot node in a completely separate anatomic region,

(i.e. submental region versus level II jugular region) that does not reach 10% of the radioactivity of the hottest node. If this second node is truly in a separate area and is significantly greater than background (two or more times background readings), it should still be harvested as a sentinel node, as it may represent a separate drainage pattern from a different portion of the tumor.

Review of the lymphoscintigraphic imaging and knowledge of basic anatomic principles will allow the surgeon to judge whether such additional areas of borderline radioactivity need to be excised. When the SLN dissections are

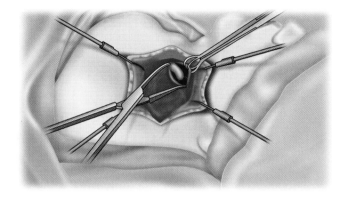

Fig. 5: The sentinel node is excised using a combination of blunt dissection and division of tissue using bipolar cautery. Unipolar cautery should be avoided when the proximity of neurovascular structure is not known

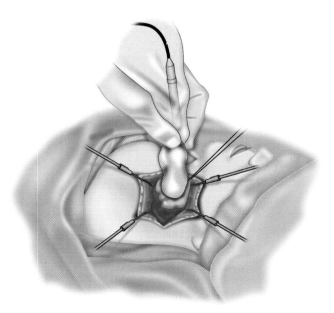

Fig. 4: Blunt dissection toward the "hot spot" is followed by reinsertion of the sentinel node into the path of dissection and angulation in various directions seeking the hot lymph node

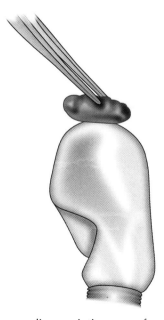

Fig. 6: Ex vivo readings pointing away from the patient should confirm whether this is the radioactive node

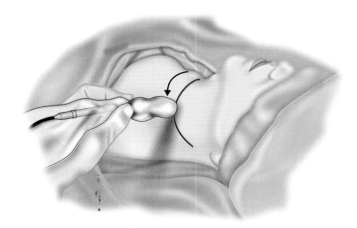

Fig. 7: The probe is drawn slowly over the neck seeking additional hot areas. This process is repeated after the hottest node(s) are removed

performed prior to resection of the oral cavity squamous cell carcinoma (OCSCC) or if significant radioactivity persists in the bed of resection, intraoral lead shields can be used to block background activity at the primary site. The presence of a collimator on the gamma probe is also recommended and most modern probes have fine tips with collimators. With tongue tumors background activity can be avoided by using a transoral suture on the tongue to pull the primary bed away from the lymphatics.

The issue of dealing with background activity at the primary site is most marked for the level one node with floor of mouth tumors. In this situation, the surgeon may need to perform some initial dissections below the level of the marginal mandibular nerve, transecting the tissues down to the level of the mylohyoid muscle. In this manner, the lymph nodes are mobilized away from the oral cavity, allowing for more accurate identification of the SLN(s) by placing the gamma probe into the tunnel, thus creating and directing the probe inferiorly away from the background radioactivity at the floor of mouth injection site. Each SLN is labeled, measured, described and recorded separately as per the location and the total ex vivo counts per second.

It is particularly important to tag the tissue adjacent to any identified marginal mandibular or spinal accessory nerve branches with permanent suture, in order to facilitate identification during a subsequent procedure, if the sentinel node is positive.

Step 6

Histopathologic Assessment of the Sentinel Node

Sentinel lymph node biopsy is gaining wide acceptance for cutaneous lesions, particularly melanoma, where formal elective lymphadenectomy is not a standard practice.

As mentioned previously, minimally invasive T1 oral lesions represent an emerging group, where the option of sentinel node biopsy might be considered. However, in any situation where sentinel node biopsy alone is performed, exhaustive histopathologic evaluation of the sentinel node with fine sectioning and sampling at thin intervals (some have advocated as thin as 150 micron intervals) and concurrent immunohistochemistry should be performed to rule out microscopic foci of cancer and allow for therapeutic neck dissection or radiation. If such an evaluation remains negative, close follow-up and consideration of serial radiological imaging (CT, MRI, or serial ultrasound) should be considered.

RISKS OF SENTINEL LYMPH NODE BIOPSY

The theoretical risk of injury to the facial nerve and spinal accessory nerve during blunt dissection through narrow exposure is one concern with SLNB in the head and neck region. The relatively few publications addressing this issue to date have reported incidences of complications that are less than 1%.[43,55] Theoretically, in the hands of an inexperienced operator, the risk of injury to the facial or spinal accessory nerves may be greater with SLNB than with formal parotidectomy and selective neck dissection. Since, the presence of sentinel node micrometastases may be recognized postoperatively, the potential risk of nerve injury related to re-exploration of an inflamed, recently operated wound needs to be considered. For this reason important structures are tagged and pathological analysis is done promptly, in order to allow for early re-exploration.

CONCLUSION

Sentinel lymph node biopsy can be used safely and with technical success for accessible head and neck squamous cell carcinomas. It offers the potential for more anatomically accurate surgery based on each patient's unique lymphatic drainage pattern. However, selective neck dissection remains the standard approach for the majority of oral cancers, particularly for larger T2, T3 and T4 lesions. SLNB can be advocated as a reasonable alternative to selective neck dissection for very early oral cancers. Unlike melanoma, where the presence of lymphatic metastases portends an extremely poor prognosis, squamous cell carcinoma with early lymphatic metastases remains curable. Thus, there is much more to lose by understaging patients or missing the involved lymph nodes.

The sentinel node concept is discarded by some, based on the misconception that selective neck dissection has no significant morbidity. Coming from a tradition of more radical neck procedures, the selective neck dissection is generally viewed as an intervention with negligible morbidity by many head and neck surgeons. In fact, although the morbidity of selective neck dissection is significantly less than that of the radical neck and modified radical neck dissections there is measurable morbidity in a variable percentage of patients, including issues with shoulder function secondary to temporary trapezius weakness followed by adhesive capsulitis of the shoulder, pain syndromes, contour changes and lower lip mobility. This has been demonstrated in numerous quality of life studies and at least two objective functional assessments.[56-58] This moderate morbidity has led some to suggest watchful waiting as an alternative for patients of lower risk. SLNB has developed as an intermediate option in response to this controversy. All of these complications are observed much less frequently with SLNB, although formal quality of life assessments have not yet been performed.

The sentinel node procedure would be more widely applicable if we develop the ability to immediately diagnose positive sentinel nodes. Frozen section, even with multiple sections, is not sufficiently accurate and may destroy valuable specimen material.[28] Thus, for the patient with the micrometastases in the sentinel node, we are potentially dealing with issues of re-exploration and dissection of functionally important nerves in a recently operated wound. Ultimately, rapid reverse transcriptase polymerase chain reaction assessment of nodes may ultimately provide immediate information regarding the status of the sentinel node.[59] As future studies are designed to safely evaluate the sentinel node biopsy technique, the opportunity should be taken to plan correlative studies to validate the role of these new technologies in tumor assessment.

SLNB ultimately may have a role in the management of oral cancer, given that there are lesions and situations where the 'wait and see' approach continues to be advocated. It may provide an intermediate approach for small but invasive T1 or smaller T2 lesions for which watchful waiting is the major alternative. It appears unlikely that this technique will ever replace selective neck dissection for larger T2 and T3N0 lesions.

Equally important is the evaluation for the significant unpredictability of lymphatic pathways observed for both cutaneous and oral lesions. In fact for lesions not involving the midline but within a few centimeters of it, lymphoscintigraphy (LS) and gamma probe guided surgery may ultimately provide the solution in these patients, for whom we often struggle with the decision regarding contralateral neck management. Increased accuracy in the identification of micrometastases will ultimately lead to more accurate staging. The sentinel node technique is likely to have an increasing role in the management of head and neck cancer in the future. Surgeons can gain experience

in the use of this technique for cutaneous malignancies, superficial oral cancers and with gamma probe guided neck dissection for invasive cancers, preferably in the context of a clinical trial. Pilot data on the use of this technique in the pharynx and larynx will continue to emerge. It is hoped that this chapter will provide a guide to surgeons as they consider the developing role of lymphoscintigraphy and sentinel node biopsy in detecting microscopic lymphatic metastases.

HIGHLIGHTS

- Sentinel node biopsy allows more accurate staging of the neck through a less invasive means than selective neck dissection. The procedure is most useful in a population with low risk of lymphatic metastases who do not have major comorbidity that precludes staged completion neck dissection and who are particularly concerned about the morbidity of selective neck dissection.
- The sentinel node technique is more accurate at diagnosing lymphatic metastases but leaves the lymphatic basins untreated, unless complete neck dissection is performed. Selective neck dissection, on the other hand, may treat lymphatic metastases that remain unrecognized, precluding the possibility of closer follow-up or adjuvant therapy. Gamma probe guided neck dissection combines the benefits of both but adds complexity to the standard selective neck dissection.
- Proper training and significant experience are necessary to perform accurate sentinel node biopsy.
- Complete, but also rapid, pathologic assessment is integral to the sentinel node procedure. Stepwise sectioning and immunohistochemistry should be completed within a few days to allow early re-exploration in the minority of patients with positive sentinel nodes, prior to onset of significant inflammatory changes in the neck.
- Proper training includes instructions on the proper injection technique, use of the gamma probe and proper pathological analysis of the sentinel nodes. Subsequently, the surgeon should develop experience through the practice of gamma probe guided neck dissection. In this procedure, the surgeon simulates sentinel node biopsy in the context of a planned selective neck dissection. This technique can lead to a more complete surgery for the patient, including better pathological identification of micrometastases and lymphatic mapping to assess contralateral drainage and include all lymph node groups at risk. It offers the surgeon the ability to develop experience in the sentinel node technique.
- The expected and potential morbidities of sentinel node biopsy are lower than the well documented morbidities of formal neck dissection.

- The concept is that an injection of a tracer will mark the first echelon lymph nodes and that the status of these lymph nodes correctly predicts the condition of a complete neck specimen, as it has been shown to apply in oral cancer, just as it does for melanoma. It is generally accepted as a standard approach for head and neck melanoma. However, practical considerations need to be addressed before this procedure can be applied in a general fashion to all N0 oral cancers as the preferred approach. Specifically, technologies are being developed to obtain early information regarding the pathological status of the sentinel node, improve patient selection, reduce background activity at the primary site and reduce marking of downstream lymph nodes. As these technologies progress, this procedure will likely progress from one that can be applied to a selected group of patients, to the one suited for all T1 and T2 N0 oral cancers.

REFERENCES

1. Morton DL, Wen DR, Wong JH, et al. Technical details of intraoperative lymphatic mapping for early stage melanoma. Arch Surg. 1992;127(4):392-9.
2. Morton DL, Wen DR, Foshag LJ, et al. Intraoperative lymphatic mapping and selective cervical lymphadenectomy for early-stage melanomas of the head and neck. J Clin Oncol. 1993;11(9):1751-6.
3. Leong SP: Selective sentinel lymphadenectomy for malignant melanoma. Surg Clin North Am. 2003;83(1):157-85.
4. Morton DL, Thompson JF, Essner R, et al. Validation of the accuracy of intraoperative lymphatic mapping and sentinel lymphadenectomy for early-stage melanoma: a multicenter trial. Multicenter Selective Lymphadenectomy Trial Group. Ann Surg. 1999;230(4):453-65.
5. Alex JC, Krag DN. The gamma-probe-guided resection of radiolabeled primary lymph nodes. Surg Oncol Clin N Am. 1996;5(1):33-41.
6. Krag DN, Meijer SJ, Weaver DL, et al. Minimal-access surgery for staging of malignant melanoma. Arch Surg. 1995;130(6):654-8.
7. Glass LF, Messina JL, Cruse W, et al. The use of intraoperative radiolymphoscintigraphy for sentinel node biopsy in patients with malignant melanoma. Dermatol Surg. 1996;22(8):715-20.
8. Albertini JJ, Cruse CW, Rapaport D, et al. Intraoperative radio-lympho-scintigraphy improves sentinel node identification for patients with melanoma. Ann Surg. 1996;223(2):217-24.
9. Ross MI, Reintgen D, Balch CM. Selective lymphadenectomy: emerging role for lymphatic mapping and sentinel node biopsy in the management of early stage melanoma. Semin Surg Oncol. 1993;9(3):219-23.
10. O'Brien CJ, Uren RF, Thompson JF, et al. Prediction of potential metastatic sites in cutaneous head and neck melanoma using lymphoscintigraphy. Am J Surg. 1995;170(5):461-6.
11. Pijpers R, Collet GJ, Meijer S, et al. The impact of dynamic lymphoscintigraphy and gamma probe guidance on sentinel node biopsy in melanoma. Eur J Nucl Med. 1995;22(11):1238-41.
12. Jesse RH, Ballantyne AJ, Larson D. Radical or modified neck dissection: a therapeutic dilemma. Am J Surg. 1978;136(4):516-9.
13. Spiro RH, Strong EW. Epidermoid carcinoma of the mobile tongue. Treatment by partial glossectomy alone. Am J Surg. 1971;122(6):707-10.
14. Spiro RH, Strong EW. Epidermoid carcinoma of the oral cavity and oropharynx. Elective vs therapeutic radical neck dissection as treatment. Arch Surg. 1973;107(3):382-4.
15. Vandenbrouck C, Sancho-Garnier H, Chassagne D, et al. Elective versus therapeutic radical neck dissection in epidermoid carcinoma of the oral cavity. Results of a randomized clinical trial. Cancer. 1980;46(2):386-90.
16. McGuirt WF, Johnson JT, Myers EN, et al. Floor of mouth carcinoma. The management of the clinically negative neck. Arch Otolaryngol Head Neck Surg. 1995;121(3):278-82.
17. Shah JP, Andersen PE. Evolving role of modifications in neck dissection for oral squamous carcinoma. Br J Oral Maxillofac Surg. 1995;33(1):3-8.
18. Kligerman J, Lima RA, Soares JR, et al. Supraomohyoid neck dissection in the treatment of T1/T2 squamous cell carcinoma of oral cavity. Am J Surg. 1994;168(5):391-4.
19. Martínez-Gimeno C, Rodríguez EM, Vila CN, et al. Squamous cell carcinoma of the oral cavity: a clinicopathologic scoring system for evaluating risk of cervical lymph node metastasis. Laryngoscope. 1995;105(7 Pt 1):728-33.
20. Ho CM, Lam KH, Wei WI, et al. Occult lymph node metastasis in small oral tongue cancers. Head Neck. 1992;14(5):359-63.
21. Urist MM, O'Brien CJ, Soong SJ, et al. Squamous cell carcinoma of the buccal mucosa: analysis of prognostic factors. Am J Surg. 1987;154(4):411-4.
22. Mohit-Tabatabai MA, Sobel HJ, Rush BF, et al. Relation of thickness of floor of mouth stage I and II cancers to regional metastasis. Am J Surg. 1986;152(4):351-3.
23. Brown B, Barnes L, Mazariegos J, et al. Prognostic factors in mobile tongue and floor of mouth carcinoma. Cancer. 1989;64(6):1195-202.
24. Spiro RH, Huvos AG, Wong GY, et al. Predictive value of tumor thickness in squamous carcinoma confined to the tongue and floor of the mouth. Am J Surg. 1986;152(4):345-50.
25. Rassekh CH, Johnson JT, Myers EN. Accuracy of intraoperative staging of the N0 neck in squamous cell carcinoma. Laryngoscope. 1995;105(12 Pt 1):1334-6.
26. Ross G, Shoaib T, Soutar DS, et al. The use of sentinel node biopsy to upstage the clinically N0 neck in head and neck cancer. Arch Otolaryngol Head Neck Surg. 2002;128(11):1287-91.
27. Shoaib T, Soutar DS, MacDonald DG, et al. The accuracy of head and neck carcinoma sentinel lymph node biopsy in the clinically N0 neck. Cancer. 2001;91(11):2077-83.
28. Civantos FJ, Gomez C, Duque C, et al. Sentinel node biopsy in oral cavity cancer: correlation with PET scan and immunohistochemistry. Head Neck. 2003;25(1):1-9.

29. Taylor RJ, Wahl RL, Sharma PK, et al. Sentinel node localization in oral cavity and oropharynx squamous cell cancer. Arch Otolaryngol Head Neck Surg. 2001;127(8):970-4.

30. Alex JC, Sasaki CT, Krag DN, et al. Sentinel lymph node radiolocalization in head and neck squamous cell carcinoma. Laryngoscope. 2000;110(2 Pt 1):198-203.

31. Stoeckli SJ, Steinert H, Pfaltz M, et al. Sentinel lymph node evaluation in squamous cell carcinoma of the head and neck. Otolaryngol Head Neck Surg. 2001;125(3):221-6.

32. Zitsch RP III, Todd DW, Renner GJ, et al. Intraoperative radiolymphoscintigraphy for detection of occult nodal metastasis in patients with head and neck squamous cell carcinoma. Otolaryngol Head Neck Surg. 2000;122(5):662-6.

33. Ross GL, Soutar DS, Gordon MacDonald D, et al. Sentinel node biopsy in head and neck cancer: preliminary results of a multicenter trial. Ann Surg Oncol. 2004;11(7):690-6.

34. Stoeckli SJ, Pfaltz M, Ross GL, et al. The second international conference on sentinel node biopsy in mucosal head and neck cancer. Ann Surg Oncol. 2005;12(11):919-24.

35. Paleri V, Rees G, Arullendran P, et al. Sentinel node biopsy in squamous cell cancer of the oral cavity and oral pharynx: a diagnostic meta-analysis. Head Neck. 2005;27(9):739-47.

36. Civantos FJ, Zitsch RP, David E, et al. Sentinel lymph node biopsy accurately stages the regional lymph nodes for T1-2 oral squamous cell carcinomas(OSCC): results of a prospective multi-institutional trial. Journal of Clinical Oncology. 2010;28(8):1395-400.

37. Werner JA, Dünne AA, Ramaswamy A, et al. Sentinel node detection in N0 cancer of the pharynx and larynx. Br J Cancer. 2002;87(7):711-5.

38. Messina JL, Reintgen DS, Cruse CW, et al. Selective lymphadenectomy in patients with Merkel cell (cutaneous neuroendocrine) carcinoma. Ann Surg Oncol. 1997;4(5):389-95.

39. Altinyollar H, Berbero lu U, Celen O. Lymphatic mapping and sentinel lymph node biopsy in squamous cell carcinoma of the lower lip. Eur J Surg Oncol. 2002;28(1):72-4.

40. Reschly MJ, Messina J, Zaulyanov LL,et al. Utility of sentinel lymphadenectomy in the management of patients with high-risk cutaneous squamous cell carcinoma. Dermatol Surg. 2003;29(2):135-40.

41. Nouri K, Rivas MP, Pedroso F, et al. Sentinel lymph node biopsy for high-risk cutaneous squamous cell carcinoma of the head and neck. Arch Dermatol. 2004;140(10):1284.

42. Devaney KO, Rinaldo A, Rodrigo JP, et al. Sentinel node biopsy in head and neck tumors-where do we stand today? Head Neck. 2006;28(12):1122-31.

43. Civantos FJ, Moffat FL, Goodwin WJ. Lymphatic mapping and sentinel lymphadenectomy for 106 head and neck lesions: contrasts between oral cavity and cutaneous malignancy. Laryngoscope. 2006;112(3 Pt 2 Suppl 109):1-15.

44. Ross GL, Soutar DS, Shoaib T, et al. The ability of lymphoscintigraphy to direct sentinel node biopsy in the clinically N0 neck for patients with head and neck squamous cell carcinoma. Br J Radiol. 2002;75(900):950-8.

45. Barzan L, Sulfaro S, Alberti F, et al. Gamma probe accuracy in detecting the sentinel lymph node in clinically N0 squamous cell carcinoma of the head and neck. Ann Otol Rhinol Laryngol. 2002;111(9):794-8.

46. Werner JA, Dünne AA, Ramaswamy A, et al. Number and location of radiolabeled, intraoperatively identified sentinel nodes in 48 head and neck cancer patients with clinically staged N0 and N1 neck. Eur Arch Otorhinolaryngol. 2002;259(2):91-6.

47. Chiesa F, Mauri S, Grana C, et al. Is there a role for sentinel node biopsy in early N0 tongue tumors? Surgery. 2000;128(1): 16-21.

48. Chiesa F, Tradati N, Calabrese L. Sentinel node biopsy, lymphatic pattern and selective neck dissection in oral cancer. Oral Dis. 2001;7(5):317-8.

49. Hyde NC, Prvulovich E, Newman L, et al. A new approach to pre-treatment assessment of the N0 neck in oral squamous cell carcinoma: the role of sentinel node biopsy and positron emission tomography. Oral Oncol. 2003;39(4):350-60.

50. Longnecker SM, Guzzardo MM, Van Voris LP. Life-threatening anaphylaxis following subcutaneous administration of isosulfan blue 1%. Clin Pharm. 1985;4(2):219-21.

51. Ionna F, Chiesa F, Longo F, et al. Prognostic value of sentinel node in oral cancer. Tumori. 2002;88(3):S18-19.

52. Mozzillo N, Chiesa F, Botti G, et al. Sentinel node biopsy in head and neck cancer. Ann Surg Oncol. 2001;8(9 suppl): S103-5S.

53. Alvi A, Johnson JT: Extracapsular spread in the clinically negative neck (N0): implications outcome. Otolaryngol Head Neck Surg. 1996;114(1):65-70.

54. Curry JM, Bloedon E, Malloy KM, et al. Ultrasound-guided contrast-enhanced sentinel node biopsy of the head and neck in a porcine model. Otolaryngol Head Neck Surg. 2007;137(5):735-41.

55. Chao C, Wong SL, Edwards MJ, et al. Sentinel lymph node biopsy for head and neck melanomas. Ann Surg Oncol. 2003;10(1):21-6.

56. Chepeha DB, Taylor RJ, Chepeha JC, et al. Functional assessment using Constant's Shoulder Scale after modified radical and selective neck dissection. Head Neck. 2002;24(5):432-6.

57. Kuntz AL, Weymuller EA. Impact of neck dissection on quality of life. Laryngoscope. 1999;109(8):1334-8.

58. Rogers SN, Ferlito A, Pelliteri PK, et al. Quality of life following neck dissections. Acta Otolaryngol. 2004;124(3):231-6.

59. Becker MT, Shores CG, Yu KK, et al. Molecular assay to detect metastatic head and neck squamous cell carcinoma. Arch Otolaryngol Head Neck Surg. 2004;130(1):21-7.

Chapter 9

Laryngopharyngectomy

Sheng-Po Hao, Shih-Wei Kuo

INTRODUCTION

Cancer of the laryngopharynx remains a major challenge to head and neck surgeons. A multidisciplinary team approach usually involves surgeons, medical and radiation oncologists as well as speech and swallow specialists. There is still an ongoing debate as how to achieve the optimal balance between the oncological cure and preservation of function. Laryngopharyngectomy has been traditionally regarded as a primary modality for the treatment of laryngopharyngeal malignancies. In recent years, combined chemoradiation therapy has been advocated for selected laryngopharyngeal cancers. However, surgery is still indicated as a primary treatment modality for selected cases as well as for salvage, after chemoradiotherapy failures. The selection of the types of treatment modalities will need to be carefully considered in accordance to the patient, disease and institutional factors in order to achieve the best oncological and functional outcomes.

ANATOMY

The hypopharynx is located between the oropharynx and the esophagus. It extends from the superior border of the hyoid bone to the lower border of the cricoid cartilage. It is a muscular tube lined with mucosa and encompasses the larynx. The hypopharynx includes the posterior pharyngeal wall, the pyriform sinuses and the postcricoid areas.

Squamous cell carcinomas are the most common type of cancer arising from these areas. They have a high tendency for submucosal spread and cervical node metastasis. Hypopharyngeal cancer has the ability for extensive submucosal spread. The cancer can also invade the paraglottic,

pre-epiglottic spaces and arytenoid joint and impair its mobility. Involvement of the above areas precludes a partial laryngopharyngectomy. However, posterior extension of the tumor to the prevertebral muscles is very uncommon. Lateral extension out of the laryngeal box through posterior cricothyroid membrane to the cervical soft tissue or carotid artery encasement with cervical nodes is also common, which also precludes partial laryngopharyngectomy.

PREOPERATIVE EVALUATION AND ANESTHESIA

Majority of the patients with hypopharyngeal cancers are chronic smokers and regular alcohol consumers, but there is no direct causal relationship to demonstrate that betel nut chewing leads to the development of cancers of the hypopharynx. Patients typically present with globus sensation, dysphagia and/or odynophagia. Referred otalgia is not uncommon and should arouse suspicion of hypopharyngeal cancers, especially in patients with the presence of the classical risk factors such as smoking and alcohol intake. Voice changes and respiratory symptoms are common, if the larynx is involved. It is not unusual to have metastatic nodes as the initial presentation. Metastatic nodes to level II and/or III are common and some forms of neck dissection are usually indicated.

Endoscopic Assessment
Flexible Endoscopy

Office based transnasal fiberoptic flexible endoscopy to assess not only the hypopharynx, but also the esophagus is mandatory as an initial evaluation. Patients are instructed to hold their breath and use Valsalva maneuver to open up the pyriform sinuses during examination. Movement of the vocal folds should be carefully evaluated. The esophageal orifice cannot be fully accessed in flexible endoscopy and unexpected second primary tumors in the esophagus are not uncommon.

Rigid Endoscopy

Direct rigid laryngopharyngoscopy is performed with the patient under general anesthesia. An extensive and thorough evaluation of the entire mucosal surface of the hypopharynx is mandatory for treatment planning.

The rigid endoscope helps to stretch the hypopharynx mucosa in order to reveal the entire tumor extent under direct vision. Rigid endoscopy has a special role in defining mucosal extension of the tumor and cannot be replaced by flexible fiberoptic endoscopy. Special care should be directed to the pyriform sinus apex and esophageal orifice where the flexible endoscopy has difficulty in getting access. Biopsy of the tumors is commonly performed after laryngopharynx mapping under rigid endoscopy.

Imaging Studies

The aim of imaging studies for cancers of laryngopharynx is to determine the three-dimensional extent of the tumors.

Computed Tomography

Computed tomography (CT) of laryngopharynx is frequently employed to evaluate the size and extent of the primary tumor in conjunction with the regional cervical nodal status. Patients are instructed to use Valsalva maneuver to open up the pyriform sinuses for dynamic evaluation during the examination.

CT is usually very useful in demonstrating cartilage destruction or extralaryngeal extensions, which are usually difficult to be evaluated with either flexible or rigid endoscopy.

Magnetic Resonance Imaging

Magnetic resonance imaging (MRI) of the hypopharynx is performed with an anterior neck coil. It allows better soft tissue resolution than CT. The MRI of hypopharynx has additional advantage that sagittal plane of examination enables accurate evaluation of vertical extent of the tumor. The MRI of hypopharynx is ideally performed before biopsy as to reduce tissue edema resulting from the biopsy, which may obscure the real tumor extent.

Positron Emission Tomography

Cancers of the laryngopharynx are notorious for their aggressive biological behavior with extensive submucosal extension, frequent lymphatic metastasis as well as early distant metastasis. Positron emission tomography (PET) is invaluable in detecting systemic dissemination and should be considered in every patient with cancer of the laryngopharynx.

Not surprisingly, an occult esophageal primary tumor can sometimes be detected by PET and thus change the entire treatment plan. But it is worthwhile noting that PET has limited ability in detecting small primary lesions, so that a negative PET cannot exclude a small second primary tumor in the esophagus, which can be detected by a transnasal flexible fiberoptic esophagoscopy.

Anesthesia

General anesthesia is generally required for surgery of the laryngopharyngeal cancer. Endotracheal intubation is the most commonly employed method of ventilation. However, tracheotomy may be necessary when tumor compromise adequate airway or when endotracheal tube itself obscures the operating field or interferes with laser excision.

In endoscopic laryngopharyngectomy, jet ventilation can be administered through a tube incorporated in the operating laryngoscope with the merit of being no tube to obscure the direct vision of the tumor. However, the passive movement of the entire operating field created by the jet ventilation precludes precise microsurgical operation with laser. Laser fire is always a major consideration. Because oxygen concentration above 30% poses an increased risk of ignition, operation should be performed while turning off the jet ventilation, i.e. operation performed under apneic phase. Another option is to use a "laser tube."

If an endotracheal intubation is selected to maintain the airway, the authors recommend a number 5 tube (inner diameter of 5 mm). The cuff should be filled with saline and protected with saline-soaked cotton balls.

The authors generally recommend tracheotomy for all large laryngopharyngeal tumors undergoing open or endoscopic laryngopharyngectomy. Unless, the tumor is relatively small and distant from the glottis, the operating field will not be interfered by the endotracheal tube.

SURGICAL TECHNIQUES

T1 or T2 hypopharyngeal cancer can be treated surgically with either open or endoscopic partial laryngopharyngectomy whereas locally advanced cases along with salvage, after radiation failures, are treated with total laryngopharyngectomy.

Transoral Endoscopic Laser Excision of Hypopharynx Cancer under Microscopy

The patient is ventilated with a size 5 endotracheal tube under general anesthesia. The cuff is filled with saline and protected with saline-soaked cotton balls. Under direct suspended laryngoscopy, the tumor in the lateral aspect of right arytenoid cartilage is fully exposed (Fig. 1). The tumor is gently palpated with forceps to evaluate the approximate depth of infiltration. Cotton balls soaked with 1% ephedrine are placed around the tumor and adjacent mucosa for vasoconstriction, which will also facilitate further delineation of the tumor extent.

The CO_2 laser is frequently chosen for tumor excision. It has a wavelength of approximately 10,600 nm and is maximally absorbed by water. It allows precise incision of the tissues by its ability to vaporize cells. A typical spot size is about 0.3–1.0 mm in diameter. Surgery is performed under the standard laser safety precautions. The patient's eyes are covered with wet eye pads and the face is protected with wet towels. The laser is delivered through an articulated arm mounted on the operating microscope. The laser is set with

continuous or superpulse mode for dissection with a power of 5–10 W. After fully exposing the tumor, the initial mucosal cut over superior aspect of arytenoid cartilage is made (Fig. 2). The mucosa is gently grasped to allow appropriate traction in order to evaluate the submucosal extent and taking care not to transect the tumor. Then, the tumor is retracted laterally away from the arytenoid cartilage. The cut mucosal surface is gently pulled away with the grasping forceps to expose the plane of dissection. En bloc laser tumor excision is then performed along with a safety resection margin (Figs 3 and 4). The resultant mucosa defect is left to heal secondarily and no mucosa resurfacing is required.

Open Laryngopharyngectomy

The patient shown in the images below has a primary pyriform sinus cancer located on the lateral wall with minimal

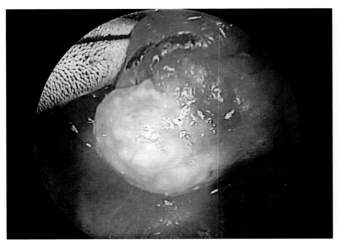

Fig. 1: The tumor in the lateral aspect of right arytenoid cartilage is fully exposed

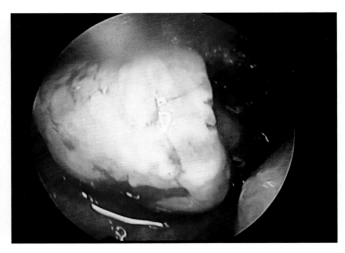

Fig. 2: Under microscopy, initial mucosal cut with laser beam over superior aspect of arytenoid cartilage is made

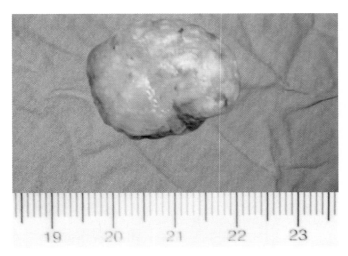

Fig. 3: Laser is applied for dissection till the entire tumor is removed using an en bloc laser with safe resection margin

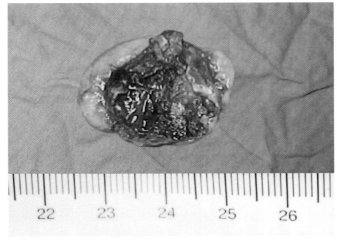

Fig. 4: The tumor is removed with enough safety margins

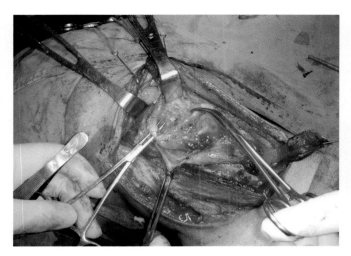

Fig. 5: The attached strap muscles are transected to create an infrahyoid pharyngotomy

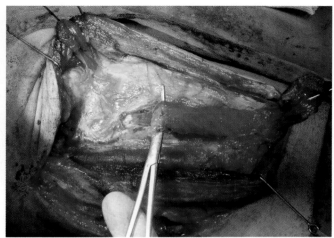

Fig. 6: A cuff of strap muscle is left attached to the under-surface of hyoid bone to facilitate subsequent closure

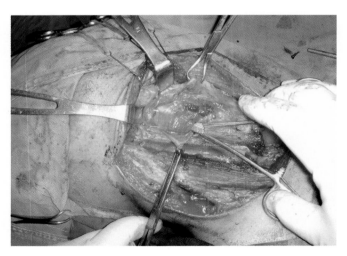

Fig. 7: Lateral pharyngotomy is performed by transection of the middle and inferior constrictor muscles

aryepiglottic fold extension. The patient is ventilated with endotracheal tube under general anesthesia. The neck is hyperextended, followed by routine preparation and draping.

A right hemiapron incision is made extending from the mastoid tip to the level of the thyroid notch. An ipsilateral selective neck dissection is carried out to remove level II, III and IV nodes. The sternocleidomastoid muscle is retracted laterally to expose the hyoid-thyroid complex. The ipsilateral thyroid lobe and superior thyroid vascular pedicles are identified and retracted laterally. Infrahyoid pharyngotomy is created after locating the hyoid bone with transection of the attached strap muscles (Fig. 5). A cuff of strap muscle is left attached to the undersurface of hyoid bone (Fig. 6) to facilitate subsequent closure. Lateral pharyngotomy is performed by transection of the middle

and inferior constrictor muscles (Fig. 7). Both the infrahyoid and lateral pharyngotomy incisions allow the full exposure of the primary tumor over the lateral hypopharyngeal wall (Figs 8A and B). Wide local excision of the tumor mass is then performed. A partial laryngectomy can also be included by incorporating the upper and lateral portion of the thyroid cartilage (Fig. 9). This maneuver opens up the larynx-hypopharynx complex in a fashion similar to opening a book (Fig. 10). The resected thyroid cartilage also serves to provide an adequate deep surgical margin (Figs 11A and B). Brisk bleeding from the branches of superior laryngeal artery can be encountered and is easily controlled with appropriate hemostasis. The resected specimen is sent to the pathology department to ensure safety margins.

A nasogastric tube is inserted and secured at the nostril (Figs 12A and B). Pharyngotomy is closed in three layers as a usual practice (Fig. 13). The strap muscles are reapproximated. Sutures are placed above and around the hyoid bone to the tongue base musculature to reinforce strap muscle closure. In cases of failure after chemoradiation therapy, an inferiorly based sternocleidomastoid muscle flap is transposed to cover and reinforce the pharyngotomy closure (Figs 14A and B). A portion of the muscular flap can be inserted between carotid artery and closed pharyngotomy prophylactically to prevent carotid blow out, should the wound be complicated by a pharyngocutaneous fistula (Fig. 15).

A close suction drain is left in place but stays some distance from the closed pharyngotomy and carotid artery. The cutaneous flap is repaired with a multiple layer closure.

Total Laryngopharyngectomy

Total excision of the larynx and hypopharynx is usually indicated in the setting of chemoradiation failures, when partial laryngopharyngectomy is considered to be inadequate.

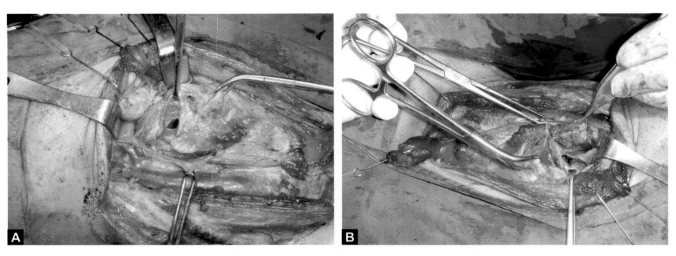

Figs 8A and B: Once the infrahyoid and lateral pharyngotomy is created, the hypopharynx is entered

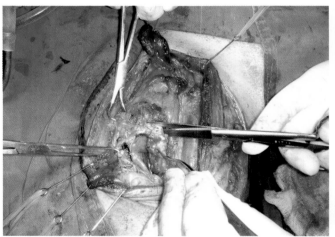

Fig. 9: A partial laryngectomy can also be performed to include the upper and lateral portion of the thyroid cartilage

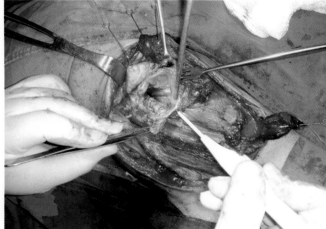

Fig. 10: This maneuver opens up the larynx-hypopharynx complex just like opening a book

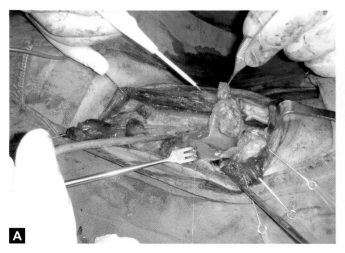

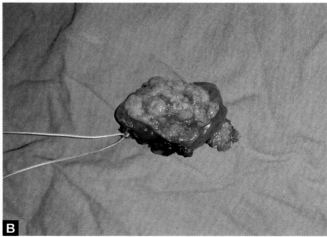

Figs 11A and B: The resected thyroid cartilage also provides adequate deep surgical margin

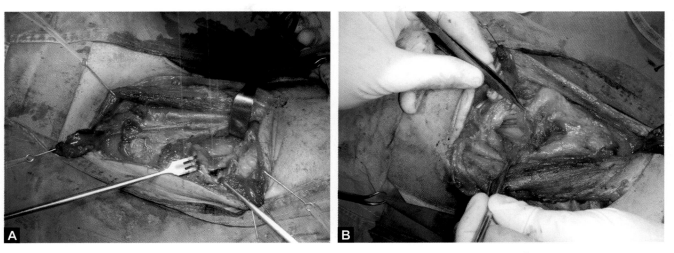

Figs 12A and B: A nasogastric tube is inserted and is secured at nostril

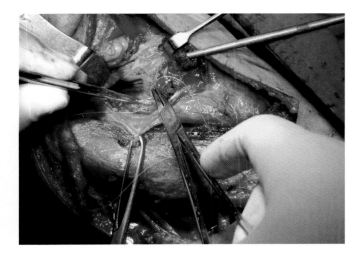

Fig. 13: The pharyngotomy is closed in three layers as usual

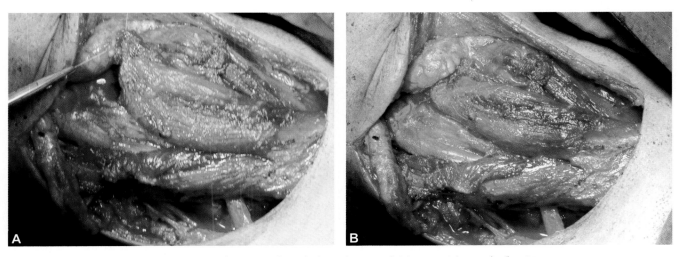

Figs 14A and B: An inferiorly based sternocleidomastoid muscle flap is transposed to cover and reinforce the pharyngotomy closure

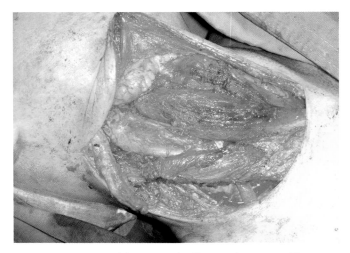

Fig. 15: A portion of the muscular flap can be inserted between carotid artery and closed pharyngostomy to prevent carotid artery blowing out once a pharyngocutaneous fistula occurs

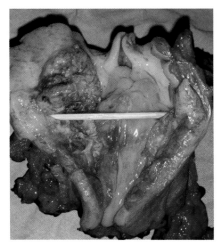

Fig. 16: The total laryngopharyngectomy is completed by doing the same above procedure on the contralateral hypopharynx

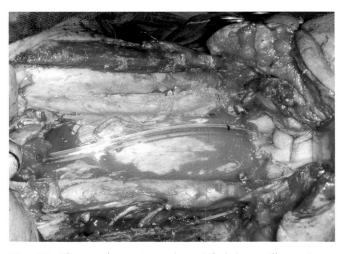

Fig. 17: The resultant circumferential defect will require to be reconstructed either with a free jejunal flap, a free radial forearm flap or a free anterolateral thigh flap

Surgery is commenced with tracheotomy performed under local anesthesia and general anesthesia is introduced via tracheotomy tube. The neck is hyperextended and is draped in the usual manner. An apron incision is created and neck flap is raised to expose the hyoid-thyroid complex. Bilateral superior thyroid vascular pedicles are identified and followed to each thyroid lobe. An ipsilateral thyroid lobectomy is usually required, especially, in advanced hypopharyngeal cancer. The contralateral thyroid lobe is intentionally preserved, however, the superior laryngeal artery needs to be transected. This is followed by the suprahyoid pharyngotomy. Lateral pharyngotomy is performed by transection of the superior and middle constrictor muscle, if not involved by the cancer. This maneuver opens the

ipsilateral hemi laryngopharynx. The tumor is inspected under direct vision, extent of resection is determined at this stage. Appropriate preservation of the contralateral hypopharyngeal mucosa and cervical esophagus is carefully considered. A total laryngopharyngectomy is mandatory if a large portion of the hypopharyngeal mucosa is involved by the cancer. Total laryngopharyngectomy is completed by repeating the above procedure on the contrateral hypopharynx (Fig. 16). A nasogastric tube is inserted through the nostril to the cervical esophagus. The resultant circumferential defect will be required to be reconstructed either with a free jejunal flap, a free radial forearm flap or a free anterolateral thigh flap (Fig. 17). In author's institution, we favor either free jejunal flap or free anterolateral thigh flap. Distant pedicle flap such as pectoralis major myocutaneous flap can be tubed as a substitute for pharynx or a gastric pull-up can be performed.

Primary tracheoesophageal puncture can be performed at this stage. A permanent tracheostoma is created by suturing the distal stump of trachea to the cervical skin below and the apron flap above. Wound is closed in layers after placement of a pair of closed suction drain.

POSTOPERATIVE TREATMENT

Transoral Endoscopic Laser Excision

Postoperatively, the patient is extubated after an intravenous dextran injection. Nutrition is initially provided through the nasogastric tube for 3–7 days. However, patient should be kept NPO within the first 24 hours postoperatively and the nasogastric tube is mainly served for gastric decompression. Fiberoptic endoscopy is used to evaluate healing and aspiration prior to commencement of oral intake. Nasogastric tube is usually removed within 5–7 days. Intravenous antibiotic is continued for 3 days and then, shifted to oral form via nasogastric tube before removing the nasogastric tube. If severe aspiration occurs, a speech and swallow therapist is invaluable for deglutition training.

Open Partial Laryngopharyngectomy with Tracheotomy

Tracheotomy cuff is inflated for the initial 8–24 hours postoperatively. Deflation is performed once absence of active wound bleeding or hematoma, is confirmed. The tracheotomy tube is removed after laryngeal swelling subsides, usually on the third postoperative day. Patient should be kept NPO within the first 24 hours postoperatively and the nasogastric tube is mainly served for gastric decompression. Nasogastric feedings is continued for 5–7 days. Longer feeding time may be necessary in cases of chemoradiation failure, for up to 10–14 days. Before removing nasogastric tube, a fiberoptic endoscopy is performed to evaluate the healing process as well as possible aspiration. Intravenous antibiotic is maintained for 3 days and then, shifted to oral form via nasogastric tube before removing the nasogastric tube. If severe aspiration occurs, speech and swallow therapist is required for the deglutition rehabilitation. Drain output is accurately recorded at 8 hours interval and removed when the cumulative drainage amount is less than 20 ml per day or less than 10 ml per 8 hours.

Total Pharyngolaryngectomy

Decannulation of the tracheotomy tube is performed in immediate postoperative setting. The patient will require nasogastric feedings for at least 5 days and longer in cases of failure, after combined chemoradiation therapy. Patient should be kept NPO for the first 24 hours postoperatively and the nasogastric tube is mainly served for gastric decompression. Intravenous antibiotic is maintained for 3 days and then, shifted to oral form via nasogastric tube before removing the nasogastric tube. Salivary leak is suspected, if bubbles are noticed in the drainage tube or bottle. It can occur, as early as, on third day postoperatively. Early recognition and prompt management is mandatory. A pharyngocutaneous fistula can be encountered in 20–30% of patients after combined chemoradiation therapy.

HIGHLIGHTS

I. Indications
- Partial laryngopharyngectomy
  - Primary tumor confined to the hypopharynx, preferably T1 or T2
  - Mobile ipsilateral arytenoid cartilage.

II. Contraindications
- Transglottic involvement
- Pyriform sinus apex involvement
- Significant tongue base involvement
- Cricopharyngeal muscle involvement
- Poor pulmonary function
- Thyroid cartilage involvement.

III. Special Preoperative Considerations
- Multidisciplinary approach
- Thorough clinical history and examination
- Accurate cancer staging with panendoscopy, biopsy and radiological imaging.

IV. Special Intraoperative Considerations
- Close collaboration with anesthetist for safe provision of airway
- Routine tracheotomy in partial laryngopharyngectomy
- Adequate laser training and exercise routine safety precautions
- Prophylactic muscle coverage of carotid artery and pharyngotomy for salvage cases following chemoradiotherapy failures.

V. Special Postoperative Considerations
- NPO for first 24 hours with nasogastric tube for gastric decompression
- Nasogastric feed for ongoing nutritional support and to facilitate wound healing
- Routine administration of perioperative antibiotics
- Quantitative and qualitative monitoring of the drainage output
- Early involvement of the speech and swallow therapist for rehabilitation
- High index of suspicion for development of complications
- Special care for salvage cases.

VI. Complications
- Salivary leak
- Pharyngocutaneous fistula
- Wound infection
- Aspiration
- Pneumonia following chemoradiotherapy failures.

ADDITIONAL READING

1. Cabanillas R, Rodrigo JP, Llorente JL, et al. Oncologic outcome of transoral laser surgery for supraglottic cancer compared with a transcervical approach. Head Neck. 2008;30(6):750-5.
2. Remacle M, Lawson G, Hantzakos A, et al. Endoscopic partial supraglottic laryngectomies: techniques and results. Otolaryngology Head Neck Surg. 2009;141(3):374-81.
3. Steiner W, Ambrosch P. Endoscopic Laser Surgery of the Upper Aerodigestive Tract. Stuttgart: Thieme; 1997.
4. Wei WI, Sham J. Cancer of the Larynx and Hypopharynx. Oxford, UK:ISIS Medical Media Ltd; 2000.

Chapter 10

Acoustic Neurinoma—Management and Surgical Approach

Tal Shahar, Yuval Shapira, Nevo Margalit

INTRODUCTION

Neurosurgeons have been excising acoustic neurinomas (AN) for over a century. The operation was characterized by high mortality and morbidity rates during the first three decades of its implementation (1895–1925). Cushing's intracapsular removal technique enabled decompression of the lesion, but preservation of nerve function was rare. From 1925–1960, Dandy demonstrated the feasibility of the total removal of AN and the first procedure in which the facial nerve was successfully preserved, was described by Carins in 1931. The House group first used the operating microscope in 1961 and together with Hitselberger, revived the translabyrinthine approach for the resection of these lesions. Yasargil used a retrosigmoid approach and revolutionized the microsurgical technique demonstrating its advantages for neurovascular preservation. From the mid 1970s, the morbidity and mortality rates have been greatly reduced with the advent of imaging studies and intraoperative monitoring techniques. Magnetic resonance imaging (MRI) studies allowed the tumor to be demonstrated in relation to adjacent neurovascular structures and also has led to early diagnosis of tumors. The use of intraoperative facial and auditory nerve monitoring enabled the surgeon to maintain the integrity of the cranial nerves (CNs) and to preserve their function. Overall, mortality associated with an AN resection surgery has been reduced from 40% in Cushing's days to 1%, while gross total resection and facial nerve preservation can be expected in 95% and 80% of cases, respectively.

For a more detailed description of the history of an AN treatment, the authors recommend acoustic neurinomas (Moskowitz et al. Historical Review of a Century of Operative Series).

CLINICAL PRESENTATION

The clinical presentation can vary widely, but the most common and early signs of ANs are unilateral sensorineural hearing loss, tinnitus and vertigo. The hearing loss is usually gradual and progressive and typically in the high frequencies. Approximately 10% of patients report a sudden loss of hearing, believed to be of vascular origin. Facial nerve compression occurs early in the course of the disease process, but facial symptoms are rarely presenting symptoms. MRI can usually diagnose ANs in early stages. However, further tumor growth can lead to compression of the brainstem and cerebellum and may cause headaches, nausea and vomiting, ataxia and other cerebellar signs. Involvement of CNs may lead to facial pain and numbness (CN V), diplopia (CN VI), facial fasciculation spasm or paresis (CN VII), and dysphagia and hoarseness (lower CNs IX, X, XII). Respiratory depression, coma and death may ensue with further increase in tumor size. Hydrocephalus followed by signs of increased intracranial pressure may be caused by obstruction of the cerebrospinal fluid flow.

PATHOLOGY

Acoustic neurinomas most commonly originate at the oligodendroglial-schwann cells transition zone (Obersteiner-Redlich's zone) of the superior division of the vestibular nerve (CN VIII) and so it would be more correct to label them "vestibular schwannomas." The site of origin is about 1 cm from the brainstem in the vicinity of the internal auditory meatus. The tumor usually grows into the internal auditory canal (IAC), eroding the surrounding bone (a radiological pathognomic finding) and then mushrooms out to the cerebellopontine cistern, compressing CNs and the adjacent brainstem (Figs 1A to C). The surrounding CNs and the adjacent blood vessels (e.g. anterior inferior cerebellar artery and posterior inferior cerebellar artery) are commonly stretched over the surface of the tumor capsule, but are rarely engulfed by the tumor mass.

The tumor is usually a slow growing benign encapsulated globoid mass. Macroscopically, the cut surface reveals a glistening mass that is greyish tan in color and a consistency varying from soft to firm. Microscopically, the tumor is composed of differentiated spindle-shaped schwann cells with a biphasic pattern. The Antoni A pattern refers to the area composed of compact elongated cells and the Antoni B pattern refers to the loose reticular hypocellular area.

Additional characteristics of the Antoni A areas are nuclear palisades and infrequently Verocay bodies (Figs 2A and B). Occasional cellular atypia, nuclear hyperchromasia and mitotic activity are demonstrated on imaging studies but these should not be misinterpreted as being indicative of malignancy.

All ANs are thought to result from the functional loss of a tumor suppressor gene that has been localized to the long arm of chromosome 22. The disease is unilateral in at least 95% of patients and the majority of cases are sporadic and result from somatic mutations. Bilateral disease is a pathognomic feature of neurofibromatosis type 2 (NF2). While the sporadic cases and the tumors associated with NF2 are cytologically identical, the ANs of NF2 tends to be multifocal and therefore, more extensively surround the nerve attached to it.

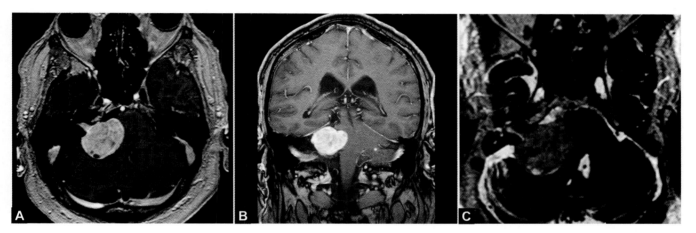

Figs 1A to C: Preoperative imaging. Magnetic resonance image showing an acoustic neurinoma. (A) Axial; (B) Coronal (T1 with gadolinium); (C) Axial T2 3D sequence. Notice the involvement of the internal auditory canal

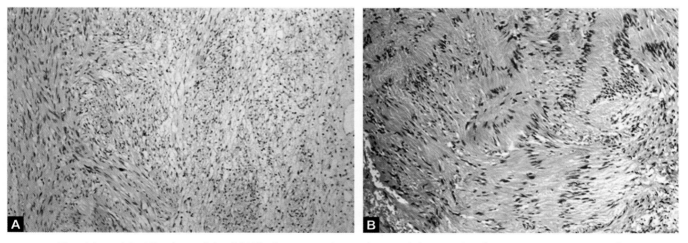

Figs 2A and B: Histology slides (H&E) of an acoustic neurinoma. (A) Example of an Antoni A pattern on the left side and an Antoni B pattern on the right side; (B) Antoni A areas with nuclear palisades and Verocay bodies

TREATMENT OPTIONS

The treatment options for ANs are various and controversial. They range from conservative observation, stereotactic radiosurgery (SRS) and three different surgical approaches. The decision of how to manage a particular AN is based on several, often complex factors, and the decision making process can become difficult. Factors that need to be considered are tumor size, tumor related neurological deficits (such as hearing loss) and documentation of tumor growth. Complicating factors are the precise location of the tumor, the presence of associated comorbid features (e.g. advanced age, chronic diseases, the presence of NF2), as well as the patient's and the surgeon's personal preferences. It is beyond the scope of this chapter to go into greater detail on the management of ANs.

Some General Guidelines for each of the Treatment Options

- Asymptomatic patients with small tumors (5–15 mm in diameter) can be monitored expectantly and periodically rescanned.
- SRS can be considered for tumors less than 25 mm in diameter and for patients who prefer SRS or who cannot tolerate surgery. In addition, SRS can be used for recurrent tumors or for residual tumor following incomplete resection.
- There are three surgical approaches commonly used for removing ANs: (i) the middle fossa approach is usually used for small sized tumors (5–10 mm in diameter) when the tumor is mostly intracanalicular and restoration of hearing is the goal. (ii) the translabyrinthine approach is used for tumors less than 3 cm in size and when there is no longer any functional hearing. (iii) the suboccipital retrosigmoid approach is used for mostly large tumors where hearing restoration is still feasible. This approach is particularly useful in large tumors that extend to the posterior fossa.

Surgical Technique

This chapter will concentrate on the suboccipital retrosigmoid approach, which is most commonly used in our practice for the removal of ANs.

The patient is placed in the sitting position. The head is fixed in a three-pin holding device and rotated toward the side of the tumor and flexed with slight lateral bending. It must be stressed at the outset that stringent measures to prevent, identify and treat air embolism must be taken by both the surgeon and the anesthesiologist. The area behind the ear and the mastoid is shaved. A straight incision is made about 2–3 cm behind the ear (Figs 3A and B). The length of the incision depends on the size of the tumor and the craniotomy to be performed. The craniotomy is planned by means of a navigation system and a preoperative computerized tomogram directed at the bony windows. The association between the asterion and the occipitomastoid suture to the transverse and the sigmoid sinuses is defined (Fig. 4). The craniotomy should be carried out in a lateral fashion if possible, without damaging the sigmoid sinus.

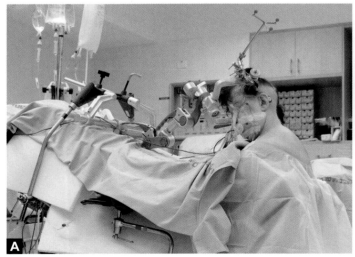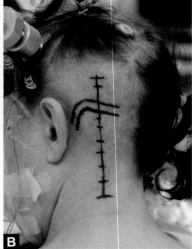

Figs 3A and B: Patient positioning. (A) Sitting position: the head is fixed and turned toward the side of the tumor with flexion and lateral bending. A facial monitor, cardiac Doppler and neuronavigation system are used; (B) Planning of the skin incision in relation to the location of the transverse and sigmoid sinuses

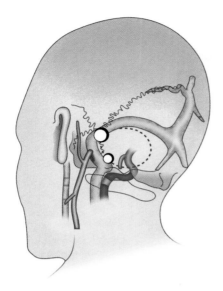

Fig. 4: Illustration of head positioning and suboccipital retrosigmoid craniotomy (dotted line) in relation to the location of the transverse and sigmoid sinuses (blue). The vertebral artery shown in red

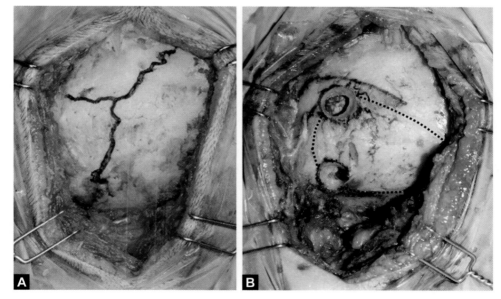

Figs 5A and B: Anatomical landmarks for burr holes and craniotomy. (A) Left retroauricular suboccipital skin incision. The asterion, lambdoid, parietomastoid and occipitomastoid sutures; (B) Outlines of a craniotomy with burr holes in place. Bone flap and burr holes for a left retrosigmoid approach. The dotted black line indicates the craniotomy line

A burr hole is made in the asterion area in order to find the transverse-sigmoid junction (Figs 5A and B). A second hole is made on the lower part of the occipitomastoid suture. The craniotomy is then performed and the bone flap is elevated. Opened air cells of the mastoid are sealed with bone wax or a piece of fat. The dura is opened and reflected medially. At this stage, the cerebellum is gently lifted up and the basal cisterns are opened to allow cerebrospinal fluid (CSF) drainage (Figs 6A and B). This facilitates relaxation of the cerebellum and allows its retraction after which the tumor is exposed

(Figs 7A and B). In small tumors, the lower CNs is visible beneath them and the tentorium can be seen above them. Using a facial nerve stimulator, the facial nerve is identified proximal to the tumor. In cases of large tumors (Figs 8A and B), the CNs are more difficult to identify. The lower nerves will be compressed, but an arachnoid layer can be found between the nerves and the tumor in most cases (Fig. 9). In this surgical approach, the facial nerve will be found on the anterior side of a large tumor or behind it and this should be verified using the stimulator. The probe is set to a high level

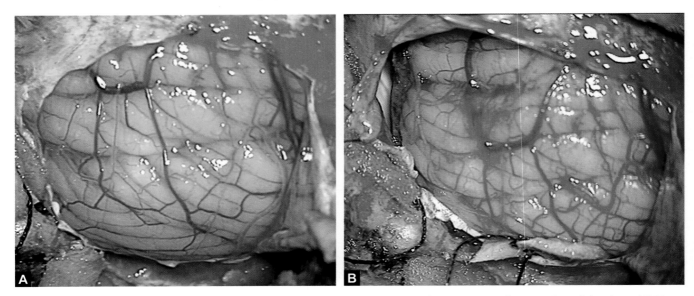

Figs 6A and B: The cerebellum before and after CSF drainage. Retrosigmoid craniotomy after opening of the dura. (A) The cerebellum before and; (B) after drainage of CSF from the cisterna magna by opening the cistern and placing a cottonoid

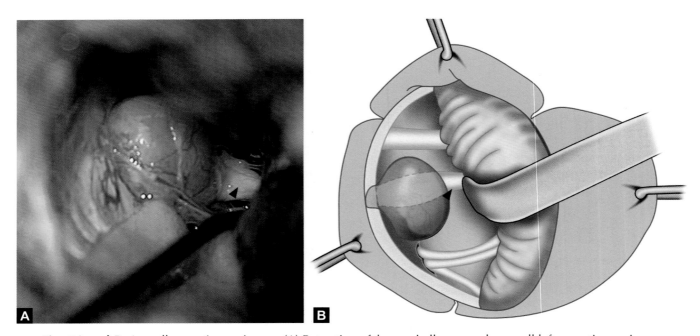

Figs 7A and B: A small acoustic neurinoma. (A) Retraction of the cerebellum reveals a small left acoustic neurinoma emerging from the internal acoustic canal and the VII–VIII cranial nerve complex medial to it (arrowhead); (B) Illustration

of stimulation and the surface of the tumor is explored to see if it will elicit any response from the facial nerve.

For small tumors, the internal auditory canal (IAC) is drilled open at this stage. This is done by using a diamond drill with irrigation to prevent heat damage to the nerves. For large tumors, the IAC is drilled after the tumor is debulked by using an ultrasonic aspirator. After drilling the IAC, the tumor is dissected from the facial nerve and from the cochlear nerve, if hearing preservation is attempted as in Figures 10A and B.

After the tumor has been removed, the air cells that had been opened in the wall of the IAC are closed with a piece of fat and glue. The dura is closed by a running suture, the bone flap is fixed and the muscles, fascia and skin are closed in a regular fashion.

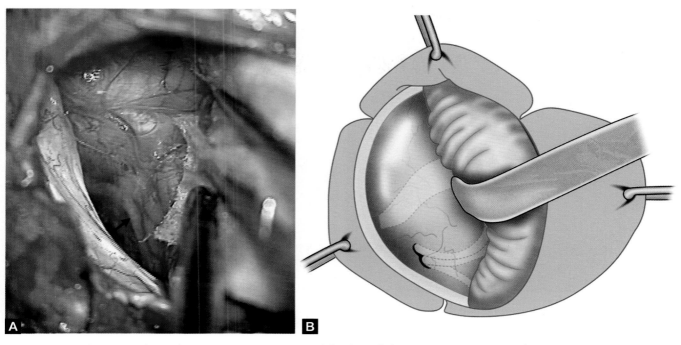

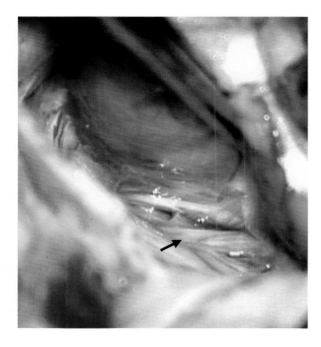

Figs 8A and B: A large acoustic neurinoma. (A) A large left acoustic neurinoma with compression of the cerebellum. The arrow indicates the anterior inferior cerebellar artery; (B) Illustration

Fig. 9: Lower cranial nerves (arrow) compressed by the tumor from above

POSTOPERATIVE CARE

In the postoperative period, the patient is placed in an intensive care setup. A computerized tomography (CT) scan is done to reveal any postoperative bleeding or other surgical complications. Rigorous monitoring of blood pressure control is critical throughout the postoperative period. In cases with facial nerve impairment, care of the eye must include eye drops and ointments to prevent dryness. Steroid treatment is given in a tapering dose for the first 7–10 postoperative days and antiemetic drugs are given for the first 3–5 postoperative days.

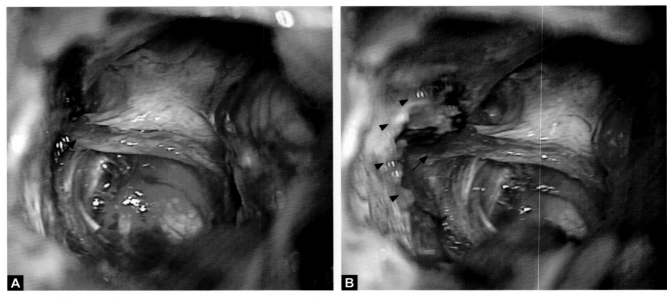

Figs 10A and B: Drilling of the left internal auditory canal (IAC). (A) After removal of the tumor from the cerebellopontine angle cistern. The arrow points to the facial nerve going into the canal; (B) After drilling of the back wall of the IAC. The arrowheads indicate the edge of the canal

HIGHLIGHTS

I. **Indications**
  - N/A
II. **Contraindications**
  - N/A
III. **Preoperative considerations**
  - Tumor size
  - Tumor-related neurological deficits
  - Documented tumor growth
  - Associated comorbidities
    – Advanced age
    – Chronic diseases
    – The presence of NF2
  - Treatment options
    – Observation with periodic scanning
    – Stereotactic radiosurgery
    – Surgical removal:
      - Middle fossa approach
      - Translabyrinthine approach
      - Suboccipital retrosigmoid approach.
IV. **Intraoperative considerations**
  - Sitting position

  - – Cardiac Doppler, central venous catheter, measurement of end-tidal CO_2 to identify and treat air embolisms
  - Neuronavigation for identification of the transverse and sigmoid sinus and enabling maximal lateral craniotomy
  - Retrosigmoid craniotomy
  - Opening of dura and CSF drainage from the basal cisterns
  - Retraction of cerebellum and tumor debulking, with continuous facial nerve and, when indicated, cochlear nerve monitoring
  - Opening of the IAC for further tumor debulking, when needed
  - Water tight closure of the dura
  - Fixation of bone flap.
V. **Postoperative considerations**
  - Intensive care unit
  - Rigorous blood pressure control
  - Postoperative CT within the first 24 hours
  - Eye care with drops and ointment for patients with facial nerve impairment
  - Steroids and antiemetic drugs.

VI. Complications

- Intraoperative air embolism
- Postoperative tension pneumocephalus
- Ipsilateral hearing loss, facial paresis or facial palsy
- Postoperative cerebellar swelling and hydrocephalus
- General neurosurgical related complications such as: bleeding, infection, CSF leak, stroke, neurological deficit, coma or death.

ADDITIONAL READING

1. Asthagiri AR, Parry DM, Butman JA, et al. Neurofibromatosis type 2. Lancet. 2009;373(9679):1974-86.
2. Burger PC, Scheithauer BW, Vogel FS. Surgical Pathology of the Nervous System and Its Coverings, 4th edition. New York: Churchill Livingstone; 2002.
3. Matthies C, Samii M. Management of 1000 vestibular schwannomas (acoustic neuromas): clinical presentation. Neurosurgery.1997;40(1):1-9.
4. Moskowitz N, Long DM. Acoustic Neurinomas. Historical Review of a Century of Operative Series. Neurosurgery Quarterly. 1991;1(1):2-18.
5. Pollock BE. Vestibular schwannoma management: an evidence-based comparison of stereotactic radiosurgery and microsurgical resection. Prog Neurol Surg. 2008;21:222-7.
6. Samii M, Matthies C, Tatagiba M. Management of 1000 vestibular schwannomas (acoustic neuromas): the facial nerve preservation and restitution of function. Neurosurgery. 1997;40(4):684-95.

Chapter **11**

The "Pterional"
(Frontotemporal) Approach

Erez Nossek, Nevo Margalit

INTRODUCTION

The frontotemporal approach, commonly known as the "pterional" approach, is actually a craniotomy used in surgery for treating pathologies in and around the anterior and middle cranial fossae. This approach was first described by Yasargil in the 1970s.[1,2] It was modified by Dolenc in the late 80s and early 90s as an attempt to reach the central skull base by an epidural approach to the cavernous sinus, Meckel's cave, the foramen ovale and the foramen rotundum for vascular lesions, meningiomas and trigeminal schwannomas.[3] The pterion is a small circular area where the frontal, parietal, greater sphenoid wing and the squamous part of the temporal bone meet[4] and the pterional is one of the most important and most frequently used approaches in neurosurgery.

A frontotemporal craniotomy consists of removing the frontal bone, the squamous part of the temporal bone and the greater wing of the sphenoid bone, and can also be extended to either the frontal or the temporal side, according to the location of the pathology.[5] A frontotemporal craniotomy allows access to several important anatomical compartments, including an approach from the anterior to the posterior part of the orbit, the planum sphenoidale, the tuberculum sella, the paraclinoidal area and the entire temporal fossa, including the petrous apex. Lesions that can be approached by means of a frontotemporal craniotomy include meningioma of the anterior cranial base, the sphenoid wing and en plaque (spheno-orbital) meningiomas. In the middle cranial fossa, this approach is used for lesions in the area of the cavernous sinus, the greater sphenoid wing and the anterior part of the petrous bone. The most common pathologies in the middle fossa for which this technique is most suitable are meningiomas, trigeminal schwannomas, malignant lesions extending from the infratemporal fossa into the temporal fossa and petrous apex lesions, such as cholesterol granulomas and chondrosarcomas.

This basic craniotomy can be modified or extended in a number of different ways. For example, a zygomatic osteotomy can be added to it for pathologies in the temporal or petrous apex area and an orbitozygomatic osteotomy can be added to it for access to the clinoid or cavernous sinus area. These osteotomies enable a lower trajectory to the base with less retraction of the frontal or temporal lobes.

SURGICAL TECHNIQUE

Various steps of surgery are illustrated in Figures 1 to 14.

Positioning

After undergoing general anesthesia, the patient is placed in the supine position, the shoulder ipsilateral to the operative field is elevated and the head is placed in a three pin holder device. The head should be elevated (to improve venous drainage), contralaterally rotated 15–20° and extended. This positioning is intended to bring the Sylvian fissure straight up and parallel to the surgeon's view, and to enable the frontal and temporal lobes to fall from the anterior and middle fossae. The extension of the head should be adequate in consideration to the tumor's location, with the rule of thumb being that the more medial and higher the lesion, the greater is the extension as in Figure 1.

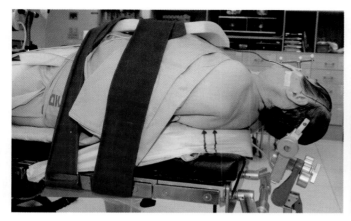

Fig. 1: The head is elevated to improve the venous drainage and contralaterally rotated 15–20 degrees with some extension

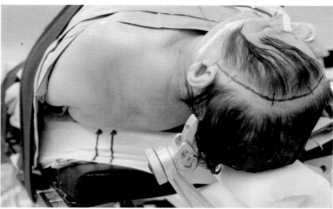

Fig. 2: The skin incision starts at the level of the zygomatic root and runs up to the superior temporal line and then turns anteriorly behind the hairline and toward the midline

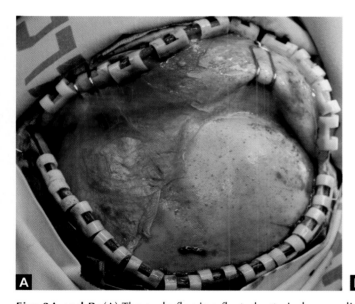

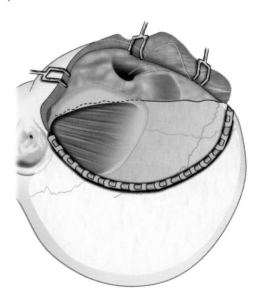

Figs 3A and B: (A) The scalp flap is reflected anteriorly, revealing the temporalis muscle with its fasciae above; (B) Illustration

Skin Incision

The skin incision starts at the level of the zygomatic root (5 mm anterior to the tragus) and runs up to the superior temporal line, staying superficial to the temporalis fascia. It then turns anteriorly behind the hairline and toward the midline. The medial extension of the incision depends on the frontal extension of the planned craniotomy (Fig. 2). An interfascial dissection is performed for cases in which a lower trajectory is needed or an osteotomy is planned in order to avoid injury to the frontal branch of the facial nerve.

Interfascial Dissection

There are three layers of the fasciae superficial to the temporal muscle and the fat pad above it. These layers relate to the frontal branch of the facial nerve, the superficial fascia and the deep fascia. The deep fascia is further divided into the "superficial deep" and the "deep deep" fascia. The "superficial deep" fascia extends along the lateral aspect of the zygomatic arch and the "deep deep" fascia extends along the medial aspect of the zygomatic arch. These two layers confine between them the temporal fat pad and the frontal branch of the facial nerve passes in its outer (superficial) part. The superficial fascia is cut parallel to the zygomatic process of the frontal bone and the lateral orbital rim in order to reach the "deep deep" layer that is deep to the fat pad (Figs 4A and B). The fat pad is then separated from the "deep deep" layer and reflected anteriorly with the scalp, thus exposing the lateral orbital rim all the way up to the zygomatic process of the frontal bone and down to the zygomatic arch (Figs 5A and B).

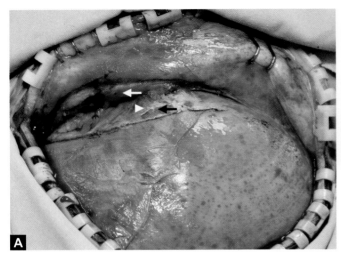

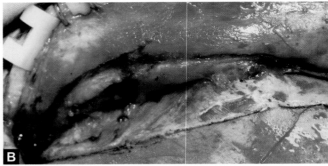

Figs 4A and B: (A) The superficial fascia is cut parallel to the zygomatic process of the frontal bone and the lateral orbital rim to reach the "deep deep" layer (white arrowhead) that is deep to the fat pad (white arrow). The temporalis muscle (black arrow) is under the "deep deep" fascia; (B) Magnified

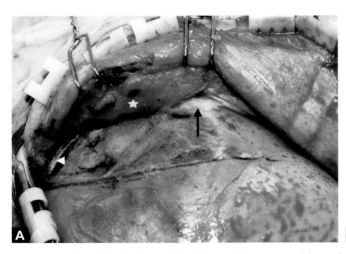

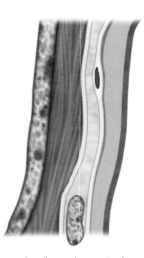

Figs 5A and B: (A) The fat pad (white star) is separated from the "deep deep" layer and reflected anteriorly with the scalp, thus exposing the lateral orbital rim (black arrow) and the zygomatic arch (white arrowhead); (B) Illustration showing a cut through the layers, including the temporalis muscle and fascia, the fat pad and the branch of the facial nerve superficial to the fat pad

The temporalis muscle is cut from the superior part of the zygomatic process of the frontal bone along the superior temporal line and then reflected inferiorly, thus becoming separated from the scalp that is reflected anteriorly (Fig. 6).

Osteotomy of the Orbital Rim, Zygoma and Orbit-Zygomatic Osteotomy (Optional)

An osteotomy may be added in cases of tumors, involving the base of the anterior or middle cranial fossa, where it is important to perform the craniotomy flush with the anterior or temporal base. These osteotomies enable a more shallow approach to the tumor and reduce the need for retraction of the frontal or temporal lobes.

Craniotomy

A craniotomy is carried out by initially making two burr holes. The first is the keyhole to the anterior end of the superior temporal line on the frontosphenoidal suture. For cases, in which an orbital osteotomy is to be done, a more anterior hole is made to expose the periorbit and the frontal lobe dura with the orbital roof between them. The second burr hole is made in the squamous part of the temporal bone just above the root of the zygomatic process (Figs 7A and B). The bony flap may extend to either the temporal side or to the frontal side, depending upon the exact location of the pathology. In cases, where the craniotomy is extended to the frontal side, it is important to note the extent of the frontal sinus on the

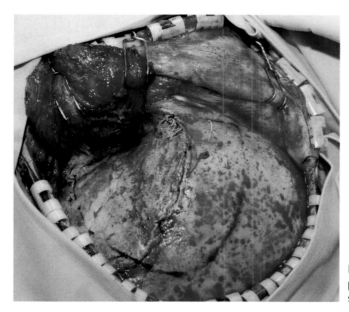

Fig. 6: The temporalis muscle is separated from the superior part of the zygomatic process of the frontal bone along the superior temporal line and is reflected inferiorly

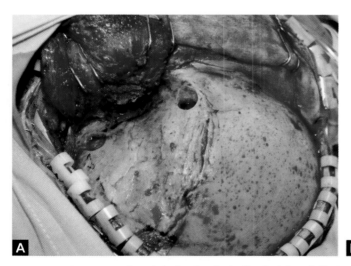

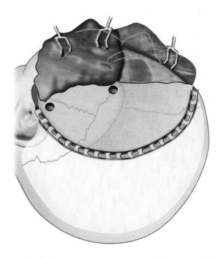

Figs 7A and B: (A) The first hole (keyhole) is drilled at the anterior end of the superior temporal line on the frontosphenoidal suture. The second burr hole is drilled in the squamous part of the temporal bone; (B) Illustration

preoperative scans in order to prevent inadvertent opening. If it is necessary to open the sinus, it must be cranialized and the mucosa must be cleaned by coagulation or drilling.

After elevating the bony flap, the bones of the skull base are drilled according to the area of interest. The posterolateral orbital roof is drilled for a flat trajectory to the tuberculum sella area. For the clinoidal cavernous sinus area, the lesser sphenoid wing is drilled (Figs 8A and B) all the way to the clinoid with the option of opening the optic canal, as is done in cases of a clinoid meningioma that extends into the canal. The temporal dura is dissected from the superior orbital fissure and cavernous sinus lateral wall, in order to drill the

clinoid. Unroofing the optic canal might sometimes open an air cell extending from the sphenoid sinus. An aerated clinoid process can be seen on the preoperative computed tomography scans and it needs to be sealed to prevent a cerebrospinal fluid (CSF) leak. This epidural drilling provides better visualization and allows better manipulation of the different structures after opening the dura.[3]

Opening of the Dura

Opening of the dura starts at the medial aspect of the craniotomy, going posteriorly and downward to the inferior part of the temporal lobe. It is then reflected anteriorly over

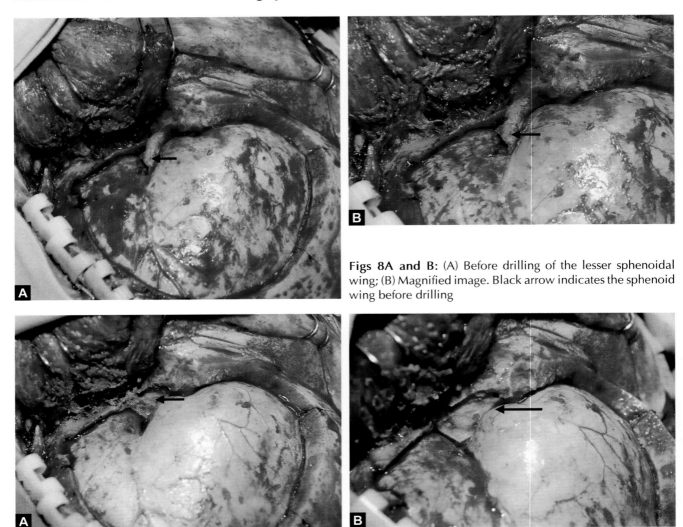

Figs 8A and B: (A) Before drilling of the lesser sphenoidal wing; (B) Magnified image. Black arrow indicates the sphenoid wing before drilling

Figs 9A and B: (A) After drilling of the lesser sphenoidal wing; (B) Magnified image. Black arrow indicates the sphenoid wing after drilling

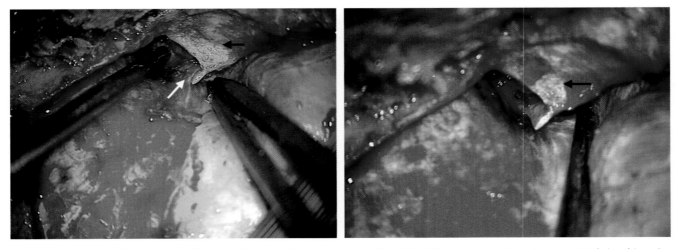

Fig. 10: Before releasing the spheno-orbital dural band (white arrow) from the sphenoidal wing (black arrow)

Fig. 11: After releasing the spheno-orbital dural band from the sphenoid wing (black arrow)

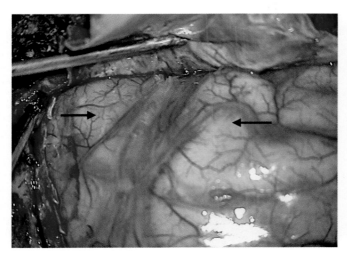

Fig. 12: Left Sylvian fissure: temporal lobe (left arrow) frontal lobe (right arrow) and Sylvian veins in between. The suction is holding the dura against the drilled sphenoidal wing

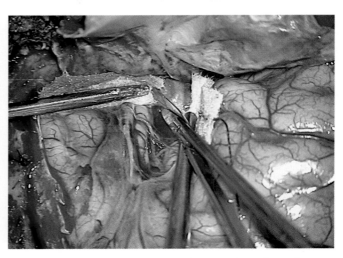

Fig. 13: Opening the arachnoid layer of the Sylvian fissure

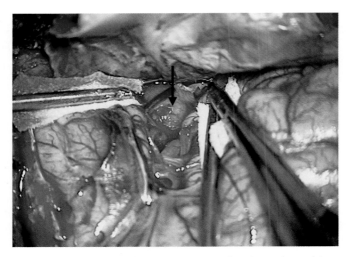

Fig. 14: The open Sylvian fissure revealing branches of the middle cerebral artery and the tumor (black arrow)

enophthalmos after surgery for the relatively fewer cases in which there is a large bony defect in the orbital wall. The osteotomies are repositioned using rigid fixation. The temporalis muscle is sutured back to the bone and the skin is closed in the usual manner.

HIGHLIGHTS

I. Indications
- Pathologies of the anterior and lateral skull base
- Pathologies involving the orbit
- Pathologies of the middle cranial fossa
- Tumors that extend from the infratemporal fossa into the middle cranial fossa
- Tumors that extend from the lateral sphenoid sinus to the medial aspect of the middle cranial fossa.

II. Contraindications
- None.

III. Preoperative Considerations:
- Obtain CT scan for bony assessment
- Positioning—Lateral rotation and extension is crucial.

IV. Intraoperative Considerations:
- Preserve the frontal branch of the facial nerve by interfascial dissection
- Avoid opening the frontal sinus
- Osteotomy
  - This will improve the trajectory to the anterior or middle cranial fossa

the sphenoid wing. The Sylvian fissure is opened either from its distal superficial part or from its proximal medial part in order to split the frontal and temporal lobes to reach medially located pathologies.

Reconstruction

When the dura needs to be replaced, we use temporalis fascia, pericranium or fascia lata (the latter if the defect is large). Effective artificial materials are also available. No reconstruction will be needed if the osseous orbital defect is small. The author uses titanium mesh to prevent

- Reconstruct the lateral orbital wall to prevent enophthalmus
- Proper closure of the dura is essential and if needed, use the pericranium and surgical glue to prevent CSF leakage.

V. Postoperative Considerations
- None.

VI. Complications
- Meningitis
- CSF leak
- Wound infection
- Diplopia
- Enophthalmus.

REFERENCES

1. Yasargil MG, Fox JL. The microsurgical approach to intracranial aneurysms. Surg Neurol. 1975;3(1):7-14.
2. Yasargil MG, Antic J, Laciga R, et al. Microsurgical pterional approach to aneurysms of the basilar bifurcation. Surg Neurol. 1976;6(2):83-91.
3. Dolenc VV. Frontotemporal epidural approach to trigeminal neurinomas. Acta Neurochir (Wien). 1994;130(1-4):55-65.
4. Williams PL. Gray's Anatomy, 38th edition. London: Churchill Livingstone; 1995.
5. Hung TW, Evandro DO, Hendler T, et al. The pterional approach: surgical anatomy, operative technique and rationale. Operative Techniques in Neurosurgery; 2001. pp.60-72.

Chapter 12

Craniofacial Resection

Dennis Kraus

INTRODUCTION

The anterior craniofacial resection was first introduced by Smith in 1954 as a technique for en bloc resection of tumors, involving the frontal sinuses and surrounding areas and was subsequently popularized by Alfred Ketcham in his landmark series of 19 patients undergoing craniofacial resection in 1963. While modifications have been made in the placement of incisions and osteotomies, more recently the use of endoscopic approaches to the paranasal sinuses, the craniofacial resection remains largely unchanged and the gold standard approach to tumors of the anterior skull base.

PREOPERATIVE EVALUATION AND ANESTHESIA

Preoperative evaluation should include clinical evaluation by a head and neck surgeon, a neurosurgeon, neuroanesthesiologist and an ophthalmologist. Clinical evaluation should include a complete head and neck examination with attention to extraocular movements and vision, facial sensation and intranasal examination with flexible or rigid nasal endoscopy. Preoperative and prebiopsy imaging should be performed, particularly for tumors medial to the middle turbinate. Coronal, axial and sagittal computed tomography (CT) and magnetic resonance imaging (MRI) are complementary and attention should be paid to the presence of orbital invasion, intracranial dural involvement, brain parenchymal, cavernous sinus, and sphenoid or clivus. Vascular tumors or tumors with intracranial involvement should be biopsied in the operating room, as cerebrospinal fluid (CSF) leak or major hemorrhage can ensue.

For a definitive surgical procedure, triple antibiotic coverage with CSF penetration should be used and a lumbar drain should be placed. Steroids and mannitol are given to decrease intracranial edema and pressure. Prophylactic anticonvulsants and antithrombotic devices should be applied.

SURGICAL TECHNIQUE

The patient is placed in the supine position in a Mayfield head frame and anesthesia is administered via standard endotracheal tube. The hair is shaved or braided out of the field of the incision and the head and face is prepped with Betadine.

Intracranial exposure is obtained by the neurosurgical team. A bicoronal incision is fashioned and brought down to, but not through the galea. The posterior flap is elevated several centimeters posteriorly to gain additional length for the galeal-pericranium flap for subsequent reconstruction of the dura and skull base. This flap has a robust dual blood supply from the supraorbital and supratrochlear arteries. The anterior flap is then elevated sharply, superficial to the galea, to the supraorbital ridge exercising caution at this level to avoid injury to the supraorbital and supratrochlear vessels. The galeal-pericranial flap is then incised at its posterior most extent and elevated in a subperiosteal plane with a freer elevator. Elevation is brought anteriorly exposing as much of the glabella, nasal bones and supraorbital ridges as possible as in Figure 1.

Osteotomies are then marked for removal of the frontal plate. Removal of the supraorbital rims improves exposure and decreases brain retraction. The supraorbital vessels can

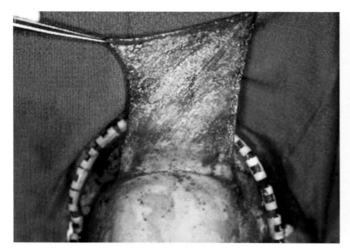

Fig. 1: Elevation of the galeal-pericranial flap is performed for reconstruction of the skull base defect

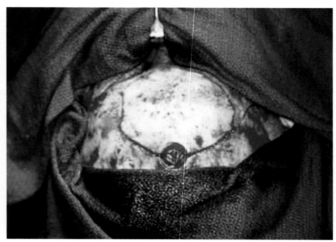

Fig. 2: Osteotomies for the frontal craniotomy is performed through a single burr hole

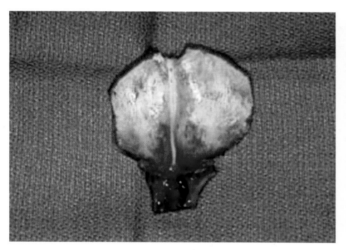

Fig. 3: The bone flap is set aside in antibiotic solution for reconstruction

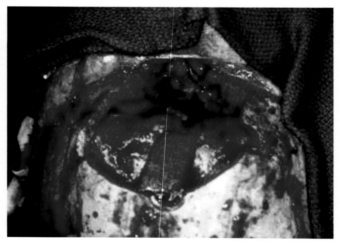

Fig. 4: Exposure is completed back to the planum sphenoidale with gentle retraction on the frontal lobe

be freed from the supraorbital notch, if necessary, to improve retraction. A single burr hole is fashioned and the remaining osteotomies are made with a Midas Rex side-cutting saw (Fig. 2). At the level of the frontal sinuses, only the anterior table is removed. The bone plate is removed and all the mucosa from the frontal sinuses on both the plates of the patient is removed. The bone from the sinuses is drilled down with a diamond burr. The frontal sinuses are plugged with bone chips, muscle, fascia, fat or a combination to prevent mucocele formation. The bone plate is placed in sterile bacitracin or gentamicin solution (Fig. 3). The dura is then gently elevated to the cribriform plate. If there is a dural invasion, the dura is sharply incised at the anterior margin and this is extended posteriorly on each side of the cribriform plate.

The author routinely excise the dura at the crista galli and reconstructs with bovine pericardium. The brain and dura are elevated posteriorly to the planum sphenoidale and held in place with self-retaining malleable retractors (Fig. 4). Osteotomies are then made around the cribriform plate with an oscillating saw completing the intracranial exposure of the tumor.

A variety of incisions can be used for the facial exposure. For the vast majority of tumors, a lateral rhinotomy incision can be used to avoid disruption of the lips. For more extensive tumors that require maxillectomy, the modified Weber-Ferguson incision may be used. The nasal component of the facial incision should lie between the junction of the dorsal nasal subunit and the lateral nasal subunit to achieve a more

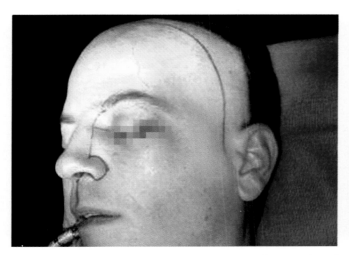

Fig. 5: Modified Weber-Ferguson incision for combined craniofacial resection with total maxillectomy. Incisions should be planned to respect facial subunits to achieve the best cosmetic result

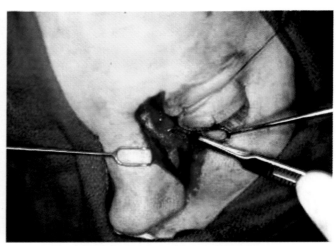

Fig. 6: The medial canthus is identified, tagged and divided sharply for resuspension to prevent telecanthus

cosmetically appealing result (Fig. 5). The most cephalad extent of the incision, if there is no need for lateral extension of the incision, should be completed with a W-plasty to prevent the formation of a web. The incision is brought through the periosteum and skin flaps are elevated medially and laterally for sufficient exposure for the osteotomies. On the lateral flap, the medial canthus is sharply divided and tagged for resuspension (Fig. 6).

Endoscopic resection offers an alternative to traditional craniofacial resection. It offers the advantage of avoiding facial incisions and improved visualization. It can be used alone or in combination with a craniotomy. Initial reports revealed high rates of CSF leak, which have decreased significantly as the technique has matured. The limits of endoscopic resection are not clearly defined, but should be clearly avoided in cases of T4a or T4b tumors and in cases involving high-grade histologies, until mature data regarding oncologic results arrive.

The facial osteotomies are dictated by the three-dimensional extent of the tumor and can include total maxillectomy and orbital exenteration or limited resection of the intranasal component. Tumors arising from the cribriform plate typically require resection of minimum of the nasal septum, ethmoid sinuses, lamina papyracea, middle turbinate and portions of the medial maxillary sinus. All soft tissue mobilization should be performed prior to the osteotomies to allow for expeditious removal of tumor after the osteotomies are completed to minimize blood loss and obstruction of the operative field. After elevation of the skin flaps, the periorbita is elevated from the inferior and medial orbital walls. The lacrimal duct is divided and marsupialized. The anterior and posterior ethmoid arteries are clipped and divided. The septal mucosa and cartilage is incised with cautery inferiorly and anteriorly. A sufficient dorsal and columellar strut is preserved on the nasal septum to preserve nasal integrity and support. Osteotomies are then made vertically through the face of the maxilla, orbital rim and nasal bone using an oscillating saw. Horizontal osteotomies are made through the nasal aperture inferiorly and superiorly from the nasal bone through the medial orbital rim with an oscillating saw. The horizontal osteotomies can then be carried posteriorly with an osteotome through the floor of the medial maxillary sinus, the vomer and the lamina papyracea. Any remaining soft tissue attachments posteriorly can be divided and mobilized with a heavy Mayo scissors.

The specimen is then delivered in concert with the neurosurgeon and the head and neck surgeon, starting anteriorly through the facial exposure. The surgical defect (Fig. 7) is then irrigated and hemostasis assured. If necessary, frozen sections are sent from the margins. The galeal-pericranial flap is placed over the cranial dural defect and sewn to the dura or suture holes at the planum sphenoidale avoiding the optic chiasm. The frontal bone flap is repositioned with titanium microplates and a drain can be placed in the extradural space (Fig. 8). The nose is packed tightly with Xeroform gauze up to the skull base defect to prevent pneumocephalus. A medial canthopexy is performed with a 3-0 prolene to a separate burr hole on the nasion. The lacrimal duct is marsupialized and stitched open, and a Jones tube is placed (Fig. 9). The incisions are then closed in a layered fashion.

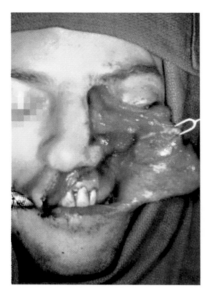

Fig. 7: Defect after craniofacial resection with total maxillectomy

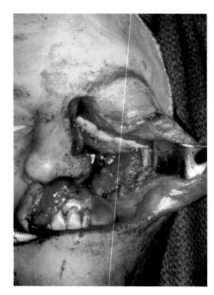

Fig. 8: Orbital support after craniofacial resection with total maxillectomy is provided with split calvarial bone grafts

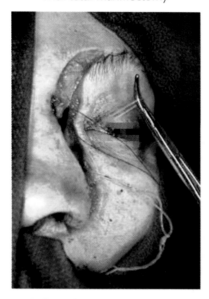

Fig. 9: The medial canthus is resuspended and Jones tubes placed through the lacrimal punctum and duct to prevent stenosis

POSTOPERATIVE TREATMENT

Packing is left in place for about 5–7 days, during which the patient is kept on antibiotics with CSF penetration. Patients are typically given a short course of anticonvulsants and steroids during which they should receive proton pump inhibitors. An aggressive bowel and antiemetic regimen should be implemented to prevent constipation and straining. Urine output, and urine and serum osmolality should be monitored for syndrome of inappropriate antidiuretic hormone (SIADH).

After the packing is removed, the patient should start saline nasal spray for one week. After the second postoperative week, the patient should begin gentle nasal saline irrigations. A noncontrast CT is typically performed on the first postoperative day to assess for pneumocephalus, hemorrhage or other intracranial pathology.

Adjuvant treatment is dictated by the histology and stage of the tumor, and can include postoperative radiation with or without chemotherapy or simply close monitoring.

HIGHLIGHTS

I. Indications
- Benign or malignant tumors of the cribriform plate
- Benign or malignant tumors of the paranasal sinuses with superior extension to the ethmoid sinuses or cribriform plate.

II. Contraindications
- Cavernous sinus involvement
- Bilateral orbital or optic nerve invasion
- Invasion of the clivus
- Gross invasion of the brain
- Patients medically unfit to endure surgical intervention
- Distant metastatic disease.

III. Special Preoperative Considerations

- MRI and CT scan are complementary
- Multimodality evaluation by head and neck surgeon, neurosurgeon, ophthalmologist, radiation oncologist and medical oncologist, where appropriate
- Review of biopsy by dedicated head and neck pathologist.

IV. Special Intraoperative Considerations

- Perioperative antibiotic coverage with vancomycin, ceftazidime and flagyl
- Place lumbar drain
- Carefully preserve blood supply of galeal-pericranial flap
- Reapproximate medial canthal tendon to prevent pseudotelecanthus.

V. Special Postoperative Considerations

- Antibiotics, steroids, proton pump inhibitors and bowel regimen
- Monitor serum/urine osmolality and limit intravenous fluid replacement
- Rigorous nasal care after removal of packing
- Frequent neurological evaluation.

VI. Complications

- CSF leakage
- Meningitis
- Pneumocephalus
- Anosmia (expected)
- Wound infection
- Brain injury, edema or hemorrhage
- Diplopia, ocular restriction, blindness
- Facial hypesthesia
- SIADH, diabetes insipidus.

ADDITIONAL READING

1. Gil Z, Patel SG, Bilsky M, et al. Complications after craniofacial resection for malignant tumors: are complication trends changing? Otolaryngol Head Neck Surg. 2009;140(2):218-23.
2. Ketcham AS, Wilkins RH, Vanburen JM, et al. A combined intracranial facial approach to the paranasal sinuses. Am J Surg. 1963;106:698-703.
3. Kraus DH, Gonen M, Mener D, et al. A standardized regimen of antibiotics prevents infectious complications in skull base surgery. Laryngoscope. 2005;115(8):1347-57.

Chapter **13**

Per Oral Glossectomy

Dennis Kraus

INTRODUCTION

Per oral glossectomy is the treatment of choice for T1 and selected T2 squamous cell carcinoma of the oral tongue, as well other benign and malignant pathologies of the oral tongue. Per oral glossectomy requires no external incisions and even large defects can often be reconstructed without the use of free tissue transfer with superb functional results.

PREOPERATIVE EVALUATION AND ANESTHESIA

Preoperative evaluation should include clinical evaluation by a head and neck surgeon. Clinical evaluation should include a complete head and neck examination with particular attention to the involved sites of the tumor and its depth, as well as the draining lymphatics. The characteristics of the tumor should be closely noted as a variety of benign and malignant processes can involve the oral tongue and have similar presentations. The presence of involvement of the tonsil, tongue base, floor of mouth, deep infiltration into the extrinsic musculature or mandible may preclude per oral resection. Numbness of the tongue or limited tongue mobility may suggest perineural spread and may clue the clinician to tumors with predilection for such spread, such as adenoid cystic carcinoma. The presence of trismus should be noted as this may limit exposure or resectability. Punch biopsy in the office can be performed in most patients. It allows pathological evaluation of the depth of tumor in suspected squamous cell carcinoma. Routine imaging is not required in superficial lesions, but can help to assess the presence of cervical lymphadenopathy. For deep or large lesions, magnetic resonance imaging gives better soft tissue details and allows for better assessment of bone marrow invasion, but computed tomography gives better bone details for suspected periosteal invasion. Clinical examination is a paramount in determining the need for mandibular resection.

Anesthesia via a nasotracheal tube allows the best unobstructed access to the oral cavity. Preoperative antibiotics are typically administered. Intravenous steroids can help with postoperative swelling and pain. A tracheostomy is rarely required, but may be needed with tumors that involve the tongue base or require extensive reconstruction.

SURGICAL TECHNIQUE

The patient is placed in the supine position and the anesthesia is administered via a nasotracheal tube. Intravenous antibiotics should be administered and intraoperative corticosteroids should be used to reduce operative edema. If a neck dissection is to be performed, the patient is prepped in a sterile fashion and this can be performed first. Once the oral portion of the procedure is performed, complete paralysis should be used to facilitate exposure. A bite block or side-biting mouth gag is placed between the molars contralateral to the tumor. For posterior or lateral tumors, the tip of the tongue is grasped with an Adair forceps or a figure-of-eight silk suture to facilitate exposure as in Figure 1.

Mucosal and deep margins should be planned, minimum of 10 mm, around the tumor. It can be marked with electrocautery or hand-held CO_2 laser (Fig. 2). One should anticipate about 30–50% shrinkage of the mucosal margins after excision and adequate tissue should be resected to

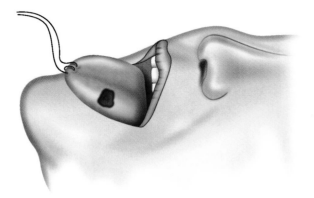

Fig. 1: A figure-of-eight stitch through the tongue facilitates exposure of T1 and small T2 tumors to be excised transorally

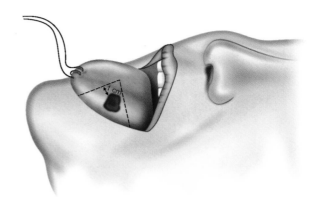

Fig. 2: A minimum of 10 mm margins should be planned around the lesion and consideration to be given to the planned reconstruction. For medium defects, a transverse wedge provides excellent functional results

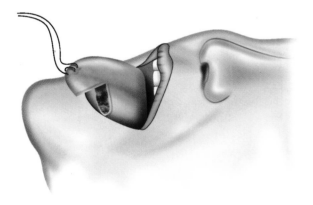

Fig. 3: The defect after transverse wedge excision of a laterally located oral tongue lesion

avoid the appearance of a positive or close margin on the final pathology report. A planned reconstruction should be considered while designing the excision. Small superficial lesions can be excised in a standard elliptical fashion and left open to granulate or closed primarily with excellent functional results. Lesions that require a deeper excision, but are less than one fifth of the total width of the tongue, can be reconstructed with a split thickness skin graft or acellular dermal matrix. One should avoid the temptation to close lateral defects in a superior to inferior dimension, as this will create a long, thin tongue, which provides less dexterity for articulation and oral preparation for swallowing. Deep lateral excisions can be best closed with a transverse wedge technique (Fig. 3). This allows a generous deep margin, approximating

the anterior aspect of the defect to the posterior aspect, keeping the natural width of the tongue intact. The tongue will initially appear foreshortened and canted toward the side of resection, but will provide excellent speech and swallowing results.

Once the lesion is fully excised, the primary surgeon should orient the specimen in the pathology suite. Mucosal margins from the anterior, superior, inferior and posterior aspect as well as a deep muscular margin should be sent for frozen section analysis. The transverse wedge closure should be performed in a layered fashion with deep 2-0 vicryl horizontal mattress sutures in the muscle (Fig. 4) and 3-0 interrupted vicryl sutures in the mucosa (Fig. 5). If the Wharton's duct is transected and a neck dissection is not performed, the duct can be dilated with a lacrimal duct probe, marsupialized and reimplanted in the floor of mouth with two 4-0 chromic sutures. Defects that are reconstructed with a skin graft or an allograft should be secured with chromic sutures using either deep tacking sutures or a Xeroform bolster.

POSTOPERATIVE TREATMENT

Typically patients can start a clear liquid diet on the first or second postoperative day. More extensive resections may require placement of a temporary feeding tube until postoperative swelling and pain subsides. Oral irrigations with sodium bicarbonate should be started on the first postoperative day and continued after every meal at

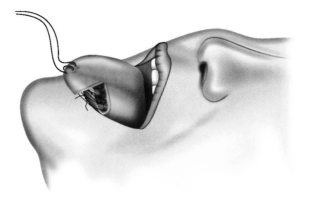

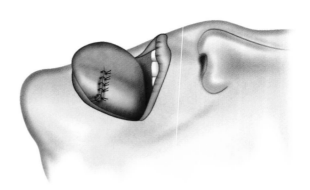

Fig. 4: The intrinsic musculature of the tongue is reapproximated using buried 2-0 vicryl horizontal mattress sutures

Fig. 5: The muscosa is then reapproximated with interrupted 3-0 vicryl sutures. Eversion is essential for preventing buried mucosa, which can lead to a wound breakdown

bedtime, until healing is complete. A liquid diet is often continued for one to two weeks as determined by the progress of healing in the presence of a bolster and tolerance of the patient.

Adjuvant treatment is dictated by the histology, the stage of the primary tumor and its nodal status. It can also include the postoperative radiation with or without chemotherapy or simply by close monitoring.

HIGHLIGHTS

I. Indications
- T1 and selected T2 squamous cell carcinoma of the oral tongue
- Benign or malignant minor salivary gland neoplasms of the oral tongue
- Other benign or malignant neoplasms of the tongue (hemangioma, low grade sarcoma, granular cell tumors).

II. Contraindications
- Invasion of the mandible, pterygoid muscles, extensive tongue base involvement
- Trismus limiting exposure
- Bilateral hypoglossal nerve invasion.

III. Special Preoperative Considerations
- Palpation for depth of tumor guides extent of resection and need for elective nodal treatment

- Review of biopsy by dedicated head and neck pathologist.

IV. Special Intraoperative Considerations
- Perioperative antibiotic coverage
- Intraoperative steroids
- Transverse wedge closure of deep lateral defects.

V. Special Postoperative Considerations
- Oral irrigations
- Pured diet for 7–14 days.

VI. Complications
- Bleeding
- Airway obstruction
- Lingual/hypoglossal nerve injury
- Wound dehiscence
- Wound infection.

ADDITIONAL READING

1. Huang SH, Hwang D, Lockwood G, et al. Predictive value of tumor thickness for cervical lymph node involvement in squamous cell carcinoma of the oral cavity: a meta-analysis of reported studies. Cancer. 2009;115(7):1489-97.
2. Spiro RH, Strong EW. Epidermoid carcinoma of the mobile tongue. Treatment by partial glossectomy alone. Am J Surg. 1971;122(6):707-10.

Chapter **14**

Parathyroidectomy

Manish D Shah, Jeremy L Freeman

INTRODUCTION

Hyperparathyroidism (HPT) is characterized by the excessive secretion of parathyroid hormone (PTH) and can be classified as primary, secondary or tertiary. Surgical management plays an essential role in the treatment of HPT and can be challenging at times, due to variable anatomy, ambiguous preoperative investigations and subtle intraoperative findings.

Numerous surgical approaches have been described for the treatment of HPT, such as bilateral four-gland parathyroid exploration, minimal access parathyroidectomy (limited exploration), radioguided parathyroidectomy and endoscopic parathyroidectomy. The approach used in an individual case is influenced by several factors, the most important of which include the etiology of the HPT (primary, secondary or tertiary), the results of preoperative localization studies and intraoperative findings (appearance of the glands and serum PTH level measurement). This chapter will provide a detailed description of the above mentioned techniques. The majority of this chapter will concentrate on the evaluation and management of primary hyperparathyroidism (PHPT). Secondary hyperparathyroidism (SHPT) and tertiary hyperparathyroidism (THPT) are discussed separately below.

PREOPERATIVE EVALUATION AND ANESTHESIA

Careful preoperative evaluation of patients with PHPT is essential to a successful surgical management. A thorough history and physical examination is important. Any patient with the classic skeletal, renal, neuromuscular, neuropsychiatric, gastrointestinal or cardiovascular manifestations of HPT should be considered for surgical intervention. There is controversy regarding the role of surgery in asymptomatic patients. The National Institute of Health recommends criteria that are regarded by many, to be too conservative (Table 1). There is evidence that all patients with PHPT benefit from successful surgical interventions (Eigelberger et al. 2004). Palpable parathyroid glands are very rare, however, coexistent thyroid pathology may be discovered with a careful examination of the neck. Vocal cord mobility should also be evaluated.

Biochemistry

Serum ionized calcium and intact parathyroid hormone (iPTH) levels should be documented abnormal on at least three separate measurements. They are as follows:
1. A 24-hour urine collection should be obtained to rule out benign familial hypocalciuric hypercalcemia.

Table 1: National Institute of Health guidelines for surgical intervention in asymptomatic primary hyperparathyroidism (Bilezikian et al. 2002)

- Serum calcium >1 mg/dl above the upper limits of normal 24-hour urine calcium excretion >400 mg
- Creatinine clearance reduced by >30% compared to age-matched controls
- Bone mineral density of the lumbar spine, hip or distal radius that is >2.5, standard deviations below peak bone mass (t-score <-2.5)
- Age <50 years; patients in whom surveillance is not desirable or possible.

2. Serum vitamin D levels should be measured to rule out vitamin D deficiency.

3. Serum phosphate and creatinine levels should be measured to document renal function.

Imaging

Technetium-99 (99Tc) sestamibi parathyroid scans are obtained for all patients with primary hyperparathyroidism and are very helpful with regards to preoperative localization of parathyroid adenomas. These scans have a positive predictive value of approximately 80% in the setting of a single adenoma. This number drops substantially in the setting of a double adenoma (30%) and may be entirely negative in multigland hyperplasia.

Our preference is also to obtain a neck ultrasound (US) to help confirm the 99Tc sestamibi scan results, identify abnormal parathyroid glands not detected by 99Tc sestamibi scanning, identify intrathyroidal parathyroid glands and examine for coexistent thyroid pathology. Retroesophageal, intrathymic and mediastinal parathyroids will be missed by US.

If the 99Tc sestamibi scan and the US do not identify abnormal parathyroid gland(s), a computed tomography (CT) or magnetic resonance imaging scan of the neck may be helpful in the identification of potentially abnormal parathyroid glands.

Selective venous sampling for serum iPTH levels can also be helpful. However, the authors do not routinely employ this technique due to its invasive nature, except for selected revision cases.

US-guided fine needle aspiration biopsy can be performed on ectopic or suspected intrathymic parathyroid glands to confirm the diagnosis. The aspirate should be evaluated for cytology and PTH measurement. These cases are rare.

Anesthesia

All procedures are carried out under general anesthesia with oral endotracheal intubation. To allow for maximal retraction and exposure, muscle relaxants are used throughout the procedure. This prevents the use of intraoperative monitoring of the recurrent laryngeal nerve (RLN), which is not routinely used at the author's institution except in revision cases.

Intraoperative Parathyroid Hormone Measurement

After the induction of anesthesia, a peripheral intravenous or arterial line is established for obtaining repeated nondiluted blood samples. Peripheral blood may be taken from foot/leg to avoid an arterial line. A baseline sample is obtained at tumor excision followed by samples at 10 minutes and 15 minutes post excision of the abnormal gland(s). There is some controversy in the literature as when to obtain blood samples. Some authors prefer to expose the abnormal glands and then draw a blood sample prior to gland excision. Operations are deemed successful once the serum iPTH level has decreased to at least 50% of the baseline value and is within the normal range specific to the author's hospital laboratory. In cases, when the baseline iPTH level is extremely high, it may take much longer than 15 minutes for the iPTH level to reach 50% post gland excision. In such instances, a trend of decreasing iPTH levels may be used as an evidence of a successful operation. Usually iPTH is not helpful in hyperplasia cases as a normal looking gland that is left on the background of appropriate fall of iPTH may soon undergo hyperplasia (and then hyperfunction). iPTH may be helpful in this situation in that it may not fall in a undetected hyperplasia situation alerting the surgeon to the correct diagnosis.

SURGICAL TECHNIQUE

Anatomy

A detailed understanding of the embryology and anatomy of the parathyroid glands is important for successful parathyroid surgery as in Figures 1A and B.

The majority of people have four parathyroid glands. However, autopsy studies have shown that up to 13% of people have more than four glands and 3% have fewer than four glands (Akerstrom et al.1984).

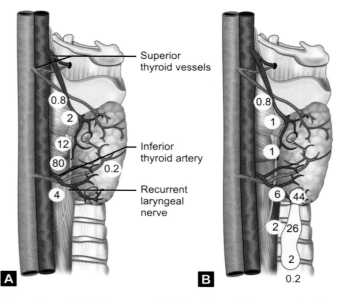

Figs 1A and B: The anatomical locations of the superior (A) and inferior (B) parathyroid glands. Adapted from Akerstrom, et al. 1984

The superior parathyroids arise from the fourth branchial arch and migrate caudally with the thyroid gland. Their typical position is behind the superior pole of the thyroid gland, just lateral and posterior to the recurrent laryngeal nerve (RLN).

The inferior parathyroid glands, which arise from the third branchial arch and migrate along with the thymus, have much more variable anatomy, when compared to the superior glands. They tend to be located around the inferior pole of the thyroid gland.

Ectopic or supernumerary glands can have variable positions. The superior glands can be found within the thyroid gland (intrathyroidal), retroesophageal space or in the posterior mediastinum. The most common location for ectopic inferior parathyroids is within the thymus, which also develops from the third branchial arch. However, they can be found anywhere from the inferior border of the submandibular gland to the anterior mediastinum, including within the carotid sheath (Butterworth et al. 1998).

Bilateral Parathyroid Exploration

Bilateral parathyroid gland exploration (BPGE) has been the gold standard surgical approach for treatment of primary hyperparathyroidism. All four glands are identified with only the abnormal glands being removed.

Indications for Bilateral Parathyroid Gland Exploration

Etiology of hyperparathyroidism: Patients with known multigland hyperplasia (multiple endocrine neoplasia syndromes, SHPT, THPT).

Results of preoperative localization investigations: Lack of clear localization on preoperative investigations is not an absolute indication for BPGE. However, one should be prepared for prompt conversion to BPGE from a more limited approach in these instances.

Intraoperative findings: Failure to identify an abnormal gland on a limited exploration must increase one's suspicion of multigland disease or incorrect preoperative localization. In addition, failure of the intraoperative iPTH level to normalize should prompt suspicion of multiple adenomas or multigland hyperplasia. Knowing that the majority of second adenomas will be contralateral (Milas et al. 2003), either of these situations requires conversion to a BPGE.

The patient should be positioned supine with a rolled blanket beneath the shoulders to provide gentle extension of the neck. The endotracheal tube should be positioned away from the operative field.

A midline transverse incision approximately one fingerbreadth below the cricoid cartilage is made, ideally in a pre-existing skin crease. The length of the incision required will vary depending on the patient's body habitus and the size of the thyroid gland, typically a 3–5 cm incision should be sufficient. Flaps are then raised in the subplatysmal plane, both superiorly to the level of the thyroid notch and inferiorly to the clavicles. The midline raphe of the infrahyoid strap muscles is identified and divided vertically from the thyroid notch to the sternal notch. The sternohyoid and sternothyroid muscles are dissected off the surface of the thyroid gland, allowing them to be retracted laterally and exposing the carotid artery. The middle thyroid vein will be seen crossing the carotid artery. It should be ligated and divided as this will facilitate medial rotation of the thyroid lobe.

A combination of blunt and sharp dissection in the perithyroidal and paratracheal tissue is used, looking for a subtle bulge or color variation (brown/blue discoloration). Unless, extremely large parathyroid glands are typically not palpable. Care must be taken to be as atraumatic as possible. Any bleeding may stain the perithyroidal tissue, making appreciation of color variations more difficult. Furthermore, rupture of the parathyroid gland can lead to seeding of the neck causing parathyromatosis, a condition that is extremely difficult to manage.

With the thyroid lobe rotated medially (Fig. 2), the authors begin to search for the parathyroid gland in the area suggested to be abnormal by the preoperative localization investigations. If these investigations are negative, the authors begin by searching for the inferior parathyroid gland. Once the inferior gland has been identified, the ipsilateral superior gland should be identified in the position described above. Further medial rotation of the thyroid lobe will be required to provide adequate exposure. A similar technique should be used on the contralateral side. Despite, the often variable anatomic locations of the parathyroid glands, there tends to be a substantial symmetry between the right and left sides. This can be used to the surgeon's advantage during BPGE.

It is not absolutely necessary to identify the RLN during BPGE. However, it may provide a useful landmark when a parathyroid gland is not initially readily identified. If the RLN is not clearly identified, care must be taken throughout to ensure that the dissection does not injure the nerve.

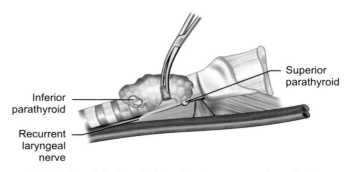

Fig. 2: The left thyroid lobe has been rotated medially, exposing both parathyroid glands and the RLN

If any of the four glands cannot be identified and there is a suspicion that the missing gland may be abnormal, one must search in the possible ectopic locations to identify the gland. It is important to recognize that "what was thought to be a "low" positioned superior parathyroid may indeed be the inferior parathyroid (or vice versa for a "high" positioned inferior gland)." This should prompt an appropriately revised search strategy.

The thymus can be bluntly mobilized and retracted superiorly into the neck (Fig. 3A). Dissection within the thymus may identify the gland. Alternatively, the portion of the thymus ipsilateral to the missing gland can be removed, if the gland is not found elsewhere. The entire tracheoesophageal groove should be inspected and the retroesophageal space can then be opened (Fig. 3B). In this situation, the RLN should be identified before the space is opened. The carotid sheath should be opened along its entire length (Fig. 3C). A high superior parathyroid gland may be difficult to identify with the superior thyroid vessels intact. These vessels can be safely ligated and divided without devascularizing the thyroid gland. This may identify a superior gland located in such a

position (Fig. 3D). Finally, intrathyroidal parathyroids must be suspected. Preoperative US reports should be reviewed and the thyroid gland palpated. Oftentimes, the gland can be safely identified and removed without conducting a thyroid lobectomy. However, the latter may be required.

Once all four glands have been identified, a decision must be made about which glands are to be removed. It is important to remember that only abnormal appearing glands should be removed as patients may have two or three adenomas as opposed to multigland hyperplasia. There is considerable variation in what is considered a normal appearing parathyroid gland (Wang et al. 1982). Typically, glands are 7–8 mm in length and weigh 20–50 mg. Except in SHPT; single adenomas are generally larger than individual glands in patients with multigland hyperplasia. There is an inconsistent correlation between preoperative serum iPTH levels and adenoma size. Therefore, iPTH levels are not reliable in predicting if a gland is indeed abnormal.

In the case of multigland hyperplasia, the authors prefer to do a total excision. The authors prefer a total parathyroidectomy with reimplantation of all or part of

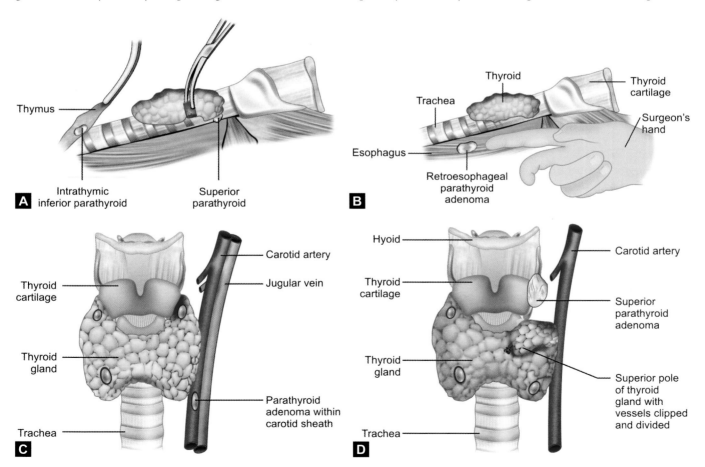

Figs 3A to D: Potential locations for ectopic parathyroid glands: (A) Intrathymic; (B) Retroesophageal;
(C) Carotid sheath; (D) High position behind the superior thyroid pole

one gland into the upper pectoralis major muscle (with appropriate marking with surgical clips) through a small infraclavicular incision. This reimplantation site mitigates against hand dysfunction in the event that a previously transplanted gland into the forearm needs removal due to hyperfunction. In dealing with HPT of the multiple endocrine neoplasia (MEN) syndromes and that of chronic renal failure, it may be advantageous to remove all four of the diseased glands and reimplant or cryopreserve one-half gland. There is a higher risk of persistent or recurrent HPT in these patients. This technique may help to prevent reoperation in the neck and its associated potential complications.

Wound drains are not routinely placed. The sternohyoid muscles are reapproximated in the midline using a running 3-0 absorbable suture. The inferiormost aspect of the strap muscles are left open to allow for decompression of the neck wound, in the case of a postoperative hematoma. The platysma muscle is then reapproximated using 4-0 absorbable suture and the skin is closed separately in a running subcuticular fashion.

Minimal Access Parathyroidectomy

The vast majority (90%) of cases of PHPT are as a result of a single parathyroid adenoma. Multiple adenomas account for 2–5% of cases and multigland hyperplasia accounts for the remaining cases (Ruda et al. 2005). This knowledge combined with the ability to predict and localize single gland disease with preoperative investigations, and the ability to predict the removal of all diseased parathyroid glands using intraoperative iPTH measurement has led to the development of limited, minimal access parathyroid explorations. The success of such procedures is similar to BPGE when patients are appropriately selected (Ruda et al. 2005).

Minimal access procedures are indicated in patients with PHPT who have preoperative 99Tc sestamibi scan localization that suggests a single adenoma. The procedure may also be used in patients with negative 99Tc sestamibi scans with convincing US or CT scan evidence of a parathyroid adenoma. In this latter instance, the surgeon and patient should be aware that conversion to a BPGE is more likely to be necessary.

A 2 cm incision is made approximately with one fingerbreadth below the cricoid cartilage, ideally in a preexisting skin crease, on the side of the localization. It is designed such that it can be extended, should conversion to a bilateral procedure be required. Flaps are then raised in the subplatysmal plane to provide exposure. The anterior border of the sternocleidomastoid (SCM) muscle is identified and dissection medial to this will identify the carotid sheath. A plane is then developed medial to the carotid sheath and lateral to the strap muscles. The strap muscles and underlying thyroid lobe are retracted medially, while the carotid sheath contents are gently retracted laterally (Figs 4A and B). This exposes the paratracheal tissue and should allow for exploration and identification of the abnormal gland, whether it is superior or inferior as in Figure 4C.

If removal of the abnormal gland does not result in correction of the serum iPTH level, the remaining ipsilateral gland should be identified. If it also appears abnormal, the possibility of a double adenoma or multigland hyperplasia must be considered. If it appears normal, a contralateral double adenoma is likely. In either situation, the procedure should be converted to a BPGE to maximize the possibility of a successful operation.

No wound drains are required and the incision is closed in a similar manner to that described for a BPGE.

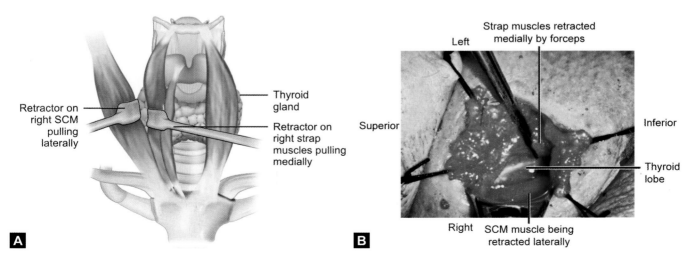

Figs 4A and B: Minimal access approach lateral to the strap muscles and medial to the carotid sheath. (A) Relevant anatomy illustrated; (B) Intraoperative approach

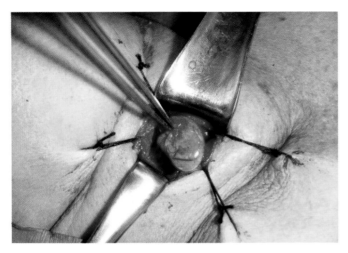

Fig. 4C: Delivery of a parathyroid adenoma

Novel Techniques

Radioguided parathyroidectomy is a minimal access procedure that is indicated in patients with PHPT and in patients with preoperative 99Tc sestamibi scan that suggests a single adenoma. Technetium-99 is administered again preoperatively on the day of surgery. A minimal access approach is used and the adenoma is removed. A background radioactivity count is obtained using a gamma probe over a neutral location (e.g. the patient's shoulder). An ex vivo count of the removed adenoma is also obtained and the operation is deemed successful if the adenoma count is at least 20% of the background count (Murphy et al. 1999). Intraoperative iPTH measurement is not used; thus, this technique offers a significant time saving advantage. A recent meta-analysis suggests similar success rates compared to BPGE in carefully selected patients (Ruda et al. 2005).

Endoscopic or video-assisted parathyroidectomy allows for a smaller skin incision to be used for access. No differences in postoperative pain or recovery have been found. This technique has yet to gain widespread acceptance and as such, the reader is referred to other references for a detailed description of this technique (Miccoli et al. 2004).

REIMPLANTATION AND CRYOPRESERVATION

Devascularized or hyperplastic parathyroid tissue can be reimplanted into any well vascularized muscle (e.g. SCM, pectoralis, deltoid, forearm, etc.). The parathyroid tissue should be cut into several tiny pieces to maximize the probability of revascularization and then reimplanted into pockets created in the muscle. The reimplantation sites should be marked with a surgical clip or a nonabsorbable suture to allow for easy identification at a later date if required. Our technique is to reimplant it in the ipsilateral pectoralis major muscle through a small infraclavicular incision. The authors prefer this technique for several reasons as it is easily accessible for later removal and avoids reoperation in the neck, it can be removed under local anesthesia and it avoids the morbidity of removal associated with tissue reimplanted in the forearm musculature.

Cryopreservation involves freezing parathyroid gland remnants for later reimplantation, if permanent hypoparathyroidism develops. This allows for more aggressive resection in the setting of multigland hyperplasia. Unfortunately, few centers have cryopreservation programs available.

SECONDARY AND TERTIARY HYPERPARATHYROIDISM

Secondary hyperparathyroidism develops when there is excessive production of PTH due to a chronic abnormal stimulus for its production. Serum calcium levels are typically low or normal. Although there are numerous causes, chronic renal failure is by far the most common. THPT involves excessive production of PTH after longstanding SHPT, resulting in hypercalcemia. It is most commonly seen following successful renal transplantation.

While the treatment of PHPT is almost exclusively surgical management, treatment of SHPT and THPT involves both medical and surgical aspects. There is no universally accepted set of indications for parathyroidectomy in these patients. However, surgery should only be considered if persistent or progressive disease is evident despite maximal medical therapy (Defechereux et al. 2009).

Preoperative localization studies are of limited value in these patients as they all have multigland disease. Preoperative US or CT scanning may be helpful in identifying ectopic glands. However, their routine use cannot be justified.

Intraoperative PTH also has a limited role in SHPT and THPT. The half-life of iPTH in renal failure is much longer, leading to a more gradual decrease in serum iPTH levels after gland excision. There is no consensus in the literature on appropriate time frames or iPTH levels for useful prediction of a successful operation.

The operative technique employed is the standard BPGE described above.

POSTOPERATIVE TREATMENT

Serum iPTH levels are checked again on the first postoperative day and serum calcium levels are monitored every 12 hours until stabilized. Oral and/or intravenous calcium replacement is used, if symptomatic hypocalcemia develops. Patients are discharged home once the calcium levels have stabilized. Serum iPTH and calcium levels are checked again after one month postoperatively and should be monitored yearly thereafter to detect recurrences.

HIGHLIGHTS

   I. Indications
- Symptomatic primary hyperparathyroidism
- Asymptomatic primary hyperparathyroidism (controversial indications)
- Secondary and tertiary hyperparathyroidism (not controlled with medial treatments).

  II. Contraindications
- Medically unfit for surgery.

 III. Special Preoperative Considerations
- Biochemical confirmation of disease (serum calcium, iPTH, creatinine and 24-hour urine calcium measurement)
- 99Tc sestamibi parathyroid scan
- Neck ultrasound or CT scan.

 IV. Special Intraoperative Considerations
- Detailed knowledge of anatomy and embryology of parathyroid glands is required
- Atraumatic technique to prevent bleeding and parathyroid gland rupture.

  V. Special Postoperative Considerations
- Serum iPTH and calcium measurements
- Long-term follow-up to monitor for recurrent disease.

 VI. Complications
- Hypoparathyroidism (transient or permanent)
- Persistent or recurrent hyperparathyroidism

- RLN injury (transient or permanent)
- Hematoma or seroma formation
- Wound infection.

ADDITIONAL READING

1. Akerström G, Malmaeus J, Bergström R. Surgical anatomy of human parathyroid glands. Surgery. 1984;95(1):14-21.
2. Bilezikian JP, Potts JT, Fuleihan Gel-H, et al. Summary statement from a workshop on asymptomatic primary hyperparathyroidism: A perspective for the 21st century. J Clin Endocrinol Metab. 2002;87(12):5353-61.
3. Butterworth PC, Nicholson ML. Surgical anatomy of the parathyroid glands in secondary hyperparathyroidism. J R Coll Surg Edinb. 1998;43(4):271-3.
4. Defechereux T, Meurisse M. Renal hyperparathyroidism: current therapeutic approaches and future directions. Oper Tech Otolaryngol Head Neck Surg. 2009;20:71-8.
5. Eigelberger MS, Cheah WK, Ituarte PH, et al. The NIH criteria for parathyroidectomy in asymptomatic primary hyperparathyroidism: Are they too limited? Ann Surg. 2004;239(4):528-35.
6. Miccoli P, Berti P, Materazzi G, et al. Results of video-assisted parathyroidectomy: single institution's six-year experience. World J Surg. 2004;28(12):1216-8.
7. Milas M, Wagner K, Easley KA, et al. Double adenomas revisited: nonuniform distribution favors enlarged superior parathyroids (fourth pouch disease). Surgery. 2003;134(6):995-1004.
8. Murphy C, Norman J. The 20% rule: a simple, instantaneous radioactivity measurement defines cure and allows elimination of frozen sections and hormone assays during parathyroidectomy. Surgery. 1999;126(6):1023-9.
9. Ruda JM, Hollenbeak CS, Stack BC. A systematic review of the diagnosis and treatment of primary hyperparathyroidism from 1995 to 2003. Otolaryngol Head Neck Surg. 2005;132(3):359-72.
10. Wang CA, Castleman B, Cope O. Surgical management of hyperparathyroidism due to primary hyperplasia. Ann Surg. 1982;195(4):384-92.

Chapter **15**

Substernal Goiter

Manish D Shah, Jeremy L Freeman

INTRODUCTION

Substernal goiter was first described by Haller in 1749. Klein was credited for having performed the first successful removal of a substernal goiter in 1820 (White et al. 2008). A goiter is defined as a thyroid gland that has enlarged to twice its normal size or greater than 40 grams (Newman et al. 1995). Although various definitions have been proposed, the two most commonly accepted definitions for substernal goiter are: any thyroid mass that extends below the plane of the thoracic inlet or has greater than 50% of its volume below the thoracic inlet (White et al. 2008).

Substernal goiters can present a challenge to surgeons. However, the authors will outline a stepwise approach in this chapter that will provide an effective technique for safe removal of such goiters.

PREOPERATIVE EVALUATION AND ANESTHESIA

A thorough history and physical examination are essential. Substernal goiters cause symptoms via compression of adjacent structures. The most common presenting symptoms are dyspnea, dysphagia and dysphonia. Signs of hypothyroidism (endemic iodine deficiency) or hyperthyroidism (toxic multinodular goiter) may also be present. An enlarged thyroid gland or mass may be palpable in the neck, although 20% of patients will not have a palpable abnormality (White et al. 2008). Indeed, many asymptomatic substernal goiters are discovered incidentally on cross-sectional imaging of the thorax done for other reasons. Substernal extension must be suspected when the inferior extent of the mass is not palpable above the clavicle. Preoperative laryngoscopy to assess vocal cord mobility is essential (Randolph et al. 2006).

Imaging of the thyroid gland preoperatively is important. Although ultrasound (US) imaging is excellent for evaluation of the thyroid gland, but it is unable to evaluate the substernal component. Cross-sectional imaging in the form of computed tomography (CT) or magnetic resonance imaging (MRI) provides excellent delineation of the substernal component, its relationship to important mediastinal structures, and evidence of tracheal compression (Figs 1A and B). Distinct, suspicious and accessible thyroid nodules should be subjected to fine needle aspiration biopsy (FNAB), either manually or via US guidance. Serum thyroid stimulating hormone (TSH) level should be measured in all patients.

Preoperative consultation should be obtained from a thoracic surgeon, if a sternotomy is required. Although there is no consensus in the literature with regards to definitive preoperative indications for sternotomy, it should be considered in the following circumstances (Randolph, 2003):

- Goiters extending below the level of the aortic arch
- Significant posterior mediastinal extension
- Goiter diameter considerably greater than the diameter of the thoracic inlet
- Suspicion of or confirmed invasive mediastinal malignancy
- Selected revision procedures
- Patients with a body habitus not amenable to cervical delivery of the goiter.

All procedures are carried out under general anesthesia with oral endotracheal intubation. Awake fiberoptic

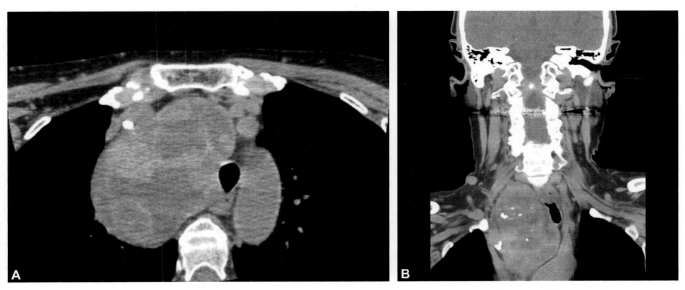

Figs 1A and B: CT images of a patient with a large substernal thyroid goiter. (A) Axial image; (B) Coronal image

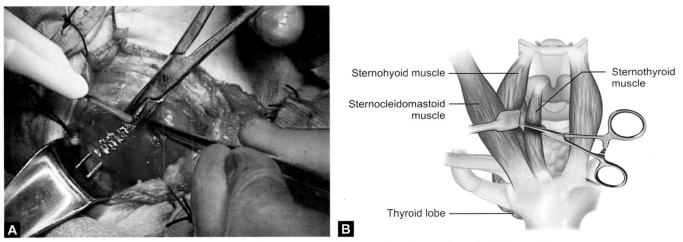

Figs 2A and B: (A) Lateral retraction of the sternohyoid muscle and division of the sternothyroid muscle at its midpoint improves exposure; (B) Illustration

intubation, may be necessary in patients with significant tracheal compression. To allow for maximal retraction and exposure, muscle relaxants are used throughout the procedure. This prevents the use of intraoperative monitoring of the recurrent laryngeal nerve (RLN), which is not routinely used at the author's institution.

SURGICAL TECHNIQUE

The patient should be positioned supine with a rolled blanket beneath the shoulders to provide gentle extension of the neck. The endotracheal tube should be positioned away from the operative field.

A midline transverse incision approximately one fingerbreadth below the cricoid cartilage is made, ideally in a pre-existing skin crease. The length of the incision required will vary depending on the patient's body habitus and the size of the goiter. Typically, a 5–7 cm incision should be sufficient. Flaps are then raised in the subplatysmal plane, both superiorly to the level of the thyroid notch and inferiorly to the clavicles. The midline raphe of the infrahyoid strap muscles is identified and divided vertically from the thyroid notch to the sternal notch. The plane between the sternohyoid and sternothyroid muscles is bluntly dissected, allowing the sternohyoid muscle to be retracted laterally. The full width of the sternothyroid muscle is then divided at its midpoint (Figs 2A and B). Next, if possible, the authors prefer to clearly delineate the anterior surface of the trachea just below the thyroid isthmus.

The authors' preference in a routine thyroidectomy is to first identify the RLN adjacent to the inferior pole of the thyroid gland. This provides for early identification of a nonrecurrent laryngeal nerve, which may be important during mobilization of the superior pole. With large goiters, however, it is usually not possible to identify the RLN at this point. Thus, the authors ligate the superior pole vessels first, which allows for mobilization of the thyroid gland and facilitates eventual delivery of the gland from the mediastinum and neck.

The superior portion of the divided sternothyroid muscle is bluntly elevated off of the thyroid gland toward its origin on the thyroid cartilage, exposing the superior pole vessels. This may also be done with cutting cautery. The avascular plane between the superior pole and the cricothyroid muscle is developed, allowing for identification of the external branch of the superior laryngeal nerve (EBSLN). Gentle inferior retraction with Allis forceps improves exposure of the superior pole vessels, which can then be appropriately ligated and divided as in Figure 3.

The next step is to deliver the substernal component of the goiter into the neck. The inferior end of the sternothyroid muscle is bluntly dissected off the gland and the carotid artery is identified laterally. The middle thyroid vein is typically encountered and should be ligated and divided. Blunt finger dissection close to the capsule of the thyroid gland along the carotid artery into the superior mediastinum allows separation of the goiter from mediastinal structures (Fig. 4). The blood supply of a goiter almost always comes from cervical vessels; rarely do mediastinal vessels supply the gland (Cho et al. 1986). Thus, this blunt dissection technique is both effective and safe. Gentle dissection around all surfaces of the substernal component facilitates mobilization. Incremental advancing steps may be required to allow the surgeon's finger to reach the inferior aspect of the goiter and deliver it into the neck. Superior retraction on the gland with Duval forceps may be beneficial in this process. Care must be taken with goiters involving posterior mediastinal extension. The RLN can be located on the ventral surface of the gland making it extremely vulnerable to injury.

If the substernal component cannot be delivered into the neck, mobilization of the contralateral thyroid lobe may increase the mobility of the larynx and trachea to facilitate delivery. Recently the authors have adopted this approach. With total dissection of the least affect side of the gland, this maneuver allows this side to act as a "handle" which, when grasped with Allis forceps, permits the less affected lobe to be a point of retraction on the substernal mass/lobe. The vectors of traction in a somewhat circular direction add an extra advantage to gently pulling the mediastinal component into the neck.

Once the substernal component has been released, from the mediastinum into the neck, the entire thyroid lobe can be delivered from the wound, exposing the paratracheal region as in Figure 5.

At this point, the RLN should be identified. This must be done carefully as the nerve may be located more anteriorly than normal or may be adherent to the undersurface of the thyroid lobe. Once identified, the nerve should be dissected free from the thyroid gland and toward its entry point into the larynx, which allows the gland to be released from the trachea and at the ligament of Berry.

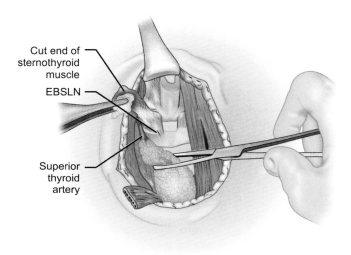

Fig. 3: Ligation of the superior thyroid pole vessels after identification of the external branch of the superior laryngeal nerve (EBSLN)

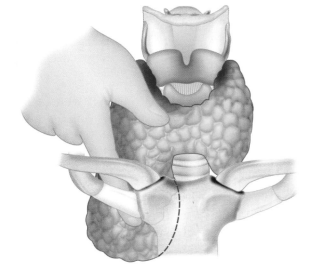

Fig. 4: Blunt mobilization of the substernal component of the thyroid gland from the mediastinum

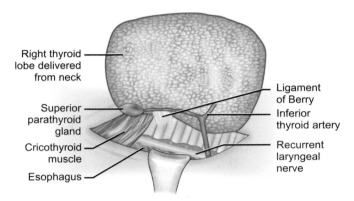

Right thyroid
lobe delivered
from neck

Superior
parathyroid
gland

Cricothyroid
muscle

Esophagus

Ligament
of Berry

Inferior
thyroid artery

Recurrent
laryngeal
nerve

Fig. 5: The thyroid gland has been delivered from the neck, exposing the recurrent laryngeal nerve (RLN), inferior thyroid artery and the superior parathyroid gland

Preservation of vascularized parathyroid gland is essential. The inferior thyroid artery will be encountered during dissection of the RLN. It should be ligated at the thyroid capsule to preserve parathyroid blood supply. The superior parathyroid glands have a more consistent position and are more easily identified during goiter surgery than the inferior glands. Once identified, the superior parathyroid gland should be dissected free from the thyroid gland while preserving its lateral based blood supply. The specimen should be closely examined before being sent for pathology and any devascularized glands should be cut into several small pieces and reimplanted into vascularized muscle.

Removal of the contralateral lobe is not always necessary in the setting of a benign disease process. If indicated, the contralateral lobe is removed in a similar fashion with care taken to identify and remove a pyramidal lobe in continuity with the specimen, if present. If a large dead space remains once the gland has been removed, the authors place a 10 mm flat Jackson-Pratt drain into the wound through a separate stab incision inferior to the operative skin incision. The sternohyoid muscles are reapproximated in the midline using a running 3-0 absorbable suture. The inferiormost aspect of the strap muscles are left open to allow for decompression of the neck wound, in the case of a postoperative hematoma. The platysma muscle is then reapproximated using 4-0 absorbable suture and the skin is closed separately in a running subcuticular fashion.

POSTOPERATIVE TREATMENT

If a total thyroidectomy has been done, serum ionized calcium and parathyroid hormone (PTH) levels are measured immediately in the postoperative recovery unit. Serum calcium levels are then checked every 12 hours until three successive stable levels are achieved. Oral and/or intravenous calcium replacement is used if serum calcium levels are low or patients are symptomatic. If total thyroidectomy is performed, all patients start with oral thyroid hormone replacement on the first postoperative day. Drains are removed when the 24-hour output is less than 30 ml. Once the neck drains have been removed and serum calcium levels are stabilized, patients are discharged from hospital. Vocal cord mobility is assessed at the patient's first postoperative office visit, approximately one week after surgery.

HIGHLIGHTS

I. **Indications**
  - Confirmed malignancy
  - Suspicion of malignancy
  - Compressive symptoms (dyspnea, dysphagia, dysphonia).

II. **Contraindications**
  - Anaplastic thyroid cancer
  - Lymphoma
  - Unresectable due to locally invasive malignancy (carotid artery/mediastinal vessels, prevertebral fascia)
  - Medically unfit for surgery.

III. **Special Preoperative Considerations**
  - Cross-sectional imaging (CT or MRI)
  - Laryngoscopy to evaluate vocal cord mobility.

IV. **Special Intraoperative Considerations**
  - Division of sternothyroid muscle to improve exposure
  - Early mobilization of the superior pole of the thyroid gland
  - Blunt finger dissection to deliver the goiter into the neck
  - RLN may be located more anteriorly or may be adherent to the undersurface of the thyroid lobe.

V. **Special Postoperative Considerations**
  - Serum PTH measurement and monitoring of serum calcium levels
  - Assess vocal cord mobility.

VI. **Complications**
  - Neural injury [RLN or EBSLN (transient or permanent)]
  - Hypoparathyroidism (transient or permanent)
  - Hematoma or seroma formation
  - Wound infection.

ADDITIONAL READING

1. Cho HT, Cohen JP, Som SL. Management of substernal and intrathoracic goiter. Otolaryngol Head Neck Surg. 1986;94(3): 282-77.
2. Newman E, Shaha AR. Substernal goiter. J Surg Oncol. 1995; 60(3):207-12.
3. Randolph GW, Kamani D. The importance of preoperative laryngoscopy in patients undergoing thyroidectomy: voice, vocal cord function, and the preoperative detection of invasive thyroid malignancy. Surgery. 2006;139(3): 357-62.
4. Randolph GW. Surgery of cervical and substernal goiter. In: Randolph GW (Ed). Surgery of the Thyroid and Parathyroid Glands. Philadelphia: Elsevier Science; 2003. pp. 70-99.
5. White ML, Doherty GM, Gauger PG. Evidence-based surgical management of substernal goiter. World J Surg. 2008;32(7): 1285-300.

Chapter 16

Thyroglossal Duct Cyst

Peter Li, Peter J Koltai

INTRODUCTION

Thyroglossal duct cysts (TGDC) are the most common nonodontogenic cysts occurring in the neck and are second only to benign lymphadenopathy of all cervical masses in childhood. They are cystic dilations of epithelial remnants of the thyroglossal duct tract formed during the migration of the thyroid during embryogenesis.

The most common clinical presentation of a TGDC is a 1–4 cm midline cystic mass below the hyoid bone in a child. Most are located below the level of the hyoid bone, although a proportion arises above the hyoid in the floor of the mouth or base of the tongue; up to 20% of cysts are noted to be slightly off the midline, with a predilection for the left and a modest proportion of cysts become clinically evident only in adulthood. Cysts below the thyrohyoid membrane are rare. There are only two reported cases: the first one reaching the suprasternal notch and the second one descending all the way to the aortic arch encroaching into the superior mediastinum. Males and females are equally affected and the cysts are usually asymptomatic, but may become infected, form abscesses and draining fistulas.

The differential diagnosis for TGDC includes submental nodes, dermoid cysts, metastatic thyroid carcinoma, pyramidal lobe nodule, branchial cleft cysts, lipomas and sebaceous cysts. Often definitive diagnosis is only made after surgical removal and pathological evaluation.

During embryogenesis, the thyroid gland arises as a midline endodermal proliferation of the pharyngeal floor at a point, between the tuberculum impar (first branchial arch derivative) and copula (second and third branchial arch derivative). This point becomes the foramen cecum and separates the anterior two thirds of the tongue from the posterior third. In the third embryonic week, the thyroglossal duct tract descends from the foramen cecum, anteroinferiorly in close relation to the hyoid bone around which it usually loops down past the thyrohyoid membrane and strap muscles, anterior to the thyroid cartilage, ending in the thyroid isthmus at approximately the 7–8th embryonic weeks (Fig. 1). The tract subsequently involutes and atrophies by the 10th week of gestational age.

Arrested migration or embryonic remnants can occur at any point along the tract. Remnants within the substance of the tongue lead to solid masses of ectopic thyroid tissue known as a "lingual thyroid". Cysts are encountered further inferiorly and are far more common, representing failure of involution of only a portion of the tract. A patent thyroglossal tract represents failure of involution of the entire tract.

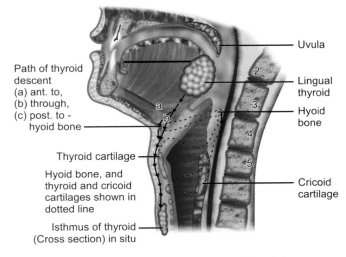

Fig. 1: Origination and descent of thyroglossal duct cyst

Many cystic remnants of the thyroglossal tract are never detected clinically. The stimulus for the expansion is not known; one hypothesis is that lymphoid tissue associated with the tract hypertrophies at the time of a regional infection, leading to occlusion of the tract with resultant cyst formation.

A concept emphasized in the literature focuses on arborization of the suprahyoid portion of the duct. In this description of the involution of the thyroglossal duct, Boyd (1950) states: "After rupture of the thyroglossal duct, the proximal portion shortens and thickens and its epithelium comes to resemble that of the tongue and frequently re-develops a lumen from which there grows out a more or less extensive system of branches."[1]

Soucy et al.[2] performed a histological review of 44 thyroglossal duct cyst specimens, which showed that the thyroglossal duct was frequently multiple and arborized into the surrounding tissues. Additionally, Horisawa et al.[3] performed anatomical reconstructions of 10 thyroglossal duct and cyst specimens. These 10 specimens showed similar patterns of multiple branches and secretory glands emerging from the thyroglossal duct at levels caudal and cranial to the hyoid bone. Finally, several authors have described thyroglossal duct cysts lateral to the midline. The arborization of the duct probably plays a significant role in the development of recurrent TGDC.

Before 1893, the removal of a TGDC included simple incision and drainage. The recurrence rate after this procedure was 50%. In 1893, Schlange proposed the excision of the cyst along with the central portion of the hyoid bone. This resulted in a drop in the recurrence rate to 20%. In 1920, Walter Sistrunk described the procedure that bears his name and which reduced the recurrence rates to between 3% and 5%.[4]

Sistrunk recommended not only taking the central portion of the hyoid bone, but also carving out a core of tissue one eighth of an inch in radius from the hyoid bone to the foramen cecum and in doing so, removing thyroglossal duct branches as well as preventing retraction of the duct remnant into the soft tissue base of tongue. Sistrunk felt there was no benefit in identifying the suprahyoid portion of the duct as there is no readily identifiable single plane of dissection in this area. Eighty years later, this remains the definitive surgical technique for this problem.

PREOPERATIVE EVALUATION AND ANESTHESIA

The preoperative evaluation of patients with a suspected TGDC consists of a history of the patient and head and neck examination with emphasis on identifying the normally positioned thyroid tissue. The incidence of ectopic thyroid tissue, in the absence of a normally positioned thyroid, is reported to be between 1% and 2% because inadvertent removal of the ectopic thyroid tissue can lead to postoperative hypothyroidism and a life long need for thyroid replacement. The goal of preoperative imaging in patients with TGDC is to assess the location of the thyroid gland as well as the nature of the lesion. Although palpation of a normal gland can be used in adults, this is more difficult in children.

There is no consensus in the literature regarding the optimal preoperative imaging modality. Ultrasound of the neck is a simple and an inexpensive test to look for the presence of the thyroid gland in its normal anatomic location and to confirm the cystic nature of the mass, but does not give functional information. Radionuclide thyroid scans provide functional information regarding thyroid tissue and rules out the possibility of the cyst containing the only functioning thyroid tissue. Computed tomography (CT) and magnetic resonance imaging (MRI) can confirm the diagnosis, provide information regarding the relationship of the cyst to the hyoid bone and identify normal orthotopic thyroid tissue. In children, the authors prefer ultrasound examination due to its availability, cost and tolerability. While thyroid function tests can be assessed preoperatively to establish baseline function, the authors resort to this in only selective patients, in whom abnormalities of thyroid function are suspected.

The incidence of thyroglossal duct cyst carcinoma is estimated to occur in 1% of all cysts and the diagnosis should always be entertained in the adult presenting with a thyroglossal duct cyst. In these cases, it is important to confirm that the carcinoma arises from within the cyst and is not a cystic metastasis to a midline lymph node from a primary thyroid cancer. Papillary thyroid carcinoma comprises the majority of TGDC carcinomas. Other variants include mixed papillary follicular carcinoma, squamous cell carcinoma and Hürthle cell carcinoma. Medullary carcinoma has not been found in any thyroglossal duct cysts. A Mayo clinic series has shown that 33% of patients with a TGDC carcinoma have a concurrent intrathyroidal malignant mass.[5]

Preoperative work-up for adults presenting with TGDC therefore, necessitates imaging of both the thyroid and TGDC. In these patients the authors advocate the use of CT, given its ability to identify calcifications and solid soft tissue elements, which are specific markers for carcinoma.[6,7]

Fine needle aspiration (FNA), although not routinely indicated, is often used to diagnose thyroglossal duct cysts or to exclude other diagnoses. The cytomorphologic features include colloid, macrophages, lymphocytes, neutrophils and ciliated columnar cells, but these are not unique to thyroglossal duct cysts.

Concurrent infection of the cyst should be treated prior to surgical excision to ensure greater surgical success. Studies by Ducic et al.[8] and by Flageole et al.[9] examined multiple variables leading to surgical failure after the Sistrunk procedure. Preoperative infection was highly associated with failure in both studies.

Routine general endotracheal anesthesia is used for all patients undergoing the Sistrunk procedure with the endotracheal tube taped to the upper lip to allow the surgeon access to the mouth. Prophylactic antibiotics are instituted perioperatively and continued throughout the immediate postoperative period.

SURGICAL TECHNIQUE

Sistrunk Procedure

After induction of general anesthesia, patients are placed in the supine position with the neck extended by placing a roll underneath the shoulders. One percent lidocaine with 1:100,000 epinephrine is injected to help with hemostasis. The anterior part of the neck is prepared and draped from the manubrium to the lower lip using a sterile technique.

A 4 cm horizontal, curvilinear incision is made at the level of the cyst in the midline of the neck (Fig. 2). The incision should be placed within a skin crease at the cervical mental junction to improve the cosmetic appearance of the subsequent scar. The incision is carried through the skin, subcutaneous tissue and platysma muscle. A subplatysmal flap is then elevated superiorly and inferiorly to expose the strap muscles, which are retracted laterally to expose the cystic lesion as in Figure 3.

The cyst is carefully dissected free from the thyroid cartilage, sternohyoid and thyrohyoid muscles and surrounding soft tissue until it is pedicled superiorly to the middle third of the hyoid bone (Fig. 4). A cuff of adjacent strap muscle is often included with the excision. The mylohyoid and geniohyoid muscles can be detached from the superior aspect of the body of the hyoid bone using an electrocautery, so that the hyoid bone is visualized at its junction between the middle and lateral thirds. Alternatively, a cuff of these muscles may be left attached to the superior aspect of the hyoid to facilitate complete excision.

Heavy Mayo scissors or bone cutters are then used to resect the middle third of the hyoid bone and the cyst (Fig. 5). This maneuver permits elevation of the body of the hyoid and dissection on the undersurface of the cyst or tract separating these structures from the thyrohyoid membrane.

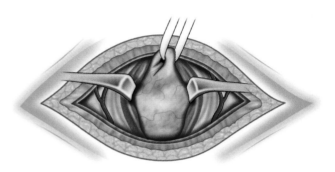

Fig. 3: The subplatysmal flaps are raised, the strap muscles are split in the midline and retracted laterally to provide exposure to the cyst

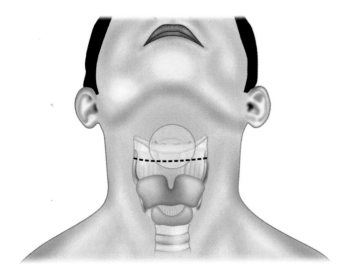

Fig. 2: Skin incision is made in the midline overlying the cyst

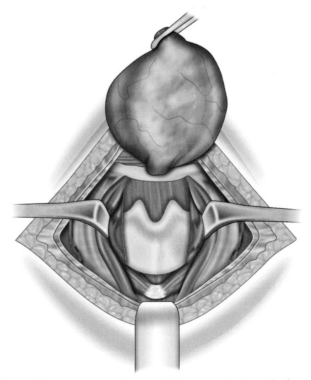

Fig. 4: The cyst is seen here pedicled superiorly to the hyoid bone once it has been freed from the surrounding soft tissues

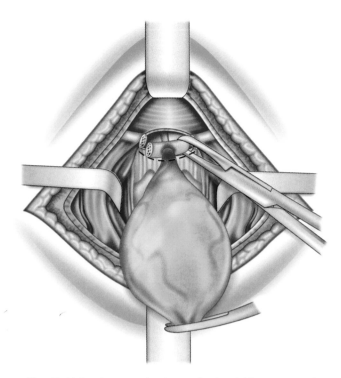

Fig. 5: Using laryngeal scissors the hyoid is transected on each side of the midline

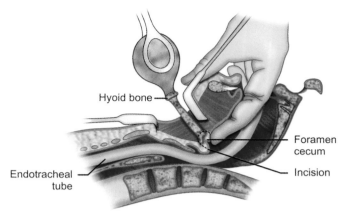

Fig. 6: A finger is placed into the vallecula to retract the base of tongue forward and upward

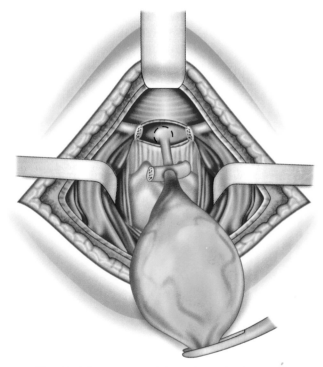

Fig. 7: A 3 mm core of tissue is excised toward the foramen cecum

With the body of the hyoid bone detached from the cornua, traction is placed on the cyst to enable the deep portion of the thyroglossal tract (if there is one) to be identified. The deep tract courses through the tongue musculature toward the foramen cecum. Only rarely, is an actual tract identified in this location. Often an ellipse of muscle tissue is excised in continuity with the hyoid bone in hope of removing the tract. If this is done, it is important that the line of excision be confined to the midline to avoid injury to the hypoglossal nerve.

To facilitate this step, the surgeon or assistant places a finger into the oral cavity, palpating the vallecula and base of tongue and pushing them forward and upwards (Fig. 6). This maneuver shortens the distance between the base of tongue and the hyoid bone. While an assistant retracts the cyst and hyoid bone, the surgeon then removes a core of tissue 3 mm on all sides extending toward the foramen cecum (Fig. 7). Some surgeons extend the excision into the pharynx but most do not.

Once the specimen in removed, the wound is irrigated and complete hemostasis is obtained. If the pharynx has been opened at the foramen cecum, it is closed with a mattressed 3-0 chromic suture (Fig. 8). Subsequent closure consists of approximation of the mylohyoid and geniohyoid muscles to the sternohyoid and thyrohyoid muscles with 3-0 vicryl

suture to reconstruct the muscular relationships that were detached from the resected hyoid bone. The transected ends of the hyoid bone are not approximated.

The strap muscles are replaced in their anatomic position, the fascia enveloping the strap muscles is closed in the vertical plane (Fig. 9). A one-fourth inch Penrose drain can be placed into the wound prior to skin closure and brought out through the corner of the wound, however, this is rarely

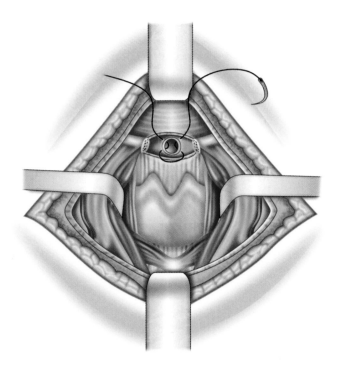

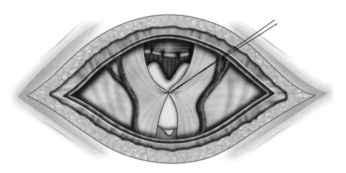

Fig. 9: The strap muscles are reapproximated in the midline

Fig. 8: The opening at the foramen cecum is then closed

necessary. The platysma muscles are then closed using 4-0 vicryl suture. The skin is closed with running subcuticular 5-0 monofilament suture. Steri-strips are applied across the incision. A compression dressing is rarely necessary.

POSTOPERATIVE TREATMENT

Most children are operated on an outpatient basis. If a drain has been placed, it is removed after 24 hours. Antibiotics are continued while the drain is in place. Oral intake is not restricted, but discomfort is common and may prevent the patient from eating a normal diet for 24–48 hours. Pain is controlled with an alternating regimen of acetaminophen and ibuprofen.

RECURRENT LESIONS

While the Sistrunk procedure has an admirably low recurrence rate, nevertheless given the variable pathways that the tracts can have, reoperation may be necessary even in the best of hands. Higher recurrence rates have been attributed to preoperative infection. Young age of the patient and rupture of the cyst, at the time of operation, renders dissection more difficult.

Review of the patient's previous operative record, paying particular attention to treatment of the hyoid bone and proximal tissue, and assessment of the pathology report is valuable when working on revision cases. Preoperative imaging with CT or MRI can be useful for surgical planning. Recurrent lesions are best managed with wide resection of the affected area, further excision of the hyoid bone and removal of a generous cuff of surrounding tissue leading to the base of tongue. Hirosawa recommends excision of at least 15 mm of the base of tongue musculature around the presumed location of the thyroglossal duct to assure that all proximal branches of the duct are included in the resection. Perkins et al. recommend a suture-guided transhyoid pharyngotomy.[10] In this procedure, a spinal needle is initially passed percutaneously through the neck adjacent to the recurrent cyst tract into the oropharynx at the foramen cecum. A suture is then passed through the spinal needle and brought out intraorally and secured to a red rubber catheter, which is then pulled into the oral cavity via traction on the transcutaneous portion of the suture. Using the suture as a traction device, the tongue base musculature can be pulled directly into the operative field allowing complete excision of a 1–1.5 cm core of the tongue base musculature in continuity with the foramen cecum mucosa.

THYROGLOSSAL DUCT CYST CARCINOMA

If noninvasive papillary cancer is found in a thyroglossal duct specimen with no demonstrated thyroid abnormalities on either palpation or on ultrasound evaluation, a Sistrunk procedure alone has been found to be an effective treatment in the majority of cases. Close follow-up is necessary along with thyroid suppression. Total thyroidectomy is necessary if there is metastasis from the thyroid gland. Some authors recommend prophylactic total thyroidectomy given the high incidence of thyroid carcinoma in this patient population.

THYROGLOSSAL DUCT CYST IN THE TONGUE BASE

Thyroglossal duct cysts can rarely, present in the tongue base looking very much like a vallecular cyst. Typically, the definitive diagnosis is made only after pathological examination of the excised tissue. Excision can be done using a laser via direct laryngoscopy after adequate exposure of the lesion. Alternatively, the lesion can be visualized endoscopically with a 4 mm diameter, 30° sinus telescope, after adequate tongue retraction and ablated using Coblation® technology.

HIGHLIGHTS

I. Indications
- Diagnosis of a mass present in the anterior neck
- Enlargement of the mass with pain, dysphagia and dyspnea
- Cosmetic concern
- Infection
- Fistula formation.

II. Contraindications
- A relative contraindication is a cyst representing the only functioning thyroid tissue
- Acute infection of the cyst should be treated prior to surgical excision
- Bleeding disorder
- Medical contraindications to general anesthesia.

III. Special Preoperative Considerations
- Examine the midline or lateral midline area. Elevation of the mass with swallowing or tongue protrusion is thought to be a pathognomonic sign for TGDC.
- Preoperative imaging studies include ultrasound, CT, MRI or radionuclide thyroid scans. Consider ultrasound as the first line in children and CT in adults.
- Fine needle aspiration may be considered if diagnosis is questionable.
- Antibiotics are administered to resolve acute infections before excision.

IV. Special Intraoperative Considerations
- Examine the patient for a thyroglossal duct opening on the lingual wall of the vallecula in the region of the foramen cecum.
- Identify the thyroid notch and thyrohyoid membrane intraoperatively to decrease the likelihood of entering the airway.
- The hypoglossal or internal branch of superior laryngeal nerve can be injured, if one divides the hyoid too laterally or dissects too aggressively in the superior direction. Dividing the hyoid medial to the lesser cornua and dissecting superiorly medial to the anterior digastric muscle can avoid this type of injury.
- Send a frozen section specimen from all solid masses for pathologic analysis.

V. Special Postoperative Considerations
- The surgical specimen should undergo careful histologic examination for TGDC carcinoma.
- The patient should be followed for development of recurrence.

VI. Complications
- Recurrence secondary to incomplete excision. Higher recurrence rates have been attributed to preoperative infection, young age of the patient and rupture of the cyst at the time of operation rendering dissection more difficult.
- Wound infection, abscess, hematoma, seroma formation
- Entry into larynx or pharynx
- Nerve injury (internal branch of superior laryngeal nerve or hypoglossal nerve)
- Hypothyroidism can be avoided with proper preoperative evaluation to determine the presence of a normal thyroid.
- Need for tracheotomy.

REFERENCES

1. Boyd, JD. Development of the thyroid and parathyroid glands and the thymus. Ann R Coll Surg Engl. 1950;7(6):455-71.
2. Soucy P, Penning J. The clinical relevance of certain observations on the histology of the thyroglossal tract. J Pediatr Surg. 1984;19(5):506-9.
3. Horisawa M, Niinomi N, Ito T. Anatomical reconstruction of the thyroglossal duct. J Pediatr Surg. 1991;26(7):766-9.
4. Sistrunk WE. Technique of removal of cysts and sinuses of the thyroglossal duct. Surg Gynecol Obstet. 1928;46:109-12.
5. Heshmati HM, Fatourechi V, van Heerden JA, et al. Thyroglossal duct carcinoma: report of 12 cases. Mayo Clinic Proc. 1997;72(4):315-9.
6. Brousseau VJ, Solares CA, Xu M, et al. Thyroglossal duct cysts: presentation and management in children versus adults. Int J Pediatr Otorhinolaryngol. 2003;67(12):1285-90.
7. Glastonbury CM, Davidson HC, Haller JR, et al. The CT and MR imaging features of carcinoma arising in thyroglossal duct remnants. Am J Neuroradiol. 2000;21(4):770-4.
8. Ducic Y, Chou S, Drkulec J, et al. Recurrent thyroglossal duct cysts: a clinical and pathologic analysis. Int J Pediatr Otorhinolaryngol. 1998;44(1):47-50.
9. Flageole H, Laberge JM, Nguyen LT, et al. Reoperation for cysts of the thyroglossal duct. Can J Surg. 1995;38(3):255-9.
10. Perkins JA, Inglis AF, Sie KC, et al. Recurrent thyroglossal duct cysts: a 23-year experience and a new method for management. Ann Otol Rhinol Laryngol. 2006;115(11):850-6.

Chapter **17**

Tracheal Resection for Locally Advanced Thyroid Cancers

N Gopalakrishna Iyer, Ashok R Shaha

INTRODUCTION

Extrathyroidal extension is recognized by most staging systems as a poor prognostic factor for well-differentiated thyroid cancer and is seen in 10–15% of patients. Based on a series of patients treated at Memorial Sloan-Kettering Cancer Center, the local recurrence rate in these patients were 48%, while 41% and 37% had metastasis to regional nodes and distant sites respectively. Structures most commonly involved include strap muscles, recurrent laryngeal nerve, trachea, esophagus and larynx. Tracheal invasion rates have been estimated to range from 2% to 20%; the variability is probably due to the expertise of the different reporting centers. A combined analysis of over 10,000 patients with thyroid cancers showed that airway invasion occurs in approximately 5% of cases. Invasion of the airway is associated with a significant reduction in local control and survival. Furthermore, several studies have shown that these patients have more aggressive histological subtypes, including poorly-differentiated, tall cell and insular variants. Depth of tracheal invasion appears to correlate with the outcome and hence, can be used as a guide for surgical decision. Most patients with tracheal invasion or adherence are asymptomatic, incidentally diagnosed during preoperative imaging or discovered during surgery. Occasionally, patients present with airway obstruction or bleeding due to transmural invasion.

As most patients are asymptomatic, tracheal invasion may only be discovered at the time of surgery hence, it demands that the surgeon takes the critical decision intraoperatively. Surgical options include a shave resection of thyroid tumor or an en bloc resection of the required tracheal segment along with other parts of the airway complex, if necessary and primary repair/reconstruction. Tangential shave resections should be limited to patients with superficial involvement of the trachea. Intraoperative assessment for depth of invasion is usually inaccurate and this accounts for the higher rates of local recurrence and mortality, after a tangential shave procedure. For patients, where the pathology report after shave procedure, suggest residual disease on the trachea, a more formal resection should be considered. It is important to note that immediate en bloc airway resection results in longer, disease-free survival than resection at the time of tumor recurrence. However, these procedures should only be performed by surgeons with adequate experience in airway resection and reconstruction. Occasionally, patients may present with previously managed thyroid cancer and tumor recurrence with airway involvement. This could represent actual recurrence in the thyroid bed or persistence/recurrence of nodal involvement in the central compartment. Surgery in this group of patients is difficult; most patients would have previously been treated with radioiodine and/or external beam radiation, leaving a hostile neck with poor vascularity and healing capacity. Apart from a difficult dissection, these patients may require additional reconstruction to introduce fresh, vascularized tissue into the surgical repair. It is crucial that the surgeon reviews the original surgical procedure and pathology, as well as excludes distant metastases in these patients before embarking into a major surgical resection.

PREOPERATIVE EVALUATION AND ANESTHESIA

A significant proportion of patients are asymptomatic and airway invasion is incidentally discovered during surgery. As such, preoperative evaluation is limited to routine imaging

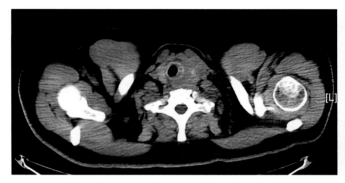

Fig. 1: CT scan images showing a large left sided thyroid mass with tracheal invasion and submucosal disease

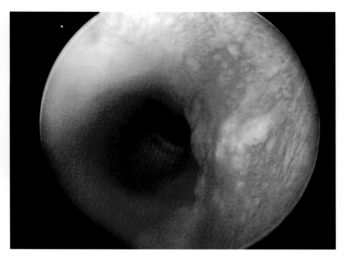

Fig. 2: Endoscopic image of the same patient in Figure 1 showing submucosal disease

of thyroid nodules, ultrasound and fiberoptic laryngoscopy. Patients who are symptomatic or present with extensive tumor, based on clinical evaluation (e.g. compressive symptoms or vocal cord palsy) or ultrasound should undergo cross-sectional imaging, usually a computed tomography (CT) scan with or without contrast. The accuracy for ultrasound scans to predict airway invasion is between 40% and 80%, depending on the experience of the sonographer. Computed tomography scans are more accurate, especially when there is frank mucosal invasion, destruction of cartilage rings or cricoid involvement (Fig. 1). Fiberoptic laryngoscopy is essential to evaluate the vocal cords and subglottic mucosa. If a patient presents with unilateral vocal cord paralysis, utmost care should be taken to preserve the contralateral recurrent laryngeal nerve, as the ipsilateral nonfunctional nerve may be resected together with the tumor. This may necessitate the use of nerve monitoring devices such as the nerve integrity monitoring system (NIM Response® 2.0). Luminal compression, erythema, edema, neovascularity and frank mucosal ulceration are indicators of airway involvement. Rigid bronchoscopy is often more accurate than flexible scopes and should be used prior to resection in patients suspected of tracheal invasion. In this situation, the purpose of rigid endoscopy (Fig. 2) is to diagnose advanced invasion and estimate luminal extent and resectability. Elderly and high-risk patients, in whom extensive resection is planned, should undergo positron emission tomography (PET) scans to rule out the possibility of extensive distant metastases, although primary tumor resection offers the best palliation even in the presence of distant disease. Patients should also undergo a preoperative fine needle or core biopsy to exclude an anaplastic thyroid case, in which all parties should be aware of the guarded prognosis.

Patients diagnosed to have airway invasion, should be counseled preoperatively for the extent and consequence of surgery and major complications, including the possible need for a tracheostomy, laryngectomy, sternal split (rarely) and a staged second procedure.

Surgery should be performed under general anesthesia, with intubation by a skilled anesthesiologist or the surgeon using fiberoptic laryngoscopy. This is to avoid trauma to any existing mucosal tumor involvement or edema to the tracheal mucosa. A small endotracheal tube is preferable, such as a size 6 mm or 6.5 mm, and the cuff should be positioned well below the vocal cords. Routine intravenous antibiotics are used, when there is an expected breach of the airway mucosa. The patient is positioned supine with the neck extended. Recurrent laryngeal nerve monitoring is a useful adjunct to avoid injury to the functioning nerve(s), especially when there is an extensive tracheoesophageal groove involvement from the previous surgery or prior unilateral vocal cord paralysis, although there is a high false-negative rate associated with these devices. If there is a preoperative evidence of an extensive disease, the chest and abdomen should also be prepped, in case there is a need for sternotomy or a gastric pull-up; although this is rarely required.

SURGICAL TECHNIQUE

Stages of Tracheal Involvement

Shin et al. proposed a staging system to guide surgical decision making, based on depth of the tracheal involvement (Fig. 3). For well-differentiated thyroid cancer with involvement of the tracheal perichondrium only, a shave resection is adequate. Any patient with deeper cartilaginous involvement, submucosal extension or extension through the tracheal wall will require full thickness resection of the airway. The major caveat to this approach is that the intraoperative assessment can underestimate the depth of tracheal invasion and this may only be appreciated, when the pathology is reviewed.

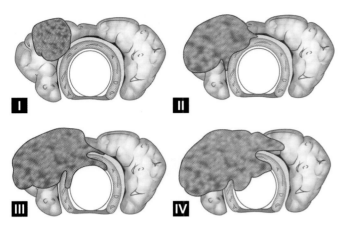

Fig. 3: Classification of tracheal invasion. Stage I involves outer perichondrium only; Stage II invades the cartilage; Stage III invades through the cartilage with submucosal involvement and Stage IV shows full thickness involvement with mucosal disease

Furthermore, there is evidence to suggest that patients undergoing shave resection have higher local recurrence and disease-specific mortality rates. Hence, some surgeons suggest that all patients should undergo full thickness tracheal resection at the time of the primary surgery.

Surgical Considerations

Total Thyroidectomy with Tracheal Resection

Total thyroidectomy with tracheal resection can be performed for curative or palliative intent; the latter is to relieve airway obstruction or hemorrhage. The aim in all these procedures is en bloc resection of the thyroidectomy specimen or recurrent tumor with the involved airway segment. A standard 6–8 cm thyroidectomy incision is fashioned in an appropriate skin crease and platysmal flaps are raised. This can be extended, if there is a need for additional lateral neck dissection. The standard approach for a thyroidectomy is employed and in almost all cases, a total thyroidectomy is performed and the specimen is left attached to the trachea. If a central compartment clearance is performed, the recurrent laryngeal nerve should be carefully dissected free and reflected laterally from the tracheoesophageal groove prior to any tracheal resection. Parathyroid glands should be preserved in situ. If the viability is in doubt, these should be removed, confirmed to be a parathyroid on frozen section, minced and reimplanted in a dry pocket in the contralateral sternocleidomastoid muscle. During the tracheal resection, the surgeon must constantly communicate with the anesthesiologist and convey his intent or plan and instructions. This process also necessitates that the anesthesiologist understands the maneuvers he needs to undertake and has easy access to the endotracheal tube.

Shave Procedure

As stated before, this is the procedure of choice when there is minimal involvement of the perichondrium. The thyroid or residual tumor is dissected, leaving it attached at the point of tracheal invasion. Using a fresh number 10 scalpel blade the thyroidectomy specimen or tumor together with the attached perichondrium, and a portion of underlying cartilage is cut tangentially. The specimen is resected and removed en bloc and the base of the resection is examined to ensure no mucosal breach. The neck is then closed in layers with or without a drain, as per routine thyroidectomy.

Full Thickness Airway Resection

Minimal tracheal involvement: Isolated involvement of a small portion of the trachea can be managed with a window or wedge resection. The thyroidectomy specimen or tumor is dissected out leaving the point of tracheal invasion attached. Prior to placing an incision on the trachea, the cuff of the endotracheal tube should be deflated and the tube is advanced, such that the cuff is situated more distal to the arc of resection. A sharp number 15 blade is used to enter the membranous trachea above and below the tracheal ring to be excised and the incision is extended transversely to include the width of invasion. A sharp, curved metzenbaum or tenotomy scissor is then used to cut across the cartilaginous ring on either side and connect the previous incisions, and the specimen is removed. The cuff of the endotracheal tube is reinflated and correctly positioned. There are a number of methods generally employed to close the defect, depending on the lateral extent of the resection. Small window defects can be closed by interposing the strap muscles or mobilizing and rotating the sternocleidomastoid and suturing it as a buttress to close the defect. Periosteal flaps attached to the sternocleidomastoid muscle may also be used. Placing a tracheostomy tube in the small tracheal defect is another easy option. Wider defects or wedge resections should be closed primarily by placing interrupted absorbable sutures such a vicryl or monocryl 2-0 sutures. For this technique, full thickness stitches are placed around the tracheal rings above and below the defect, starting in the middle of the defect and working laterally. Once all the sutures have been placed, they are tied leaving the knots extraluminally. At the end of the repair, the wound is irrigated with saline and a Valsalva maneuver is performed with the cuff deflated to confirm no air leakage through the repair. The wound is usually closed over a Penrose drain in a layered fashion. A tracheostomy is best avoided after a window or wedge resection, as it delays healing and is often a source of infection.

Sleeve Resection

Tumor involvement of multiple tracheal rings necessitates a more extensive tracheal resection, i.e. a sleeve resection, which involves removing a circumferential segment of the trachea (Figs 4A to E). Prior to undertaking a sleeve resection, it is crucial to evaluate the extent of intraluminal disease and proximity to the subglottis and carina. If the tumor involves more than 5–7 tracheal rings or extends to the carina, the tumor may be deemed inoperable. The upper limit of the resection should also be at least 1 cm below the subglottis for primary tracheal anastomosis.

Before resecting the involved segment of trachea, the thyroidectomy specimen or tumor should be dissected completely and left attached to the trachea. Central compartment clearance should be completed, where required, for carefully preserving the recurrent laryngeal nerves bilaterally. During dissection, it is important not to devascularize the trachea by avoiding excessive circumferential dissection. The nerves should be retracted laterally from the tracheoesophageal groove. The plane between the trachea and esophagus is initially developed by blunt dissection taking care not to injure the esophageal musculature or mucosa.

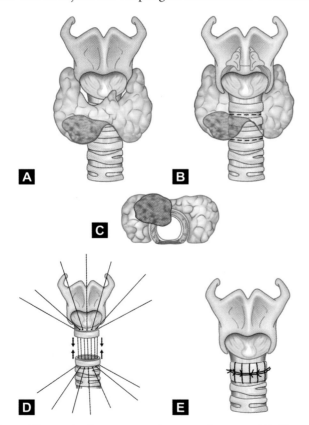

Figs 4A to E: Sleeve resection step-by-step. (A) Thyroid cancer (shaded) with full thickness (stage IV) tracheal invasion showing anterior and transverse views; (B) Dashed lines show extent of sleeve resection; (C) Intraluminal extent of disease on transverse section; (D) After resection and placement of sutures; (E) Sutures tied extraluminally

A Penrose drain is passed across the plane and around the entire trachea to separate it from the esophagus, only as far as the segments to be resected. Prior to placing an incision on the trachea, the endotracheal tube should be advanced beyond the site of resection. Using a sharp number 15 blade, the membranous trachea is incised along the superior border of the planned segment of resection, contralateral to the site of tracheal invasion. This will allow visualization of the tumor during the remainder of the resection. The incision is extended transversely to the contralateral side, keeping an adequate margin above the tumor. The incision is then extended circumferentially around the initial point of entry, mobilizing the upper limit of the 'sleeve'. Similarly, the inferior incision should be placed in the membranous trachea contralateral to the tumor, extending across and circumferentially, while ensuring an adequate margin between the tumor and the line of resection. A heavy nylon suture is used to stabilize the distal tracheal stump and prevent retraction into the mediastinum. The cuff of the endotracheal tube is deflated and the tube is withdrawn into the larynx allowing the specimen to be removed. The tube is then readvanced into the distal trachea and cuff is reinflated.

End-to-end tracheal anastomosis should be tension free and performed with interrupted sutures, usually monocryl or vicryl 2-0 sutures. If only short tracheal segments (< 3 cm) are removed, then these can be anastomosed primarily without any mobilization of the trachea or larynx. Segments longer than 3–4 cm require further mobilization.

Further mobilization: Figure 5 shows the various maneuvers and length of trachea that can be mobilized by each maneuver. Suprahyoid release of the larynx is performed by detaching the suprahyoid muscles (geniohyoid, mylohyoid and hyoglossus) from the hyoid bone using electrocautery. This should be performed carefully, especially along the lateral edge of the hyoid to prevent injury to the hypoglossal nerve and lingual artery. Detachment of the strap muscles attached to the hyoid (infrahyoid release) is also very helpful for the 'laryngeal drop'. The neck should then be placed in flexion. This usually requires removal of shoulder rolls or flexion of the head plate from the surgical table. If additional length is required, the hilum may have to be released and even further mobilization may necessitate bronchial reimplantation, although these are rarely used and excessive mediastinal mobilization may devascularize the trachea. The trachea is then anastomosed using interrupted monocryl or vicryl 2-0 suture, starting in the midline posteriorly and working laterally. The stitch is placed around the superior and inferior tracheal rings and knots are tied extraluminally. It may be necessary to withdraw the endotracheal tube proximally to facilitate suturing of the posterior wall. Once the posterior anastomosis is complete, the endotracheal tube is advanced and the anterior wall is anastomosed by placing

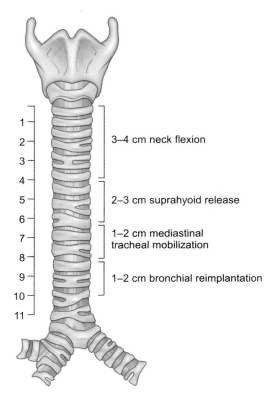

Fig. 5: Tracheal length gained by maneuvers. Neck flexion and suprahyoid release may be performed to close large tracheal defects. Mediastinal mobilization and bronchial reimplantation should be performed with caution in selected cases

the sutures, but not tying them, until all sutures have been placed. Occasionally, a segment of cricoid needs to be excised together with the sleeve resection. In this case, a sharp Mayo scissor may be used to make the cuts across the cricoid. The inferior tracheal stump can then be fashioned to rotate and fit into the cricoid defect like a piece of a puzzle as in Figures 6A to C.

Once the anastomosis is completed, the wound is flooded with saline and a Valsalva maneuver is performed with the cuff deflated to exclude air leaks. The strap muscles can be used as a buttress over the anastomotic line and the wound is closed in layers over a Penrose drain. After skin closure, a heavy nylon suture is placed through the submental and presternal skin of tissues to keep the neck in flexion and avoid inadvertent neck extension for a period of 10 days postoperatively.

Reoperative or Postradiotherapy Surgery

There are a number of important considerations when dealing with a neck, which has been operated or irradiated before. Dissection can be difficult with an increased risk of injury to the recurrent laryngeal nerve. Hence, nerve monitoring systems may be invaluable. Tracheal dissection should be minimized in order to limit devascularization. It has been suggested that fresh vascularized tissue can be used to wrap around and protect the tracheal anastomosis. The most popular flap in this scenario is a pedicled omentum, although other pedicled and free flaps have been described.

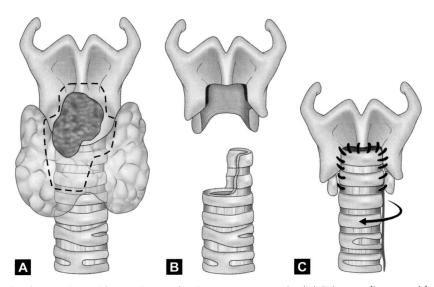

Figs 6A to C: Cricotracheal resection with rotation and primary anastomosis. (A) Primary disease with cricotracheal invasion with dashed line showing extent of resection; (B) Lower segment of trachea fashioned to fit the cricoid defect; (C) Lower segment rotated and anastomosis performed to reconstruct cricoid defect

POSTOPERATIVE TREATMENT

After satisfactory tracheal anastomosis, the patient may be extubated in the operating room under optimal circumstances or left intubated overnight and extubated with minimal laryngeal irritation the next day. The submental suture is usually kept in place for 10–14 days, after which it is removed. Drains remain for 2–3 days or until the drainage is less than 30 ml a day. There is usually no need for postoperative antibiotics and the patient can start on a liquid diet, progressing to soft diet within 2–3 days. The patient is monitored for hypocalcemia with serial serum calcium levels and treated accordingly. Thyroxine replacement is commenced the day after surgery.

Most patients require adjuvant treatment to improve local control. While radioiodine is commonly used, many of these tumors are less-differentiated and hence, tend not to be iodine avid. As such, they may not respond to radioiodine therapy. External beam radiotherapy is an alternative adjuvant radiotherapy, which can be used to augment the local control, but is no substitute for complete tumor resection with the adequate margins. Moreover, radiation greatly increases the risk of future airway resection, even when vascularized tissue such as omentum is used to bolster the anastomosis. Several studies have been undertaken to study different methods of tracheal reconstruction in experimental animals, specifically replacement using tracheal transplants. However, their applicability in human beings is still under investigation.

HIGHLIGHTS

I. Indications
- Primary or recurrent thyroid cancer with tracheal invasion
- Recurrent or persistent central compartment nodal disease with tracheal invasion.

II. Contraindications
- Inoperable primary tumor
  - Extensive tracheal invasion of < 5–7 cm involving carina
  - Prevertebral muscle invasion
  - Carotid encasement
  - Anaplastic thyroid cancer.
- Extensive distant metastasis
- Medically unfit for tracheal resection.

III. Special Preoperative Considerations
- Evaluate airway with fiberoptic laryngoscopy for intubation with senior anesthesiologist
- Preoperative imaging to define extent of invasion
- Preoperative biopsy to exclude anaplastic thyroid cancer
- PET scan to exclude extensive metastatic disease.

IV. Special Intraoperative Considerations
- Fiberoptic intubation by experienced anesthesiologist or surgeon with small endotracheal tube
- Constant communication between surgeon and anesthesiologist
- Protect recurrent laryngeal nerve using nerve monitoring system, careful dissection and retraction, when mobilizing trachea.
- Minimize tracheal dissection to avoid devascularization
- Avoid injury to hypoglossal nerve and lingual artery when performing suprahyoid release.

V. Special Postoperative Considerations
- Avoid traumatic extubation
- Maintain chin stitch to keep neck flexed for 10–14 days
- Watch for subcutaneous emphysema as an early warning to anastomotic breakdown.

VI. Complications
- Anastomotic breakdown
- Subcutaneous emphysema
- Hematoma
- Recurrent laryngeal nerve injury
- Hypoparathyroidism.

ADDITIONAL READING

1. Gilbert RW, Neligan PC. Microsurgical laryngotracheal reconstruction. Clin Plast Surg. 2005;32(3):293-301,v.
2. Grillo HC, Suen HC, Mathisen DJ, et al. Resectional management of thyroid carcinoma invading the airway. Ann Thorac Surg. 1992;54(1):3-10.
3. Grillo HC. Tracheal blood supply. Ann Thorac Surg. 1977;24(2):99.
4. Honings J, Stephen AE, Marres HA, et al. The management of thyroid carcinoma invading the larynx or trachea. Laryngoscope. 2010;120(4):682-9.
5. Kim AW, Maxhimer JB, Quiros RM, et al. Surgical management of well differentiated thyroid cancer locally invasive to the respiratory tract. J Am Coll Surg. 2005;201(4):619-27.
6. Park CS, Suh KW, Min JS, et al. Cartilage-shaving procedure for the control of tracheal cartilage invasion by thyroid carcinoma. Head Neck. 1993;15(4):289-91.
7. Price DL, Wong RJ, Randolph GW, et al. Invasive thyroid cancer: management of the trachea and esophagus. Otolaryngol Clin North Am. 2008;41(6):1155-68, ix–x.
8. Shin DH, Mark EJ, Suen SJ, et al. Pathologic staging of papillary carcinoma of the thyroid with airway invasion based on the anatomic manner of extension to the trachea: a clinicopathologic study based on 22 patients who underwent thyroidectomy and airway resection. Hum Pathol. 1993;24(8):866-70.

Chapter 18

Excision and Reconstruction of Recurrent Pleomorphic Adenoma of the Parotid Gland

Adam S Jacobson, Mark L Urken

INTRODUCTION

Pleomorphic adenoma, also known as benign mixed tumor (BMT), is the most common tumor of the parotid gland. It is a benign neoplasm, which is nontender to palpation, firm and slow growing. The current standard treatment for a pleomorphic adenoma of the parotid gland is surgical resection through excision of the superficial lobe, deep lobe or the total parotid with facial nerve identification and preservation. Historically, local excision procedures, i.e. enucleation were associated with local recurrence rates ranging from 20% to 45%.[1-3] With the introduction of the more comprehensive procedure of parotidectomy with facial nerve identification and preservation, the local recurrence rates have decreased between 1% and 5%.[2,4-6] Although, the rate of recurrence is very low using contemporary surgical techniques, these benign tumors can and do still recur; either because of capsule rupture with tumor spillage, incomplete resection of microscopic extensions beyond the pseudocapsule or due to occult multifocal disease.[1,3,7] Recurrence can occur up to 30 years after the initial surgery.[8]

Regardless of the etiology of the recurrence, the treatment of recurrent pleomorphic adenomas remain a challenge and with each successive surgery further recurrence becomes increasingly likely.[9-11] Unfortunately, these recurrences are often multifocal and intimately involved with the facial nerve. Temporary and permanent weakness or paralysis of the facial nerve is not uncommon, while treating this disease. Reported control rates after treatment of recurrent pleomorphic adenomas range from 37% to 90%.[4,9,11-15]

External beam radiation therapy (XRT) has been utilized in the setting of a recurrent BMT as adjuvant therapy, but remains controversial. While some studies have reported improved local control with adjuvant radiotherapy when compared with historic controls treated with surgery alone, others have shown no significant improvement in outcome.[16-23]

Reoperative parotidectomy is a challenge because the function of the facial nerve remains extremely important to patients on a variety of different levels (cosmesis, oral competence and eye hygiene). Yet, adequate resection of a recurrent BMT takes precedence over concerns about the facial nerve function because of the potential for malignant transformation. Some series report an incidence of carcinoma ex pleomorphic adenoma, as high as 9% with each local recurrence.[8,11,24,25]

PREOPERATIVE EVALUATION AND ANESTHESIA

All patients scheduled for the surgery are evaluated preoperatively by a head and neck surgeon. If a facial nerve sacrifice is planned, the patient is extensively counseled on the sequela of this decision and a facial reanimation procedure is planned in combination with the resection.

Radiological evaluation includes axial and coronal computed tomography (CT) or magnetic resonance imaging (MRI) of the head and neck. Figure 1 shows a typical preoperative axial MRI scan of a patient with multiple recurrent BMTs of the parotid gland.

If the recurrent mass appears to have grown rapidly or has overlying skin changes (erythema, fixation to underlying mass), a fine needle aspiration biopsy is performed to evaluate the possibility of malignant transformation. Additionally, if there is a new onset of facial nerve paresis or paralysis, malignant transformation is most likely, developed. All the procedures of surgery, for this disease, are performed under general anesthesia without muscle relaxation so that the facial nerve activity can be monitored intraoperatively.

SURGICAL TECHNIQUE

The surgical techniques in three different case studies (case 1, 2 and 3) has been illustrated in Figures 2 to 4 respectively.

After the induction of anesthesia the patient's neck and face are cleaned, prepped and draped in the standard surgical fashion. The old incision line from the prior resection of the BMT is examined. If there is recurrence at the incision line, a new incision is drawn around the old scar and the skin with the underlying tumor is removed en bloc. If the recurrence (Fig. 2A) is distant from the original incision line, then it is safe to reincise through the original scar. A skin flap is elevated in a plane deep to the subcutaneous fat as in Figure 2B. If the recurrence is a subcutaneous nodule, very superficial skin flap is elevated. Once the entire parotid gland or bed is exposed, the sites of recurrence are identified and then, the facial nerve is identified as in Figure 2F. Facial nerve identification and dissection can be performed anterograde or retrograde as in Figure 3C. The traditional technique of anterograde dissection involves, exposing the tympanomastoid suture line and identifying the main trunk of the facial nerve (Fig. 4C) as it exits the stylomastoid foramen. If this cannot be accomplished because the tumor is obstructing its identification, then the mastoid can be drilled down to allow for identification of the vertical segment of the facial nerve (Fig. 4D) within the temporal bone. The

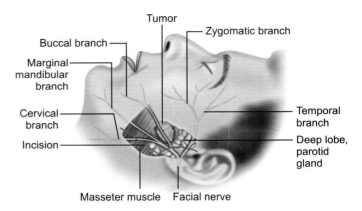

Fig. 2A: Case #1. Illustration showing recurrent tumor deep to the buccal branch of the facial nerve

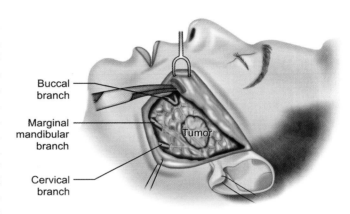

Fig. 2B: Case #1. Illustration showing skin flap elevated with exposure of the entire parotid gland. The distal branches of the facial nerve have been identified

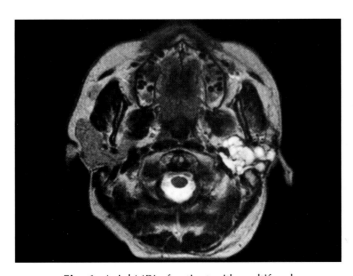

Fig. 1: Axial MRI of patient with multifocal recurrence of BMT

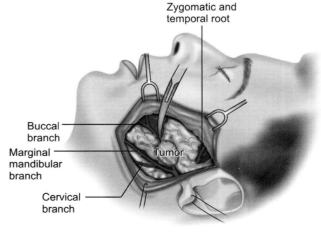

Fig. 2C: Case #1. Illustration of retrograde dissection of the buccal branch of CN VII with a Jacobson Mosquito

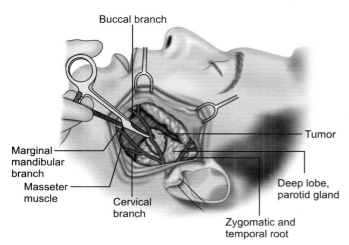

Fig. 2D: Case #1. Illustration of dissection of the tumor from the deep surface of buccal branch of the facial nerve

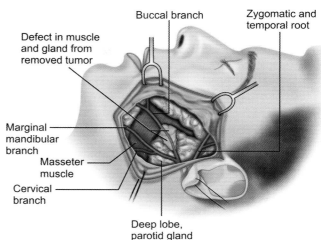

Fig. 2E: Case #1. Illustration of the tumor removed and preservation of all branches of the facial nerve with resultant defect deep to the nerve

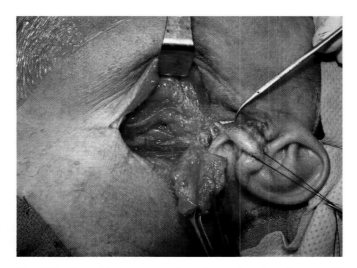

Fig. 2F: Case #1. Intraoperative photo showing the parotid bed after tumor removal with preservation of the marginal and buccal branches of the facial nerve

nerve can then be traced anterograde from that point toward the tumor. A Jacobson mosquito forcep (Fig. 2C) is used to trace the nerve and dissect the overlying tissue for complete exposure. If the tumor is intimately associated with the facial nerve (Fig. 3A) and either obstructs anterograde dissection or the main trunk cannot be identified, the surgeon can locate each individual distal branch (Fig. 3B) of the facial nerve (temporal, zygomatic, buccal, marginal and cervical) and dissect in a retrograde fashion with the Jacobson mosquito forcep.

Once identification of the main trunk of the nerve and the five terminal branches has been performed, the decision must be made to sacrifice (Fig. 3D) or preserve the nerve. If

the nerve is to be sacrificed, preservation of the nondiseased nerve, as much as possible, is crucial for performing a successful interpositional nerve graft. If the nerve is able to be preserved (Fig. 3E), all of the overlying parotid tissue, which is lateral to the facial nerve is removed en block with the tumor. If the tumor is deep to the facial nerve, then the nerve branches are gently dissected free from the underlying tissue (Fig. 2D) and the tumor is delivered (Fig. 2E). A facial nerve monitor is used throughout this procedure to facilitate the identification of the nerve.

If a section of the facial nerve is resected, interposition of a nerve graft is performed, when the proximal and distal ends of the nerve cannot be coapted in a tension-free manner. Neurorrhaphies are performed under microscopic visualization with 9-0 nylon suture, approximating epineurium of the native facial nerve to the epineurium of the interposed nerve graft. The greater auricular nerve or the sural nerve can easily be harvested and used as an interpositional (aka) cable graft as in Figure 4F. The sural nerve is a good nerve graft for facial nerve reconstruction because it has a good diameter match for this cranial nerve and it has sufficient length to bridge the extensive nerve gaps. Since this is a sensory nerve, the neurological deficit that results from the harvest of this nerve causes little morbidity. The key landmark for locating the sural nerve is the lateral malleolus. The initial incision is placed posterior to the lateral malleolus and the nerve is located medial to the short saphenous vein. The nerve is dissected from distal to proximal until a sufficient length and sufficient branching pattern is obtained. In an effort to prevent neuroma formation, the proximal stump of the sural nerve is sutured into the gastrocnemius muscle.

Since nerve grafting (Fig. 4G) results in an acute facial paralysis and the effects of nerve regeneration takes months to realize, there must be both a short and long-term plan to rehabilitate these patients. In addition to having significant cosmetic implications, facial paralysis affects patient's ability to maintain oral competence, articulate and maintain adequate eye protection.

When approaching a patient, who has a facial nerve paralysis, one must take a segmental approach to facial rehabilitation by reanimating the forehead, eye and the mouth independently. The most important complication of facial nerve paralysis is the avoidance of exposure keratitis and corneal ulceration, which can lead to decreased visual acuity and blindness. Reanimation may require surgery on the upper eyelid alone and/or in combination with lower eyelid surgery. Gold weight implantation into the upper eyelid remains the most popular upper lid procedure. Lower lid ectropion can be addressed by a horizontal lid shortening procedure or a lower lid sling using a tarsal strip technique.

Lower facial rehabilitation can be approached with a static or dynamic reanimation procedure. The goal of both these approaches is to return facial symmetry and achieve oral competence. Dynamic reanimation is accomplished by transposition of the temporalis or masseter muscles. A temporalis transposition is performed by harvesting a 2 cm wide strip of temporalis muscle from the central one third of the muscle belly, pedicling it proximally and transposing it to the corner of the mouth. Prolene sutures are then used to attach

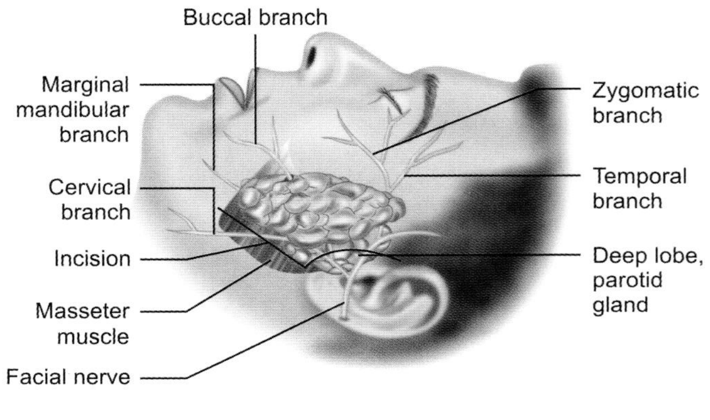

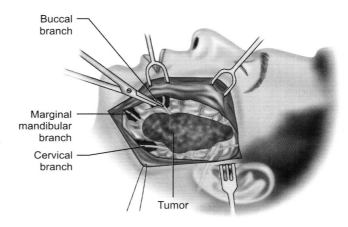

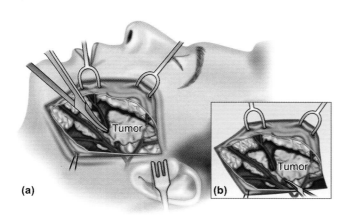

Fig. 3A: Case #2. Illustration showing a large tumor involving multiple branches of the facial nerve

Fig. 3B: Case #2. Illustration showing identification of the distal branches of the facial nerve and retrograde dissection along the branches

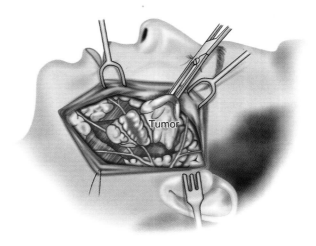

Fig. 3C: Case #2. Illustration with two parts. Part a shows retrograde dissection along the branches of the facial nerve, which are involved with the tumor. Part b shows anterograde dissection from the main trunk of the facial nerve toward the tumor

Fig. 3D: Case #2. Illustration showing all branches of the facial nerve skeletonized and delivery of the tumor from deep to the nerves

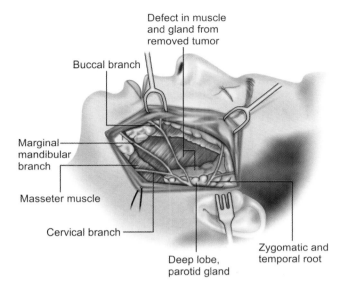

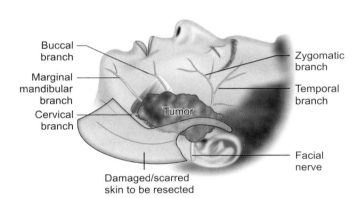

Fig. 4A: Case #3. Illustration showing a large recurrence intimately involved with all branches of the facial nerve. Additionally, the overlying skin is severely damaged and scarred by multiple prior surgeries. The skin is to be resected en bloc with the tumor and the facial nerve

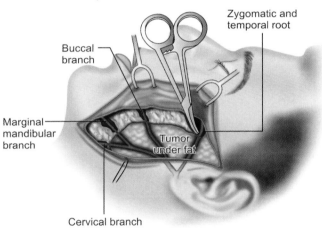

Fig. 3E: Case #2. Illustration showing preservation of all branches of the facial nerve with resultant defect from tumor removal from deep to the nerves

Fig. 4B: Case #3. The initial incision is made and the distal branches of the facial nerve are identified

POSTOPERATIVE TREATMENT

After a recurrent BMT is resected the postoperative care can range from simple to complicated, depending on whether a facial nerve sacrifice is performed or not. In the case of resection of a recurrent BMT without facial nerve sacrifice, Penrose drains are utilized for passive drainage. A Barton's dressing is often placed to decrease postoperative fluid collection. In the case of a resection of a BMT with facial nerve sacrifice, meticulous postoperative care is critical to prevent exposure keratitis. Artificial tears are placed in the affected eye every 3–4 hours. Additionally, lacrilube is utilized at night to obtain a long-lasting lubrication of the affected eye.

The role of adjuvant radiotherapy remains questionable. Jackson et al. recommend postoperative radiotherapy in cases with positive resection margins or with suspected intraoperative tumor spillage.[26] Renehan et al. recommend adjuvant XRT for multifocal recurrences.[19,27]

the muscle to the orbicularis oris. The defect left by harvest of the middle third of the temporalis muscle can be filled with a temporoparietal fascia flap, raised prior to the temporalis muscle transfer. Static rehabilitation techniques restore facial symmetry and improve oral competence, but does not allow dynamic change during facial expression (smiling). Autologous tissue, such as fascia lata can be used to perform a static sling from the zygoma to the orbicularis oris muscle. Alloplastic materials such as Gore-Tex® can also be utilized, but should be avoided if radiation therapy is considered as a treatment strategy, due to the increased risk of infection and extrusion. Overcorrection during placement is important due to stretching, which occurs over time of the static sling.

Douglas et al. recommend radiotherapy for selected cases, i.e. when complete extirpation is not possible and sacrifice of the facial nerve is necessary or after multiple recurrences.[18] Finally, Glas et al. recommend adjuvant XRT for difficult cases, in which further surgical treatment of recurrent disease is not recommended for technical reasons.[28] Most of the literature consists of retrospective analysis of patient's outcome with and without the use of adjuvant XRT. Prospective trials with and without XRT are necessary to determine the efficacy of XRT in obtaining local control.

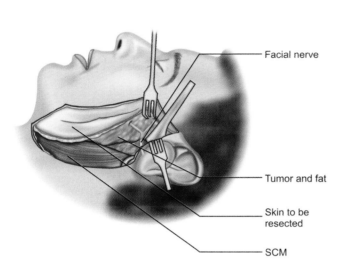

Fig. 4C: Case #3. The main trunk of the facial nerve is identified

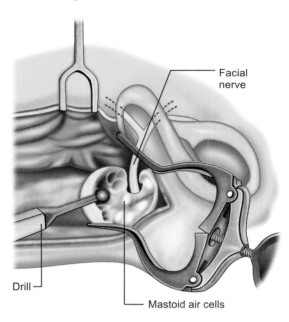

Fig. 4D: Case #3. The mastoid is drilled down to identify the vertical segment of the facial nerve to gain extra length of the nerve

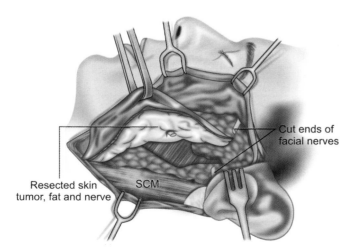

Fig. 4E: Case #3. The radical parotidectomy is completed, leaving the distal branches of the facial nerve and the main trunk

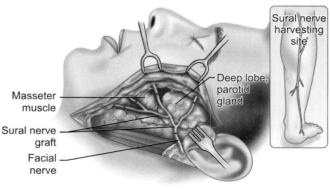

Fig. 4F: Case #3. The sural nerve is harvested and used as a cable graft between the main trunk of the facial nerve and the distal branches

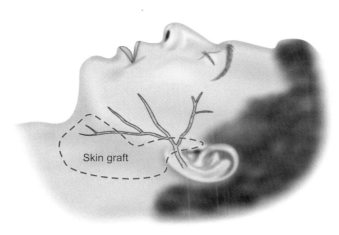

Fig. 4G: Case #3. Illustration showing the nerve graft in place and the skin graft replaces the resected skin segment

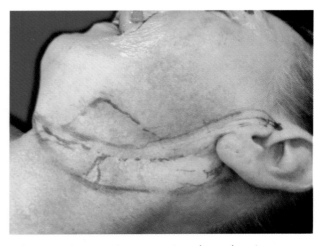

Fig. 4H: Case #3. Intraoperative photo showing extent of skin to be resected

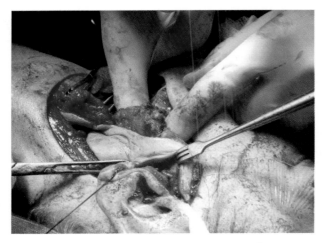

Fig. 4I: Case #3. Intraoperative photo showing skin resection and identification of styloid process by palpation

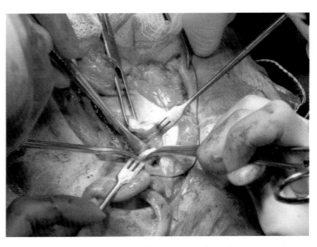

Fig. 4J: Case #3. Intraoperative photo showing identification of the main trunk of the facial nerve

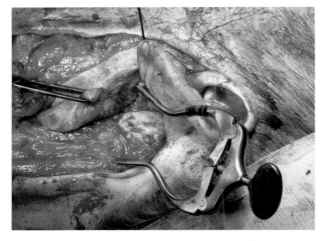

Fig. 4K: Case #3. Intraoperative photo showing exposure of mastoid

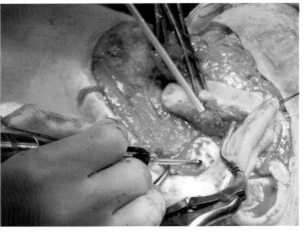

Fig. 4L: Case #3. Intraoperative photo showing drilling of mastoid

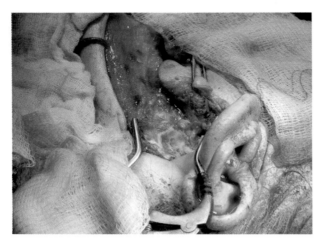

Fig. 4M: Case #3. Intraoperative photo showing identification of the vertical segment of the facial nerve

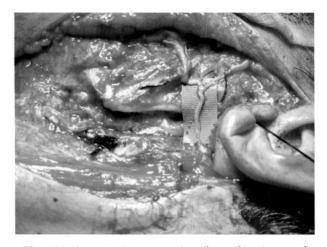

Fig. 4N: Case #3. Intraoperative photo showing sural cable graft in place

HIGHLIGHTS

I. Indications
- First recurrence
  - Facial nerve identification and preservation
  - En bloc resection of tumor and involved structures (i.e. skin, facial nerve).
- Second recurrence or more
  - Facial nerve identification and preservation, if possible
  - Facial nerve sacrifice, if tumor is intimately involved with nerve
  - En bloc resection of tumor and involved structures (i.e. skin, facial nerve)
  - Adjuvant external beam radiotherapy.

II. Contraindications
None.

III. Special Preoperative Considerations
- Facial nerve function
- Number of previous recurrences.

IV. Special Intraoperative Considerations
- Multifocal vs unifocal disease
- Intimacy of recurrence with facial nerve
- Involvement of overlying skin.

V. Special Postoperative Considerations
- Meticulous eye care
- Facial rehabilitation
- Margin status.

VI. Complications
- Facial nerve sacrifice

- Exposure keratitis
- Oral incompetence
- Facial asymmetry
- Future recurrences with increasing likelihood of malignant transformation.

REFERENCES

1. Donovan DT, Conley JJ. Capsular significance in parotid tumor surgery: reality and myths of lateral lobectomy. Laryngoscope 1984;94(3):324-9.
2. Leverstein H, van der Wal JE, Tiwari RM, et al. Surgical management of 246 previously untreated pleomorphic adenomas of the parotid gland. Br J Surg. 1997;84(3):399-403.
3. Witt RL. The significance of the margin in parotid surgery for pleomorphic adenoma. Laryngoscope. 2002;112(12):2141-54.
4. Foote FW, Frazell EL. Tumors of the major salivary glands. Cancer. 1953;6(6):1065-133.
5. Woods JE, Chong GC, Beahrs OH. Experience with 1,360 primary parotid tumors. Am J Surg. 1975;130(4):460-2.
6. Krolls SO, Boyers RC. Mixed tumors of salivary glands. Long-term follow-up. Cancer. 1972;30(1):276-81.
7. Stennert E, Guntinas-Lichius O, Klussmann JP, et al. Histopathology of pleomorphic adenoma in the parotid gland: a prospective unselected series of 100 cases. Laryngoscope. 2001;111(12):2195-200.
8. Zbären P, Tschumi I, Nuyens M, et al. Recurrent pleomorphic adenoma of the parotid gland. Am J Surg. 2005;189(2):203-7.
9. Maran AG, Mackenzie IJ, Stanley RE. Recurrent pleomorphic adenomas of the parotid gland. Arch Otolaryngol. 1984;110(3):167-71.

10. O'Dwyer PJ, Farrar WB, Finkelmeier WR, et al. Facial nerve sacrifice and tumor recurrence in primary and recurrent benign parotid tumors. Am J Surg. 1986;152(4):442-5.

11. Phillips PP, Olsen KD. Recurrent pleomorphic adenoma of the parotid gland: report of 126 cases and a review of the literature. Ann Otol Rhinol Laryngol. 1995;104(2):100-4.

12. Fee WE, Goffinet DR, Calcaterra TC. Recurrent mixed tumors of the parotid gland—results of surgical therapy. Laryngoscope. 1978;88(2 Pt 1):265-73.

13. Myssiorek D, Ruah CB, Hybels RL. Recurrent pleomorphic adenomas of the parotid gland. Head Neck. 1990;12(4):332-6.

14. Samson MJ, Metson R, Wang CC, et al. Preservation of the facial nerve in the management of recurrent pleomorphic adenoma. Laryngoscope. 1991;101(10):1060-2.

15. Niparko JK, Beauchamp ML, Krause CJ, et al. Surgical treatment of recurrent pleomorphic adenoma of the parotid gland. Arch Otolaryngol Head Neck Surg. 1986;112(11):1180-4.

16. Carew JF, Spiro RH, Singh B, et al. Treatment of recurrent pleomorphic adenomas of the parotid gland. Otolaryngol Head Neck Surg. 1999;121(5):539-42.

17. Gleave EN, Whittaker JS, Nicholson A. Salivary tumors—experience over thirty years. Clin Otolaryngol Allied Sci. 1979;4(4):247-57.

18. Douglas JG, Einck J, Austin-Seymour M, et al. Neutron radiotherapy for recurrent pleomorphic adenomas of major salivary glands. Head Neck. 2001;23(12):1037-42.

19. Renehan A, Gleave EN, McGurk M. An analysis of the treatment of 114 patients with recurrent pleomorphic adenomas of the parotid gland. Am J Surg. 1996;172(6):710-4.

20. Chen AM, Garcia J, Bucci MK, et al. Recurrent pleomorphic adenoma of the parotid gland: long-term outcome of patients treated with radiation therapy. Int J Radiat Oncol Biol Phys. 2006;66(4):1031-5.

21. Friedrich RE, Li L, Knop J, et al. Pleomorphic adenoma of the salivary glands: analysis of 94 patients. Anticancer Res. 2005;25(3A):1703-5.

22. Liu FF, Rotstein L, Davison AJ, et al. Benign parotid adenomas: a review of the Princess Margaret Hospital experience. Head Neck. 1995;17(3):177-83.

23. Dawson AK. Radiation therapy in recurrent pleomorphic adenoma of the parotid. Int J Radiat Oncol Biol Phys. 1989;16(3):819-21.

24. Olsen KD, Lewis JE. Carcinoma ex pleomorphic adenoma: a clinicopathologic review. Head Neck. 2001;23(9):705-12.

25. Lewis JE, Olsen KD, Sebo TJ. Carcinoma ex pleomorphic adenoma: pathologic analysis of 73 cases. Hum Pathol. 2001;32(6):596-604.

26. Jackson SR, Roland NJ, Clarke RW, et al. Recurrent pleomorphic adenoma. J Laryngol Otol. 1993;107(6):546-9.

27. Renehan A, Gleave EN, Hancock BD, et al. Long term follow-up of over 1000 patients with salivary gland tumours treated in a single centre. Br J Surg. 1996;83(12):1750-4.

28. Glas AS, Vermey A, Hollema H, et al. Surgical treatment of recurrent pleomorphic adenoma of the parotid gland: a clinical analysis of 52 patients. Head Neck. 2001;23(4):311-6.

ADDITIONAL READING

1. Carew JF, Spiro RH, Singh B, et al. Treatment of recurrent pleomorphic adenomas of the parotid gland. Otolaryngol Head Neck Surg. 1999;121(5):539-42.

2. Chen AM, Garcia J, Bucci MK, et al. Recurrent pleomorphic adenoma of the parotid gland: long-term outcome of patients treated with radiation therapy. Int J Radiat Oncol Biol Phys. 2006;66(4):1031-5.

3. Donovan DT, Conley JJ. Capsular significance in parotid tumor surgery: reality and myths of lateral lobectomy. Laryngoscope. 1984;94(3):324-9.

4. Leverstein H, van der Wal JE, Tiwari RM, et al. Surgical management of 246 previously untreated pleomorphic adenomas of the parotid gland. Br J Surg. 1997;84(3):399-403.

5. Olsen KD, Lewis JE. Carcinoma ex pleomorphic adenoma: a clinicopathologic review. Head Neck. 2001;23(9):705-12.

6. Phillips PP, Olsen KD. Recurrent pleomorphic adenoma of the parotid gland: report of 126 cases and a review of the literature. Ann Otol Rhinol Laryngol. 1995;104(2):100-4.

7. Samson MJ, Metson R, Wang CC, et al. Preservation of the facial nerve in the management of recurrent pleomorphic adenoma. Laryngoscope. 1991;101(10):1060-2.

8. Zbären P, Tschumi I, Nuyens M, et al. Recurrent pleomorphic adenoma of the parotid gland. Am J Surg. 2005;189(2):203-7.

Chapter 19

Parotidectomy with Facial Nerve Resection

Jose P Zevallos, Ehab Y Hanna

INTRODUCTION

Parotidectomy with facial nerve resection is indicated in the treatment of aggressive malignancies of the parotid gland or surrounding structures that have infiltrated the facial nerve. Several primary salivary gland malignancies have a propensity toward perineural invasion, including adenoid cystic carcinoma, salivary duct carcinoma and high-grade mucoepidermoid carcinoma. Additionally, aggressive cutaneous malignancies or tumors arising from other adjacent structures can require partial or complete facial nerve sacrifice in order to establish negative margins.

The extent of resection is dictated by the primary tumor site and its invasion into surrounding structures, and can include the mandible, temporomandibular joint, the temporal bone, the infratemporal fossa and the skin. Adjuvant procedures are often required when treating these tumors, including resection of facial or cervical skin, mandibulectomy or lateral temporal bone resection. In addition, a neck dissection may be indicated when regional metastasis is present or suspected. (Vicentis, 2005)

Re-establishing facial nerve continuity should be considered after resection, whenever oncologically sound. Primary end-to-end anastomosis is the preferred technique, although a cable nerve graft is an acceptable alternative. Patients undergoing radical parotidectomy with facial nerve sacrifice often require complex reconstruction that may include local skin flaps, myocutaneous flaps or free tissue transfer [(Bova, 2004) (Teknos, 2003)]. Postoperative radiotherapy to the parotid bed and ipsilateral cervical lymph nodes is offered to most patients undergoing radical parotidectomy.

PREOPERATIVE EVALUATION

A thorough history and physical examination is crucial in all patients undergoing parotidectomy with possible facial nerve sacrifice. Pain and impaired facial nerve function are ominous signs of malignancy with nerve infiltration and patients should be counseled on the possible need for facial nerve sacrifice. The degree and distribution of facial nerve impairment should be well documented prior to surgery. Patients should undergo a complete medical evaluation prior to surgery, particularly if significant comorbidities are present. Preoperative imaging studies are also important in identifying the extent of tumor and formulating a surgical plan. Magnetic resonance imaging (MRI) is particularly useful in detecting neurotropic spread, which will often be detected as enhancement or widening of the facial nerve. Additionally, MRI allows accurate tumor delineation and degree of infiltration into surrounding structures. Computed tomography (CT) is useful preoperatively to evaluate the skull base, invasion of the mandible of maxilla and involvement of the temporal bone. Fine needle aspiration biopsy and skilled cytological assessment is very helpful in the preoperative evaluation of aggressive tumors with characteristics of malignancy.

The treatment plan for patients with advanced parotid malignancies requires a complete multidisciplinary evaluation, including head and neck surgery, medical oncology and radiation oncology. The patient requiring a lateral temporal bone resection or mastoidectomy should also be evaluated by an otologic surgeon preoperatively. A CT of the temporal bone with thin cuts may be helpful in identifying tumor invasion as well as in defining intratemporal facial nerve anatomy. A preoperative baseline audiogram should also be considered. Dental extractions can be planned at the time of tumor resection, if radiation therapy is required postoperatively. Also, a medical oncologist should assist in determining the need for induction or postoperative chemotherapy and a reconstructive surgeon should evaluate patients in which large defects are anticipated. Finally, an ophthalmologist may be required to address eye care postoperatively.

SURGICAL TECHNIQUE

After induction of anesthesia, the patient is prepped and draped in sterile fashion. The choice of parotidectomy incision depends on the extent of tumor and the need for adjuvant procedures, such as neck dissection, lateral temporal bone resection or mastoidectomy (Fig. 1A). The incision is carried down through skin and subcutaneous tissues. If the overlying facial and neck skin are to be preserved, subplatysmal flaps are raised in the neck and a supraparotid flap is raised on the face. Tumors involving the skin require a large cutaneous resection (Fig. 1B). The posterior border of the parotid gland is identified and dissected free from the cartilaginous external auditory canal. Key surgical anatomic landmarks are identified, including the sternocleidomastoid

and posterior digastric muscles, the greater auricular nerve (Fig. 2) and the tragal pointer of the cartilaginous external auditory canal (Fig. 3). The main trunk of the facial nerve can be identified reliably approximately 1 cm inferior to the tragal pointer and at the depth of the posterior digastric muscle (Figs 4A and B). If tumor extends posteriorly into the external auditory canal or mastoid, a lateral temporal bone resection is required. In this case, the mastoid segment of the facial nerve is identified intratemporally (Fig. 5). The stylomastoid foramen is identified and the nerve is traced peripherally into the parotid gland.

Once the facial nerve is identified, the surgeon must determine the extent of tumor infiltration and assess whether all or part of the facial nerve is to be sacrificed. The nerve is typically traced from proximal to distal and all branches that are grossly involved with tumor are resected along with the specimen. If the main trunk of the facial nerve is grossly infiltrated by tumor, the nerve can be traced intratemporally and resected. Distal cut branches of the facial nerve are identified and tagged. It is important to rule out microscopic tumor invasion by frozen section of all preserved proximal and distal facial nerve remnants.

The tumor is resected circumferentially with a wide margin of normal tissue. The medial limit of the dissection is the parapharyngeal space, masseter muscle and mandible, while the lateral limit extends to and may include facial skin.

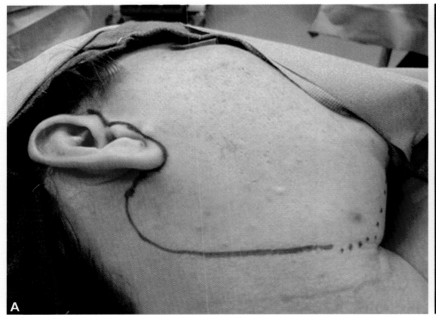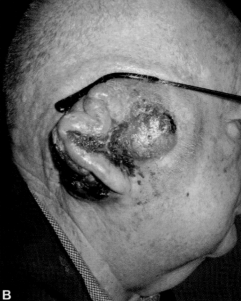

Figs 1A and B: The planned incision depends on the extent of tumor invasion and the need for adjuvant procedures. (A) Standard preauricular parotidectomy incision with extension for neck dissection; (B) Advanced tumors can involve significant cutaneous resection

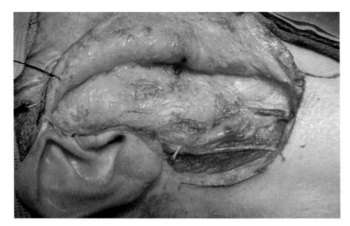

Fig. 2: Supraparotid and subplatysmal flaps are raised. Note important superficial landmarks: the external jugular vein, sternocleidomastoid, and greater auricular nerve

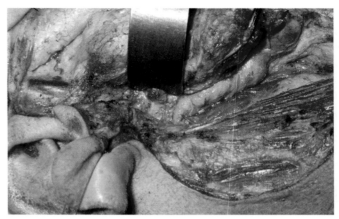

Fig. 3: The tragal pointer of the external auditory canal and posterior digastric muscle serve as landmarks for identification of the facial nerve

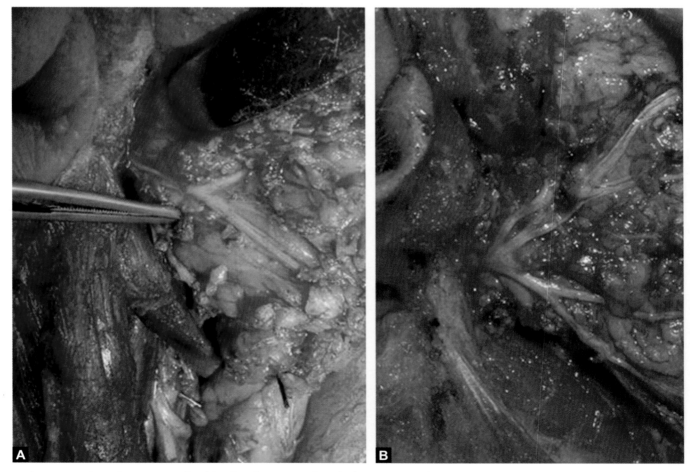

Figs 4A and B: The main trunk of the facial nerve is identified approximately 1 cm inferior to the tragal pointer and at the depth of the posterior digastric muscle. The nerve branches can be traced distally and assessed for tumor infiltration

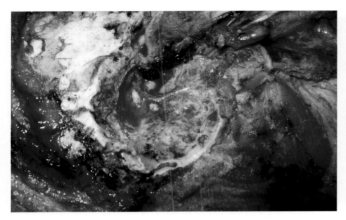

Fig. 5: The nerve can be identified intratemporally in the setting of mastoidectomy or lateral temporal bone resection. Note the resected end of the facial nerve at the stylomastoid foramen

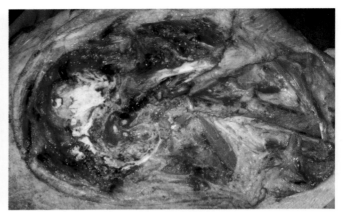

Fig. 6: A large defect after radical parotidectomy, mandibulectomy, lateral temporal bone resection and neck dissection

The superior extent of dissection is the zygomatic process, infratemporal fossa and skull base. Inferiorly, the dissection extends to the sternocleidomastoid and posterior digastric muscles. The surgeon must be cognizant of the several important structures as this dissection progresses, including the internal carotid artery and internal jugular vein medially, the hypoglossal nerve inferiorly and the skull base superiorly as in Figure 6.

After tumor extirpation and hemostasis has been achieved, attempt should be made at re-establishing facial nerve continuity. After frozen section has determined that the proximal and distal nerve remnants are free of tumor, nerve ends can be reapproximated using 9-0 prolene under microscopic visualization. If a large segment of nerve has been resected, a cable nerve graft using the greater auricular or sural nerve can be used (Figs 7A to C). It is important to assure that the greater auricular nerve is free of tumor prior to harvest. In many cases, the distal cut nerve ends are of insufficient size and length, precluding the possibility of neurorrhaphy.

The surgeon may elect to place a gold weight in the ipsilateral upper eyelid, if the upper branches of the facial nerve have been resected. This simple reanimation technique allows prevention of dry eye symptoms and protection of the cornea from exposure keratitis. After placement of a corneal shield, an incision is made in the supratarsal crease. The gold weight is inserted deep to the orbicularis muscle, inferior to the insertion of the levator palpebrae superioris and is sutured to the superficial tarsal capsule with 8-0 nylon placed through preformed holes in the gold weight. Consideration can also be given for tarsorrhaphy or a lower eyelid shortening procedure in order to provide additional corneal protection and rehabilitation of the lower eyelid.

Two bulb suction drains are then placed in the wound bed with care not to impinge on the facial nerve repair. If closure of the parotidectomy incision site is possible, inverted 3-0 vicryl sutures are used for platysmal reapproximation and 4-0 nylon for the skin. Larger defects require locoregional, pedicled or free flap reconstruction as in Figure 8.

POSTOPERATIVE CARE

The majority of patients undergoing parotidectomy with facial nerve resection can be transferred to surgical floor after a period of observation in the postoperative anesthesia care unit. The need for admission to the surgical intensive care unit (SICU) is dictated by the extent of surgery, the need for tracheostomy and the type of reconstruction. Patients undergoing microvascular reconstruction often require at least an overnight stay in the SICU for ventilator support and flap checks. Patients with a significant history of alcohol abuse must be monitored closely for signs of withdrawal and appropriate consultations should be sought for patients with significant medical comorbidities.

Postoperative eye care is essential in patients with complete loss of eye closure secondary to facial nerve resection. Lack of adequate care can result in corneal injury, eye dryness, exposure keratitis and blindness. In the early postoperative period, artificial tear solution should be applied several times throughout the day to the affected eye and a sterile ointment should be placed on the cornea prior to sleep. Additionally, many patients require tape to secure the eye closure during sleep and prevent corneal abrasions. Long-term eye protection can be provided by gold weight placement, tarsorrhaphy and/or lower lid shortening procedures as described above. Also, facial reanimation procedures can be considered after resection of the facial nerve.

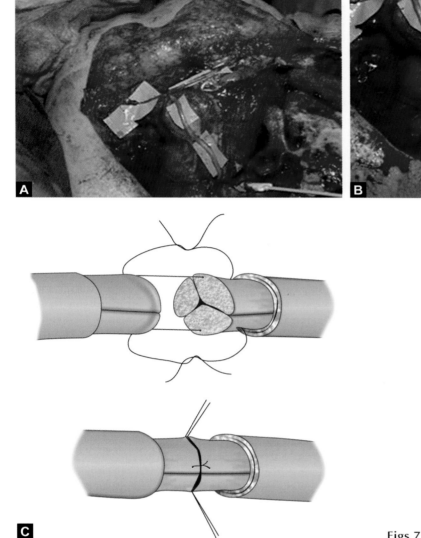

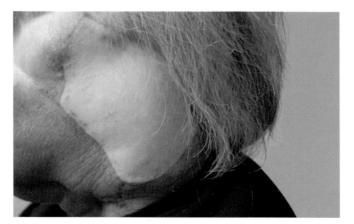

Figs 7A to C: Facial nerve repair using a cable graft

Fig. 8: A rectus abdominus flap is used for reconstruction after resection of a large cutaneous malignancy and radical parotidectomy

HIGHLIGHTS

I. Indications

- Indicated in the treatment of aggressive malignancies of the parotid gland or surrounding structures that have infiltrated the facial nerve.
- Adjuvant procedures are often required when treating these tumors, including resection of facial or cervical skin, mandibulectomy or lateral temporal bone resection.
- Re-establishing facial nerve continuity should be considered after resection whenever oncologically sound.
- Radical parotidectomy with facial nerve sacrifice often require complex reconstruction that may include local skin flaps, myocutaneous flaps or free tissue transfer.

II. Contraindications
- None.

III. Special Preoperative Considerations
- MRI and CT are complementary in the preoperative evaluation
- A complete multidisciplinary evaluation, including head and neck surgery, medical oncology and radiation oncology is required.

IV. Special Intraoperative Considerations
- Surgical technique
  - The choice of parotidectomy incision depends on the extent of tumor and the need for adjuvant procedures such as neck dissection, lateral temporal bone resection or mastoidectomy.
  - The main trunk of the facial nerve can be identified reliably, approximately 1 cm inferior to the tragal pointer and at the depth of the posterior digastric muscle.
  - Once the facial nerve is identified, the surgeon must determine the extent of tumor infiltration with frozen section.
  - Every attempt at facial nerve preservation should be made without compromising a sound oncologic resection.

- Primary neurorrhaphy or a cable graft can be used for nerve reanastomosis
- A gold weight in the ipsilateral upper eyelid and tarsorrhaphy can be considered for postoperative eye protection, if the upper branches of the facial nerve have been resected.

V. Special Postoperative Considerations
- Postoperative care
  - The need for admission to the surgical intensive care unit (SICU) is dictated by the extent of surgery, the need for tracheostomy and the type of reconstruction.
  - Patients with a significant history of alcohol abuse must be monitored closely for signs of withdrawal.
  - Postoperative eye care is essential; long-term eye protection can be provided by gold weight placement, tarsorrhaphy and/or lower lid shortening procedures.
  - Facial reanimation procedures can be considered after resection of the facial nerve.

VI. Complications
- Lack of adequate care can result in corneal injury, eye dryness, exposure keratitis and blindness
- Corneal abrasions.

Chapter 20

Salivary Gland Endoscopy

Oded Nahlieli

INTRODUCTION

Obstructive sialadenitis, with or without sialolithiasis, represents the main inflammatory disorder of the major salivary glands. The diagnosis and treatment of obstructions and inflammations of salivary glands can, at times, be problematic due to the limitations of the standard imaging techniques. Satisfactory treatment depends on the ability to reach a precise diagnosis and in the case of sialoliths, to accurately locate the obstruction. Until recently, many of these glands required complete removal under general anesthesia.

The symptomatic group of patients admitted to hospital each year has been estimated as 57 cases per million per annum in the British population representing 3,420 patients per annum. If this incidence is applied to the European or American population (300 million), then approximately 17,100 patients per annum will require hospital treatment for sialolithiasis and its complication sialadenitis. This data does not include patients who were treated as ambulatory (outpatient) cases. There is a male preponderance and the peak incidence is between 30 years and 60 years.

Sialolithiasis is a common finding accounting for 50% of major salivary gland diseases. The submandibular gland is the most prone to sialolithiasis. In various studies, it was found that approximately 80% of all sialolithiasis cases occurs in the submandibular glands, 19% occurs in the parotid gland and around 1% is found in the sublingual gland.

Sialolithiasis is most often found in adults, but it may be diagnosed in children as well. Sialoliths may vary in size, shape, texture and consistency. They may occur as a single stone or may be multiple in numbers. Bilateral submandibular stones are rare conditions (5% of submandibular sialolithiasis cases). Sialolithiasis of submandibular and parotid gland together are not reported in the literature. The amount of symptomatic and asymptomatic sialolithiasis cases, found in the autopsy material, is 1% of the population.

Sialoliths grow by deposition and range in size from 0.1 mm to 30 mm. Presentation is typically with a painful swelling of the gland at meal times, when the obstruction caused by the calculus becomes most acute. During the past decade, with the introduction of salivary gland endoscopy there has been a major step forward, not only in providing an accurate means of diagnosing and locating intraductal obstructions, but also in permitting minimally invasive surgical treatment that can successfully manage those blockages not accessible intraorally.

In this section, the author reviews the modern methods developed for salivary gland obstructions. The rapid developments in technology (especially optical miniaturization, lithotripsy equipment and micro instruments), the influence from other surgical fields and the author's knowledge about the regeneration potential of the salivary glands directed them to develop new methods of treatment, which are noninvasive, minimally invasive and less invasive.

PRE-ENDOSCOPY ASSESSMENT

Following the clinical evaluation, plain X-rays, which include panorex, occlusal, occlusal oblique view are recommended for submandibular stones (Figs 1A and B). In parotid stones located in the middle or posterior parts, computed tomography (CT) scan is indicated (Figs 1C and D). Prior to sialendoscopy, it is helpful to map the ductal system by

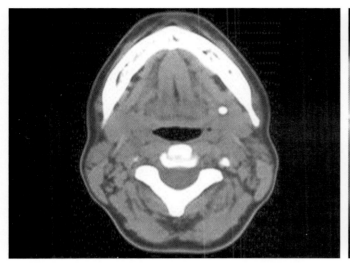

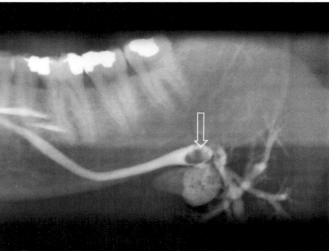

Fig. 1A: CT (axial cut) of a 42-year-old female suffering from meal time syndrome (swelling before or during meals) demonstrating 5 mm stone in the hilum of the left submandibular gland

Fig. 1B: Sialogram of 57-year-old male suffering from recurrent swelling of the left submandibular region. The arrow is pointed toward the stone located in the hilum region

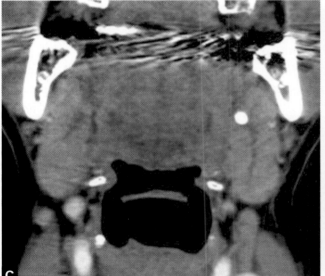

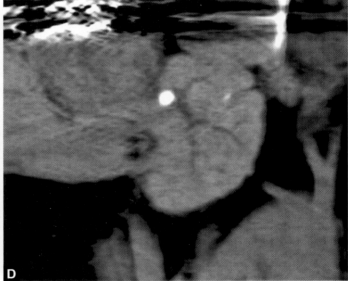

Figs 1C and D: (C) Coronal image; (D) Sagittal image of the same patient demonstrating the hilar location of the stone

sialography or ultrasound examination in order to check variations in duct diameter, stricture and to establish whether the duct has the ability to dilate under pressure.

ENDOSCOPIC SIALOLITHOTOMY

Methods Available for Endoscopic Sialolithotomy

- Endoscopic intraductal approach
- Endoscopic extraductal approach.

The intraductal approach is a pure endoscopic technique. The extraductal approach involves endoscopic-assisted techniques.

PREOPERATIVE EVALUATION AND ANESTHESIA

The evaluation of the affected gland includes patient history, clinical evaluation and imaging methods. The main data essential for the procedure is the exact location of the obstruction, the diameter and configuration of the stone, and the information on mobility or fixation of the stone.

Most of the endoscopic procedures can be done under local anesthesia in the ambulatory care centers. For submandibular gland, lingual block and infiltration around the Wharton's duct orifice with lidocaine 2% and adrenaline 1:200,000 are essential.

For parotid gland, infiltration of local anesthesia around the Stensen's duct papilla is needed. For both the glands, irrigation with lidocaine 2% into the ductal system with small diameter vein line numbs the entire gland. If general anesthesia is indicated, nasotracheal intubation is the preferred technique.

SURGICAL TECHNIQUES

I. Indications
- Diagnostic purposes
- Diagnosis and inspection of salivary ducts, in recurrent episodes of salivary gland swelling without obvious cause.
- Sialolithotomy
- Removal of deeply located small to medium (< 5 mm) stones in the middle and posterior portion of the Wharton's or Stensen's ducts.
- Exploration of the duct system for secondary stones or strictures following calculi removal from the anterior or middle part of the submandibular or parotid ducts.
- Treatment of submandibular and parotid sialadenitis.

II. Contraindications
- Acute sialadenitis.

III. Complications
- Strictures
- Ranula formation (in submandibular sialendoscopic cases)
- Sialadenitis
- Lingual paresthesia (in submandibular sialendoscopic cases).

III. Special Preoperative Considerations
- Preoperative imaging
- Localization of the obstruction site
- Assessment of the stone size and mobility.

IV. Special Intraoperative Considerations
- Identification of the duct orifice
- Identification of the duct direction
- Identification of the location of obstruction
- Assessment of the possibility of the connection of the stone to the duct
- Identification of additional stones and strictures in the main and secondary salivary ducts.

V. Special Postoperative Considerations
- All patients are to be treated postoperatively with amoxicillin (submandibular) or cephalosporin/augmentin (parotid gland) for 7 days.
- Intravenous dexamethasone (12 mg) is to be administered before the procedure. Following the procedure hydrocortisone (100 mg) is flashed into the duct.
- The patient is encouraged for hydration greater than 2 liters per day with no sialogogues and to massage the affected gland three times a day.

INTRADUCTAL VERSUS EXTRADUCTAL PROCEDURE

Basically, there are two different approaches: (i) intraductal approach and (ii) extraductal approach. The intraductal approach involves pure endoscopic diagnostic or surgical procedures via the ductal lumen. The extraductal approach is based on endoscopic-assisted techniques, which can be performed intraorally (in submandibular glands) or extraorally (in parotid cases).

Irrigation During Sialendoscopy

Irrigation is a crucial prerequisite for any sialendoscopic procedure for the duct, which is usually deflated. Consequently, the lumen must be filled with isotonic saline to allow adequate visualization of the lumen. The duct system is sensitive to lumenal pressure (much like the kidney). So, before irrigating, the duct should be washed with 2–4 ml of 2% lignocaine. Irrigation is performed with the aid of an elongation tube connected to a 20 cc syringe filled with normal saline or a self-filling syringe or simply a 20 ml syringe connected by a short (60 cm) tube to the endoscope. The syringe should not be connected directly to the endoscope because pressing the plunger moves the endoscope and the image will be lost. Stones can be removed by the intraductal approach, if they are smaller than 5 mm.

Intraductal Pure Endoscopic Procedure

The first step for the pure endoscopic approach is orifice dilatation of the duct with a duct dilator (Fig. 2A). Following the dilatation procedure, the endoscope with the blunt obturator is used. The anterior part of the duct is to be held with the aid of a fine hemostat in order to straighten the duct for easier manipulation of the endoscope. The endoscope is moved forward with the aid of constant irrigation of saline as in Figures 2B and C.

When a sialolith is encountered, its diameter is estimated using caliber of the endoscope as a reference. The calculus may be retrieved with wire baskets or being grasped by forceps.

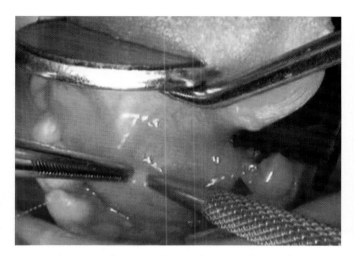

Fig. 2A: Dilatation of the Wharton's duct orifice with duct dilator

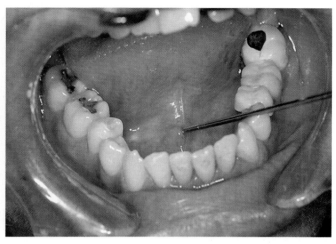

Fig. 2B: Introduction of the sialendoscope through the orifice of the Wharton's duct (following the dilatation) into the submandibular gland. Note the transillumination effect

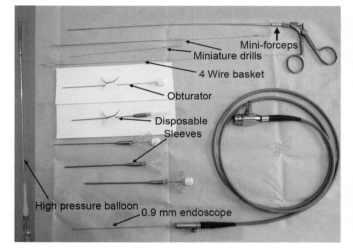

Fig. 2C: The modular endoscopic system for sialendoscopy procedures, including the 0.9 mm endoscope, disposable sleeves, mini forceps drills and balloons

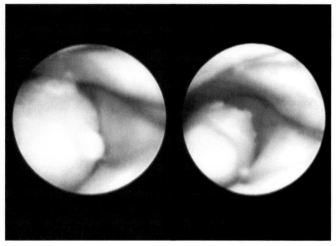

Fig. 2D: Endoscopic view of basket retrieval of the stone from the submandibular hilum

The basket needs to bypass the stone, when the stone is mobile. Otherwise, the procedure cannot be successful. The basket maneuver is to bypass the stone and then to rotate the basket clockwise. When the stone is entrapped and is inside the basket, a backward movement toward the duct orifice is indicated (Fig. 2D). If the stone is not mobile and/or cannot be bypassed by the basket, then the surgeon should not try to use this technique and should switch to the use of mini forceps. The mini forceps has the advantage that there is no need to bypass the stone and the practitioner can hold the stone in the frontal region. The prongs of the forceps can be controlled from the handle as in Figures 2E and F.

An alternative method can be of crushing the calculus with the mini forceps and then removing the fragments. Extracorporeal shockwave lithotripsy (Sialo Technology Ltd. Ashkelon, Israel) can be applied before the endoscopic procedure in order to disconnect the stone for further easier procedure (Figs 3A and B). The ideal goal is to remove the calculus in one piece.

When the sialolith is retrieved and located near the orifice, a small incision is performed above the location of the stone to prevent the soft tissue damage. An alternative and preferred technique is to expose and explore the anterior part of the duct and to perform ductal section in the anterior part (Fig. 4). Following the stone removal, a sialodrain is inserted and secured to the oral mucosa and the ductal walls with 4-0 vicryl sutures for 28 days.

Extraductal Sialolithotomy

The following two extraductal approaches are available:
1. *Intraoral technique:* This technique can be used for the removal of submandibular stones.

2. *Extraoral technique:* This technique is exclusively reserved for the removal of impacted parotid stones.

Intraoral Sialolithotomy

This approach or the so called "ductal stretching technique" (Figs 5A and B) is applied in the event of stones, which are not accessible via pure endoscopic techniques. In our experience, indications for this technique include:

• Large-sized calculi, measuring more than 5 mm
• Narrowness of the duct effectively rules out the option of attempting an intraductal approach
• Failures of the intraductal pure endoscopic procedure.

The ductal stretching technique involves the following seven steps:

1. Introduction of a miniature endoscope for accurate stone localization and lavage in order to disconnect the calculus from its ductal attachment.
2. Introduction of a lacrimal probe into the duct and incision above the duct using a free beam of CO_2 laser in a noncontact technique. The other options are electro surgery or the usage of a cold blade.
3. Dissecting and isolating the duct from the surrounding tissue as far as to the first molar (submandibular) as in Figure 5C.

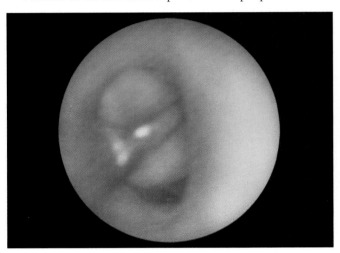

Fig. 2E: Endoscopic view of mini forceps retrieval of the same sialolith from the submandibular hilum

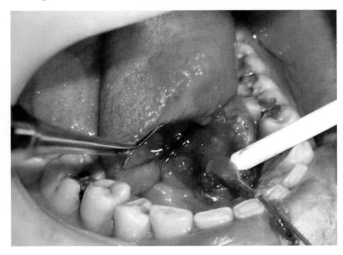

Fig. 2F: The same stone between the prongs of mini forceps on its way out from the gland

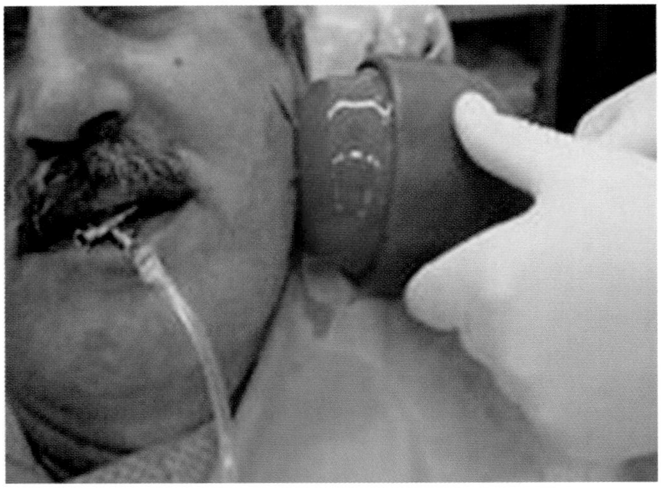

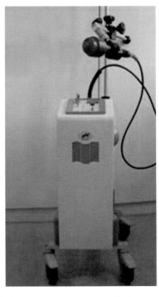

Fig. 3A: Extracorporeal shock wave lithotripsy. The lithotripter probe is applied to parotid stone

Fig. 3B: The miniature extracorporeal shock wave lithotripter (Sialo Technology Ltd. Ashkelon, Israel)

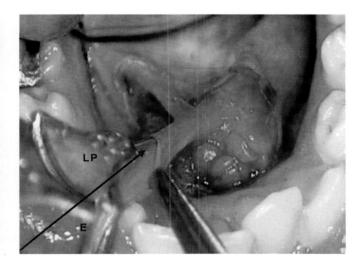

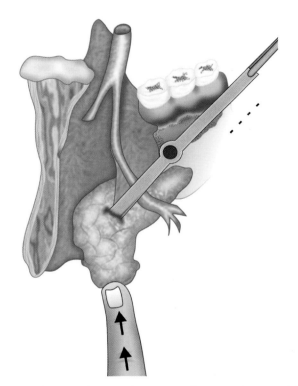

Fig. 4: Exploration of the Wharton's duct in the anterior region. Note the diameter of the duct, sufficient for insertion of large sized endoscope and removal of medium to large sized stone. Lacrimal probe (LP) is in the duct for showing the correct location. Note the position of the endoscope (E) for accurate insertion

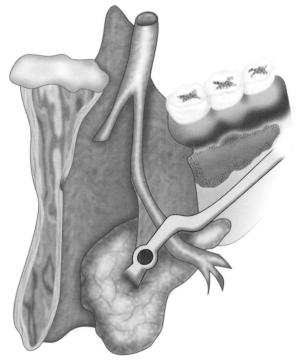

Fig. 5A: This diagram demonstrates the stretching technique. The stone is located in the submandibular hilum region

4. *Digital pressure:* The gland is shifted toward the mouth by applying mild digital pressure to the submandibular region as in Figure 5D.
5. Ductal section above the calculus and sialolithotomy are performed as in Figure 5E.
6. Endoscopic exploration for removal of additional calculi and lavage are needed.
7. Temporary placement of the sialodrain (Sialo Technology Ltd. Ashkelon, Israel) should be done for 28 days as in Figures 5F to H.

Fig. 5B: The stretching technique itself. Note the stretching and the digital manual pressure on the gland that brings the stone to a more favorable anterior location (anterior to the lingual nerve)

Extraoral Sialolithotomy

This approach is exclusively reserved for the removal of impacted parotid stones.

The indications for the extraoral approaches are:
• Calculi that have failed to respond to other methods of extraction. These calculi are usually large (> 5 mm) and typically there is a history of acute infection.

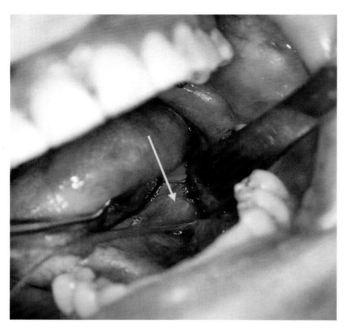

Fig. 5C: The duct is exposed and stretched and the stone is brought from the hilum to the floor of the mouth

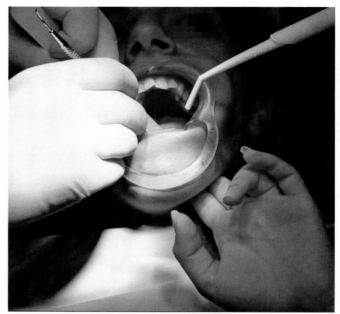

Fig. 5D: The procedure performed under local anesthesia, note the patient assist with digital pressure on the submandibular gland

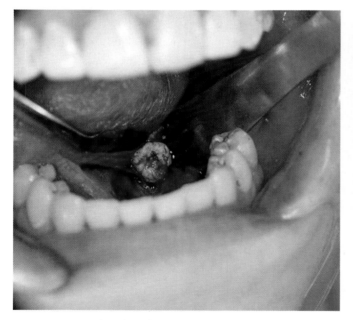

Fig. 5E: After ductal section, the stone is removed

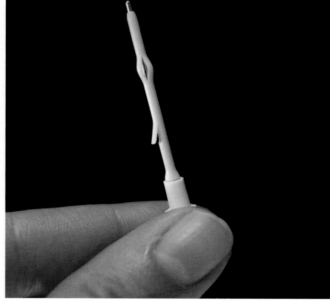

Fig. 5F: Sialodrain (Sialo Technology Ltd. Ashkelon, Israel)

- Stricture of the proximal or middle third of Stensen's duct that can make calculus removal problematic.
- Intraparenchymal stones.

There are two options for the removal of the sialolith: (i) via modified rhytidectomy approach or (ii) via cheek incision.

Surgery is performed with the aid of magnifying loupes (magnification 2.5–3.5X).

MODIFIED RHYTIDECTOMY APPROACH

Under general anesthesia without muscle relaxants and with continuous nerve monitoring, the first step is to dilate parotid duct orifice with lacrimal probes. The sialendoscope is then introduced in the duct. Once the stone is located, the light of the endoscope transmitted through the skin allows a mark to be made extraorally that will aid to locate the stone

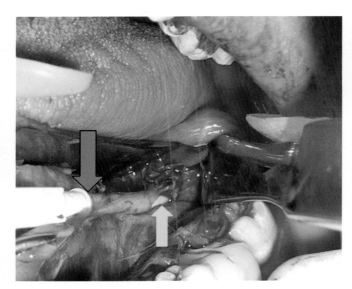

Fig. 5G: Intraoperative view following removal of submandibular hilar stone. Sialodrain (blue arrow) introduced to the gland via the duct. The yellow arrow points to the location of the stone

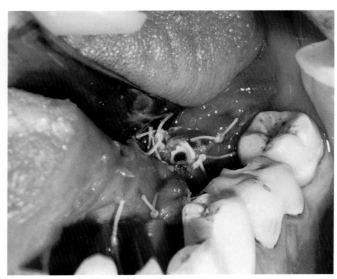

Fig. 5H: The sialodrain sutured following the endoscopic procedure

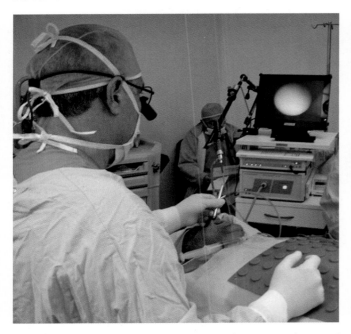

Fig. 6A: Position of the surgeon during the extraoral parotid sialolithotomy approach. Note the insertion of the endoscope and the position of the endoscopic unit

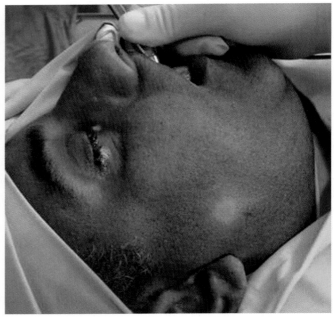

Fig. 6B: Transillumination by the endoscope through the cheek. The endoscope lies in the parotid duct. The exact position of the stone can be seen and marked on the skin

(Figs 6A to F). Another option in the absence or narrowness of the duct or in cases with intraparenchymal stone is to locate the stone with the aid of ultrasound. The stone location is marked with biopsy marker or injection of methylene blue to the stone location under continuous ultrasound as in Figures 6G to I.

The sialendoscope is temporarily removed while the patient is prepared and draped for the parotidectomy procedure. A preauricular incision with postauricular and short vertical extension, till the edge of the ear lobe, is made long enough to allow the skin flap to be raised a few millimeters anterior to the position of the stone.

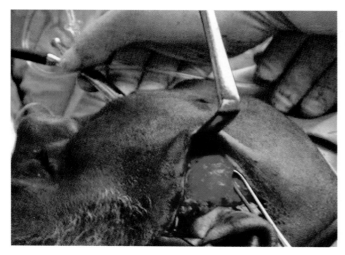

Fig. 6C: Exposure of the parotid gland via rhytidectomy approach. Note the transillumination effect

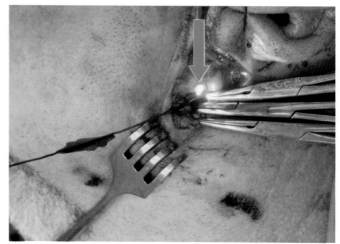

Fig. 6D: The tip of the endoscope (arrow) points to the exact location of the stone

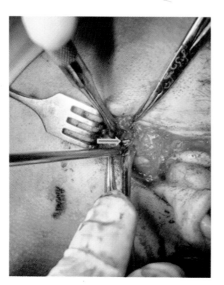

Fig. 6E: Extraction of the same stone (arrow) following the endoscopic identification

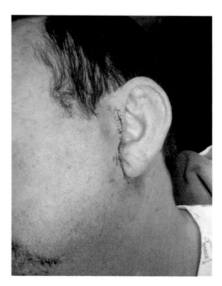

Fig. 6F: The same patient following the rhytidectomy approach

The flap is raised in subcutaneous tissue over the parotid fascia. The skin flap is retracted by an assistant or held in position with temporary stay sutures. The endoscope is now repositioned in the duct with the tip being located close to the stone. Transillumination from the scope directs the dissection, first through the parotid fascia and then by careful blunt dissection through the parotid until the duct is exposed. The buccal branch of the facial nerve is closely related to the duct and is usually identified at this point in the procedure. The duct is slowly defined by careful blunt dissection. The parotid duct is opened longitudinally with a fresh number 11 blade and the stone is delivered with fine

dental curettes and excavators. The endoscope is advanced to check for any residual stone and strictures in the proximal and distal part of the duct. After removal of the stone, a parotid sialodrain is inserted into this region directed from the location of the stone intraorally. The sialodrain is fixated with 4-0 vicryl sutures to the oral buccal mucosa. The parotid duct is sutured with 4-0 nylon sutures and the capsules are sutured with 4-0 vicryl sutures. Subcutaneous tissue and skin are sutured in the usual manner and pressure dressing is applied for 48 hours. The sialodrain is removed at fourth week. Antibiotic coverage is followed after the procedure with augmentin 1.5 gm per day for 1 week.

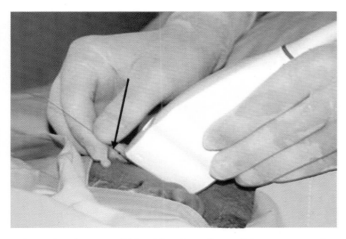

Fig. 6G: Ultrasound identification of parotid stone, note the biopsy marker (arrow) directed to the stone

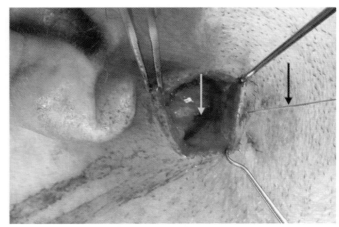

Fig. 6H: Intraoperative view during the stone removal with the aid of the biopsy marker (arrows)

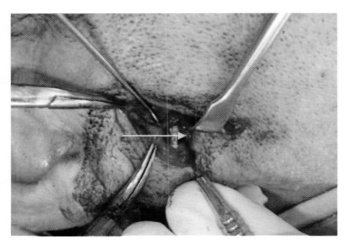

Fig. 6I: Removal of the stone (arrow)

CHEEK APPROACH

Under general anesthesia without muscle relaxants and with continuous nerve monitoring, the first step is to locate a sialolith and mark its position on the skin of the cheek. Normally, the calculus is identified by an endoscopic inspection of the salivary duct. The calculus is then identified and its location is pinpointed by the transillumination effect of the sialendoscope (Fig. 7A). If the calculus cannot be identified this way or there is no patent duct, one can resort to high resolution ultrasound examination. The stone location is marked with a biopsy marker or injection of methylene blue to the stone location under continuous ultrasound.

An incision of 1 cm is made along the course of the facial lines. Sharp and blunt dissection will expose the stone. If it proves difficult to localize the sialolith during dissection, an ultrasound probe is used intraoperatively. If an endoscope

is in the duct, it can be moved up and down the lumen to demonstrate the position of the duct.

When the stone is encountered, the duct may be hypertrophied over its surface. Scalpel with number 11 blade is used to open the duct in a longitudinal direction to expose the stone, which is removed with the aid of a curette (Fig. 7B). A guidewire is advanced into the cavity that is formed upon removal of the stone and the 1.1 mm modular sialendoscope is inserted to screen the area and remove the residual fragments. A thorough lavage under direct vision must be performed. Then, the sialodrain (Sialo Technology Ltd. Ashkelon, Israel) is introduced via an intraoral approach to lie across in the incised duct. A stent is fixed to the oral mucosa with 4-0 silk sutures.

If the anterior part of the duct is found to be obliterated and no passage can be obtained to the oral cavity, then consideration can be given to ligating the proximal duct as long as all stone fragments have been removed (the stone acts as a source of infection) or a 1.7 mm vein line is introduced from the previous location of the stone to the oral mucosa. The needle is removed, the shaft is incised using 4-0 silk suture and the vein line is fixed to the oral mucosa as in Figure 7C.

Limitations of the technique are as follows:
- The stone should not be located deeper than 6 mm from the outer skin surface.
- Screening of the surrounding tissue for large blood vessels and for phleboliths is mandatory.
- In the presence of deeply located calculi or close proximity to a large-sized blood vessel, the author recommends exploring this region using a modified rhytidectomy approach.

After completion of the procedure, antibiotic coverage is provided (augmentin) and a pressure dressing is applied for 24 hours.

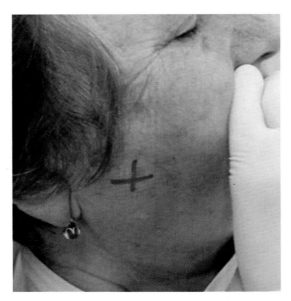

Fig. 7A: Cheek approach, transillumination by the endoscope through the cheek for exact location

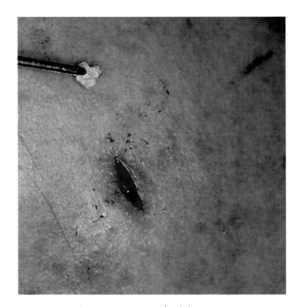

Fig. 7B: Removal of the same stone via cheek incision

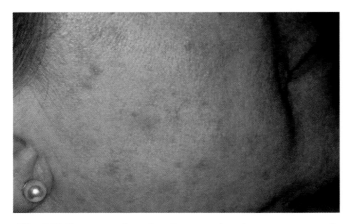

Fig. 7C: Postoperative view 2 years after the stone removal

CONTRAINDICATION

There is only one absolute contraindication to sialendoscopy, namely acute sialadenitis. This should be eliminated by a course of antibiotics before undertaking endoscopy.

POSTOPERATIVE MANAGEMENT AND FOLLOW-UP CARE

Following interventional sialendoscopy, a temporary sialodrain (Sialo Technology Ltd. Ashkelon, Israel) is introduced into the duct and kept in place as long as the tissues and the patient can tolerate its presence. Ideally, a 28-day period of retention is most desirable.

HIGHLIGHTS

I. **Indications**
   - Diagnostic purposes
     – Diagnosis and inspection of salivary ducts, in recurrent episodes of salivary gland swelling without obvious cause.
   - Sialolithotomy
     – Removal of deeply located small to medium (< 5 mm) stones in the middle and posterior portion of the Wharton's or Stensen's ducts.
   - Exploration of the duct system for secondary stones or strictures following calculi removal from the anterior or middle part of the submandibular or parotid ducts.
   - Treatment of submandibular and parotid sialadenitis.

II. **Contraindications**
   - Acute sialadenitis.

III. **Special Preoperative Considerations**
   - Preoperative imaging
   - Localization of the obstruction site
   - Assessment of the stone size and mobility.

IV. **Special Intraoperative Considerations**
   - Identification of the duct orifice
   - Identification of the duct direction
   - Identification of the location of obstruction
   - Assessment of the possibility of the connection of the stone to the duct
   - Identification of additional stones and strictures in the main and secondary salivary ducts.

V. Special Postoperative Considerations

- All patients are to be treated postoperatively with amoxicillin (submandibular) or cephalosporin/augmentin (parotid gland) for 7 days.
- Intravenous dexamethasone (12 mg) is to be administered before the procedure. Following the procedure hydrocortisone (100 mg) is flashed into the duct.
- The patient is encouraged for hydration greater than 2 liters per day with no sialogogues and to massage the affected gland three times a day.

VI. Complications

- Strictures
- Ranula formation (in submandibular sialendoscopic cases)
- Sialadenitis
- Lingual paresthesia (in submandibular sialendoscopic cases).

ADDITIONAL READING

1. Iro H, Zenk J, Escudier MP, et al. Outcome of minimally invasive management of salivary calculi in 4691 patients. Laryngoscope. 2009;119(2):263-8.
2. Karavidas K, Nahlieli O, Fritsch M, et al. Minimal surgery for parotid stones: a 7-year endoscopic experience. Int J Oral Maxillofac Surg. 2010;39(1):1-4.
3. Nahlieli O, Iro H, McGurk M, Zenk J (Eds). Modern Management Preserving the Salivary Glands Isradon 2007.
4. Nahlieli O, Shacham R, Zaguri A. Combined external lithotripsy and endoscopic techniques for advanced sialolithiasis cases. J Oral Maxillofac. Surg. 2010;68(2):347-53.
5. Nahlieli O, Shacham R, Zaguri A, et al. The ductal stretching technique: an endoscopic assisted technique for submandibular stones. Laryngoscope.2007;117(6);1031-5.
6. Nahlieli O. Advanced sialoendoscopy techniques rare findings and complications. Otolaryngol Clinic of North Am. 2009;42(6):1053-72.

Chapter **21**

Modified Radical Neck Dissection

Fernando L Dias, Roberto A Lima, Fernando Walder

INTRODUCTION

Originally developed as a technique of monoblock lymph-adenectomy for head and neck malignancies, radical neck dissection (RND) has been increasingly modified to minimize morbid dysfunction and disfigurement while preserving its oncological "sense". Radical neck dissection was first described by George Crile in 1906 and further popularized by Hayes Martin who standardized the procedure to become the standard of care for metastatic carcinoma of the lateral neck for much of the 20th century.

Several authors attempted to reduce the morbidity by developing a surgical technique to preserve the form and function, while preserving its therapeutic integrity. Oswaldo Suarez was the first to describe the technique of "functional neck dissection". It was popularized by Ettore Bocca who recommended this technique for comprehensive clearance of regional cervical lymph nodes in the lateral neck in a monoblock fashion preserving the sternocleidomastoid muscle, the internal jugular vein and the spinal accessory nerve. The classical RND entails clearance of essentially all of the fibrofatty and lymphatic tissue in the lateral neck (cervical lymph nodes at all five levels) as well as resection of non-lymphatic structures such as the spinal accessory nerve, the sternocleidomastoid muscle, the internal jugular vein and the submandibular gland in a monoblock fashion (Figs 1A and B). Anything less than a classical RND is considered a "modified" or "selective" neck dissection.

With the development of the many modifications of the classical RND, there has been a proliferation of terms to describe these various procedures, resulting in a nonuniform and confusing nomenclature. To facilitate communication and to ensure standardization, the American Academy of Otolaryngology-Head and Neck Surgery has proposed a classification scheme for neck dissection. In this scheme, modified radical neck dissection (MRND) consists of preservation of one or more non-lymphatic structures normally removed in RND. This nomenclature is described in greater detail in Table 1.

The surgical treatment of regional lymph nodes for carcinoma of the head and neck region is based on the understanding of anatomy of regional lymphatics and on the predictable patterns of lymphatic spread of squamous cell carcinoma (SCC) of the primary tumor. Current indications for classic RND include N3 neck disease, gross apparent extranodal spread with invasion of the spinal accessory nerve and or internal jugular vein and skin involvement by metastatic disease. However, when appropriate indications exist, a function-preserving comprehensive neck dissection sparing one or more vital anatomic structures should be considered as long as it does not compromise satisfactory clearance of metastatic disease.

The term comprehensive neck dissection is applied to all surgical procedures on the lateral neck, which comprehensively removes the cervical lymph nodes from level I through level V. Under this broad category, MRND are included and classified as follows:

1. Modified radical neck dissection Type I (MRND-I): This procedure selectively preserves the spinal accessory nerve.
2. Modified radical neck dissection Type II (MRND-II): This procedure preserves the spinal accessory nerve and the sternocleidomastoid muscle but sacrifices the internal jugular vein.

Table 1: Nomenclature describing types of neck dissection

Type of neck dissection	Nodal levels dissected	Structures preserved
Radical neck dissection (RND)	I–V	None
Type I Modified radical neck dissection (MRND I)	I–V	SAN
Type II Modified radical neck dissection (MRND II)	I–V	SAN SCM
Type III Modified radical neck dissection (MRND III)	I–V	SCM IJV SAN
Supraomohyoid neck dissection (SOHND)	I–III	SCM IJV SAN
Lateral neck dissection (LND)	II–IV	SCM IJV SAN
Anterolateral neck dissection (ALND)	I–V	SCM IJV SAN
Posterolateral neck dissection (PLND)	II–V	SCM IJV SAN

SAN: Spinal accessory nerve; SCM: Sternocleidomastoid muscle; IJV: Internal jugular vein

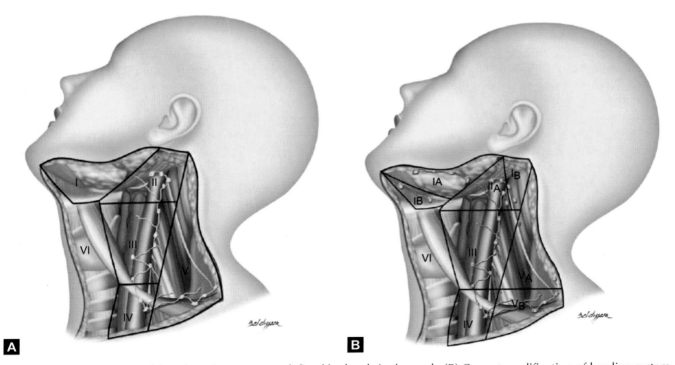

Figs 1A and B: (A) Cervical lymph node groups are defined by levels in the neck; (B) Current modification of leveling system. Modified radical neck dissection encompasses the nodes in levels I–V

3. Modified radical neck dissection Type III (MRND-III): This procedure requires preservation of the spinal accessory nerve, internal jugular vein and sternocleidomastoid muscle.

PREOPERATIVE PREPARATION

No specific preoperative preparation is required for patients undergoing neck dissection other than the usual clinical/anesthesiological evaluation for a major surgical procedure. Planning of the incision for neck dissection should be carefully made, particularly if the primary tumor is to be resected simultaneously or if any reconstructive effort is required to repair the surgical defect created following the excision of the primary tumor.

SURGICAL TECHNIQUE

Modified Radical Neck Dissection (Type I)

After the induction of general endotracheal anesthesia with adequate muscle relaxation, the patient is placed in a supine position. The head and the chest are elevated at 30°, the neck is hyperextended and turned to the contralateral side. The operative field is scrubbed with surgical sponges containing chlorhexidine solution (0.05% w/v) and draped in a standard and sterile fashion. It is very important, particularly in elderly patients, with limited extension of the neck that the occiput should be palpated when putting the neck in extension. This ensures that the head is not hanging. This situation has the potential to cause cervical spine complications.

Although the skin incision will be affected by the planned resection of the primary tumor and subsequent reconstruction, adequate exposure and preservation of

cutaneous vascular supply must be achieved. Most commonly, a trifurcate incision is used (Figs 2A and B). A transverse incision is made at least two fingerbreadths below the angle of the mandible, extending from the ipsilateral mastoid tip along the upper neck skin crease up to the midline, at the level of the thyrohyoid membrane. A curvaceous vertical limb begins at the point posterior to the carotid artery and ends at the midclavicular point. Skin and platysma flaps are elevated to expose the whole operative field. The superior skin flap is carefully elevated, close to the inner aspect of the platysma muscle, up to the lower border of the body of the mandible identifying and preserving the mandibular branch of the facial nerve, as well as facilitating dissection of the prevascular facial group of lymph nodes. The posterior skin flap is then elevated well over the anterior border of the trapezius muscle to expose at least 1 cm of its anterolateral surface.

At this point, meticulous attention should be paid as elevation of the lateral aspect of the skin flap approaches the anterior border of the trapezius muscle in the lower part of the neck, since the accessory nerve enters the muscle in this region. The medial skin flap is then elevated to expose the lower end of the sternocleidomastoid muscle as in Figures 3A and B.

Countertraction is applied and the soft tissue is divided from the anterior border of the trapezius muscle and elevated off the floor of the posterior triangle of the neck. At this point, the spinal accessory nerve is identified as it enters the trapezius muscle along the lower one-third of its anterior border, dissecting one layer of fibroadipose tissue at a time, until the nerve is visualized. Caution at this time is advisable, if the electrical cautery is used to incise tissue in order to minimize direct stimulation and/or injury of the nerve. A tissue spreading technique with a hemostat is advisable to dissect the fascia and soft tissue over the nerve to prevent its

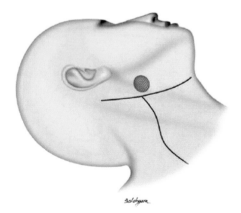

A

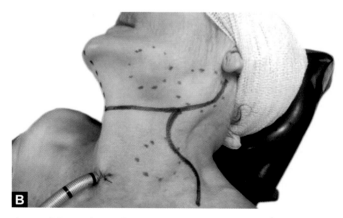

B

Figs 2A and B: (A) The single trifurcate incision is most commonly used for unilaterally modified radical neck dissection. It can be extended to accommodate resection of the primary tumor; (B) The location of the palpable lymph node is outlined on the patient (dashed circles), as well as the mark is extended to the patient's chin

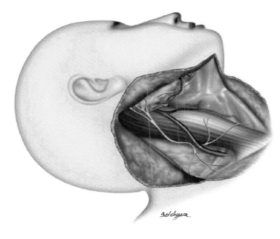

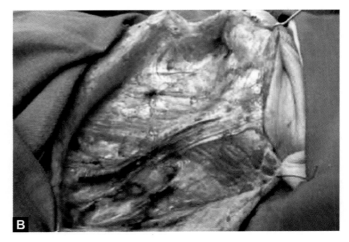

Figs 3A and B: (A) Skin and platysma flaps are elevated to expose the whole operative field. The superior limit is the lower border of the mandible, the posterior limit is the anterior border of the trapezius muscle and the anterior limit is composed of the anterior belly of the omohyoid muscle and the strap muscles; (B) Aspect of the surgical field after raising the cutaneous flap

injury. The nerve is traced up to its exit from the posterior border of the sternocleidomastoid muscle. Although not considered as consistent as some anatomy texts proclaim (due to its possible confusion with cutaneous branches of the cervical plexus), the Erb's point (i.e. the point where the greater auricular nerve curves forward around the posterior border of the sternocleidomastoid muscle) can also be used as an anatomical point for the identification of the nerve. Additionally, preservation of the innervation to the levator scapulae and the cervical nerve root contributions to the accessory nerve may help support the shoulder and preserve function.

Dissection of the posterior triangle continues with sequential and partial exposure of splenius capitis, levator scapulae and scalene muscles. During this dissection, the peripheral cutaneous branches of the cervical plexus are divided, as well as the posterior belly of the omohyoid muscle and the spinal accessory nerve in its lower part is dissected free from the rest of the specimen. Components from the cervical roots, such as the nerve supply to the posterior compartment muscles as well as the descending fibers contributing to the phrenic nerve are carefully preserved, while cutaneous roots are ligated along with the accompanying small blood vessels as in Figures 4A and B.

The transverse cervical artery and vein are identified, divided between clamps and ligated inferiorly. Once again, care is taken to identify the phrenic nerve (lying over the anterior scalene muscle) as well as the brachial plexus (between the middle and anterior scalene muscles). It is important to mention that the cervical rootlets are divided leaving small stumps on the phrenic nerve to assure its preservation. This is usually facilitated by division of the posterior belly of the omohyoid muscle and its retraction medially. The surgical specimen is then flipped medially

and the inferior skin flap is elevated to expose the lower insertion of the sternocleidomastoid muscle. With the use of the electrocautery, the sternal and the clavicular heads of the sternocleidomastoid muscle are divided near their insertion.

A layer of fibrofatty tissue, which is always present between the undersurface of the sternocleidomastoid muscle and the carotid sheath, serves as a limitation for the use of the electrocautery. At this juncture, lymphatics between the deep jugular lymph nodes at the lateral aspect of the internal jugular vein are carefully identified, divided and ligated with particular attention to controlling the thoracic duct on the left side of the neck.

The transverse cervical artery and vein are also divided and ligated. The lower end of the jugular vein is circumferentially dissected free carefully, protecting the common carotid artery, the vagus nerve, the sympathetic chain and the phrenic nerve, which are previously identified by meticulous sharp and blunt dissection. The vein is doubly ligated, divided and its stump is suture ligated as in Figures 5A and B.

Further dissection of the accessory nerve requires splitting of the sternocleidomastoid muscle in its upper-half, keeping the nerve in constant view at all times (Fig. 6). The sternocleidomastoid muscle is divided up to the posterior belly of the digastric muscle to expose the spinal accessory nerve in its entirety from the jugular foramen cephalad, until its entry into the trapezius muscle caudad. At this time, mobilization of the specimen provides exposure of the internal jugular vein from the posterior belly of the digastric muscle cephalad to the root of the neck caudad, as well as the splenius capitis and levator scapulae muscles in its entirety.

Dissection continues cephalad within the carotid sheath all the way up to the lower border of the digastric muscle with division of the superior thyroid vein, preservation of the

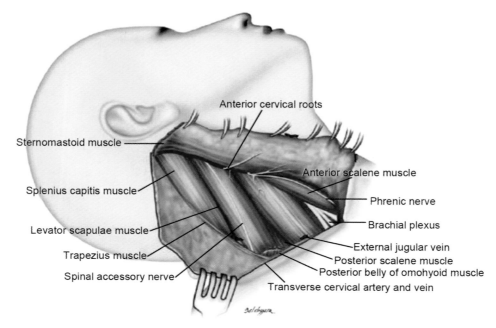

Anterior cervical roots

Sternomastoid muscle

Splenius capitis muscle

Levator scapulae muscle

Trapezius muscle

Spinal accessory nerve

Anterior scalene muscle

Phrenic nerve

Brachial plexus

External jugular vein

Posterior scalene muscle

Posterior belly of omohyoid muscle

Transverse cervical artery and vein

A

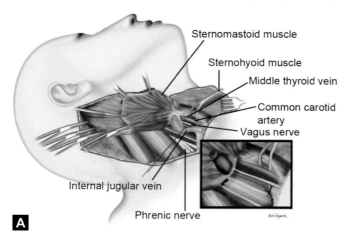

B

Figs 4A and B: (A) The spinal accessory nerve is identified at its point of entry in the trapezius muscle. Elevation of the fibro-fatty and lymphatic tissue of the floor of the posterior triangle also reveals the phrenic nerve and its cervical nerve rootlets on the surface of the anterior scalene muscle and the brachial plexus between the middle and anterior scalene muscles; (B) The spinal nerve is being dissected in the posterior triangle of the neck, until its entry in the sternocleidomastoid muscle

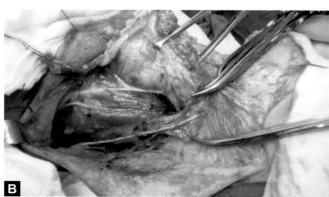

Sternomastoid muscle

Sternohyoid muscle

Middle thyroid vein

Common carotid artery

Vagus nerve

Internal jugular vein

Phrenic nerve

A

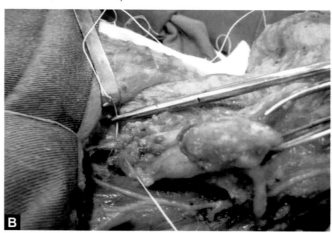

B

Figs 5A and B: (A) With the sternocleidomastoid muscle retracted superiorly and the strap muscles retracted medially, the carotid sheath is entered. The internal jugular vein is divided and doubly ligated after the vagus nerve has been identified and protected (inset). The lymphatic ducts at the root of the neck are equally divided and ligated; (B) Detail on the double ligation of the internal jugular vein superior thyroid artery and identification of the hypoglossal nerve after the carotid bifurcation, where it may loop around the occipital branch of the external carotid artery. Often, the descendens hypoglossi to the strap muscles is a good guide, leading up to the hypoglossal nerve. The dissection proceeds medially, along the superior belly of the omohyoid muscle up to the hyoid bone, from where it is detached. The anterior belly of the omohyoid muscle is the anterior limit of the dissection. Several minor bleeding points along the branches of the descendens hypoglossi are divided and eletrocoagulated, and the common facial vein and several pharyngeal veins crossing the digastric muscle are divided to expose the posterior belly and tendon of the digastric muscles. Once the lower border of the diagastric muscle is completely exposed, the surgical specimen is allowed to rest over the lower part of the neck as in Figures 7A and B.

Attention is then turned to the submandibular/submental region already exposed by the elevation of the superior skin/platysma flap. The marginal mandibular branch of the facial nerve is identified as it crosses the facial artery and vein, directly overlying the submandibular gland. Identification of the facial artery and vein, which are good landmarks, can help to identify the nerve. The vein runs almost parallel to the cervical branch of the facial nerve (Figs 8A and B). The facial artery and vein are then divided and ligated with retraction of the superior stumps of these vessels to protect the nerve. This is due to the fact that the posterior facial vein lies deep to the mandibular branch of the facial nerve, thus dividing the vein low and retracting its upper stump cephalad. This would also protect the already dissected and mobilized nerve on the upper skin flap. This surgical maneuver is known as "Hayes Martin maneuver" as in Figures 9A and B.

Dissection continues anteriorly along the border of the mandible. The submental group of lymph nodes are dissected from the midline and brought toward the right-hand side. At this point, the superomedial limit of dissection is the anterior belly of the contralateral digastric muscle. The nerve and blood supply of the mylohyoid muscle is divided and ligated. With the mylohyoid muscle retracted toward the chin of the patient and the submandibular gland gently retracted to the opposite side, the undersurface of the floor of the mouth is brought into view and it is then possible to identify the secretomotor fibers to the submandibular gland, as they come off the lingual nerve as in Figures 10A and B.

The lingual nerve is identified and its paraganglionic secretomotor fibers are divided, as is the Wharton's duct with accessory salivary tissue along the duct. The facial artery and vein on the posterior aspect of the gland proceeding toward

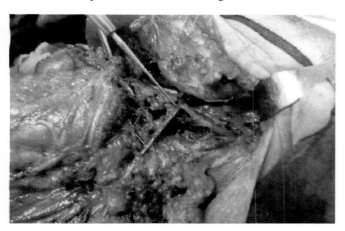

Fig. 6: Further dissection of the spinal nerve after splitting the sternocleidomastoid muscle

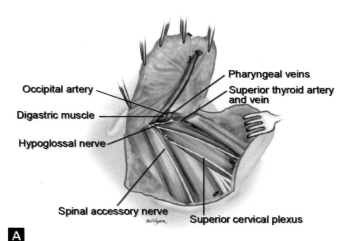

Occipital artery

Digastric muscle

Hypoglossal nerve

Spinal accessory nerve

Pharyngeal veins

Superior thyroid artery and vein

Superior cervical plexus

A

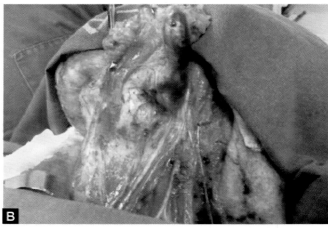

B

Figs 7A and B: (A) Dissection of the spinal accessory nerve up to the posterior belly of the digastric muscle is shown. Dissection continues cephalad along the carotid sheath exposing the hypoglossal nerve and descendens hypoglossi. The pharyngeal venous plexus and occipital artery are identified and are divided between clamps and ligated; (B) Photographic version of the same aspect

the body of the mandible are dissected next. In most cases the facial artery must be individually clamped, divided and ligated with the facial vein as well. Division of the facial vessels allows the caudal retraction of the submandibular gland, providing full exposure of the underlying mylohyoid muscle. During this dissection, the hypoglossal nerve is seen in a deeper plane to Wharton's duct and should be carefully protected. Any remaining veins of the pharyngeal venous plexus accompanying the hypoglossal nerve must be divided between clamps and ligated as in Figures 11A to C.

After the posterior belly of the digastric is exposed and retracted superiorly, which may require transection of the tail of the parotid gland (Fig. 12); the internal jugular vein

is identified and skeletonized circumferentially. The internal jugular vein is divided between clamps and doubly ligated, allowing delivery of the specimen as in Figures 13A and B.

Meticulous hemostasis is achieved and the wound is closed over two suction drains: (i) the posterior drain is allowed to rest along the anterior border of the trapezius muscle and; (ii) the anterior drain is placed parallel to the strap muscles. The surgical field following removal of the specimen can also be seen in the Figures 14A and B. Care must be taken to achieve an airtight closure and to initiate suction on the drains during closure to prevent clots from forming within the drains. Postoperatively, the drains are removed when there is minimal serous drainage. The skin

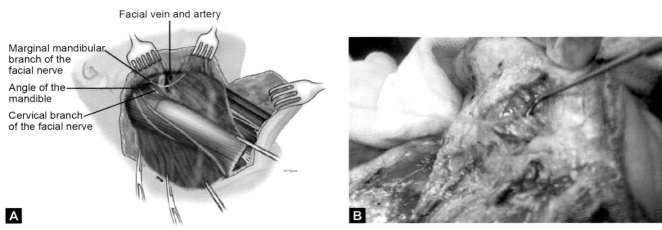

Figs 8A and B: (A) The marginal mandibular branch of the facial nerve is identified as it crosses superficially to the facial artery and vein. The cervical branch of the facial nerve may be divided; (B) Dissector pointing to the mandibular branch of the facial nerve. Facial vein already identified

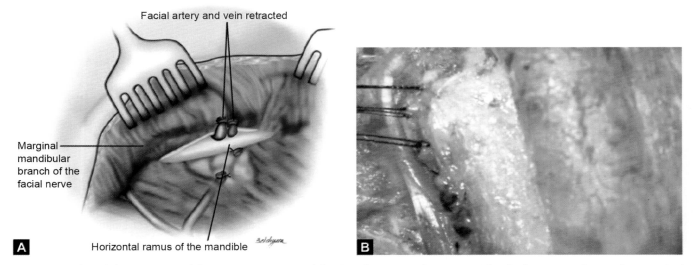

Figs 9A and B: (A) Retraction of the superior stumps of the facial artery and vein provides further protection to the marginal mandibular branch of the facial nerve, which is thereafter elevated with the skin flap; (B) Detail on the nerve already identified and the facial artery and vein stumps ligated

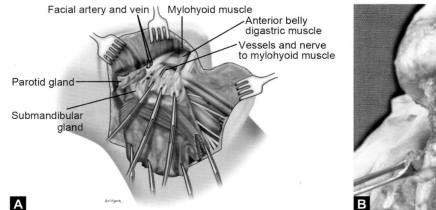

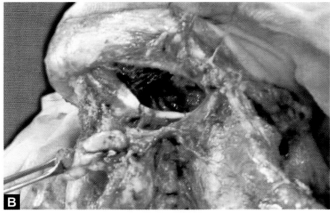

Figs 10A and B: (A) The vessels and nerve to the mylohyoid muscle are identified, divided and ligated as the contents of the submental triangle are retracted; (B) Aspect of the submental and submandibular triangles dissected from its contents

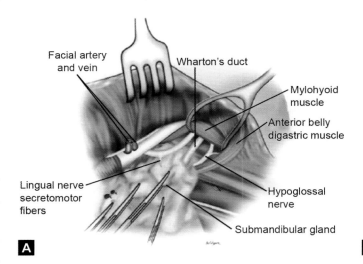

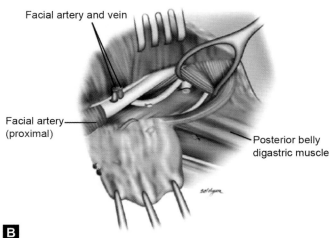

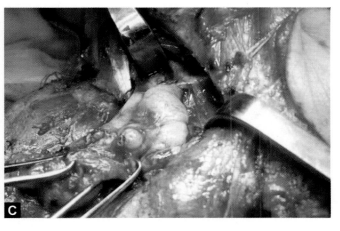

Figs 11A to C: (A) Retraction of the mylohyoid muscle medially and the submandibular gland inferolaterally allows the identification; (B) Division and ligation of the lingual nerve secretomotor fibers and Wharton's duct with the proximal portion of the facial artery identified; (C) Lingual nerve and its secretomotor fibers in detail

incision is thereafter closed in two layers using 3-0 vicryl interrupted sutures for platysma and 4-0 nylon sutures or staples for skin closure as in Figure 15.

Modified radical neck dissection in its three versions: (i) Type I; (ii) Type II and; (iii) Type III are shown in the Figures 16A to C.

Regarding the control of disease in the neck, adjuvant radiation therapy still stands as the therapy of choice with proven efficacy, according to the international literature. Risk factors for failure in the neck include the presence of extracapsular extension (ECS) of the disease, the presence of multiple positive nodes, as well as the size of the metastatic lymph nodes. Administration of radiation therapy for regional control of the disease should be reserved for patients with the adverse prognostic factors mentioned above. On the other hand, if radiotherapy is indicated for the primary tumor as adjuvant therapy, then the neck should be irradiated as well.

Fig. 12: The tail of the parotid gland may require transection between the angle of the mandible and the tip of the mastoid to adequately expose the upper end of the internal jugular vein

HIGHLIGHTS

I. **Special Operative Considerations**
  - Include platysma muscle in skin flaps unless adherent or invaded by tumor
  - Use superior belly of omohyoid muscle as medial guide
  - Use scalenus muscle fascia as a guide for depth
  - Critical areas and structures include:
    - Carotid vessel
    - Vagus nerve
    - Internal jugular vein superiorly and inferiorly
    - Subclavian vein
    - Posterior facial vein hidden in tail of parotid
    - Superior laryngeal nerve deep to external and internal carotid arteries.
    - Thoracic duct on left side and accessory duct on the right side
    - Apical pleura
    - Phrenic nerve
    - Sympathetic chain

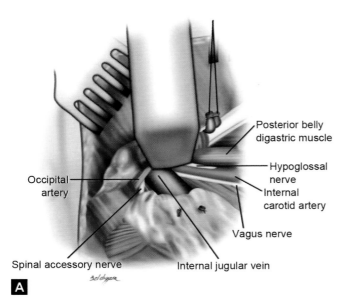

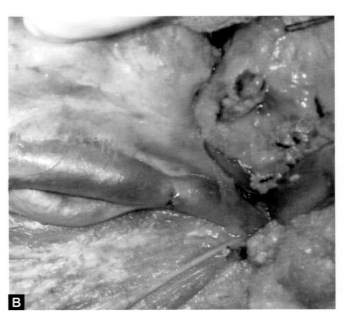

Figs 13A and B: (A) At the skull base with the retractor pulling the posterior belly of the digastric muscle up, the spinal nerve is identified and carefully dissected/preserved. The occipital artery and vein are ligated to allow visualization and skeletonization of the upper end of the jugular vein. The specimen is delivered with division and double ligation of the internal jugular vein; (B) The upper portion of the internal jugular vein and its close relation with the spinal accessory nerve

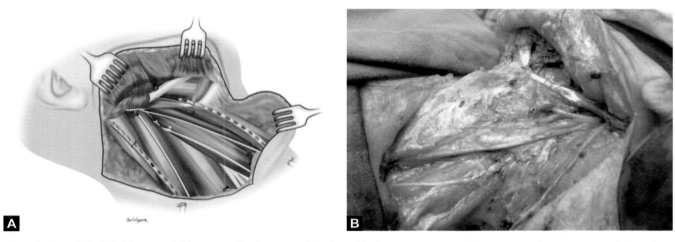

Figs 14A and B: (A) After careful hemostasis, the wound is closed in layers over two drains, one at the anterior and the other at the posterior region; (B) Final aspect of the surgical field after completion of a modified radical neck dissection Type I

Fig. 15: Final aspect of the neck with the skin incision closed in layers

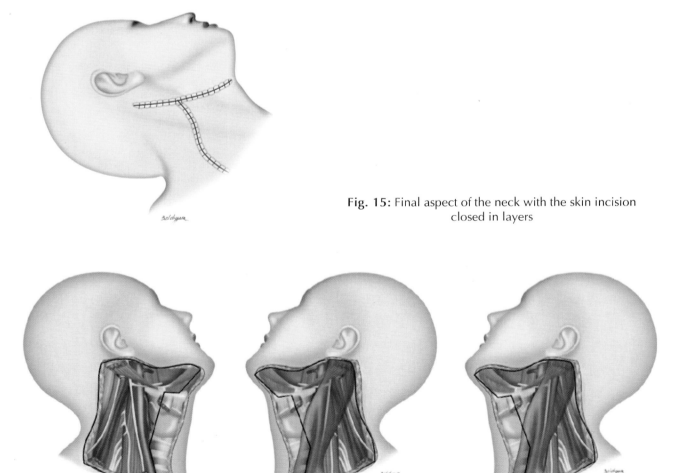

Figs 16A to C: Modified radical neck dissection. (A) Type I; (B) Type II; (C) Type III

- Spinal accessory nerve
- Marginal mandibular branch of the facial nerve
- Place incision so that bifurcation does not overlie carotid vessels.

II. Complications

- During the operation
  - Injury to uninvolved nerves
  - Laceration of internal jugular vein near base of skull or at the thoracic inlet
  - Injury to thoracic duct
  - Injury to subclavian vein causing air embolism
  - Injury to pleura causing pneumothorax
  - Danger of ventricular fibrillation with undue pressure on carotid sinus in patient heavily digitalized
- Postoperative
  - Hemorrhage, especially from posterior facial vein if not occluded with a tie and a suture ligature
  - Severe hemorrhage from the stump of internal jugular vein during struggling after a severe stormy reaction from anesthesia
- Skin slough
- Carotid artery blowout
- Wound infection
- Chylous fistula
- Pneumothorax
- Pain referred to shoulder and arm
- Drainage
  - Erosion of a major vessel by the suction tube or skin necrosis due to excessive pressure
- Deformity
  - Superior tenting of the lower lip due to injury to either the mandibular branch of the facial nerve or the platysma muscle via innervation from the cervical branch of the facial nerve.

- Edema of the face, especially with bilateral neck dissection
- Intracranial complications with bilateral neck dissection (blindness and cerebral edema)
- Myositis ossificans
- Transection of the phrenic nerve in an infant may result in scoliosis and in elderly patients or patients with pulmonary obstructive disease may result in atelectasis.

ADDITIONAL READING

1. Crile G. Landmark article: excision of cancer of the head and neck with special reference to the plan of dissection based on one hundred and thirty two operations. JAMA. 1987;258(22):3286-93.
2. Dias FL, Lima RA, Cernea CR. Cancer of the floor of the mouth. Oper Tech Otolaryngol Head Neck Surg. 2005;16:10-7.
3. Dias FL, Lima RA. N0 neck in oral cancer: elective neck dissection. In: Cernea CR, Dias FL, Fliss D, Lima RA, Myers EN, Wei WI (Eds). Pearls and Pitfalls in Head and Neck Surgery. Basel: Karger; 2008. pp.38-9.
4. Lindberg R. Distribution of cervical lymph node metastases from squamous cell carcinoma of the upper respiratory and digestive tracts. Cancer. 1972;29(6):1446-9.
5. Martin H, Del Valle B, Ehrlich H, et al. Neck dissection. Cancer. 1951;4(3):441-99.
6. Robbins KT, Medina JE, Wolfe GT, et al. Standardizing neck dissection terminology. Official report of the Academy's Committee for Head and Neck Surgery and Oncology. Arch Otolaryngol Head Neck Surg. 1991; 117(6):601-5.
7. Shah JP, Kraus DH. Radical neck dissection and its modifications. In: Donohue JH, Herdeen JA, Monson J (Eds). Atlas of Surgical Oncology. Cambridge Massachussetts: Blackwell Science; 1995. pp. 61-80.
8. Shah JP, Patel SG. Cervical lymph nodes. In: Shah JP, Patel SG (Eds). Head and Neck Surgery and Oncology, 3rd edition. Edinburgh: Mosby; 2003. pp. 353-94.

Chapter 22

Treatment of Benign Cysts of the Jawbones

Benjamin Shlomi, Ilana Kaplan

INTRODUCTION

The majority of benign lesions affecting the jaws are odontogenic cysts, which vary considerably in their microscopic characteristics and biological behavior.

CYSTS OF THE JAWS

Epithelium-lined cysts of bone are found almost exclusively in the jawbones, originating in the majority of cases, from odontogenic epithelium and less frequently from epithelial remnants along embryonic fusion lines. Features of selected cysts of the jaws are listed in Table 1.

Enucleation is the treatment of choice for most of these cysts. However, in large diameter cysts if the cortical plate integrity is compromised or when the cyst is close to vital structures, marsupialization (or decompression) is an option. Following irrigation through a patent opening for a period of time sufficient for significant reduction in lesion size, second phase enucleation is performed.

Glandular odontogenic cyst (GOC) and odontogenic keratocyst (OKC) (which is also called keratocystic odontogenic tumor in the 2005 WHO classification) are more aggressive in nature than the above mentioned cysts. They often reach large sizes and tend to perforate through the cortical plates. In both OKC and GOC enucleation alone is associated with a relatively high recurrence rate, therefore additional interventions such as peripheral ostectomy, freezing or chemical cauterization of the surrounding bone after enucleation are recommended. Marginal resection may also become an option in unusually large lesions.[1-3]

PREOPERATIVE ASSESSMENT AND ANESTHESIA

The preoperative standard of care for enucleation of cysts of the jaws includes patient history, physical examination, panoramic X-ray and computed tomography (CT) scans of the jaw as in Figures 1 and 2 respectively.

In large lesions, multilocular lesions, those with obvious expansion or if perforation of cortical plates is recognized during preoperative imaging, a biopsy for diagnosis is recommended prior to enucleation.

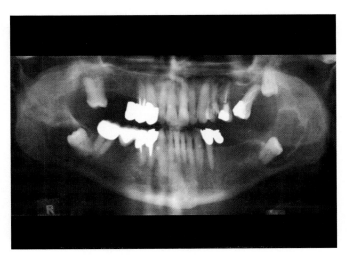

Fig. 1: Panoramic radiograph exhibiting two mandibular pericoronal well-defined radiolucent lesions surrounding the wisdom teeth. The lesion on the left shows scalloping margins

Table 1: Clinical and radiographic features of odontogenic cysts of the jaws with treatment recommendations

Type	Periapical (radicular)	Residual	Buccal bifurcation
Inflammatory/ Developmental	Inflammatory	Inflammatory	Inflammatory
Location	Periapical/periradicular Nonvital tooth	Site of a previous extraction	Buccal bifurcation and root, first permanent molar
Frequency	Most common cyst of jaws	Not rare	Rare, one-third cases bilateral
Age	Any age	Adults	Children, 1st –2nd decade
Characteristics	May be small or large cortical expansion, displacement of teeth, root for resorption are typical	May be small or large	1–2.5 cm, swelling may be associated with proliferative periostitis
Treatment requirements	Root canal treatment, enucleation If large, marsupialization, second phase enucleation	Enucleation	Enucleation, extraction not required

Type	Dentigerous		Lateral periodontal
Inflammatory/ Developmental	Developmental, may be secondarily infected		Developmental
Location	Surrounding crown of unerupted tooth, mandible> maxilla		Inter-radicular area, vital teeth Mandibular premolar lateral incisor
Frequency	Common, ~20% of jaw cysts		Rare, < 2% of jaw cysts
Age	Any, most frequently 1st–3rd decade		5th– 7th decade
Characteristics	May be small or large Expansion and displacement of teeth may be present		Usually < 1 cm, may displace adjacent roots A rare multilocular variant called Botryoid cyst
Treatment requirements	Enucleation with or without extraction of the tooth If large, marsupialization second phase enucleation		Enucleation, extraction not required

Type	Odontogenic keratocyst (keratocystic odontogenic tumor)		Glandular odontogenic cyst
Inflammatory/ Developmental	Developmental (cystic tumor as per WHO classification)		Developmental odontogenic
Location	mandible> maxilla posterior, not necessarily tooth related		mandible> maxilla, anterior, not necessarily tooth related
Frequency	3–11% of all jaw cysts		Uncommon, < 1% of all jaw cysts
Age	Any, majority 1st–3rd decade		Middle-aged adults, rare under 20
Characteristics	Potentially aggressive, tendency for cortical perforation and recurrence Expansion and root resorption uncommon Multiple OKC in nevoid basal cell carcinoma syndrome (Gorlin syndrome)		Potentially aggressive, expansion, frequent cortical perforation, high recurrence rate
Treatment requirements	Enucleation complemented by peripheral ostectomy or chemical cauterization with Carnoy's solution Marsupialization, second phase enucleation		Enucleation, peripheral ostectomy, or en bloc resection in large cysts, marsupialization, second phase enucleation

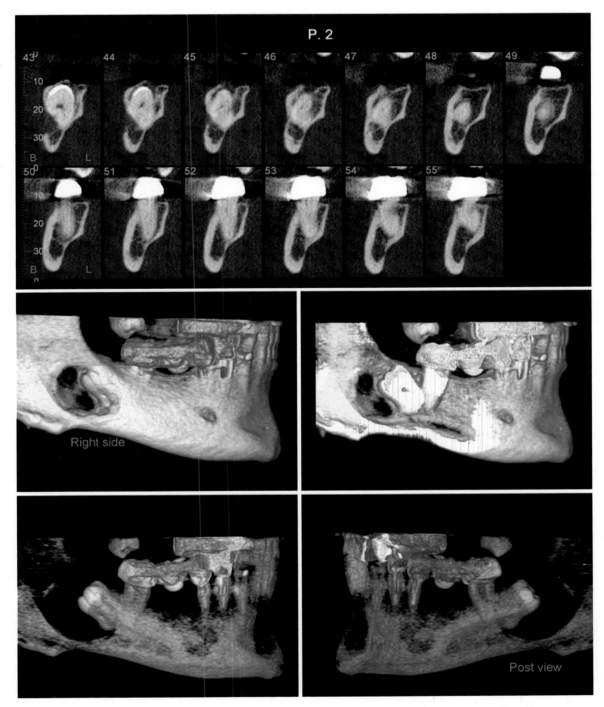

Fig. 2: CT imaging with 3D reconstructions demonstrates thinning of the cortical wall

General medical condition and the age of patient, as well as the size and location of the lesion are the factors considered in the choice of either enucleation or marsupialization as the surgical approach. In large size lesions, if the width of the cortical plates is compromised or in cases of proximity to vital structures marsupialization with second phase enucleation should be considered.

The same factors are important in the decision concerning the need for postoperative immobilization and reconstruction. Some of the procedures are better performed under general anesthesia, while others can be safely conducted in the office, under local anesthesia.

When general anesthesia is chosen, nasotracheal intubation with pharmacological muscle relaxation is preferred, to enable mouth opening and access to the posterior regions.

SURGICAL TECHNIQUE

For posterior mandibular lesions, local inferior alveolar nerve block is achieved by injecting 2% lidocaine with 1:100,000 adrenalin. The mouth is kept wide open with the aid of a molt mouth gag.

The buccal tissues and the tongue are retracted and protected. The incision is started at the crest of the ridge and is carried posteriorly, along the anterior border of the ascending ramus. A mucoperiosteal full-thickness flap is elevated, using a number 9 molt periosteal elevator (Fig. 3). The bony undersurface should be clearly visualized, often exposing incidental perforations caused by expansion of the cyst underneath. The bone should be removed judiciously, facilitating the separation of the cyst lining from the encasing wall and at the same time preserving the thick buccal bone of the external oblique ridge to prevent inadvertent jaw fractures.

If an impacted tooth is present attached to the cyst, it is carefully sectioned with a drill and removed as in Figures 4A and B.

The cyst lining is then removed (Figs 5A and B) with an appropriate surgical curette and the residual cavity is thoroughly irrigated and inspected for any remaining fragments of lining.

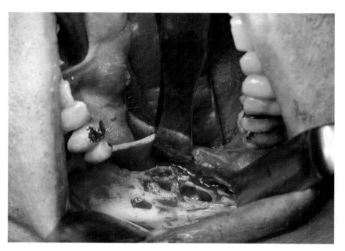

Fig. 3: Following a crestal incision, a mucoperiosteal flap is elevated exposing the underlying bone. Multiple perforations of the cortex are evident

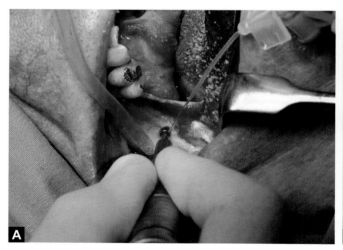
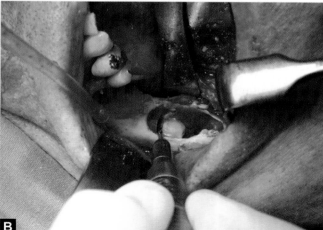

Figs 4A and B: Using a round burr and irrigation bone is carefully removed allowing for adequate exposure of the embedded tooth. The tooth is then sectioned and removed

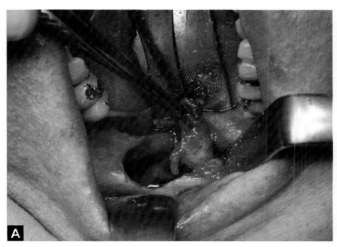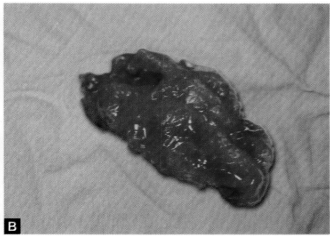

Figs 5A and B: Enucleation of the cyst

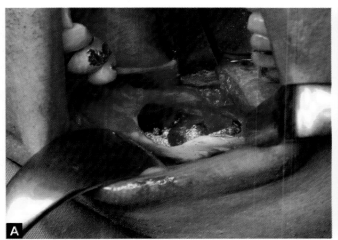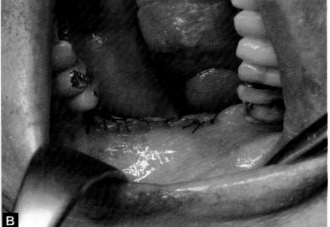

Figs 6A and B: (A) Packing of the cavity with Surgicel
followed by (B) Closure and suturing of the flap

To help prevent the blood clot from disintegration, prior to suturing, resorbable hemostatic material (e.g. Surgicel or Gelfoam) can be packed into the cavity (Fig. 6A). The mucosa is then closed tightly with interrupted sutures over the blood clot created as in Figure 6B.

POSTOPERATIVE TREATMENT

Perioperative antibiotics (penicillin and metronidazole or penicillin/clavulanate or cindamycin) are administered. Ice packs and systemic steroids (dexamethasone 2 mg PO BID for 3 days or 16–20 mg IV single dose) are helpful in reducing postoperative edema and pain. Postoperative pain is also controlled with IM pethidine (for inpatients) or PO percocet for outpatients. In addition, diclofenac 50–75 mg IM Q 4 hours or ketrolac 15–30 mg IM or 10 mg PO are helpful in pain control. Nausea and vomiting are controlled with metoclopramide, 5–10 mg IM.

The patient is instructed to start frequent mouth rinses with either warm saline or chlorhexidine 0.2 % BID, the day after surgery. Soft diet is prescribed for a few days.

Postoperative X-rays are taken 1 week and 3 months post surgery to assess the degree of bone fill of the cavity. A follow-up period of 3–6 months is usually sufficient for most types of odontogenic cysts. Prolonged follow-up is advised for OKC and GOC, as they may recur even years after treatment.

The histopathological diagnosis of the case presented was OKC (keratocystic odontogenic tumor). Follow-up is continued after every 6 months.

HIGHLIGHTS

- In large lesions and multilocular lesions, those with obvious expansion or if perforation of cortical plates is recognized during preoperative imaging. A biopsy for diagnosis is recommended prior to enucleation.
- In large size lesions, if the width of the cortical plates is compromised or in cases of proximity to vital structures marsupialization with second phase enucleation should be considered.
- In OKC and GOC, it is recommended to complement enucleation with peripheral ostectomy or chemical cauterization by Carnoy's solution as a method to reduce the frequency of recurrent disease.
- Prolonged follow-up is advised for OKC and GOC, whereas 3–6 months are sufficient in all other types of odontogenic cysts.

REFERENCES

1. Kaplan I, Gal G, Anavi Y, et al. Glandular odontogenic cyst: treatment and recurrence. J Oral Maxillofac Surg. 2005;63(4): 435-41.
2. Kuroyanagi N, Sakuma H, Miyabe S, et al. Prognostic factors for keratocystic odontogenic tumor (odontogenic keratocyst): analysis of clinico-pathologic and immunohistochemical findings in cysts treated by enucleation. J Oral Pathol Med. 2009;38(4):386-92.
3. Tolstunov L, Treasure T. Surgical treatment algorithm for odontogenic keratocyst: combined treatment of odontogenic keratocyst and mandibular defect with marsupialization, enucleation, iliac crest bone graft, and dental implants. Oral Maxillofac Surg. 2008;66(5):1025-36.

Chapter **23**

Base of Tongue Surgery

Carol M Lewis, Randal S Weber

CHAPTER OVERVIEW

The tongue is one of the most common sites of head and neck malignancy. The anterior two-thirds of the tongue is considered oral cavity, with the posterior one-third being oropharynx. Roughly one-third of all tongue squamous cell carcinomas (SCC) occur in the tongue base. In India, however, the reverse is true; the incidence of oral tongue SCC is one-third that of tongue base SCC.[1] Of tongue base cancers, nearly 90% are SCC, with lymphoma and minor salivary gland malignancies comprising the majority of the remaining 10%.[2] For tongue base SCC, the age range at presentation is 30–90 years,[1] with a median age of 63 years and a male to female ratio of 2.7:1.[2] Prolonged use of tobacco and alcohol are major risk factors with mounting evidence for human papillomavirus (HPV) as the etiologic agent in a younger population of patients who are nonsmokers and nondrinkers.[3]

Anatomically, the tongue base extends from the circumvallate papillae anteriorly to the vallecula inferoposteriorly, with the glossopalatine sulcus as the lateral limit. It therefore includes the lingual tonsils and glossopharyngeal and glossoepiglottic folds. Local extension is common given this location and it may be difficult to determine whether the tumor's primary site of origin is the tongue base, oral tongue, tonsil, or retromolar trigone.

Most patients present with the complaint of persistent sore throat; other symptoms may include dysarthria, weight loss, neck mass, dysphagia, foreign body sensation and otalgia.[1] When taking a history, it is important to elicit tobacco and alcohol exposure, pain, and functional impairments such as dysphagia and dysarthria. Physical examination should include direct or indirect inspection and palpation to assess the extent of the tumor. In addition to evaluating the tumor on physical exam, tongue mobility, trismus, and cranial nerve deficits should also be assessed. Since 60% of patients present with N1 disease and up to 20% of patients present with bilateral neck disease,[1] assessment for cervical lymphadenopathy is mandatory.

Imaging ought to include a contrast computed tomography (CT) or magnetic resonance imaging (MRI) of the head and neck for delineation of the primary lesion and lymphadenopathy, including retropharyngeal lymphadenopathy which has poor prognostic significance. Additionally, a chest X-ray is indicated for evaluation for potential metastases. Laboratory studies should include liver function tests, as well as other indicated preanesthesia tests. Depending on the patient's specific comorbidities, a preanesthesia evaluation and medical clearance should be obtained. An examination under anesthesia is recommended to determine the full extent of the tumor, including mucosal invasion and submucosal spread, tumor fixation, and whether there may be a synchronous primary tumor.

A multidisciplinary assessment including head and neck surgery, radiation oncology, medical oncology, speech and language pathology, and dental oncology is essential for formulating the most appropriate individual management plan. The best treatment for tongue base malignancy is still debated with the goal being oncologic cure with preservation of function. Recent trends in treatment have been toward radiotherapy with or without chemotherapy,[4,5] although between 1985 and 1996, the most common management strategy combined surgery and radiotherapy.[2] There does not seem to be a clear advantage of surgery or radiotherapy for unilateral T1 or T2 tumors. For lesions involving the midline, root of tongue, or larynx, surgery with postoperative radiotherapy may offer the highest probability of local and regional control, but can inflict profound functional impairment.[6] Nonetheless, combined modality therapy is indicated for T3 and T4 tumors.

This chapter describes the surgical approaches to the tongue base,[7] which may be categorized as follows:
- Transmandibular
  - Mandibular swing approach
  - Composite resection
  - Midline labiomandibular glossotomy.
- Transpharyngeal
  - Transhyoid pharyngotomy
  - Lateral pharyngotomy.
- Transoral
  - Transoral lateral oropharyngectomy.
- Combination transoral-transcervical
  - Mandibular lingual release.

Although, the technique of neck dissection is not detailed here, cervical lymphadenectomy should be part of the surgical management of every oropharyngeal SCC. This may be unilateral for unilateral lesions and bilateral for lesions involving the midline. Depending on the extent of anticipated resection, reconstructive options should be considered in surgical planning.

REFERENCES

1. Weber PC, Myers EN, Johnson JT. Squamous cell carcinoma of the base of tongue. Eur Arch Otorhinolaryngol. 1993;250(2):63-8.
2. Zhen W, Karnell LH, Hoffman HT, et al. The National Cancer Data Base report on squamous cell carcinoma of the base of tongue. Head Neck. 2004;26(8):660-74.
3. Fakhry C, Gillison ML. Clinical implications of human papillomavirus in head and neck cancers. J Clin Oncol. 2006;24(17):2606-11.
4. Koch WM. Head and neck surgery in the era of organ preservation therapy. Semin Oncol. 2000;27(4 Suppl 8):5-12.
5. Han P, Hu K, Frank DK, et al. Management of cancer of the base of tongue. Otolaryngol Clin North Am. 2005;38(1):75-85, viii.
6. Weber RS, Gidley P, Morrison WH, et al. Treatment selection for carcinoma of the base of the tongue. Am J Surg. 1990;160(4):415-9.
7. Holsinger FC, Laccourreye O, Weber RS. Surgical approaches for cancer of the oropharynx. Operative Techniques in Otolaryngology. 2005;16:40-8.

Part A: Transmandibular Approaches

Mandibular Swing Approach

INTRODUCTION

Roux is credited with being the first to divide the lip and mandible to access the floor of mouth and tongue in 1836. Subsequent surgeons proposed a similar technique with modifications, including Sédillot in 1844 and Syme in 1857.[8,9] In 1862, Billroth made two mandibular osteotomies and retracted the free mandibular segment with the soft tissue flap while the tumor was resected; then the segment was replated.[9] Trotter offered his modifications in 1913 and Kremen espoused this approach in conjunction with concurrent cervical lymphadenectomy in 1951.[8]

In 1902, Kocher advocated Sédillot's symphyseal mandibulotomy for all but the smallest of the tongue tumors.[9] Current indications include tumors of the lateral tongue base, including those involving the tonsillar fossa and glossopharyngeal sulcus.

PREOPERATIVE EVALUATION AND ANESTHESIA

As discussed in the chapter overview, the work-up involves a thorough history and physical examination, appropriate imaging and laboratory studies, and examination under anesthesia with biopsy after obtaining appropriate preanesthesia medical clearance. Multidisciplinary evaluation is imperative, including speech pathology evaluation of the patient's level of function and dental oncology for indicated dental extractions. Depending on the extent of anticipated resection, reconstructive options should be considered in surgical planning.

Tracheotomy is routinely performed with this procedure. If tracheotomy will be performed after the oncologic resection, nasotracheal intubation will facilitate this approach by eliminating the hindrance of an oral endotracheal tube. Perioperative intravenous antibiotics are initiated an hour before incision.

SURGICAL TECHNIQUE

Beginning with an examination under anesthesia, the tumor is reassessed to confirm anticipated margins of resection and to assess tumor fixation. If mandibular involvement is indeterminant, the mandibulotomy should be placed more posteriorly in case the mandibulotomy is converted to a mandibulectomy. The tracheotomy is generally performed next, but may be performed after tumor resection. This eliminates the endotracheal tube from potentially interfering with the surgical field. The appropriate neck dissection(s) is performed prior to resection of the tumor.

The lip-splitting incision is then made in the midline. The vertical mental incision may be somewhat camouflaged by the use of a stair step design or W or M-plasty (Fig. 1). Intraorally, a gingivolabial incision is extended toward the ipsilateral side to the first premolar, ensuring that the incision remains anterior to the mental foramen. This incision is made with at least 1 cm of mucosa between the gingiva and the incision to facilitate closure. The mandibular periosteum is elevated both medially and laterally. The subperiosteal elevation should only continue laterally, inferior to the mental foramen and exposing just enough mandible as is needed for the plate reconstruction. Once adequate mandibular exposure is obtained, a reconstructive plate is bent to fit the contour of mandible and plated, taking care not to disrupt dental roots. The plate is then removed. If necessary, a tooth may be removed at the anticipated osteotomy site

to facilitate the cut. The authors review the preoperative panorex. If there is a room for the mandibulotomy between adjacent tooth roots, then the authors do not extract the tooth. However, if this is not the case, then tooth extraction at the mandibulotomy site is necessary. The mandibulotomy is then made with an appropriate motor saw as in Figure 2.

A mucosal incision is then made in the line of the mandibulotomy on the lingual surface of the mandible, aimed posterolaterally on the ipsilateral side (Fig. 3). The mucosal incision continues posteriorly parallel to the mandible, leaving at least a 1 cm cuff of mucosa between the gingiva and the incision to facilitate closure. The floor of mouth musculature, including the mylohyoid and anterior digastric muscles, are divided. If necessary, for exposure or for obtaining adequate margins, this paralingual incision can be continued through the glossopharyngeal fold and inferiorly along the pharynx to the level of the hyoid. While performing this extension, care must be taken to identify and preserve the lingual artery and hypoglossal nerve; the authors usually divide the lingual nerve. If the tumor involves the soft palate and tonsillar fossa, the incision can be carried superiorly to enable an en bloc extirpation. Once adequate exposure is obtained, the tumor is reassessed and removed with adequate margins.

After removal of the tumor, surgical margins are assessed by frozen section analysis to confirm the adequacy of resection. A nasogastric tube is then placed. Rarely

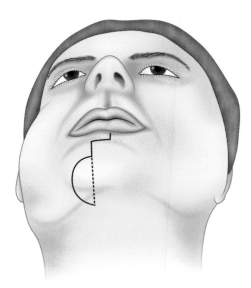

Fig. 1: The lip-split incision can be straight, fashioned as a W or M-plasty, stair stepped, or curved around the pogonion in the mental crease

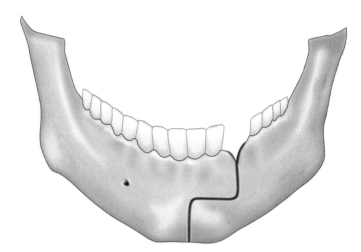

Fig. 2: The mandibular osteotomy can be straight or stair stepped

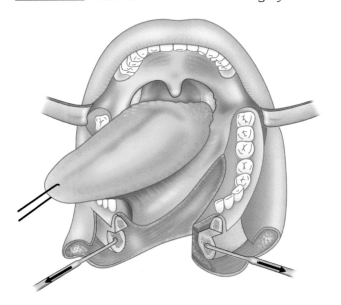

Fig. 3: A mucosal incision is then made on the lingual surface of the mandible, aimed posterolaterally and planned parallel to the mandible, leaving at least a 1 cm cuff of mucosa between the gingiva and the incision to facilitate closure

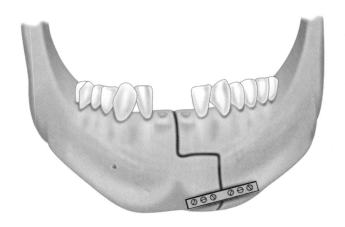

Fig. 4: Replating the osteotomy

can these defects be closed primarily, and when possible, primary closure is usually obtained to the detriment of form and function. Reconstruction usually takes the form of regional or microvascular free flaps, the details of which are beyond the scope of this chapter. After the flap inset, watertight closure is achieved along the paralingual incision by approximating the cuff of mucosa on the lingual aspect of the mandible to the tongue and floor of mouth. The mandible is then plated (Fig. 4), followed by closure of the anterior floor of mouth and gingiva. The gingivolabial incisions are then reapproximated. The transected floor of mouth musculature may be reapproximated through the cervical incision. The lip-split incision is closed in three layers (mucosal, muscular/soft tissue and skin), with careful realignment of the vermilion border. The neck incision is then closed in layers over bulb-suction drains.

POSTOPERATIVE TREATMENT

Postoperative management includes nasogastric tube feeding and routine tracheotomy care. Ideally, the patient should be decannulated prior to initiating oral intake. Speech pathology plays a critical role in evaluating the safety of oral intake and teaching patients swallowing maneuvers. Broad-spectrum antibiotics are recommended at least in the early postoperative period and gastroesophageal reflux prophylaxis should be instituted. Oral care may be taken in the form of salt and soda rinses.

HIGHLIGHTS

I. Indications
- Tumors of the lateral tongue base, including those involving the tonsillar fossa and glossopharyngeal sulcus.

II. Contraindications
- Mandibular involvement should convert the mandibulotomy to a mandibulectomy
- Prohibitive medical comorbidities.

III. Special Preoperative Considerations
- Imaging
- Multidisciplinary evaluation, including speech pathology and dental oncology
- Medical evaluation and preanesthetic clearance
- Reconstructive planning as indicated.

IV. Intraoperative Considerations
- When making the gingivobuccal or paralingual incisions, leave a cuff of mucosa between the incision and the mandible to facilitate closure.
- Fitting the mandibular plate, prior to making the osteotomies assists in maintaining postoperative occlusion and mandibular contour.
- The mandibular plate should be placed inferior to the mental foramen, taking care not to disrupt tooth roots.
- The osteotomy should be made anterior to the mental foramen when possible.
- Closure of the lip incision should include careful realignment of the vermilion border.

V. Postoperative Considerations
- Enteral feeding by nasogastric tube

- Tracheotomy care
- Broad-spectrum antibiotics in the initial post-operative period
- Gastroesophageal reflux prophylaxis
- Oral care, which may include salt and soda rinses.

VI. **Complications**
- Dysphagia
- Aspiration with or without pneumonia
- Dysarthria
- Poor mastication
- Lip scarring/cosmetic deformity
- Malocclusion
- Nonunion
- Temporomandibular joint pain

- Hemorrhage
- Wound infection, including osteomyelitis
- Chronic pain
- Pharyngocutaneous fistula
- Risks of anesthesia.

REFERENCES

8. Kremen AJ. Cancer of the tongue; a surgical technique for a primary combined en bloc resection of tongue, floor of mouth, and cervical lymphatics. Surgery. 1951;30(1):227-40.
9. Spiro RH, Gerold FP, Strong EW. Mandibular "swing" approach for oral and oropharyngeal tumors. Head Neck Surg. 1981;3(5):371-8.

Composite Resection

INTRODUCTION

The term "composite resection" was first coined by Ward and Robben in 1951 to reflect en bloc removal of an oral cavity or oropharyngeal tumor with involved mandible and associated lymphatics.[10,11] En bloc resection has long been advocated for the extirpation of malignancy. In 1880, Kocher reported removing an oral cavity primary tumor in contiguity with the cervical lymphadenectomy specimen. In a chapter published in 1927, Semken described an en bloc resection of the neck dissection specimen with a primary lesion involving either the buccal mucosa, oral commissure or mandible.[10] In 1949, Slaughter et al. expanded this to include mandibulectomy.[12]

Historically, composite resection involving a segmental or hemimandibulectomy was felt to be necessary for the resection of oral cavity and oropharyngeal tumors, even without mandibular invasion due to the widespread belief that these tumors seeded via periosteal lymphatics.[11] However, Marchetta et al. disproved this notion of tumor spread.[13] Currently, this approach is utilized for advanced oral cavity or oropharyngeal malignancies in which mandibular invasion is either overt or cannot be excluded.

PREOPERATIVE EVALUATION AND ANESTHESIA

As discussed in the chapter overview, the work-up involves a thorough review of the history and physical examination, appropriate imaging and laboratory studies, and examination under anesthesia with biopsy after obtaining appropriate preanesthesia medical clearance. Multidisciplinary evalua-tion is imperative, including speech pathology evaluation of the patient's level of function and dental oncology for indicated dental extractions. Depending on the extent of anticipated resection, reconstructive options should be considered in surgical planning.

Tracheotomy is routinely performed with this procedure. If tracheotomy is performed after the oncologic resection, nasotracheal intubation will facilitate this approach by eliminating the hindrance of an oral endotracheal tube. Perioperative intravenous antibiotics are initiated an hour before incision.

SURGICAL TECHNIQUE

Beginning with an examination under anesthesia, the tumor is reassessed to confirm anticipated margins of resection. The tracheotomy is generally performed next. This eliminates the endotracheal tube from potentially interfering with the surgical field.

The tumor resection can either be performed through a visor incision, which is more cosmetic but puts the contralateral mental nerve at risk, or with a lip-splitting incision, which risks cosmetic deformity, but affords a broader exposure. If the lip-splitting approach is chosen, the vertical mental incision may be somewhat camouflaged by the use of a stair step design (Fig. 5) or by placing it along the curve of the chin pad. The cervical component of either incision should take care to avoid contiguity with the tracheotomy site. Once the incision is designed, the appropriate neck dissection(s) is performed.

A supraperiosteal plane is then elevated over the mandible, anterior to the masseter. The inferior mandibular

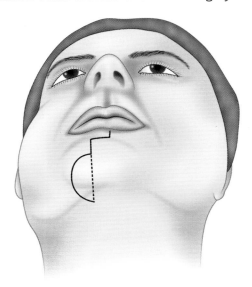

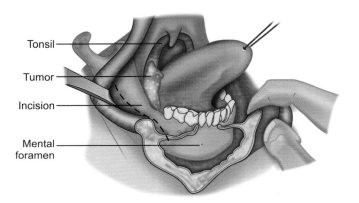

Fig. 6: The intraoral incision is then made along the gingivobuccal sulcus, taking care to ensure an adequate soft tissue margin around the tumor and modifying this incision as indicated

Fig. 5: If the lip-splitting approach is chosen, the vertical mental incision may be somewhat camouflaged by the use of a stair step design, or by placing it along the mental crease, curving around the pogonion

attachment of the masseter is then divided and the muscle is elevated off the mandible. The marginal mandibular branch of the facial nerve is thereby included in the soft tissue superior flap. If the tumor extends through the mandible and involves the overlying soft tissue, elevation of this flap should be modified to ensure oncologically sound margins, possibly involving the sacrifice of the marginal mandibular nerve, the masseter muscle or the skin.

If a lip-splitting incision is made, it is then divided in the midline. The skin flaps are elevated in continuity with the elevated superior soft tissue flap, dividing the mental nerve in the process. The intraoral incision is then made along the gingivobuccal sulcus, taking care to ensure an adequate soft tissue margin around the tumor and modifying this incision as indicated (Fig. 6). The gingivobuccal incision is then made contiguous with the cervical incision.

If a lip-splitting incision is not performed, the gingivobuccal incision is made transorally. If extension of this incision along the contralateral gingivolabial sulcus is required to improve exposure, care must be taken to identify and preserve the contralateral mental nerve. The gingivobuccal incision is then made contiguous with the cervical incision. Penrose drains may then be passed between the lips and threaded through the passage connecting the gingivobuccal and cervical incision to facilitate retraction of the superior soft tissue flap.

The osteotomies are then planned and marked on the mandible at least 2 cm away from grossly or radiographically apparent tumor. Depending on the extent of the tumor,

this may involve the removal of the coronoid process or the entire condyle. Division of the temporalis muscle mandibular attachments and/or disarticulation of the temporomandibular joint should be performed as indicated. If tumor does involve the ascending ramus, resection of adjacent pterygoid musculature and/or plates should be considered to ensure adequate margins.

Once the osteotomies are marked, the mandibular reconstruction plate may be contoured and screw holes drilled to facilitate later boney reconstruction and to assist in maintaining postoperative occlusion and facial contour. If dental extractions do not occur at the start of the procedure, they may be performed at this juncture. If necessary, a tooth may be removed at the anticipated osteotomy sites to facilitate the cuts. The osteotomies are then made with an appropriate powered saw or Gigli saw (Fig. 7). Performing the osteotomy procedure before the soft tissue resection, facilitates soft tissue incisions by allowing lateral retraction of the free mandibular segment. Soft tissue incisions are then made around the tumor. Portions of the soft palate may be included in the resection specimen as indicated. If the posterior incision requires superolateral extension in the oropharynx, consideration should be given to divide the medial pterygoid, as well as branches of the mandibular branch of the trigeminal nerve and of the internal maxillary artery.

After en bloc removal of the tumor, surgical margins are assessed by frozen section analysis to confirm the adequacy of resection. A nasogastric tube is then placed. Rarely can these defects be closed primarily and when possible, primary closure is usually obtained to the detriment of form and function. Reconstruction usually takes the form of regional or microvascular free flaps, the details of which are beyond the scope of this chapter. After flap inset, the gingivobuccal incisions are reapproximated for a watertight closure.

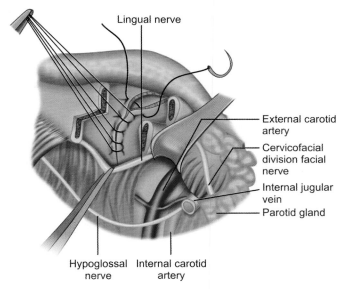

Lingual nerve

External carotid artery

Cervicofacial division facial nerve

Internal jugular vein

Parotid gland

Hypoglossal nerve   Internal carotid artery

Fig. 7: The osteotomies are then made with an appropriate powered saw or Gigli saw roughly 2 cm away from the tumor edge. Performing these before the soft tissue resection facilitates soft tissue incisions by allowing lateral retraction of the free mandibular segment

The lip-split incision is closed in three layers (mucosal, muscular/soft tissue and skin), with careful realignment of the vermilion border. The neck incision is then closed in layers over bulb-suction drains.

POSTOPERATIVE TREATMENT

Postoperative management includes nasogastric tube feeding and routine tracheotomy care. Ideally, the patient should be decannulated prior to initiating oral intake. Speech pathology plays a critical role in evaluating the safety of oral intake and teaching patients swallowing maneuvers. Broad-spectrum antibiotics are recommended at least in the early postoperative period and gastroesophageal reflux prophylaxis should be instituted. Oral care may take the form of salt and soda rinses.

HIGHLIGHTS

I. Indications
- Oral cavity or oropharyneal malignancies in which mandibular invasion is either overt or cannot be excluded.

II. Contraindications
- Prohibitive medical comorbidities.

III. Special Preoperative Considerations
- Imaging

- Multidisciplinary evaluation, including speech pathology and dental oncology
- Medical evaluation and preanesthetic clearance
- Reconstructive planning as indicated.

IV. Special Intraoperative Considerations
- When extending the intraoral incision contralaterally to improve exposure, the contralateral mental nerve should be identified and preserved.
- Mandibular osteotomies should be placed at least 2 cm from grossly or radiographically apparent tumor.
- Fitting the mandibular plate prior to making the osteotomies assists in maintaining postoperative occlusion and mandibular contour.
- The procedure should be tailored to the individual tumor and incisions should be modified to ensure the oncologic integrity of this procedure.
- If a lip-splitting incision is used, closure should involve careful realignment of the vermilion border.

V. Special Postoperative Considerations
- Enteral feeding by nasogastric tube
- Tracheotomy care
- Broad-spectrum antibiotics in the initial postoperative period
- Gastroesophageal reflux prophylaxis
- Oral care, which may include salt and soda rinses.

VI. Complications
- Dysphagia
- Aspiration (with or without pneumonia)
- Dysarthria
- Poor mastication
- Facial deformity/depression over mandibulectomy
- Lip scarring/cosmetic deformity
- Malocclusion
- Temporomandibular joint pain
- Hemorrhage
- Wound infection, including osteomyelitis
- Chronic pain
- Pharyngocutaneous fistula
- Risks of anesthesia.

REFERENCES

10. Ward GE, Robben JO. A composite operation for radical neck dissection and removal of cancer of the mouth. Cancer. 1951;4(1):98-109.
11. Holsinger FC, Laccourreye O, Weber RS. Surgical approaches for cancer of the oropharynx. Operative Techniques in Otolaryngology. 2005;16:40-8.
12. Slaughter DP, Roeser EH, Smejkal WF. Excision of the mandible for neoplastic diseases; indications and techniques. Surgery. 1949;26(3):507-22.
13. Marchetta FC, Sako K, Badillo J. Periosteal lymphatics of the mandible and intraoral carcinoma. Am J Surg. 1964;108: 505-7.

Midline Labiomandibular Glossotomy

INTRODUCTION

The earliest report of splitting the mandible to access the oral cavity was by Roux in 1836, who used this technique to access anterior tongue neoplasms.[14] In 1929, Trotter extended the application of this approach to include lesions of the tongue base, epiglottis and posterior pharyngeal wall through what he termed a "median (anterior) translingual pharyngotomy". This involved removing the central portion of the hyoid bone.[15] This approach remained unpopular until 1959, when Perzik et al. reported success using this technique to remove a posterior pharyngeal wall tumor in an infant.[16] Martin et al. then popularized this procedure in 1961, renaming it as "median labiomandibular glossotomy".[17] Since this approach does not provide adequate lateral exposure, the indications have been narrowed to small midline tongue base tumors and posterior pharyngeal wall lesions not extending too far inferiorly to the arytenoids. It also has applicability to midline, bulky but benign and noninfiltrating minor salivary gland lesions, as well as to certain soft palate lesions. When combined with a transpalatal approach, it may also be used to access selected lesions of the nasopharynx and skull base.

PREOPERATIVE EVALUATION AND ANESTHESIA

As discussed in the chapter overview, the work-up involves a thorough history and physical examination, appropriate imaging and laboratory studies, and examination under anesthesia with biopsy after obtaining appropriate preanesthesia medical clearance. Special attention should be given to patient's pulmonary status, since postoperative aspiration may occur. Multidisciplinary evaluation is imperative, including speech pathology evaluation of the patient's level of function. Depending on the extent of anticipated resection, reconstructive options should be considered in surgical planning.

Tracheotomy is routinely performed and patients should be counseled appropriately. If tracheotomy will be performed after the oncologic resection, nasotracheal intubation will facilitate this approach by eliminating the hindrance of an oral endotracheal tube. Perioperative intravenous antibiotics are initiated an hour before incision.

SURGICAL TECHNIQUE

Beginning with an examination under anesthesia, the tumor is reassessed for anticipated margins of resection and to ensure it is still a reasonable candidate for resection via median labiomandibular glossotomy, since this approach does not provide adequate lateral exposure and is best suited for midline lesions. The anticipated margins can be marked out during the endoscopy. The tracheotomy is generally performed next. This eliminates the endotracheal tube from potentially interfering with the surgical field. In designing the lip-split incision, the vertical mental incision may be somewhat camouflaged by the use of a stair step design, or W or M-plasty (Fig. 8). This incision extends down through the midline submentum to the level of the hyoid. If neck dissection(s) is planned, the submental incision can be made contiguous with this incision. The appropriate neck dissection(s) is performed prior to resection of the tumor.

The lip-splitting incision is then made in the midline to mandibular periosteum. The periosteum of the anterior mandible is then elevated and the planned osteotomy marked (Fig. 9). A medial incisor may be removed to avoid damage to neighboring tooth roots. Once adequate mandibular exposure is obtained, a reconstructive plate is molded to the contour of mandible and plated along the inferior aspect of the anterior mandible, taking care not to disrupt the dental roots. The plate is then removed and appropriately sized screws are placed aside for closure. Next, the osteotomy is made with an appropriate powered saw (Fig. 10).

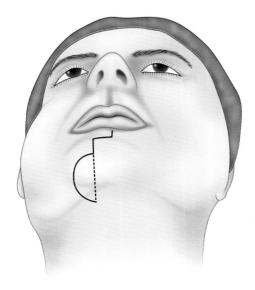

Fig. 8: The vertical mental incision may be somewhat camouflaged by the use of a stair step design, or by placing it along the mental crease, curving around the pogonion

The oral tongue and floor of mouth musculature is then divided along the median raphe with electrocautery as in Figures 11A and B.

If the tumor is in the tongue base, this lingual incision serves as the anterior margin, which emphasizes the importance of starting with an examination under anesthesia. Great care should be taken to ensure deep muscular margins. When taking lateral margins, the hypoglossal nerve and lingual artery should be identified and preserved.

After removal of the tumor, surgical margins are assessed by frozen section analysis to confirm the adequacy of resection. A nasogastric tube is then placed. If the resection area is small, the defect may be closed primarily in layers, such that the tongue and floor of mouth muscles and mucosa are reapproximated in the midline (Fig. 12).

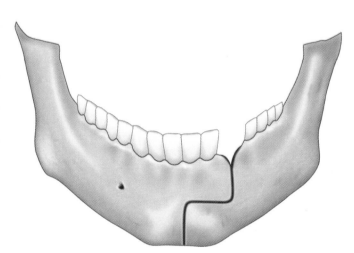

Fig. 9: The mandibular osteotomy can be straight or stair stepped

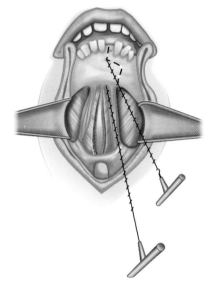

Fig. 10: The osteotomy is made with an appropriate powered saw or Gigli saw

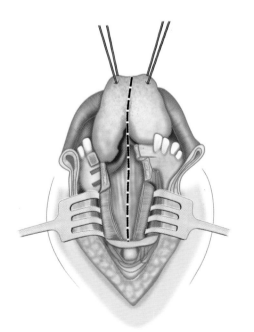

A

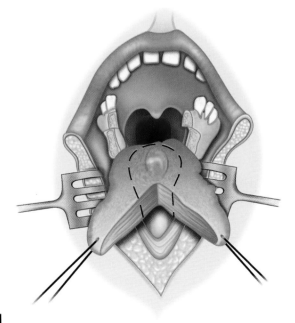

B

Figs 11A and B: The oral tongue and floor of mouth musculature is then divided along the median raphe with electrocautery

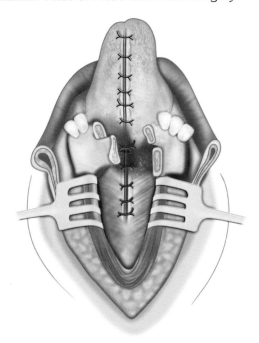

Fig. 12: If the resection area is small, the defect may be closed primarily in layers such that the tongue and floor of mouth muscles and mucosa are reapproximated in the midline

If primary closure is not possible, local tongue flaps,[14] regional muscle or myocutaneous flaps or microvascular free flaps are the reconstructive options; the details of these are beyond the scope of this chapter. Once the primary defect is closed, the oral tongue and floor of mouth musculature should be reapproximated in muscle and mucosal layers. The mandible should be replated in the midline with the prefitted plate. The lip-split incision is closed in three layers (mucosal, muscular/soft tissue and skin), with careful realignment of the vermilion border. The submental incision is then closed in layers over bulb-suction drains.

POSTOPERATIVE TREATMENT

Postoperative management includes nasogastric tube feeding and routine tracheotomy care. Ideally, the patient should be decannulated prior to initiating oral intake. Speech pathology plays a critical role in evaluating the safety of oral intake and teaching patients swallowing maneuvers. Broad-spectrum antibiotics are recommended at least in the early postoperative period and gastroesophageal reflux prophylaxis should be instituted. Oral care may take the form of salt and soda rinses.

HIGHLIGHTS

I. Indications
- Small midline tongue base tumors and posterior pharyngeal wall lesions not extending too far inferiorly to the arytenoids
- Midline, bulky but benign and noninfiltrating minor salivary gland lesions, including certain soft palate lesions
- When combined with a transpalatal approach, this may also be used to access selected lesions of the nasopharynx and skull base.

II. Contraindications
- Involvement of the lateral tongue base such that resection with adequate margins would require sacrifice of the hypoglossal nerve and/or lingual artery
- Mandibular fixation
- If the tumor is on the posterior pharyngeal wall, or has extension inferior to the arytenoids
- Prohibitive medical comorbidities.

III. Special Preoperative Considerations
- Imaging
- Multidisciplinary evaluation including speech pathology and dental oncology
- Medical evaluation and preanesthetic clearance
- Reconstructive planning as indicated.

IV. Special Intraoperative Considerations
- Fitting the mandibular plate prior to making the osteotomies assists in maintaining postoperative occlusion and mandibular contour.
- The mandibular plate should be placed inferiorly on the anterior mandible, taking care not to disrupt tooth roots.
- A medial mandibular incisor may be removed, prior to osteotomy to avoid injury to neighboring tooth roots.
- Divide the tongue and floor of mouth muscles along the median raphe.
- When removing tongue base lesions, great care must be taken to adequately estimate deep muscle margins. In addition, for resection margins that involve the lateral tongue base, the lingual artery and the hypoglossal nerve should be identified and preserved.
- Closure of the lip incision should include careful realignment of the vermilion border.

V. Postoperative Considerations
- Enteral feeding by nasogastric tube
- Tracheotomy care
- Broad-spectrum antibiotics in the initial postoperative period
- Gastroesophageal reflux prophylaxis
- Oral care, which may include salt and soda rinses.

VI. Complications
- Dysphagia
- Aspiration/pneumonia
- Dysarthria
- Poor mastication
- Lip scarring/cosmetic deformity
- Malocclusion
- Nonunion
- Temporomandibular joint pain
- Hemorrhage
- Wound infection, including osteomyelitis
- Chronic pain
- Pharyngocutaneous fistula
- Risks of anesthesia.

REFERENCES

14. Alperin KM, Levine HL, Wood BG, et al. Approach to and reconstruction for lesions of the posterior third of the tongue via midline labiomandibular glossotomy. Head Neck Surg. 1984;6(3):744-50.

15. Trotter W. Operations for malignant disease of the pharynx. British Journal of Surgery. 1929;16:485-95.

16. Perzik SL, Rubin HJ, Schorr R. Excision of obstructing retropharyngeal tumor in an infant; excision by sagittal jaw splitting approach. AMA Arch Surg. 1959;78(3):503-6.

17. Martin H, Tollefsen HR, Gerold FP. Median labiomandibular glossotomy. Trotter's median (anterior) translingual pharyngotomy. Am J Surg. 1961;102:753-9.

Part B: Transpharyngeal Approaches

Transhyoid Pharyngotomy

INTRODUCTION

The concept of employing a suprahyoid approach to the tongue base dates back to 1826, when it was suggested by the anatomist Vidal de Cassis. In 1834, Malgaigne reported autopsy studies which revealed access to the hypopharynx, tongue base and epiglottis through a suprahyoid incision. In 1895, Jeremitsch observed that in a patient who had attempted suicide, the suprahyoid wound bled minimally, did not disrupt the nerves and provided excellent access to the pharynx. The first successful suprahyoid pharyngotomy was performed by Grunwald in 1906, but he disparaged the procedure when his patients developed "sagging of the larynx". Despite the success by subsequent surgeons, the approach remained unpopular. In reviewing the history of this procedure, Blassingame indicates that this complication resulted from failure to resuspend the larynx.[18] Even with Blassingame's defense, this procedure did not gain popularity until 1980s. Moore and Calcaterra reported success using a transhyoid approach in 13 patients with T3 tongue base tumors. In some patients, this was combined with a supraglottic laryngectomy.[19] Weber et al. advocated a suprahyoid approach for T1 or T2 tongue base neoplasms.[20] Since then, many other authors have reported success with this approach. Studies comparing this approach with the more traditional mandibulotomy have found fewer complications and better functional outcomes after transhyoid pharyngotomy with similar oncologic outcomes.[21-23]

PREOPERATIVE EVALUATION AND ANESTHESIA

As discussed in the chapter overview, the work-up involves a thorough history and physical examination, appropriate imaging and laboratory studies, and examination under anesthesia with biopsy after obtaining appropriate preanesthesia medical clearance. Special attention should be given to patient's pulmonary status, since postoperative aspiration is an expected occurrence. Multidisciplinary evaluation is imperative, including speech pathology evaluation of the patient's level of function. Depending on the extent of anticipated resection, reconstructive options should be considered in surgical planning. Tracheotomy is routinely performed and patients should be counseled appropriately. Perioperative intravenous antibiotics are initiated an hour before incision.

SURGICAL TECHNIQUE

Beginning with an examination under anesthesia, the tumor is reassessed to ensure it is a reasonable candidate for resection via transhyoid pharyngotomy. The tracheotomy is generally performed next. This eliminates the endotracheal tube from potentially interfering with the surgical field. The appropriate neck dissection(s) is then performed through a superiorly based apron flap that is carefully designed to avoid contiguity with the tracheotomy site.

The suprahyoid musculature is transected at the hyoid bone, leaving a 5 mm cuff of muscle on the hyoid to assist with resuspension at the time of closure (Fig. 13). Bilateral hypoglossal nerves, superior laryngeal nerves and lingual arteries are identified and preserved. Superior retraction of the divided suprahyoid muscles will delineate the hyoepiglottic ligament. Zeitels et al. advocate identification of this ligament, which fans out from a narrow epiglottic insertion to a broad hyoid attachment to facilitate precise medicine entry at the median glossoepiglottic fold.[24] To provide an additional margin of mucosa in the vallecula, the mucosa of the vallecula may be bluntly dissected off the lingual surface of the epiglottis to its tip and the pharyngotomy is made just superior to the tip of the epiglottis. Previously identified hypoglossal nerves, superior laryngeal nerves and lingual arteries are retracted laterally. The tongue base is then grasped with a tenaculum or Allis clamp and delivered through the pharyngotomy (Figs 14A and B). If exposure is limited, the central hyoid bone can be excised. The tumor is once again evaluated, appropriate margins are determined and the tumor is resected taking care not to disrupt the lingual arteries or hypoglossal nerves.

After the confirmation of surgical margins by frozen section analysis, a layered closure may be used to close the wound primarily after placement of a nasogastric tube. Tongue base mucosa can be approximated to vallecula and/or epiglottis mucosa using inverted sutures for a watertight closure. The tongue base musculature can be sewn to hyoid periosteum. Suprahyoid muscles are then reapproximated in the midline. The neck incision is then closed in layers over bulb-suction drains. More extensive resections may require flap reconstruction, the details of which are beyond the scope of this chapter.

POSTOPERATIVE TREATMENT

Postoperative management includes nasogastric tube feeding and routine tracheotomy care. Ideally, the patient should be decannulated prior to initiating oral intake. Speech pathology plays a critical role in evaluating the safety of oral intake and teaching patients swallowing maneuvers. Broad-spectrum antibiotics are recommended at least in the early postoperative period and gastroesophageal reflux prophylaxis should be instituted.

HIGHLIGHTS

I. Indications
- Small T1–T2 tongue base lesions not extending anterior to the circumvallate papillae or involving the epiglottis
- Salivary neoplasms of the tongue base
- T1–T2 lesions of the posterior pharyngeal wall and hypopharynx.

II. Contraindications
- Extension anterior to the circumvallate papillae, which prevents primary closure, creates a more uncertain anterior margin of resection and augments postoperative functional deficits.
- Extension to the vallecula/lingual surface of the epiglottis, which prohibits oncologically sound pharyngotomy at these sites.
- Prohibitive medical comorbidities.

III. Special Preoperative Considerations
- Imaging
- Multidisciplinary evaluation, including speech pathology
- Medical evaluation and preanesthetic clearance, including evaluation of pulmonary status since aspiration is an expected postoperative occurrence.
- Reconstructive planning as indicated.

IV. Special Intraoperative Considerations
- Identify and preserve bilateral hypoglossal and superior laryngeal nerves to preserve safe postoperative swallowing.

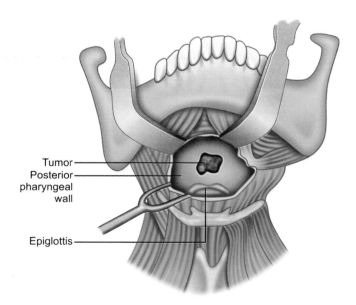

Tumor
Posterior pharyngeal wall
Epiglottis

Fig. 13: The suprahyoid musculature is transected at the hyoid bone, leaving a 5 mm cuff of muscle on the hyoid to assist with resuspension at the time of closure

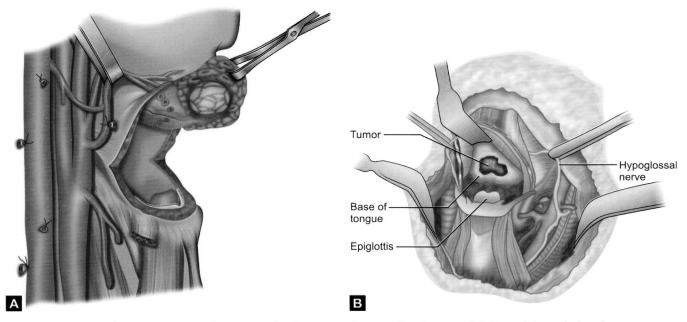

Figs 14A and B: The tongue base is then grasped with a tenaculum or Allis clamp and delivered through the pharyngotomy

- Identify and preserve bilateral lingual arteries to ensure adequate perfusion to the remaining tongue
- Resuspend the larynx by reapproximating the suprahyoid musculature to limit postoperative dysphagia.

V. Special Postoperative Considerations
- Enteral feeding by nasogastric tube
- Tracheotomy care
- Broad-spectrum antibiotics in the initial postoperative period
- Gastroesophageal reflux prophylaxis
- Close involvement of speech pathology with initiation of oral intake.

VI. Complications
- Wound infection
- Dysphagia
- Aspiration with or without pneumonia
- Dysarthria
- Hemorrhage
- Chronic pain
- Pharyngocutaneous fistula
- Risks of anesthesia.

REFERENCES

18. Blassingame CD. The suprahyoid approach to surgical lesions at the base of the tongue. Ann Otol Rhinol Laryngol. 1952;61(2):483-9.
19. Moore DM, Calcaterra TC. Cancer of the tongue base treated by a transpharyngeal approach. Ann Otol Rhinol Laryngol. 1990;99(4 Pt 1):300-3.
20. Weber PC, Johnson JT, Myers EN. The suprahyoid approach for squamous cell carcinoma of the base of the tongue. Laryngoscope. 1992;102(6):637-40.
21. Agrawal A, Wenig BL. Resection of cancer of the tongue base and tonsil via the transhyoid approach. Laryngoscope. 2000;110(11):1802-6.
22. Azizzadeh B, Enayati P, Chhetri D, et al. Long-term survival outcome in transhyoid resection of base of tongue squamous cell carcinoma. Arch Otolaryngol Head Neck Surg. 2002;128(9):1067-70.
23. Nasri S, Oh Y, Calcaterra TC. Transpharyngeal approach to base of tongue tumors: a comparative study. Laryngoscope. 1996;106(8):945-50.
24. Zeitels SM, Vaughan CW, Tommey JM. A precision technique for suprahyoid pharyngotomy. Laryngoscope. 1991;101(5):565-6.

Lateral Pharyngotomy

INTRODUCTION

First described by Cheever in 1869, the lateral pharyngotomy was initially reported as a method for removing a tonsil tumor.[25] Trotter popularized the procedure in 1913 by describing its utility as an approach to the pharynx. He detailed both: (i) A superior lateral pharyngotomy, which involved an accompanying mandibulotomy and provided access to the oropharynx and (ii) An inferior lateral pharyngotomy, which necessitated removal of the greater cornu of the hyoid and the lateral thyroid ala for access to the supraglottis.[26] Despite many modifications since that time, this procedure remains an effective approach to the oropharynx and hypopharynx.[27-29] In a 1994 description by Byers, the indications for a lateral pharyngotomy are noted to be T1 or T2 lesions in the tongue base, oropharyngeal wall or soft palate, or localized recurrence in these sites after primary radiotherapy.[28] Importantly, unlike the transhyoid pharyngotomy, this procedure may be used for tumors involving the vallecula. This approach may also be used for benign supraglottic lesions. Recently, Laccourreye et al. reported on an extended lateral pharyngotomy used in patients with lateral tongue base tumors ranging from T1–T4a, suggesting that this approach may have application in broader patient population.[30]

PREOPERATIVE EVALUATION AND ANESTHESIA

As discussed in the chapter overview, the work-up involves a thorough history and physical examination, appropriate imaging and laboratory studies, and examination under anesthesia with biopsy after obtaining appropriate preanesthesia medical clearance. Special attention should be given to patient's pulmonary status, since postoperative aspiration is common. Multidisciplinary evaluation is imperative, including speech pathology evaluation of the patient's level of function. Depending on the extent of anticipated resection, reconstructive options should be considered in surgical planning. Tracheotomy is routinely performed and patients should be counseled appropriately. Perioperative intravenous antibiotics are started within an hour before incision.

SURGICAL TECHNIQUE

Beginning with an examination under anesthesia, the tumor is reassessed to ensure it is a reasonable candidate for resection via lateral pharyngotomy. In order to ensure precisely placed mucosal incisions, the appropriate surgical margins may be tattooed at the time of direct laryngopharyngoscopy. The tracheotomy is generally performed next. This eliminates the endotracheal tube from potentially interfering with the surgical field. The appropriate neck dissection(s) is performed first through a superiorly based apron flap that is carefully designed to avoid contiguity with the tracheotomy site. If a neck dissection is not indicated, some authors report that the incision may be midline and horizontal, hidden in a skin crease near the level of the thyrohyoid membrane. In the authors' experience however, an upper neck dissection is necessary to provide adequate exposure.

The pharyngotomy is planned on the side with the most extensive mucosal involvement. The hypoglossal nerve is identified and traced along its course posteriorly to the occipital artery and anteriorly into the lingual musculature. To optimize exposure, the overlying vena comitans hypoglossi are carefully ligated and the digastric, stylohyoid, hyoglossus and mylohyoid muscles are divided. The hypoglossal nerve can then be mobilized after transecting the ansa cervicalis nerve and the hypoglossal branch to the stylohyoid muscle and retracted out of harm's way with a vessel loop.

The facial and lingual arteries are then identified close to the external carotid artery. The lingual artery is mobilized and retracted to allow access to the lateral pharyngeal space. This is done with vessel loops, which additionally serve as potential hemostatic control. The first two branches of the lingual artery are ligated.

The superior laryngeal nerve is identified; either it lies under the superior thyroid artery at the greater cornu of the hyoid or as it bisects the angle between the external carotid artery and the take-off of the lingual artery. The superior laryngeal nerve is then dissected along its course, which necessitates ligation of the common facial vein and associated branches. This dissection allows for inferior retraction and preservation of the nerve.

Muscular attachments are then divided off the lateral aspect of the hyoid bone, allowing the hyoid to be retracted anteromedially and facilitating dissection of lateral oropharyngeal mucosa off the hyoid. The hyoid is divided at the midline and the ipsilateral lateral hyoid, including the greater and lesser cornu, is removed. The pharynx is then entered in an area not within the margin of resection for the tumor. A pharyngotomy made between the superior laryngeal and the hypoglossal nerves allows visualization of the tongue base, vallecula and suprahyoid epiglottis (Fig. 15). If oncologically indicated, this incision can be extended superiorly into the oral cavity and along the floor of mouth, nearly to midline.

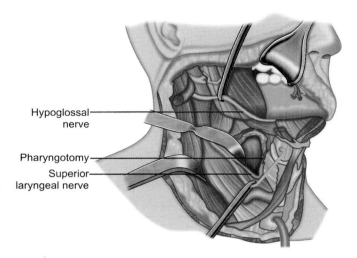

Fig. 15: A pharyngotomy made between the superior laryngeal and the hypoglossal nerves allows visualization of the tongue base, vallecula and suprahyoid epiglottis

The tongue is then delivered under the body of the mandible and through the pharyngotomy. If exposure is limited or if oncologically indicated, the pharyngotomy can be extended inferiorly through the lateral wall of the pyriform sinus to the postcricoid region. The lateral aspect of the thyroid ala may be removed, if further exposure is necessary.

Once the tumor has been resected with appropriate margins, as confirmed by frozen section analysis, a layered closure may be used to close the wound primarily after placement of a nasogastric tube. Mucosa is reapproximated using inverted sutures for a watertight closure. Muscle layers are then closed primarily. The neck incision is then closed in layers over bulb-suction drains. More extensive resections may require flap reconstruction, the details of which are beyond the scope of this chapter.

POSTOPERATIVE TREATMENT

Postoperative management includes nasogastric tube feeding and routine tracheotomy care. Ideally, the patient should be decannulated prior to initiating oral intake. Speech pathology plays a critical role in evaluating the safety of oral intake and teaching patients swallowing maneuvers. Broad-spectrum antibiotics are recommended at least in the early postoperative period and gastroesophageal reflux prophylaxis should be instituted.

HIGHLIGHTS

I. **Indications**
   - Small T1–T2 lesions in the tongue base, oropharyngeal wall and soft palate
   - Localized recurrences in the tongue base, oropharyngeal wall and soft palate after primary radiotherapy
   - Benign supraglottic lesion
   - Foreign bodies that cannot safely be removed transorally.

II. **Contraindications**
   - Direct extension of tumor into cervical soft tissues
   - Tumor involvement of greater than one-third of the oropharyngeal wall
   - Neoplasms requiring a supraglottic or total laryngectomy
   - Prohibitive medical comorbidities.

III. **Special Preoperative Considerations**
   - Imaging
   - Multidisciplinary evaluation, including speech pathology
   - Medical evaluation and preanesthetic clearance, including evaluation of pulmonary status, since aspiration is an expected postoperative occurrence
   - Reconstructive planning as indicated.

IV. **Special Intraoperative Considerations**
   - Tattooing the appropriate surgical margins at the time of laryngopharyngoscopy ensures precise mucosal incisions
   - Identify and preserve the hypoglossal and superior laryngeal nerves to preserve safe postoperative swallowing
   - Identify and preserve the lingual artery to ensure adequate perfusion to the remaining tongue.

V. **Special Postoperative Considerations**
   - Enteral feeding by nasogastric tube
   - Tracheotomy care
   - Broad-spectrum antibiotics in the initial postoperative period
   - Gastroesophageal reflux prophylaxis
   - Close involvement of speech pathology with initiation of oral intake.

VI. **Complications**
   - Wound infection
   - Dysphagia
   - Aspiration with or without pneumonia
   - Dysarthria
   - Hemorrhage
   - Pharyngocutaneous fistula
   - Risks of anesthesia.

REFERENCES

25. Cheever DW. Cancer of the tonsil: removal of the tumor by external incision (second case). The Boston Medical and Surgical Journal. 1878;99(5):183-9.

26. Trotter W. A method of lateral pharyngotomy for the exposure of large growths in the epilaryngeal region. Proc R Soc Med. 1920;13(Laryngol sec):196-8.

27. Orton HB. Lateral Transthyroid Pharyngotomy: Trotter's Operation for Malignant Conditions of the Laryngopharynx. Arch Otolaryngol Head Neck Surg. 1930;12:320-38.

28. Byers RM. Anatomic correlates in head and neck surgery. The lateral pharyngotomy. Head Neck.1994;16(5):460-2.

29. Holsinger FC, Motamed M, Garcia D, et al. Resection of selected invasive squamous cell carcinoma of the pyriform sinus by means of the lateral pharyngotomy approach: the partial lateral pharyngectomy. Head Neck. 2006;28(8):705-11.

30. Laccourreye O, Seccia V, Menard M, et al. Extended lateral pharyngotomy for selected squamous cell carcinomas of the lateral tongue base. Ann Otol Rhinol Laryngol. 2009;118 (6):428-34.

Part C: Transoral Lateral Oropharyngectomy

INTRODUCTION

Huet is credited with describing the first transoral approach to an oropharyngeal cancer in 1951, when he published a case report detailing a transoral technique for surgical salvage in a patient with recurrent tonsil SCC.[31] Since then, transoral approaches have evolved with technology. In 2003, Steiner et al. identified resectable tongue base tumors and performed transoral laser microsurgery with curative intent. This approach involves cutting the tumor into manageable pieces. Reported limitations of this technique are the functional outcomes in lesions involving cervical soft tissue and extensive adjacent spread.[32] In 2006, O'Malley et al. described the feasibility of transoral robotic surgery for the management of tongue base neoplasms, as trialed in preclinical canine and cadaver studies, as well as in three patients.[33]

Alongside these technologically and skill-specific advances, head and neck surgeons have continued to utilize the transoral approach Huet proposed, although the technique has evolved. In 2000, Galati et al. reported a series of 84 tonsil SCC patients, in which a transoral approach was used.[34] Watskinson et al. described the use of a transoral extended radical tonsillectomy in small (T1, T2) tonsil and tongue base SCC in 2002.[35] More recently, a large series of patients who underwent transoral lateral oropharyngectomy for tonsil and tonsillar fossa SCC was reported, providing sound anatomic foundation for the approach with acceptable oncologic outcomes.[31,36]

PREOPERATIVE EVALUATION AND ANESTHESIA

As discussed in the chapter overview, the work-up involves a thorough history and physical examination, appropriate imaging and laboratory studies, and examination under anesthesia with biopsy after obtaining appropriate preanesthesia medical clearance. Multidisciplinary evaluation is imperative, including speech pathology evaluation of the patient's level of function. If neoadjuvant therapy is anticipated, consideration should be given to tattoo the appropriate surgical margin during the examination under anesthesia. Depending on the extent of anticipated resection, reconstructive options should be considered in surgical planning.

Nasotracheal intubation and/or tracheotomy will facilitate this approach by eliminating the obstructive potential of an oral endotracheal tube. Perioperative intravenous antibiotics are started within an hour before incision.

SURGICAL TECHNIQUE

This procedure is performed under general anesthesia, either before or after the accompanying neck dissection(s). It may be helpful to perform the neck dissections first in order to locate the carotid artery prior to the transoral lateral oropharyngectomy. According to the literature, tracheotomy does not need to be routinely performed and this decision can be made on an individual patient basis.

Beginning with an examination under anesthesia, the tonsillar fossa is evaluated for mobility and the tumor is reassessed to ensure that it is a reasonable candidate for transoral resection. An oropharyngeal retractor is introduced and the patient is placed into suspension. The mucosal and submucosal raphe between the superior constrictor and buccinator muscle is identified by palpation and divided using electrocautery. This incision is then extended superiorly toward maxillary dentition and inferiorly to the extreme floor of mouth as in Figure 16.

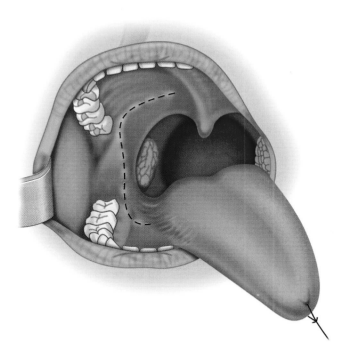

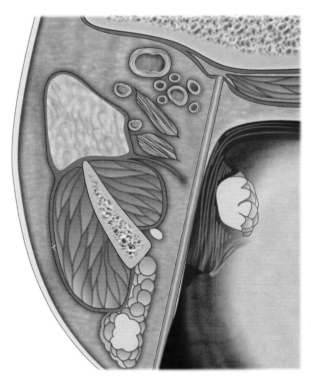

Fig. 16: The incision begins at the raphe between the buccinator and superior constrictor muscles, extending superiorly to the maxillary dentition and inferiorly to the extreme floor of mouth

Fig. 17: The submuscular plane of dissection is illustrated by the black bar. The superior constrictor muscle and anterior and posterior tonsillar pillars are medial to this plane of dissection, which marks the lateral oncologic margin. Note the relationship of the internal carotid artery to the dissection plane

A tenaculum is then used to grasp the ipsilateral tonsil for medial retraction. This enables medial retraction of the superior constrictor muscle, which opens the submuscular plane of dissection (Fig. 17). The lateral oncologic margins of resection are therefore the superior constrictor muscle and anterior and posterior tonsillar pillars. This plane of dissection is then bluntly developed posteriorly to the prevertebral fascia. The internal carotid artery can then be identified in the posterolateral wound bed, deep to fascia and fat.

The anterior tonsillar pillar and ipsilateral soft palate are then transected superiorly as determined by the extent of tumor and appropriate margins. As oncologically indicated, this can be extended to involve the entire ipsilateral or complete soft palate, with portions of the hard palate and buccal mucosa. This defines the superior limit of resection. The posterior tonsillar pillar is then transected and separated from the posterior pharyngeal wall. This can be extended as oncologically necessary to include the posterior oropharyngeal wall. At this point, the anterior, superior and posterior limits of resection have been defined.

Inferiorly, the anterior tonsillar pillar is divided at its junction with the tongue base, but can be extended to include the tongue base, as oncologically indicated. The specimen is then removed along the glossopharyngeal fold leaving only the inferomedial margin attached. The styloglossus and stylopharyngeal muscles are identified and divided. The inferior margin is then made contiguous with the lateral and posterior margins.

Depending on the size and extent of the surgical defect, it may be left to heal by secondary intent or may be reconstructed. Options for reconstruction are beyond the scope of this chapter. Prior to waking the patient from anesthesia, a nasogastric feeding tube should be placed.

POSTOPERATIVE TREATMENT

Postoperative management includes nasogastric tube feeding and routine tracheotomy care, if one is performed. Ideally, the patient should be decannulated prior to initiating oral intake. Broad-spectrum antibiotics are recommended at least in the early postoperative period and gastroesophageal reflux prophylaxis should be instituted. Oral care may take the form of salt and soda rinses.

HIGHLIGHTS

I. Indications
- Small T1–T2 and selected T3 oropharyngeal tumors.

II. Contraindications
- Trismus, suggestive of invasion deep to the plane of dissection and involving the parapharyngeal space
- Fixation of the tonsil or tonsillar fossa to the lateral oropharyngeal wall or mandible
- Invasion of the nasopharynx, glossopharyngeal fold, vallecula, pharyngoepiglottic fold and/or low pyriform sinus, all of which are inadequately visualized with this approach
- Poor exposure due to individual patient anatomy
- Prohibitive medical comorbidities.

III. Special Preoperative Considerations
- Imaging
- Multidisciplinary evaluation, including speech pathology
- Medical evaluation and preanesthetic clearance
- If neoadjuvant therapy is planned, pretreatment tattoo of appropriate surgical margins
- Reconstructive planning as indicated.

IV. Special Intraoperative Considerations
- Mucosal and muscular incisions should be made layer by layer with electrocautery to ensure complete hemostasis.
- Continuous and strong medial retraction with the tonsil tenaculum is essential for developing the appropriate submuscular plane and ensuring a safe distance from the carotid artery.
- If ipsilateral soft palate is extensively resected, rotational and transpositional myomucosal pharyngeal flaps are indicated for prevention of velopharyngeal insufficiency. If the soft palate is resected subtotally, no reconstructive attempts are warranted, as the patient can be fit with a palatal obturator postoperatively.

V. Special Postoperative Considerations
- Enteral feeding by nasogastric tube
- Tracheotomy care
- Broad-spectrum antibiotics in the initial postoperative period
- Gastroesophageal reflux prophylaxis
- Oral care, which may include salt and soda rinses.

VI. Complications
- Trismus
- Dysphagia
- Aspiration with or without pneumonia
- Dysarthria
- Hemorrhage
- Wound infection
- Chronic pain
- Velopharyngeal insufficiency
- Pharyngocutaneous fistula
- Risks of anesthesia.

REFERENCES

31. Holsinger FC, McWhorter AJ, Ménard M, et al. Transoral lateral oropharyngectomy for squamous cell carcinoma of the tonsillar region: I. Technique, complications, and functional results. Arch Otolaryngol Head Neck Surg. 2005;131(7): 583-91.

32. Steiner W, Fierek O, Ambrosch P, et al. Transoral laser microsurgery for squamous cell carcinoma of the base of the tongue. Arch Otolaryngol Head Neck Surg. 2003;129(1): 36-43.

33. O'Malley BW, Weinstein GS, Snyder W, et al. Transoral robotic surgery (TORS) for base of tongue neoplasms. Laryngoscope. 2006;116(8):1465-72.

34. Galati LT, Myers EN, Johnson JT. Primary surgery as treatment for early squamous cell carcinoma of the tonsil. Head Neck. 2000;22(3):294-6.

35. Watkinson JC, Owen C, Thompson S, et al. Conservation surgery in the management of T1 and T2 oropharyngeal squamous cell carcinoma: the Birmingham UK experience. Clin Otolaryngol Allied Sci. 2002;27(6):541-8.

36. Laccourreye O, Hans S, Ménard M, et al. Transoral lateral oropharyngectomy for squamous cell carcinoma of the tonsillar region: II. An analysis of the incidence, related variables, and consequences of local recurrence. Arch Otolaryngol Head Neck Surg. 2005;131(7):592-9.

Part D: Combination Transoral-Transcervical Approach

Mandibular Lingual Release

INTRODUCTION

The release of the tongue into the cervical operative site can be performed by delivering only the affected part of the tongue, in conjunction with a composite resection[37] or as a mandibular lingual release (also referred to as the "delivery" or "pull-through" approach in the literature), which delivers the entire tongue. The latter will be described below.

In 1838, Regnoli described a submental approach to a benign tongue lesion, which delivered the entire tongue through a T-shaped submental incision.[38] This was later modified by Billroth in 1874 and by Kocher in 1880.[39] Historically, composite resection was felt to be necessary for the resection of oral cavity and oropharyngeal tumors, even without mandibular invasion due to the widespread belief that these tumors seeded via periosteal lymphatics.[40] After Marchetta et al. disproved this notion of tumor spread, the mandibular lingual release became more widely accepted.[41] More recently, Stanley described this procedure with emphasis on the importance of a patient's dentition in the design of an intraoral incision. In addition, he highlighted the advantage of avoiding the morbidities of a mandibulotomy, while removing the lesion en bloc with the neck dissection specimen.[38] This approach is best suited for tongue base lesions confined to the tongue base, without lateral extension to the tonsillar region or glossopharyngeal sulcus.

PREOPERATIVE EVALUATION AND ANESTHESIA

As discussed in the chapter overview, the work-up involves a thorough history and physical examination, appropriate imaging and laboratory studies, and examination under anesthesia with biopsy after obtaining appropriate pre-anesthesia medical clearance. Multidisciplinary evaluation is imperative, including speech pathology evaluation of the patient's level of function. If neoadjuvant therapy is anticipated, consideration should be given to tattoo the appropriate surgical margin during the examination under anesthesia. Depending on the extent of anticipated resection, reconstructive options should be considered in surgical planning.

Tracheotomy is routinely performed with this procedure. If tracheotomy is performed after the oncologic resection, nasotracheal intubation will facilitate this approach by eliminating the obstructive potential of an oral endotracheal tube. Perioperative intravenous antibiotics are started within an hour before incision.

SURGICAL TECHNIQUE

Beginning with an examination under anesthesia, the tumor is reassessed to ensure that it is a reasonable candidate for resection via mandibular lingual release, since lateral extension to the tonsillar region or glossopharyngeal sulcus will affect the posterior aspect of the releasing incisions and may affect the posterior margin of resection. Additionally, the tumor should be assessed for fixation to the mandible, as this necessitates at least an accompanying marginal mandibulectomy. The tracheotomy is generally performed next. This eliminates the endotracheal tube from potentially interfering with the surgical field. The appropriate neck dissection(s) is then performed through a superiorly based modified visor flap that is carefully designed to avoid contiguity with the tracheotomy site. This flap is not elevated superior to the inferior border of the mandible.

If bilateral neck dissections are performed, the periosteum overlying the inferior border of the mandible is incised from one angle of the mandible to the other. If bilateral neck dissections are not performed, this periosteal incision may extend from medial to the facial artery and vein on the uninvolved side to the angle of the mandible with the division of the facial artery and vein on the involved side. The attachments of the anterior bellies of bilateral digastric muscles are divided off the mandible, leaving a small cuff of muscle on the bone, and elevation continues in a subperiosteal plane superiorly to the level of the floor of mouth musculature. Laterally, the pterygomasseteric sling is released. The mandibular attachments of the geniohyoid, mylohyoid and genioglossus muscles are then transected leaving a small cuff of muscle attached to the mandible to facilitate closure.

The transoral incisions are then addressed. If the patient has dentition and the lingual mucoperiosteum is included in the resection specimen for oncologic margins, the mucosal incision extends around the inner table of the mandible from one glossopharyngeal fold to the other, just inferior

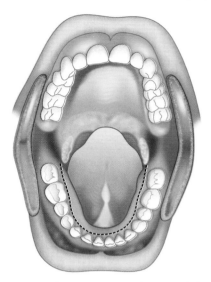

Fig. 18: The mucosal incision extends around the inner table of the mandible from one glossopharyngeal fold to the other, just inferior to the teeth. The lingual mucoperiosteal flap is then elevated inferiorly, releasing the tongue and floor of mouth

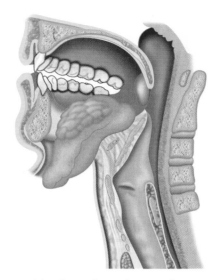

Fig. 19: Division of the floor of mouth musculature and elevation of the mandibular mucoperiosteum allows for delivery of the tongue through the cervical incision

to the teeth (Fig. 18). This lingual mucoperiosteal flap is then elevated inferiorly, releasing the tongue and floor of mouth.

If oncologic margins do not dictate the need for mucoperiosteal margins, the releasing incisions extend from one glossopharyngeal fold to another at a paralingual level, which provides adequate mucosa for closure while allowing for complete mobilization. In edentulous patients, this intraoral incision is placed at the level of the mandibular crest. For tongue base lesions, this incision can be extended posteriorly and inferiorly along the pharyngeal wall on the involved side. If this extension is performed, great care must be taken to identify and preserve the hypoglossal nerve and lingual artery.

Once the tongue is released into the cervical incision (Fig. 19), the tumor is once again evaluated, appropriate margins are determined, and the tumor is resected with preservation of the lingual artery and hypoglossal nerve. After the confirmation of surgical margins by frozen section analysis, a layered closure may be used to close the wound primarily, after placement of a nasogastric tube. Residual tongue may be reapproximated to the lingual mucoperiosteum. Depending on the level of the mucosal incision, interdental sutures may be necessary to achieve closure. The floor of mouth musculature is then reapproximated to the mandible. The neck incision is then closed in layers over bulb-suction drains. More extensive resections may require flap reconstruction, the details of which are beyond the scope of this chapter.

POSTOPERATIVE TREATMENT

Postoperative management includes nasogastric tube feeding and routine tracheotomy care. Ideally, the patient should be decannulated prior to initiating oral intake. Speech pathology plays a critical role in evaluating the safety of oral intake and teaching patients swallowing maneuvers. Broad-spectrum antibiotics are recommended at least in the early postoperative period and gastroesophageal reflux prophylaxis should be instituted. Oral care may take the form of salt and soda rinses.

HIGHLIGHTS

I. **Indications**
   • Tongue base lesions confined to the tongue base without lateral extension to the tonsillar region or glossopharyngeal sulcus.
   • Patients in whom mandibulotomy is not possible or should be avoided (e.g. after radiotherapy).

II. **Contraindications**
   • Lateral extension to the tonsillar region or glossopharyngeal sulcus, which will affect the posterior aspect of the releasing incisions and may also affect the posterior margin of resection
   • Prohibitive medical comorbidities.

III. **Special Preoperative Considerations**
   • Imaging
   • Multidisciplinary evaluation, including speech pathology

- Medical evaluation and preanesthetic clearance
- If neoadjuvant therapy is planned, pretreatment tattoo of appropriate surgical margins
- Reconstructive planning as indicated.

IV. **Special Intraoperative Considerations**
- The patient's dentition and appropriate oncologic margins determine the placement of the intraoral incision
- If the intraoral incision is extended posteroinferior to the glossopharyngeal fold, the ipsilateral hypoglossal nerve and lingual artery should be identified and preserved
- Reapproximation of the floor of mouth musculature must be carefully performed to recreate the muscular sling.

V. **Special Postoperative Considerations**
- Enteral feeding by nasogastric tube
- Tracheotomy care
- Broad spectrum antibiotics in the initial postoperative period
- Gastroesophageal reflux prophylaxis
- Oral care, which may include salt and soda rinses.

VI. **Complications**
- Dysphagia
- Aspiration with or without pneumonia
- Dysarthria
- Hemorrhage
- Wound infection
- Chronic pain
- Pharyngocutaneous fistula
- Risks of anesthesia.

REFERENCES

37. Ward GE, Robben JO. A composite operation for radical neck dissection and removal of cancer of the mouth. Cancer. 1951;4(1):98-109.
38. Stanley RB. Mandibular lingual releasing approach to oral and oropharyngeal carcinomas. Laryngoscope. 1984;94(5 Pt 1): 596-600.
39. Kremen AJ. Cancer of the tongue; a surgical technique for a primary combined en bloc resection of tongue, floor of mouth, and cervical lymphatics. Surgery. 1951;30(1):227-40.
40. Holsinger FC, Laccourreye O, Weber RS. Surgical approaches for cancer of the oropharynx. Operative Techniques in Otolaryngology. 2005;16:40-8.
41. Marchetta FC, Sako K, Badillo J. Periosteal lymphatics of the mandible and intraoral carcinoma. Am J Surg. 1964;108: 505-7.

Chapter **24**

Laryngotracheoplasty and Laryngotracheal Reconstruction

Ari DeRowe

INTRODUCTION

Increased awareness to prevention of intubation injuries has lowered the incidence of glottic and subglottic stenosis. However, the treatment of damage to the laryngeal structures with resulting scar formation still presents a challenge to the surgeon.

The aim of the surgery is to attain a patent airway, while preserving swallowing and speech functions.

The surgical technique that is chosen for each case depends on many factors: (i) degree of stenosis; (ii) laryngeal involvement; (iii) location of the stenosis; (iv) length of stenotic segment; (v) synchronous lesions; and (vi) coexisting tracheostomy. Endoscopic approaches have gained popularity in recent years. However, for the more difficult cases of stenosis or when endoscopic approaches fail, laryngotracheoplasty (LTP) and laryngotracheal reconstruction (LTR) will provide optimal results.

PREOPERATIVE EVALUATION

- Microscopic direct laryngoscopy and rigid bronchoscopy
  - Timing of the procedure and surgical approach are determined by examination under anesthesia.
- Flexible awake nasopharyngolaryngoscopy
  - Assessment of vocal cord mobility prior to surgery is imperative. Lack of mobility of one or both vocal cords has a great impact on which surgery is performed and on results.
- Imaging
  - Computed tomography (CT), magnetic resonance imaging (MRI), 3D reconstruction, virtual endoscopy.

Not necessary in all cases, but may be helpful in difficult and unusual cases.
- pH metry
  - Gastroesophageal reflux (GER) must be treated preoperatively. In all cases, a proton pump inhibitor should be administered postoperatively for at least 1 month.
- Speech and swallowing evaluation in all cases
  - Videofluoroscopic—swallow study, when swallowing problems exist or when aspirations are suspected.
- Culture of tracheostomy secretions
  - Perioperative antibiotics can be determined based on bacterial sensitivity.
- Pulmonary consultation, especially in the neonatal intensive care unit (NICU) graduate with lung disease.

SURGICAL TECHNIQUES

One Stage Laryngotracheal Plasty Anterior Cartilage Graft

The typical candidate for anterior cartilage graft LTP will be a graduate of the NICU, weighing over 8 kg at surgery, with a tracheostomy performed for failed extubation and subglottic stenosis. The scarring will be mostly anterior Myer-Cotton grade III, without vocal cord involvement. The surgical steps are as follows:
- Surgery begins with a direct laryngoscopy (DL) and rigid bronchoscopy (Fig. 1) to evaluate the lesion and plan the surgery. Even if such an exam was performed recently, this exam is important in verifying that correct procedure is being performed and also assists in making intraoperative decisions as in Figures 2A and B.

2. The patient is prepped for the surgical field to include the chest wall for rib cartilage graft harvest. The head is placed in an extension and the tracheotomy tube is replaced with a cuffed armored endotracheal tube, which is secured by suturing it to the skin. An uncuffed nasotracheal tube is placed so that the tip is situated above the vocal cords to facilitate insertion during surgery. Sizing of the nasotracheal tube is important. A preoperative CT or MRI can be used to measure the diameter of the normal trachea and correlate it to the nasotracheal tube diameter. A small leak is desirable and has to be kept in mind.

3. A horizontal incision that includes excision of the stoma around the tube is performed. Subplatysmal flaps are raised with the superior flap reaching above the thyroid notch and the inferior flap reaching the sternal notch.

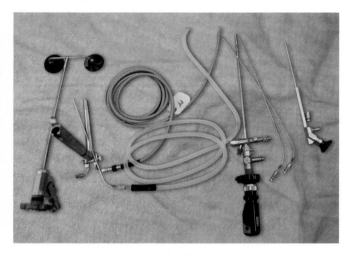

Fig. 1: Tray set-up for direct laryngoscopy and rigid bronchoscopy

4. Vertical midline dissection superior to the stoma is performed revealing the laryngeal and superior tracheal framework (Fig. 3). Care is taken to preserve the perichondrium.

5. A vertical midline incision of the laryngotracheal framework based on the approximate location of the stenotic segment, are performed as determined by the preoperative DL and bronchoscopy. This can extend from the tracheal stoma superiorly through tracheal cartilage, cricoid ring, cricothyroid membrane and inferior half of the thyroid cartilage. With the help of a headlight, direct visualization of the stenotic segment is performed. Care must be taken to make sure that the whole stenotic segment is included in the incision. It is important not to damage the anterior commissure. It is also possible to simultaneously perform direct laryngoscopy to accurately perform the laryngofissure. The length of the incision is measured for preparation of rib graft harvest.

6. A horizontal incision is made on the anterior chest wall, over the rib, just below the nipple. The rib cartilage is dissected very carefully to prevent pneumothorax. A curved rib dissector can be helpful. The length of the rib cartilage is measured before removal to assure adequate cartilage for the reconstruction. The cartilage is excised and the wound is irrigated, while positive ventilation pressure is applied by the anesthesiologist to make sure there is no air leak from the pleura. If a leak is discovered, positive pressure is applied and primary mattress suture closure is performed. The wound is closed without a drain.

7. The graft is carved into a shape. Usually the thickness of the cartilage requires splitting in half (filleting), before

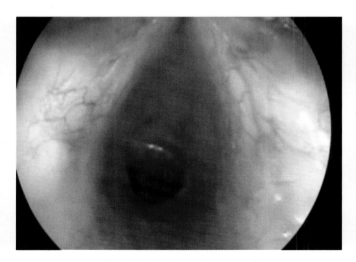

Fig. 2A: Endoscopic view of subglottic stenosis

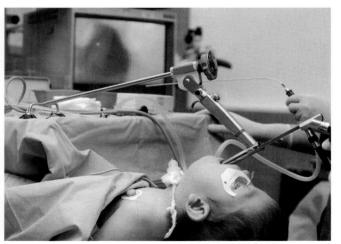

Fig. 2B: Child in suspension for the endoscopy. Larynx and trachea viewed and recorded on video monitor

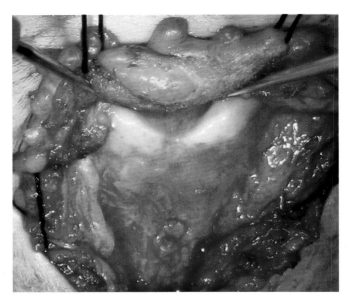

Fig. 3: Laryngeal framework exposed

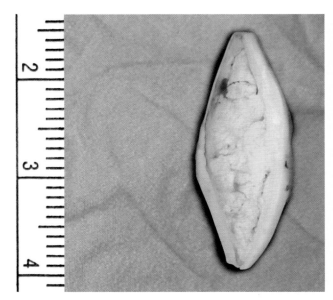

Fig. 4: Carved anterior graft. Note beveled edges

carving. The shape of the cartilage should be like the shape of a boat (Fig. 4). Care is taken to preserve the perichondrium on one side, which will be the internal side of the graft. A step is carved out surrounding the graft with the narrower part on the perichondrial side. Repeatedly, the graft is measured and placed on the laryngotracheal incision to ensure accurate sizing. When finished, the graft is placed in an antibiotic solution (e.g. cefamezin).

8. While retracting the laryngotracheal incision, the nasotracheal tube is advanced by the anesthesiologist and when observed in the tracheal lumen, the armored tracheal tube is removed. The nasotracheal tube is advanced further below the stomal area avoiding a one lung intubation. Attention is paid to the depth of insertion and the tube is secured.

9. The graft is sutured using polydiaxanone (PDS) 4-0 mattress sutures, with the perichondrium facing intraluminally, so that the groove of the carved cartilage sits on the cartilage of the laryngotracheal incision. The sutures are tied down after placement of all the sutures. The wound is irrigated and again positive ventilation pressure is applied by the anesthesiologist. Additional sutures are applied, if a leak is observed.

10. The wound is closed in layers. A Penrose drain is secured. Dressing is applied and soft bandage is wrapped around the neck with minimal pressure. The patient is transferred to the pediatric intensive care unit (PICU). A chest X-ray is performed to ensure the tube depth and evaluate the possibility of pneumothorax.

11. The duration of intubation is about 1–7 days based on the surgeon's preference. It is better to have the patient

awake and mildly sedated. However, this is not always possible. In that case, the patient is deeply sedated and placed on a ventilatory support.

12. Extubation is performed in the PICU and the patient is placed on steroids and humidification mask. One week post surgery, or if breathing difficulties appear, the patient is taken to the operation room for MDL and bronchoscopy, for evaluation and wound care. This could include removal of granulation tissues, mild dilatation or mytomycin application. Additional MDL and bronchoscopy will need to be scheduled to follow the laryngotracheal wound healing process. These follow-up evaluations are extremely important in attaining a successful LTP.

One Stage Posterior Graft Laryngotracheoplasty

The typical patient is a NICU graduate with posterior glottic scarring caused by prolonged or traumatic intubation. It may be difficult to differentiate the posterior glottic adhesion of the vocal cords to that of the bilateral vocal cord paralysis. Preoperative MDL with direct visualization and palpation are required to make differential diagnosis. The patient is most likely tracheostomy-dependent. The surgical steps are as follows:

1. Steps 1–4 are performed as in the anterior graft.

2. The vertical incision in the laryngotracheal framework is modified to include first tracheal ring, cricoid and thyroid cartilage. A complete laryngofissure (Fig. 5) enables good visualization. However, it is suggested initially not to advance beyond the anterior commissure.

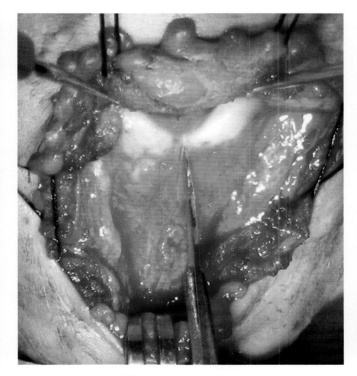

Fig. 5: Laryngofissure

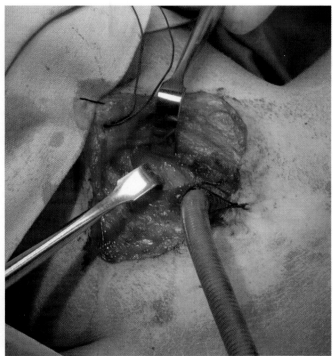

Fig. 6: Posterior cricoid split

3. Cottonoid pledgets soaked with adrenaline 1:1,000 are placed on the posterior commissure and cricoid, and removed after a few minutes to decrease bleeding. With great care, a midline incision starting from the inferior portion of the cricoid advancing cephalad through the scarred interarytenoid area is made. The incision must split the posterior cricoid plate and the scar completely (Fig. 6). A subperichondrial pocket is dissected on both sides of the split posterior cricoid to enable insertion of the cartilaginous wings of the graft as in Figure 7.

4. During this stage and during graft placement, accuracy and visualization can be increased by an assistant performing direct laryngoscopy with rigid videoendoscopy. The site of surgery is simultaneously viewed on a monitor screen.

5. The posterior cricoid incision is measured for the preparation of a rib cartilage graft harvest (Fig. 8) as described in step 6 of the anterior graft.

6. The cartilage is then carved in a rectangular shape with wings (Fig. 9) beveled "butterfly". Perichondrium is preserved on the intraluminal side.

7. Under direct and endoscopic vision the split cricoid is retracted laterally and the wings of the graft are pushed under the cricoid ring. If placed correctly, the graft snaps into place and no sutures are necessary as in Figure 10.

8. The nasotracheal tube can now be advanced and the tracheal tube can be removed (Fig. 11). The laryngotracheal

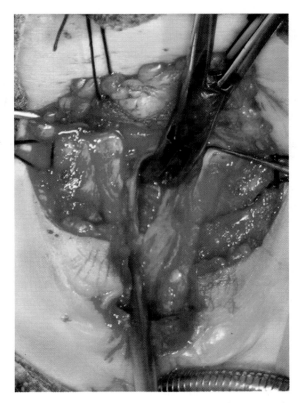

Fig. 7: Dissection posterior to cricoid cartilage to make a pocket for the wings of the posterior graft

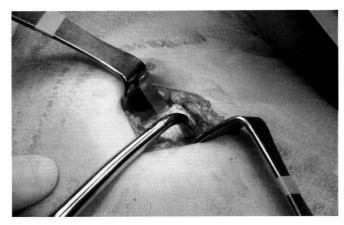

Fig. 8: Harvesting of costal cartilage using curved rib dissector

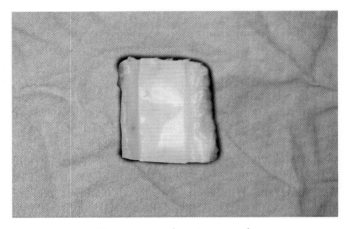

Fig. 9: Carved posterior graft. Note wings

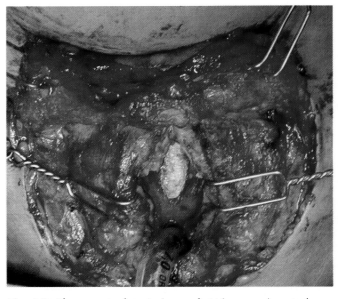

Fig. 10: Placement of posterior graft. Wings are inserted posteriorly to the cricoid plate and snapped into place. Sutures are not necessary

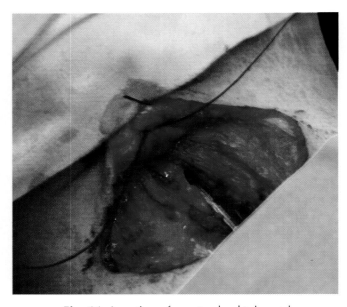

Fig. 11: Insertion of nasotracheal tube and removal of tracheal armored tube

incision is sutured with 4-0 PDS and attention is paid to accurate approximation, especially if the anterior commissure is violated. The stomal opening is also closed.

9. Wound closure and follow-up are similar to steps 10–12 of the anterior graft.

Anterior and Posterior Graft

Two Stage Laryngotracheal Reconstruction

In severe cases of subglottic stenosis, when subglottic and glottic stenosis coincide, an anterior and posterior graft may be required. This can be done as a one stage procedure.

However, in extensive cases, it may be preferable to perform the procedure in two stages. Laryngotracheal reconstruction is preferred when anterior glottic scar or congenital fusion exists because the prolonged stenting is superior in preventing readhesion of the vocal cords. The two stage procedure requires stent placement. The tracheostomy is left in place for the first stage of surgery. The stent is left in place for 6 weeks, although optimal stenting time is controversial. In the observation room, the stent is removed under MDL and granulation is removed. A few weeks later, MDL along with rigid bronchoscopy are performed and if the airway appears patent, decannulation can be initiated. The authors

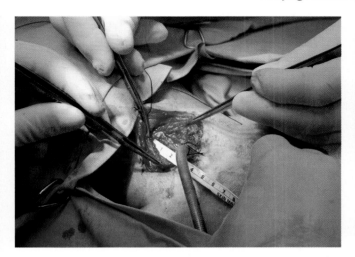

Fig. 12: Measurement of anterior and posterior graft beds

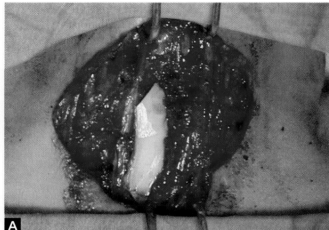

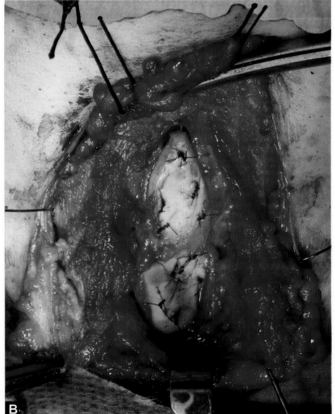

have found the Montgomery T-tube to be an optimal stenting material. In older children and adults, the T-tube is modified to fit the dimensions of the patient's airway. If there is a need to place it superior to the vocal cords, as in glottic stenosis, the proximal arm can be suture-closed to prevent aspiration. In that case, while the stent is in place, speech is impossible. In smaller children, the proximal arm is cut and used as a stenting material. The chosen diameter of the stent is important and can be determined by preoperative imaging or intraoperative measurement. The surgical steps are as follows:

1. Steps 1–5 are performed as in the posterior graft.
2. Rib graft harvest is performed as in step 6 of the anterior graft. Sufficient graft is prepared for both posterior and anterior grafts based on the measurements (Fig. 12) of the posterior and anterior laryngotracheal incisions.
3. The posterior graft is placed first as described in step 7 of the posterior graft.
4. The Montgomery T-tube is placed and an improvised connector is attached to the external arm to facilitate ventilation. If the proximal arm is not suture-closed, a Foley's catheter is placed via the laryngoscope and inflated with saline to temporarily close the proximal arm. In smaller child, a standard tracheotomy tube is placed with the cut proximal arm of the T-tube above.
5. The anterior graft is sutured in place (Figs 13A and B). In a smaller child, a nylon 2-0 suture is passed through the skin, larynx and through the stent and then out through the skin to secure the stent from migration. The suture ends are then tied externally to the skin with plastic buttons to prevent any pull-through of the suture.

Figs 13A and B: (A) Placement of anterior graft. The sutures are tied as seen in illustration; (B) Anterior graft sutured in place

6. The wound is closed as in the anterior graft.
7. Since, the patient remains with a tracheostomy, he or she can be awakened from anesthesia and standard tracheostomy care can be performed on the ward.

PITFALLS OF LARYNGOTRACHEAL RECONSTRUCTION AND LARYNGOTRACHEOPLASTY

- Immature scar
  - Surgery on an incompletely healed larynx is doomed for failure. An inflamed larynx, when seen on preoperative MDL and bronchoscopy is a contraindication to surgical repair.
- Unnoticed synchronous airway lesion
  - Thus, the importance of preoperative awake flexible and MDL with bronchoscopy. Operating on a sub-glottic stenosis, while an unnoticed bilateral vocal cord paralysis or peritracheostomal collapse exists, will result in failure.
- Untreated GER
  - Uncontrolled GER will have a negative effect on healing.
- Incorrect choice of surgical approach for the specific lesion

- Inadequate endoscopic follow-up for laryngotracheal wound care
- Inappropriate measurement of stents or inadequate stenting material.

ADDITIONAL READING

1. Herrington HC, Weber SM, Andersen PE. Modern management of laryngotracheal stenosis. Laryngoscope. 2006;116(9): 1553-7.
2. Lando T, April MM, Ward RF. Minimally invasive techniques in laryngotracheal reconstruction. Otolaryngol Clin of North Am. 2008;41(5):935-46.
3. Rutter MJ, Cotton RT. The use of posterior cricoid grafting in managing isolated posterior glottic stenosis in children. Arch Otolaryngol Head Neck Surg. 2004;130(6):737-9.
4. Sisk JD, Schweinfurth JM. Cartilage graft laryngotracheoplasty for anterior subglottic stenoses. Laryngoscope. 2008;118(5): 813-5.

Chapter **25**

Tracheotomy

Oshri Wasserzug, Dan M Fliss, Ziv Gil

INTRODUCTION

Tracheotomy is a surgical procedure in which an opening is made in the anterior wall of the trachea to establish an airway. It dates back to the fourth millennium BC and it has been associated with high mortality rates until the beginning of the 19th century, when Chevalier Jackson improved the efficacy and the safety of the procedure.

The most common indications for tracheotomy today are prolonged intubation and upper airway obstruction. Most tracheotomies in our institute are performed in the intensive care unit (ICU) with the use of a percutaneous tracheotomy set that had been demonstrated to lower complications rates compared with an open procedure.

In this chapter, the authors will describe a simple surgical technique for tracheostomy, which is performed in the operating room or emergency suite under local or general anesthesia.

PREOPERATIVE EVALUATION AND INDICATIONS

The patient's medical record should be reviewed for previous neck surgery, thyroid gland pathologies or lymphadenopathy. The neck is palpated thoroughly to exclude the presence of goiter or other midline neck masses, which may interfere in the procedure. Imaging studies of the neck are not routinely performed, unless a midline neck mass is suspected. Complete blood count and coagulation studies should be performed.

SURGICAL TECHNIQUE

Tracheotomy should be performed in the operating room, whenever possible thereby benefiting from an experienced team that includes an anesthesiologist, more skilled assistance, better equipments and improved lighting. When there is no cervical spine pathology, the patient is usually placed in a supine position with a rolled towel under the shoulders to hyperextend the neck. Patients with acute and severe upper airway obstruction, however, may not tolerate a supine position, whereupon the procedure would need to be carried out with the patient in a sitting position.

The lower part of the face, the neck and the shoulders are prepared with a Septal Scrub® solution and a sterile drape is placed in such a way that it enables free access to the neck. A horizontal or vertical 2–3 cm long incision is made midway between the suprasternal notch and the cricoid cartilage (Fig. 1). The incision extends through the platysma muscle. Following incision of the platysma, the operation continues in the midline superficial to the trachea. The trachea should be palpated periodically during the whole procedure, since it may be pushed laterally by a growing thyroid goiter or due to scoliosis of the vertebral column. Two Army-Navy angled retractors are positioned lateral to the midline for retraction of the skin (Fig. 2). The dissection continues in the midline. A Adson clamp is used to elevate the fibrofatty tissue over the trachea and the tissue is cut with a monopolar electrocautery. A vertical dissection using Adson clamp and monopolar cautery is continued until the trachea is exposed (Fig. 3). The thyroid isthmus can be sometimes visualized at this stage. If required, the isthmus is freed from its attachment

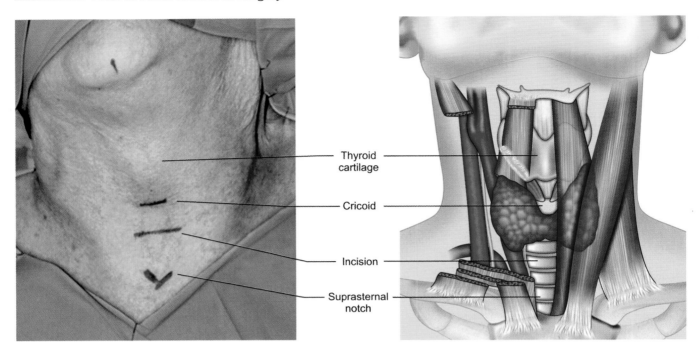

Fig. 1: Positioning and draping. The skin incision is performed midway between the suprasternal notch and the cricoid cartilage

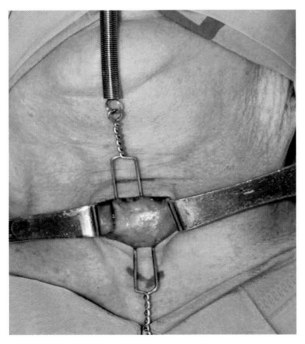

Fig. 2: Midline dissection along the fibrofatty tissue overlying the trachea. The dissection is performed with a Adson clamp and a monopolar electrocautery. The trachea should be palpated periodically during the whole procedure, since it may be pushed laterally by a growing thyroid goiter or due to scoliosis of the vertebral column

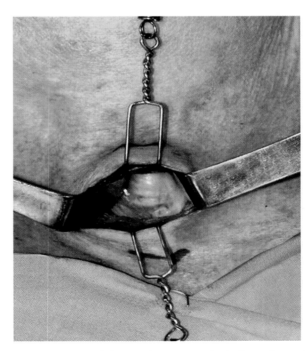

Fig. 3: Exposure of the trachea. A vertical dissection using Adson clamp and monopolar cautery is continued until the trachea is exposed

to the trachea along the Berry's ligament. This can be easily performed with a Adson clamp and a bipolar electrocautery. When the trachea has been identified, a tracheal hook is placed below the cricoid cartilage and the cricoid is retracted cephalad. This maneuver elevates the trachea superiorly, allowing exposure of the tracheal rings.

At this point of surgery, the team should be prepared for the tracheotomy procedure. This includes checking of the tracheostomy tube, ventilation with 100% oxygen and untying of the endotracheal tube by the anesthesiologist. Next, the second and the third tracheal rings are identified, and the membrane between the second and the third ring is marked with a monopolar electrocautery. After marking the area of the tracheotomy, the membrane between the second and the third or the third and the fourth tracheal rings is incised using a number 11 blade knife (Fig. 4). A wide incision should be performed, but care should be taken to avoid separation of the trachea. The incision is dilated with a Adson clamp or using a Laborde tracheal dilator. At this stage, the anesthesiologist pulls out the endotracheal tube up to the level of the cricoid cartilage. The incision is further dilated and a hook is used to retract the upper ring cephalad. The tracheostomy tube can now be inserted under vision through the stoma as in Figure 5.

When the tracheotomy is expected to be permanent or long-lasting, the anterior portion of the second or the third tracheal ring can be resected. The surgeon should recognize that tracheal rings tend to be calcified in older patients and heavy scissors are required to cut the tracheal ring in these cases.

After the tracheostomy tube has been inserted and inflated, its correct placement is verified visually and by means of auscultation and capnography measurements. Usually, it is not necessary to approximate the wound edges lateral to the tube. The flanges of the tube are sutured to the skin on both sides (Fig. 6) and the cannula is tied around the neck, leaving a one fingerbreadth gap between the tied portion and the skin.

POSTOPERATIVE TREATMENT

Ideally, the patients and their family members should be instructed on the care of a tracheostomy tube before the procedure or afterwards as soon as possible. Meticulous postoperative care of the tracheotomy site can prevent life-threatening events, such as obstruction of the cannula due to crusting. It is advisable that 24-hour continuous cold steam of 40% O_2 via a nebulizer be applied to the tracheotomy site for the first week following the procedure. This will prevent acute obstruction of the cannula from crusts. Usually, the tracheostomy tube is replaced by a double lumen cannula 7–10 days after surgery, allowing periodic cleansing of the inner tube.

TRACHEOTOMY IN THE PEDIATRIC POPULATION

There are a number of differences between tracheotomy in the adult and pediatric populations. The incision in the child's trachea should be vertical and there is no tracheal ring resection. Instead of performing a resection, two nylon traction/stay sutures are placed on both sides of the

Coronal view of the tracheotomy site

Epiglottis

Hyoid bone

Thyrohyoid membrane

Thyroid cartilage

Cricothyroid ligament

Cricothyroid muscles

Cricoid cartilage

Trachea

Area of tracheotomy

Axial view of the tracheotomy site

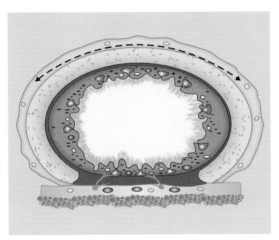

Fig. 4: Incision of the trachea. Incision is made between the second and the third tracheal rings. The incision is performed along the anterior third of the trachea

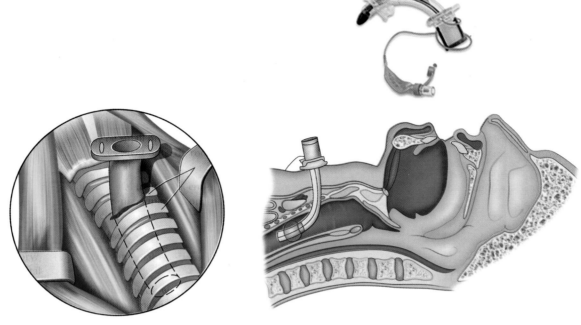

Fig. 5: Insertion of the tracheostomy tube. After the endotracheal tube is pulled above the upper ring, the tracheostomy tube can be inserted under vision through the stoma

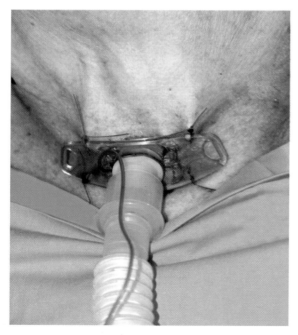

Fig. 6: The flanges of the tube sutured to the skin

trachea to enable emergent identification of the opening in the trachea in case of tracheostomy tube displacement. The internal diameter (ID) of the cufless tracheostomy tube is conveniently expressed by the formula: ID (mm) = (age in years/3) + 3.5. A chest X-ray should be performed at the end of the procedure in order to rule out a pneumothorax, which is more common in the pediatric population due to the higher pulmonary apexes.

HIGHLIGHTS

I. Indications
- Prolonged intubation
- Providing a long-term route for mechanical ventilation in cases of respiratory failure
- Upper airway obstruction not amenable to intubation
- Chronic life-threatening aspiration
- A temporary procedure after head and neck procedures with airway compromise.

II. Contraindications
- Relative contraindications include a huge or retrosternal goiter and a subglottic tumor extending into the trachea
- Tracheal stenosis above the carina
- Tumor infiltration of the trachea.

III. Special Preoperative Considerations
- Tracheotomy is most safely and easily performed in the operating room
- Perform computed tomography (CT) scan of the neck, if a goiter is suspected
- Hyperextension of the patient's neck will facilitate the procedure.

IV. Special Intraoperative Considerations
- Perform the dissection in the midline to avoid unnecessary bleeding
- Palpate the trachea periodically during the whole procedure
- Perform a vertical midline dissection using Adson clamp and a monopolar cautery, until the trachea is exposed
- Place a tracheal hook below the cricoid cartilage to elevate the trachea
- Avoid opening of the trachea with an electrocautery to prevent accidental burning
- The tracheostomy tube should be inserted under vision through the stoma.

V. Special Postoperative Considerations
- 24-hour continuous cold steam of 40% O_2 via a nebulizer should be applied to the tracheotomy site
- Periodic cleaning of the tracheostomy tube and stoma
- Replace the tube after 7–10 days with a double lumen tracheostomy tube.

VI. Complications
- Hemorrhage
- Pneumothorax
- Tracheal separation
- Tracheoesophageal fistula
- Wound infection
- Tube dislodgement
- Tube obstruction
- Subcutaneous emphysema
- False route
- Tracheal stenosis
- Stomal granulation
- Tracheoinnominate fistula.

ADDITIONAL READING

1. Cummings CW, Fredrickson JM, Harker LA, Krause CJ, Richardson MA, Schuller DE (Eds). Otolaryngology, Head and Neck Surgery, 3rd edition. St. Louis: Mosby-Year book; 1998.
2. De Leyn P, Bedert L, Delcroix M, et al. Tracheotomy: clinical review and guidelines. Eur J of Cardiothorac Surg. 2007;32(3):412-21.
3. Dierks EJ. Tracheotomy: elective and emergent. Oral Maxillofac Surg Clin North Am. 2008;20(3):513-20.
4. Freeman BD, Isabella K, Lin N, et al. A meta-analysis of prospective trials comparing percutaneous and surgical tracheostomy in critically ill patients. Chest. 2000;118(5):1412-8.
5. Grillo HC. Tracheostomy: uses, varieties, complications. In: Grillo HC (Ed). Surgery of the Trachea and Bronchi. Hamilton, London: BC Decker Inc; 2004. pp. 291-300.
6. Wright CD. Management of tracheoinnominate artery fistula. Chest Surg Clin N Am. 1996;6(4):865-73.

Chapter **26**

Marginal and Segmental Mandibulectomy

Ziv Gil, Dan M Fliss

INTRODUCTION

Tumors, which involve the mandible can be of primary origin or can invade the bone from the adjacent oral cavity or oropharyngeal mucosa. Most primary mandibular neoplasms are benign tumors, originating in the bone, teeth or dental pulp. These most frequently include, benign cysts (e.g. periapical cysts, dentigerous cysts, odontogenic keratocyst, Gorlin cyst), which require local excision and curettage. Larger and more destructive tumors, such as ameloblastoma or osteosarcoma will necessitate wider resection with free margins in order to achieve cure. The most frequent secondary tumor invading the mandible is squamous cell carcinoma (SCC). This tumor can originate in the oral cavity mucosa, tongue or oropharynx and invade the bone. Salivary gland carcinomas including adenoid cystic and mucoepidermoid carcinoma can also invade the mandible from adjacent areas. Carcinomas of the submandibular or minor salivary glands can also invade the mandible.

Patients with tumors of the mandible may complain of growing lesion in the gingiva, pain and inability to fit their dentures. Frequently, the diagnosis of mandibular cancer is achieved by the dentist, following extraction of a loose tooth. Advanced stage cancer may lead to trismus due to pterygoid muscles involvement. Lower lip numbness may occur due to inferior alveolar nerve involvement.

Resection of tumor involving the mandible can be divided according to the type of osteotomy. Malignant tumors that reach the cortex of the mandible or those with minor bone erosion, the tumor can be extirpated by marginal mandibulectomy. In this procedure, the tumor is removed in an en bloc fashion along with the cortical bone and portion of the cancellous part of the mandible (Figs 1A and B). If the tumor fully invades the cortex of the mandible or the

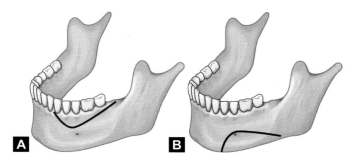

Figs 1A and B: Marginal mandibulectomy. (A) Depiction showing an upper marginal mandibulectomy for oral cavity cancer; (B) Depiction showing a lower marginal mandibulectomy for submandibular gland carcinoma

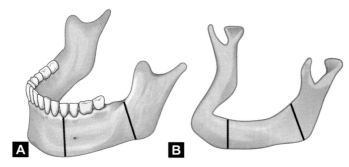

Figs 2A and B: Segmental mandibulectomy. (A) The osteotomy sites in a normal mandible and; (B) In an edentulous mandible

inferior alveolar nerve canal, segmental mandibulectomy is indicated (Fig. 2A). In edentulous patients, the ramus of the mandible is relatively narrow and marginal mandibulectomy may imminently lead to bone fracture. In these patients, segmental mandibulectomy is used for cancer ablation as in Figure 2B.

In this chapter, we shall describe in details the technique practiced by the authors for resection of tumors involving the mandible. Both the techniques of marginal and segmental mandibulectomy are described. The means for reconstruction of the mandible are also discussed.

PREOPERATIVE EVALUATION AND ANESTHESIA

All patients scheduled for operation are evaluated preoperatively by a head and neck surgeon, an anesthesiologist, an oral and maxillofacial surgeon, and a plastic surgeon. Radiological evaluation of the patients includes computed tomography (CT) with contrast, magnetic resonance imaging (MRI) and positron emission tomography-computed tomography (PET-CT). Dental scan may be also used to evaluate the level of mandibular invasion. Figure 3 shows preoperative MRI and PET-CT scan of patients with tumor infiltrating the mandible. Flexible endoscopy is used, in these cases, to examine the larynx, hypopharynx and cervical esophagus. All patients should undergo routine blood tests including complete blood count and coagulation function tests. Lower extremities CT angiography scan with contrast is indicated, if a fibula free flap is planned.

Most patients with advanced disease will require adjuvant treatment. Therefore, it is suggested to evaluate the need for teeth extraction before the operation. In addition, placement of percutaneous endoscopic gastrostomy (PEG) is indicated, if adjuvant chemoradiation is expected.

SURGICAL TECHNIQUE

The surgical approach for marginal and segmental mandibulectomy (Figs 4A to C) is planned prior to the operation. The surgical access is planned through a transoral approach (Figs 5 to 9), transcervical approach (Figs 10 to 13) or through a lip-split incision, extended to a horizontal neck incision toward the ipsilateral side of the tumor (Figs 14 to 29). Since, this is a clean-contaminated operation, prophylactic antibiotics treatment with first-generation

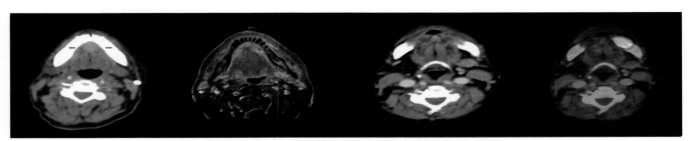

Fig. 3: Preoperative imaging of a patient with squamous cell carcinoma of the oral cavity invading the mandible. CT, MRI and CT-PET scans are shown

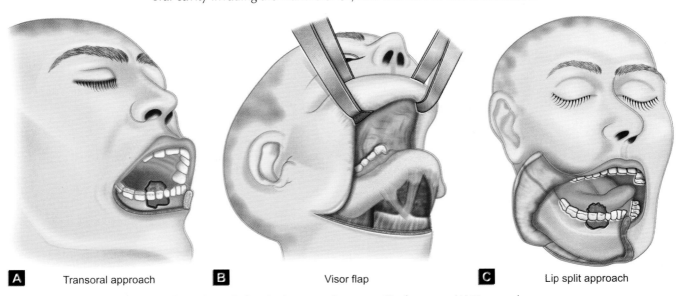

| A | Transoral approach | B | Visor flap | C | Lip split approach |

Figs 4A to C: Surgical approach to mandibulectomy. (A) Transoral; (B) Visor flap; and (C) Lower lip-split approaches may be used

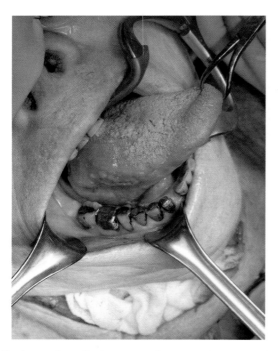

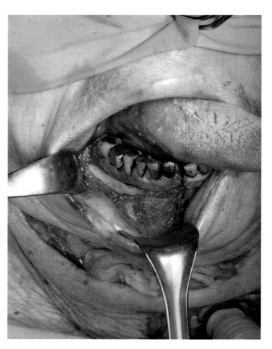

Fig. 5: An oral cavity tumor at the ventral tongue abutting the mandible. This clinical T2N0M0 squamous cell carcinoma reached the lower alveolar ridge but does not infiltrate the bone

Fig. 6: Performance of the osteotomy in marginal mandibulectomy. A smooth, rounded osteotomy, which evenly distributes the stress along the mandible, is preferred over a sharp angle osteotomy, which increases the risk of fracture

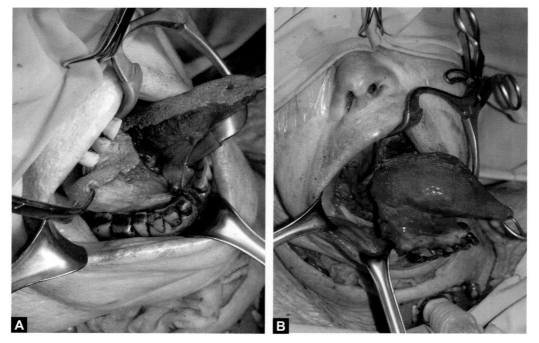

Figs 7A and B: Composite resection of the tumor. Excision of the tumor is achieved in a monoblock fashion along with the floor of mouth. Note that the tumor reaches the lower alveolar ridge but does not invade the bone

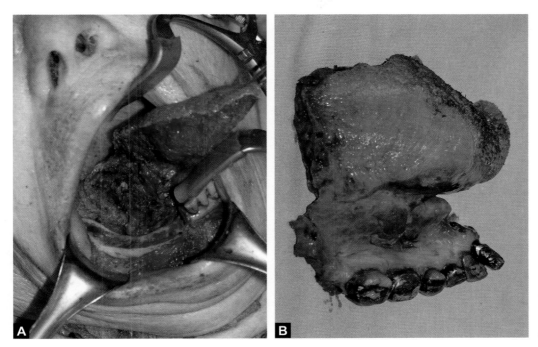

Figs 8A and B: The surgical field after tumor resection. (A) The surgical field after tumor resection; and (B) The tumor specimen. The tumor was extirpated en bloc and included partial glossectomy and marginal mandibulectomy. A selective neck dissection involving levels I–IV was also performed

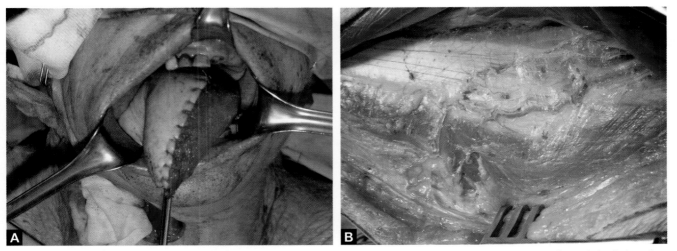

Figs 9A and B: Reconstruction of the surgical defect. The reconstruction was performed with an anterolateral thigh free flap

cephalosporin and metronidazole is indicated. Surgery is performed under general anesthesia with muscle relaxation. After endotracheal or nasal intubation, a tracheostomy is performed. The tracheostomy tube is usually inserted as low as possible in the neck to separate it from the neck flaps.

Marginal Mandibulectomy

Marginal mandibulectomy is usually performed as part of a composite resection for tumors abutting the mandible, which originate in the oral tongue and floor of mouth

(Fig. 5). In order to reassure free margins, the composite resection should include the tumor, 2 cm circumferential margins and the upper part of the body or ramus of the mandible. For tumors, which originate in the submandibular gland, the lower part of the body of the mandible can be resected as part of the marginal mandibulectomy (Fig. 10). The operation starts with a selective neck dissection, which is usually indicated in these tumors. After completing the neck dissection, attention is turned to the composite resection. We usually maintain the tumor specimen in continuity with the

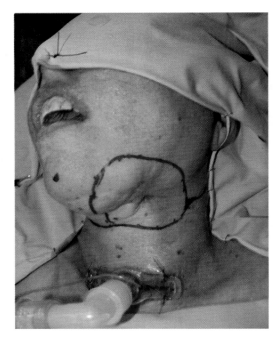

Fig. 10: Planning of the incision in a patient with recurrent adenoid cystic carcinoma of the submandibular gland. This patient had recurrent adenoid cystic carcinoma originating in the submandibular gland (clinical T3N2aM0)

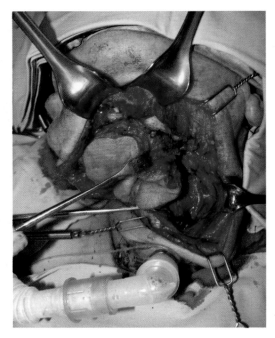

Fig. 11: Composite resection of the tumor and exposure of the mandible

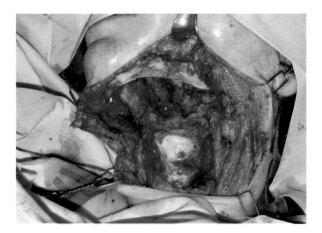

Fig. 12: The surgical field after tumor resection. The figure shows a lower marginal mandibulectomy. The composite resection including the skin, lower marginal mandibulectomy, floor of mouth, hyoid bone and selective neck dissection of levels I–IV. The lower margin of the operation was the thyroid cartilage and cricoid cartilage, which were partially drilled out to ensure negative margins

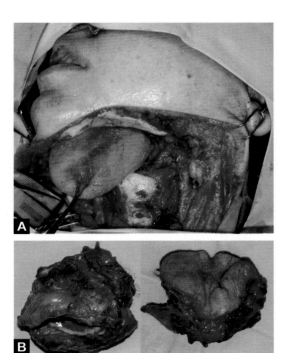

Figs 13A and B: The surgical field and specimen. (A) The picture shows resection of the tumor and floor of mouth; (B) The surgical specimen. The left picture of Fig. 13B shows the deep plane of the specimen (arrow indicates the marginal mandibulectomy) and right picture of Fig. 13B shows the superficial plane of the specimen

neck dissection. If a transoral resection is feasible, an incision is made 2 cm from the distal margin of the tumor and is extended to the level of the outer cortex of the mandible including segment of the oral tongue and the floor of mouth (Fig. 6). If amendable, without violating a total removal of the cancer, a transoral marginal mandibulectomy can be

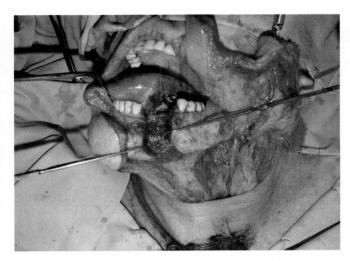

Fig. 14: Marginal mandibulectomy and mandibulotomy. This clinically T4N2bM0 tumor of the oral tongue invaded the base of tongue, and tonsillar fossa. The surgery was performed via mandibular split to allow resection of the base of tongue part of the tumor. A marginal mandibulectomy was performed as part of the composite resection

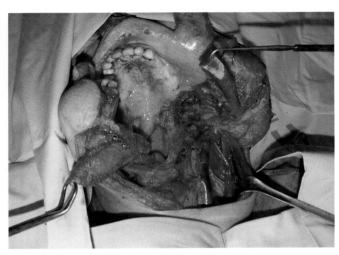

Fig.15: The surgical field after tumor resection. The resection included partial glossectomy, marginal mandibulectomy, resection of the left tonsillar fossa, hyoid bone and floor of mouth

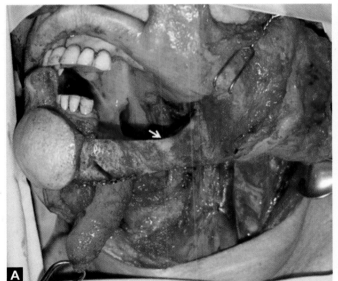

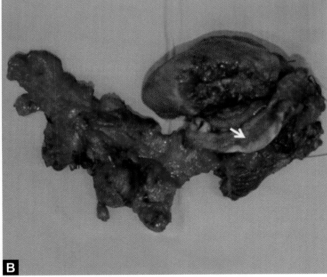

Figs 16A and B: Approximation of the mandible and its fixation. The specimen is shown on the right. The marginal mandibulectomy is indicated with an arrow. In this case, the reconstruction was performed with an anterolateral thigh free flap

performed. This eliminates the need of a lip-split incision or a visor flap, which is usually required for exposure of tumors located posteriorly or for large tumors. If a transoral composite resection is performed, the incision is continued toward the lower alveolus and the mandible is exposed proximal and distal to the tumor. Approximately, 2–3 cm on each side of the planned osteotomy should be exposed. Care is taken to maintain at least 2 cm margins from the tumor and preserve the mental nerve, which enters the mental foramen.

Attention is now turned to the osteotomy. As a general rule, a curved osteotomy should be performed in continuous fashion (Fig. 6). A smooth, rounded osteotomy, which evenly distributes the stress along the mandible, is preferred over a sharp angle osteotomy, which increases the risk of fracture. The osteotomy is performed with a reciprocal, sagittal mechanical saw with a thin blade to minimize bone loss. A flat malleable retractor is inserted deep into the bone to protect the soft tissue and vessels. Once the marginal mandible is performed, the specimen is swung medially

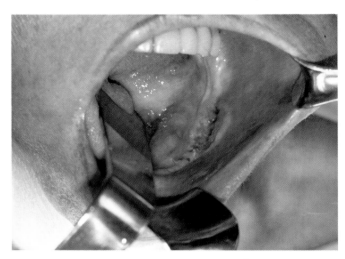

Fig. 17: A T4N0M0, stage IV oral cavity SCC invading the mandible

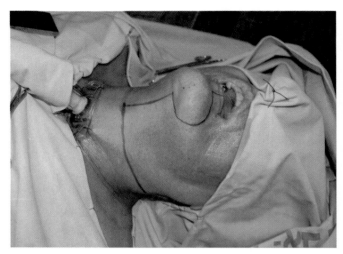

Fig. 18: Planning of the skin incision. The planned surgery is a composite resection, segmental mandibulectomy, floor of mouth resection and selective neck dissection of levels I–IV

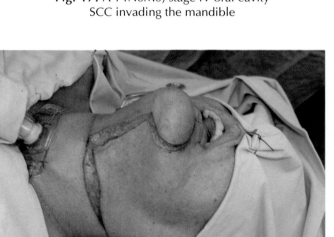

Fig. 19: Skin incision. A lip-split incision is performed and the skin flaps are elevated

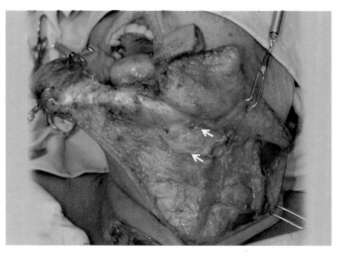

Fig. 20: Elevation of the neck flaps. The flaps are elevated in a subplatysmal plane. Care is taken to prevent injury to the marginal mandibular nerve. The fascia overlying the submandibular gland is incised (arrows) and its fascia is reflected upward. This fascia contains the marginal mandibular branch of the facial nerve

and the resection is extended toward the tongue and deep muscles of the floor of mouth (Figs 7A and B). The incision is extended toward the extrinsic muscles of the tongue and mylohyoid muscle, allowing resection of the deep portion of the specimen. If indicated, a division of the mylohyoid muscle is required to allow through and through delivery of the specimen toward the neck. Excision of the tumor is achieved in a monoblock fashion along with the floor of mouth (Figs 8A and B). After removal of the tumor, margins are evaluated by frozen section analysis. Reconstruction is performed with an anterolateral thigh free flap or with a radial forearm free flap as in Figures 9A and B.

Similar to the transoral approach, tumors of submandibular origin abutting the lower edge of the mandibular ramus can be resected via transcervical approach (Fig. 10). Figures 10 to 13, show a case of a recurrent adenoid cystic carcinoma (T4N1M0). In this case, the tumor involved the submandibular gland, strap muscles, hyoid bone and skin. Following exposure of the mandible via a transcervical approach (Fig. 11), a lower marginal mandibulectomy is performed in an en bloc fashion as in Figures 12 and 13.

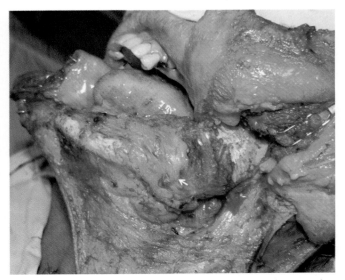

Fig. 21: Exposure of the osteotomy site. After the lip and skin of the chin are split in the midline, the incision is extended to the level of the outer cortex of the mandible. Care is taken to include the pre- and postvascular lymph node on the specimen (arrow)

Tumors, which invade the oral tongue posteriorly and the base of tongue, floor of mouth and oropharynx necessitate a mandibulotomy approach (see chapter 23). In this case, marginal mandibulectomy is indicated if the tumor reaches the cortex of the mandible, but not invade it. Figure 14 shows the approach for a T4N2bM0 SCC of the oral cavity, which required a mandibulotomy. The composite resection included a partial glossectomy, marginal mandibulectomy, resection of the floor of mouth, tonsillar fossa and base of tongue as in Figures 15 and 16.

Segmental Mandibulectomy via Lip-Split Approach

A segmental mandibulectomy via a lip-split incision is the workhorse technique for most malignant tumors with bone invasion. The patient is placed on the operating room table in a supine position. The head is stabilized with a soft donut holder and the whole operating table is then elevated in an angle with the head up in order to minimize bleeding.

In case of a lip-split approach, the incision will allow rising of a lower cheek flap, exposure of the mandibulectomy

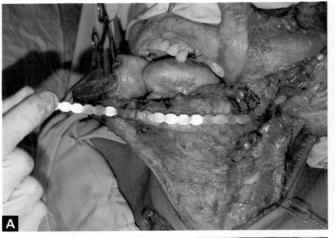

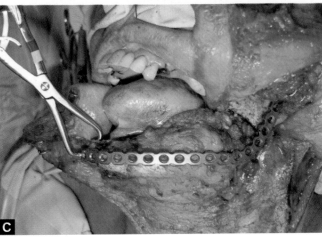

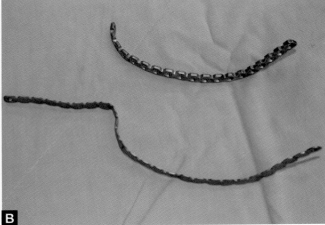

Figs 22A to C: Prebanding and fixation of the titanium miniplates. Before performing the osteotomy, an osseointegrated titanium plate is prebanded and fixed to the mandible. A malleable aluminum plate (purple) is used to employ the contour of the mandible. The titanium plate (yellow) is then banded according to the outline of the aluminum plate

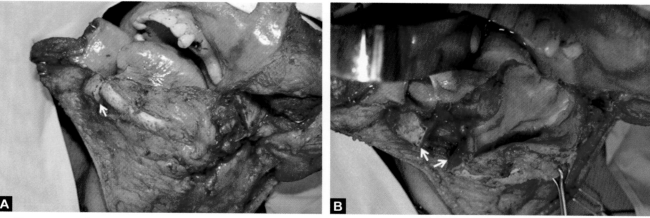

Figs 23A and B: Segmental osteotomy of the mandible. The osteotomy is performed in a straight line with a reciprocal, sagittal mechanical saw with a thin blade to minimize bone loss. The arrows indicate the osteotomy

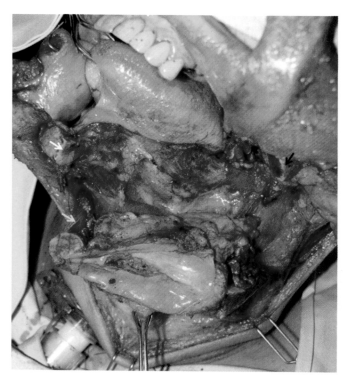

Fig. 24: Composite resection of the tumor. Excision of the tumor is achieved in a monoblock fashion along with the floor of mouth and lymph nodes of the neck. The proximal (white arrow) and distal (black arrow) osteotomies are shown. The yellow arrow indicates the mylohyoid muscle, which is divided medial to the mandible

site and neck dissection (Fig. 18). In case of a benign tumor (i.e. ameloblastoma), the operation can be performed via a visor flap. Marking of the incision is preferably performed with the neck slightly flexed in order to identify the lines of relaxed skin tension. The lip incision is performed in

the midline, circumferencing the chin toward the side of the tumor, extended caudally up to the level of the cricoid cartilage. This incision is then extended laterally to a formal collar neck incision up to the level of the mastoid bone (Fig. 18). After marking the incision, the patient is prepped and draped in a standard surgical fashion.

This operation is performed as a part of a composite resection for tumors involving the oral tongue, floor of mouth and mandible. Usually, a selective neck dissection of levels I–IV is indicated in these cases. For oral cavity squamous cell carcinomas (Fig. 17) crossing the midline, a bilateral neck dissection should be performed before approaching the primary tumor.

Elevation of Subplatysmal Flaps

The skin is incised with a number 15 blade and subsequent dissection of the subcutaneous tissue and the platysma is carried out with an electrocautery at the lowest effective setting. Subplatysmal flaps are elevated superiorly, 1 cm below the ramus of the mandible and inferiorly to the clavicle (Figs 19 and 20). This plane separates the superficial cervical fascia from the superficial layer of the deep cervical fascia. Care is taken to prevent injury to the marginal mandibular branch of the facial nerve. The nerve runs within the fascia superior to the submandibular gland. Injury to the nerve is prevented by elevation of the flap immediately below the platysma, leaving the superficial layer of the deep cervical fascia on the submandibular gland. The flap is elevated to the level of the mandible exposing the facial artery and vein. The facial vein is divided over the submandibular gland and reflected superiorly, protecting the marginal mandibular branch of the facial nerve. The lower flap should remain separate from the tracheostomy incision in order to prevent contamination of the surgical area by tracheal secretions.

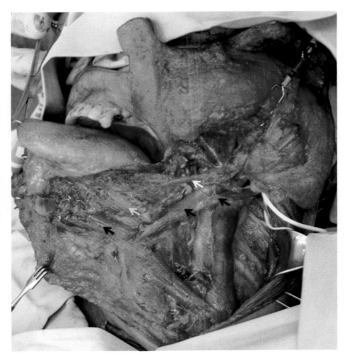

Fig. 25A: The surgical field after removal of the specimen. The arrows indicate the posterior belly of the digastric muscle and stylohyoid muscle (black arrows), the styloglossus muscle (white arrow) and the hypoglossal nerve (yellow arrow)

Osteotomies

The composite resection includes the tumor, 2 cm margin, the floor of mouth and segment of the mandible. After the lip and skin of the chin are split in the midline, the incision is extended to the level of the outer cortex of the mandible (Fig. 21). A lower cheek flap is elevated within a plane superficial to the tumor. A 2–3 cm flap is raised in the contralateral side of the planned osteotomy. Care is taken to preserve the mental nerve in the contralateral side. Before performing the osteotomy, an osseointegrated titanium plate is prebanded and fixed to the mandible (Figs 22A to C). Alternatively, titanium miniplates are used after the mandibulectomy for the bony reconstruction with a fibula free flap. Attention is now turned to the osteotomy. The osteotomy is performed in a straight line with a reciprocal, sagittal mechanical saw with a thin blade to minimize bone loss (Figs 23A and B). Once the segment of the mandible is freed, both sides of the remaining mandible are swung laterally like a book. The gingivolabial incision is extended toward the anterior pillar of the tonsil, allowing further exposure of the tumor and its circumference. After achieving adequate exposure, attention is turned to resect the lateral and posterior aspects of the tumor. Two centimeter margins are required to assure complete resection. During the resection, brisk bleeding is expected from the lingual artery and its branches, which are controlled with number 4-0 silk sutures and bipolar electrocautery.

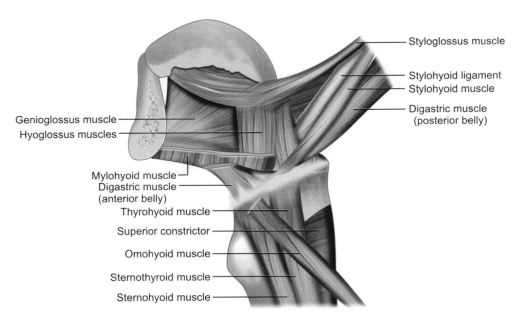

Fig. 25B: A depiction of the anatomical structures

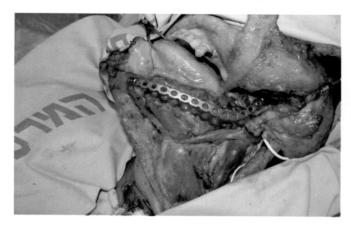

Fig. 26: Reconstruction of the defect. The picture shows the titanium plate fixed onto the mandible. The reconstruction was performed with a composite fibula free flap

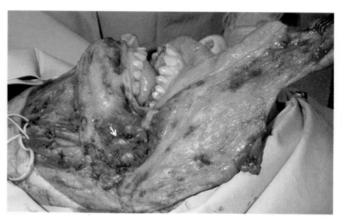

Fig. 27: A composite resection of a tumor involving the retromolar trigone. This T4N2bM0 Stage IV recurrent SCC tumor invaded the mandible, ventral tongue, floor of mouth, tonsillar fossa, pterygoid muscles and maxilla. The patient underwent multiple surgeries and chemoradiation therapy before the index operation. The picture shows exposure of the mandible and resection of the masseter (arrow)

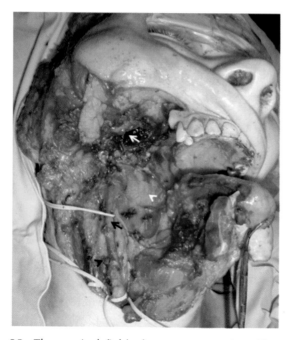

Fig. 28: The surgical field after tumor resection. The composite resection included segmental mandibulectomy, partial glossectomy, partial maxillectomy, nasopharyngectomy and extended radical neck dissection with resection of the external carotid artery. Internal carotid artery (black arrow), stump of the external carotid artery (black arrowhead), the nasopharynx (white arrowhead), the skull base and retromaxillary space (white arrow)

Excision of the tumor is achieved in a monoblock fashion along with the floor of mouth and lymph nodes of the neck (Fig. 24). After removal of the tumor (Figs 25A and B), the margins are evaluated by frozen section analysis.

After the resection, the titanium plate is fixed according to the predrilled holes as in Figure 26.

The same approach is used for larger tumors invading multiple compartments of the oral cavity, oropharynx, nasopharynx and neck. The case shown in Figures 27 to 29 show resection of a recurrent T4 tumor, originating in the retromolar trigone and invading multiple adjacent compartments, including the nasopharynx and maxilla.

Segmental Mandibulectomy via a Visor Flap

A visor flap is indicated for benign tumors or for small tumors involving the anterior segment of the mandible. This approach eliminates the splitting of the chin and lip. A bilateral apron flap is performed and the flaps are elevated as described before, exposing the cortex of the mandible as in Figures 30 to 32.

Reconstruction

The reconstruction technique is designed according to the size and location of the defect, based on radiological and intraoperative calculations. Microvascular reconstruction with a composite free flap is usually used in most patients. Free composite fibula flap or iliac crest free flap are the means of choice for reconstruction. If free flap reconstruction is contraindicated, a titanium plate and pectoralis major rotational flaps may be used. However, the main disadvantage of this method is poor functional outcome and high-rate of plate extrusion, especially in irradiated patients.

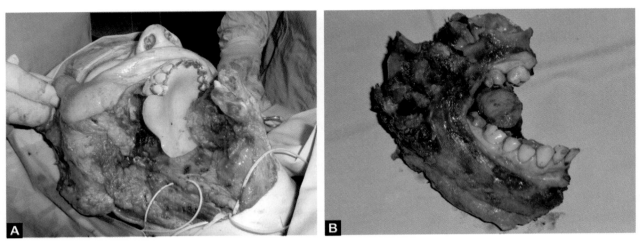

Figs 29A and B: The reconstruction and surgical specimen. (A) The reconstruction was performed with an obturator (maxillary reconstruction) and lateral thigh free flap (soft tissue reconstruction); (B) The specimen including the segmental mandibulectomy, glossectomy and maxillectomy, which was excised in an en bloc fashion

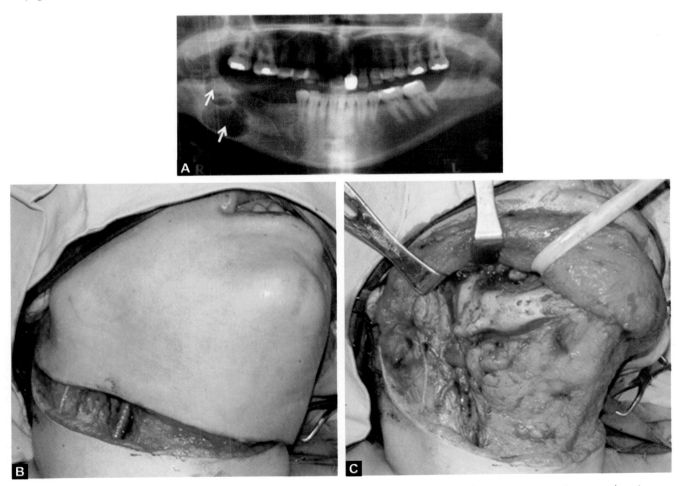

Figs 30A to C: A visor flap approach for resection of an ameloblastoma of the mandible. (A) A panoramic X-ray showing two lytic lesions in the right mandibular ramus (white arrows); (B) The neck incision is performed with an apron flap; (C) Exposure of the mandible is achieved without splitting of the lip

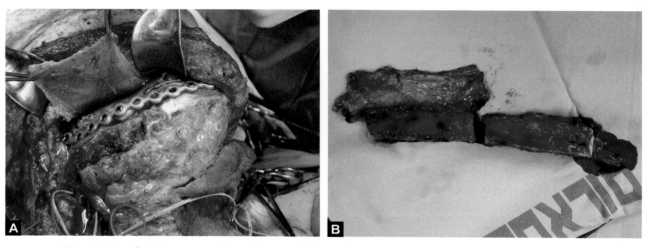

Figs 31A and B: Reconstruction of the mandible with a composite fibula free flap. A double barrel mandibular flap is used and covered with a fascia. The oral cavity is reconstructed with a skin island

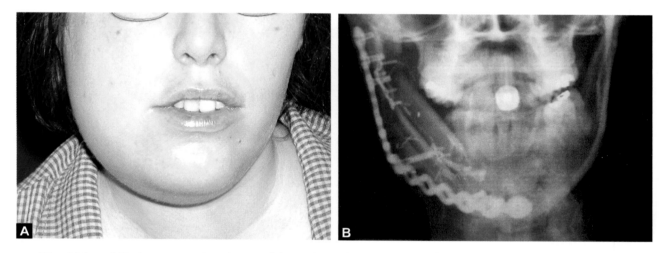

Figs 32A and B: A postoperative picture of the patient. The cosmetic result and the panoramic X-ray are shown

The specimen is oriented and submitted to the pathology laboratory for analysis. The wound is copiously irrigated, inspected and hemostasis is performed as indicated. A blood pressure above 120/80 should be confirmed prior to closure for adequate hemostasis. A Jackson-Pratt number 7 drain is left at the surgical bed. The mucosa and subcutaneous tissue are approximated and sutured with number 4-0 vicryl suture. The platysma is sutured with an absorbable stitches and the skin is closed with 5-0 nylon stitches or with clips.

HIGHLIGHTS

I. Indications
- Large oral cavity tumors with mandibular invasion

- Tumor of the oropharynx with bone invasion
- Primary submandibular gland tumors with mandibular invasion
- Large metastases to level I with extracapsular spread and bone involvement.

II. Contraindications
- Small T1–T2 oral tongue cancers without mandibular invasion
- Oropharynx or base of tongue squamous cell carcinoma amendable for chemoradiation treatment
- Tumor involving the internal or common carotid
- Tumors involving the prevertebral fascia
- Metastatic disease.

III. Special Preoperative Considerations
- Routine imaging including CT, dental scan and MRI

- Prior evaluation by a maxillofacial surgeons for teeth extraction
- Prophylactic antibiotic treatment
- Prior planning of the reconstruction means
- Percutaneous endoscopic gastrostomy in selected cases
- CT angiography of the lower extremities for fibula free flap.

IV. Special Intraoperative Considerations
- Nasal intubation in case of trismus
- Temporary tracheostomy
- Place the skin incision along a transverse skin crest in the lower neck
- Prevent injury to the marginal mandibular branch of the facial nerve
- Preserve the mental nerve in the contralateral side
- Prebanding of the titanium plate (before the osteotomy) to allow accurate repositioning of the bony reconstruction
- Leave 2 cm margins around the tumor
- Stretching of the tongue while demarcating the resection lines may lead to erroneous evaluation of the margins
- Leave a sleeve of mucosa over the lower alveolar ridge to facilitate mucosal closure
- Frozen sections are used for intraoperative evaluation of surgical margins
- Adequate reconstruction for restoration of structure and function.

V. Special Postoperative Considerations
- Nasogastric tube feeding
- Oral cleansing
- Removal of the tracheostomy tube when the airway is patent.

VI. Complications
- Bleeding
- Malunion of the mandible
- Wound infection
- Nerve injury
- Wound dehiscence
- Flap failure
- Fistula.

ADDITIONAL READING

1. Gourin CG, Johnson JT. A contemporary review of indications for primary surgical care of patients with squamous cell carcinoma of the head and neck. Laryngoscope. 2009;119(11):2124-34.
2. McGregor AD, MacDonald DG. Patterns of spread of squamous cell carcinoma to the ramus of the mandible. Head Neck. 1993;15(5):440-4.
3. Neligan PC, Gullane PJ, Gilbert RW. Functional reconstruction of the oral cavity. World J Surg. 2003;27(7):856-62.
4. Patel RS, Dirven R, Clark JR, et al. The prognostic impact of extent of bone invasion and extent of bone resection in oral carcinoma. Laryngoscope. 2008;118(5):780-5.
5. Shaha AR. Mandibulotomy and mandibulectomy in difficult tumors of the base of the tongue and oropharynx. Semin Surg Oncol. 1991;7(1):25-30.
6. Shah JP, Gil Z. Current concepts in management of oral cancer—surgery. Oral Oncol. 2009;45(4-5):394-401. Epub 2008 Jul 31.

Chapter **27**

Total Laryngectomy

Ziv Gil, Dan M Fliss

INTRODUCTION

Due to the development of organ preservation regimes for patients with laryngeal cancer, total laryngectomy is currently reserved for tumors with extensive thyroid or cricoid cartilage erosion and for tumors with extralaryngeal involvement or as salvage therapy. For these patients, tracheoesophageal prosthesis has revolutionized the rehabilitation, restoration of speech and quality of life. Despite the success of minimally invasive techniques for management of laryngeal tumors, patients who are poor surgical candidates would frequently benefit from total laryngectomy (TLR). Patients with poor laryngeal function (incompetent larynx), at the time of diagnosis, may also benefit from primary TLR because functional recovery after nonsurgical treatment is unlikely. In case of tumor persistence or recurrence after primary radiation or chemoradiation treatment, the only remaining option for cure is surgery in the form of salvage partial or total laryngectomy. The type of previous treatment, the extent of the tumor and the clinical condition of the patient typically determines the type of surgery needed.

Despite, the reproducibility of the surgical technique of TLR, this procedure still involves high-risk for postoperative pharyngocutaneous fistula (PCF), especially if performed in less than 1 year after the primary radiation treatment. Preoperative treatment with chemotherapy and radiotherapy can increase the risk of PCF formation after salvage TLR. To deal with this significant postoperative morbidity, several authors have advocated routine utilization of a pectoralis major muscle flap (PMMF) with the goal of reinforcing the primary pharyngeal suture line with vascularized tissue.

In this chapter, we shall describe in details the technique practiced by the authors for total laryngectomy. The reconstruction technique with PMMF, which is performed in selected cases, is also discussed.

PREOPERATIVE EVALUATION AND ANESTHESIA

All patients scheduled for operation are evaluated preoperatively by a head and neck surgeon and an anesthesiologist. Radiological evaluation of the patient includes computed tomography (CT) with contrast. Clinical suspicion of aggressive thyroid cancers with tracheal, vascular or esophageal involvement may necessitate magnetic resonance imaging (MRI) of the neck to assess infiltration of the tumor to neighboring structures. All patients should undergo flexible fiberoptic evaluation of the upper aerodigestive tracts and complete examination of the larynx prior to surgery. Flexible tracheoscopy and esophagoscopy may be also used in case of a subglottic extension or tumors of the upper esophagus. Positron emission tomography-CT hybrid (PET-CT), prior to the operative procedure, offers locoregional and distant metastatic work-up as well as evaluation of a second primary cancer.

Tissue Diagnosis

All patients should undergo direct laryngoscopy, upper esophagoscopy and biopsy prior to the definitive treatment. Tissue diagnosis should be confirmed by a head and neck pathologist from the treating medical institution. Evaluation

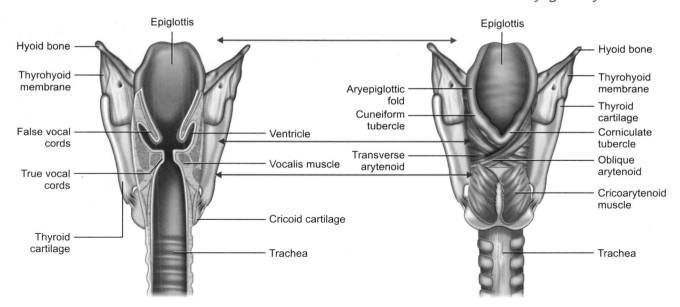

Fig. 1: Compartment of the larynx. The sites and subsites of the larynx include the supraglottis (subsites include laryngeal face of the epiglottis, aryepiglottic folds, false cords, arytenoids and ventricle), glottis (subsites include true vocal cords, anterior and posterior commissure) and subglottic area (right and left lateral walls). The purple arrows indicate the borders between the supraglottis, glottis and subglottis sites

is performed under anesthesia and should include inspection of the glottis, supraglottis, pyriform sinuses, hypopharynx and subglottis area (Fig. 1). The tumor extension to the subsites of the larynx should be documented.

Staging

Staging of laryngeal tumors is based on physical examination (vocal cord mobility), direct laryngoscopy (involvement of each laryngeal subsite) and radiologic evaluation (involvement of the pre-epiglottic space and thyroid cartilage). Each site and subsite of the larynx should be evaluated (Table 1). The primary tumor (T) staging of laryngeal tumors is shown in Table 2. Staging is crucial for tailoring of treatment. Primary laryngectomy is indicated for patients with T4 stage tumors, with high volume disease (>1 cm), base of tongue involvement and for tumors penetrating through the thyroid cartilage. Salvage TLR is performed at any stage when partial laryngectomy is not feasible and in high-risk patients. Stage T4b and the presence of distant metastases contraindicate surgery.

SURGICAL TECHNIQUE

First-generation cephalosporins and metronidazole may be used for prophylaxis treatment. Surgery is performed under general anesthesia with endotracheal intubation and muscle relaxation. If intubation is contraindicated due to imminent airway obstruction, "awake tracheostomy" is performed.

Table 1: The different sites and subsites of the larynx

Site	Subsite
Supraglottis	False vocal cords
	Arytenoids
	Suprahyoid epiglottis
	Infrahyoid epiglottis
	Aryepiglottic folds
Glottis	Vocal cord
	Anterior commissure
	Posterior commissure
Subglottis	Right lateral wall
	Left lateral wall

If total laryngectomy is performed as a primary treatment, the surgery should include extirpation of the larynx, its attached prelaryngeal muscles, the ipsilateral thyroid lobe (if indicated) and the lymph nodes of level VI bilaterally. Surgery starts with unilateral or bilateral selective neck dissection of levels II–IV.

Skin Incision

The patient is placed on the operating room table in a supine position. The head is stabilized with a soft donut holder and the whole operating table is then elevated in an angle with the head up in order to minimize bleeding.

Table 2: Primary tumor (T) staging of laryngeal tumors

TX: Primary tumor cannot be assessed

T0: No evidence of primary tumor

Tis: Carcinoma in situ

Supraglottis

T1: Tumor limited to one subsite of supraglottis with normal vocal cord mobility

T2: Tumor invades mucosa of more than one adjacent subsite of supraglottis or glottis, or region outside the supraglottis (e.g. mucosa of base of tongue, vallecula, medial wall of pyriform sinus) without fixation of the larynx

T3: Tumor limited to larynx with vocal cord fixation and/or invades any of the following:
- Postcricoid area
- Pre-epiglottic tissues
- Paraglottic space and /or inner cortex of the thyroid cartilage

T4a: Tumor invades through the thyroid cartilage, and/or extends into soft tissues of the neck, thyroid and/or esophagus

T4b: Tumor invades prevertebral space, encases the carotid artery or invades mediastinal structure

Glottis

T1: Tumor limited to vocal cord(s) (may involve anterior or posterior commissure) with normal mobility
- *T1a*: Tumor limited to one vocal cord
- *T1b*: Tumor involves both vocal cords

T2: Tumor extends to supraglottis and/or subglottis and/or with impaired vocal cord mobility

T3: Tumor limited to the larynx with vocal cord fixation and/or invades any of the following:
- Pre-epiglottic tissues
- Paraglottic space and /or inner cortex of the thyroid cartilage

T4a: Tumor invades through the thyroid cartilage, and/or extends into soft tissues of the neck, thyroid, and/or esophagus

T4b: Tumor invades prevertebral space, encases the carotid artery or invades mediastinal structure

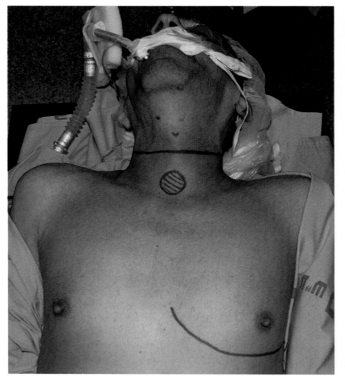

Fig. 2: Positioning and skin incision planning

The surgical access is planned through a horizontal neck incision (Fig. 2). If reconstruction with PMMF is indicated, an inframammary incision is marked. A wide bridge of skin should be left between the incision and the stoma. Therefore, the incision is performed at the level of the thyrohyoid membrane. It extends along the anterior borders of the trapezius muscles bilaterally. The stoma is performed at the suprasternal notch, with an approximate diameter of 2–3 cm, according to the size of the patient's thumb. The thumb is used to close the stoma during esophageal speech. After incision marking, a roll is placed under the shoulders to hyperextend the neck. This positioning moves the larynx anterior and cephalad. The surgeon should be aware of the possibility that extension of the neck may pull the endotracheal tube out 2–4 cm from its original location. In such cases, repositioning of the tube caudally may be required. The patient is then prepped and draped in a standard surgical fashion.

Skin Incision and Elevation of Subplatysmal Flaps

After marking, the skin is injected with lidocaine (0.06%) and epinephrine (1:1,000,000) to reduce the amount of pain after surgery and for hemostasis. The skin is incised with a number 15 blade and subsequent dissection of the subcutaneous tissue and the platysma is carried out with an electrocautery at the lowest effective setting (Fig. 3). Subplatysmal flaps are elevated superiorly above the hyoid bone and inferiorly to the sternum (Fig. 4). Care is taken to prevent injury to the anterior jugular veins, which are left on the superficial layer of the deep cervical fascia. The flaps are retracted and held using skin hooks. The anterior jugular veins are divided and ligated.

Mobilization of the Larynx

A neck dissection is performed prior to the laryngectomy (Fig. 5). After the flaps are elevated, mobilization of the larynx is preformed. This is achieved by resecting the suprahyoid muscles at the upper surface of the hyoid bone and the

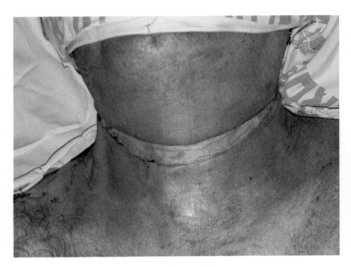

Fig. 3: Skin incision

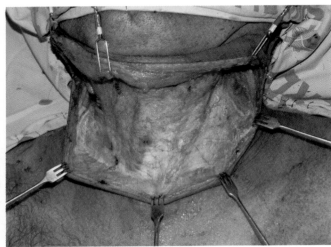

Fig. 4: Elevation of the subplatysmal flaps

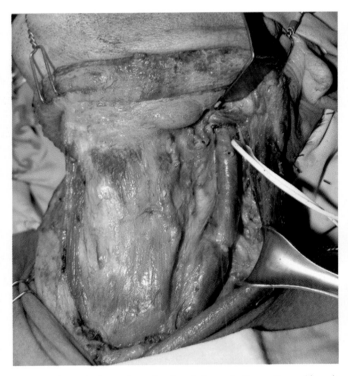

Fig. 5: Completion of a selective left neck dissection of levels II–IV for recurrent T3N0M0 left glottic tumor after failure of chemoradiation therapy

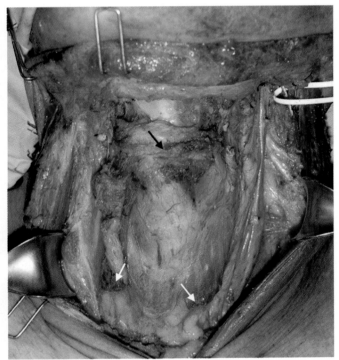

Fig. 6: Mobilization of the larynx. The hyoid bone (black arrow) is grasped with an Allis grasper and the suprahyoid muscles are transected. The sternohyoid, sternothyroid and omohyoid muscles (white arrows) are also divided low in the neck

strap muscles attachments to the clavicles and sternum (Fig. 6). The hyoid bone is grasped with an Allis clamp and retracted caudally. At the root of the neck, the sternohyoid, sternothyroid and omohyoid muscles are divided above the clavicles. The muscles are divided with a monopolar electrocautery. When dissecting along the hyoid bone, care

is taken not to injure the lingual artery and hypoglossal nerve (Fig. 7). The dissection here is performed directly on the upper edge of the bone from the midline to the greater cornua on both sides. If necessary, the tip of the great cornu may be cut with a Liston bone cutter. After releasing the hyoid bone, the superior thyroid artery and its superior laryngeal branch are identified (Fig. 8). The superior laryngeal artery is divided and ligated above its entrance to the thyrohyoid membrane.

Exposure and Resection of the Ipsilateral Thyroid Lobe

In this case, the tumor involves the left vocal cord and subglottic area. Since there is a significant risk of thyroid gland involvement in tumors with subglottic invasion, a left thyroid lobectomy is indicated. An adequate exposure of the gland is accomplished without dividing the sternothyroid muscles.

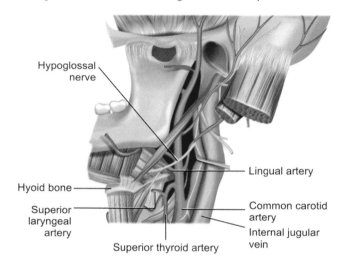

Fig. 7: Anatomical structure at the area of the hyoid bone and larynx

First the isthmus of the thyroid gland is divided (Fig. 9). Next, the superior thyroid artery is divided and the left thyroid lobe is separated and left on the specimen. The left lobe is rotated medially and retracted gently with two pediatric Babcock forceps. At this point, the dissection continues with a "subcapsular" dissection along the visceral fascia, in a cranial to caudal direction. This fascia is consistent of multiple thin layers of connective tissue that encapsulate the thyroid gland and its superficial thyroid vasculature. The fascia is striped from the underlying thyroid by spreading of a micro clamp and by cauterizing the small vessels with bipolar cautery. While the visceral fascia is reflected laterally, the terminal branches of the inferior thyroid artery are ligated distal to the parathyroid glands and the thyroid "capsule" is peeled away along with the parathyroid glands. As the dissection of the left thyroid lobe is completed, the gland is left on the trachea and the remaining right thyroid lobe is separated from the specimen and retracted laterally (Fig. 10). The right lobe and its superior and inferior blood supply are preserved along with the parathyroid glands.

Separation of the Thyroid Cartilage

Next, the inferior constrictor muscle is detached from the lateral face of the thyroid cartilage. The thyroid cartilage is now rotated medially with a double hook retractor and the muscle is separated from its attachments with Freer dissector at the level of the perichondrium (Fig. 11). Care is taken not to compromise tumor margins in case of thyroid cartilage invasion. After completion of this stage, the trachea, cricoid and thyroid cartilages are exposed and mobilized. The ipsilateral thyroid lobe and strap muscles are left in

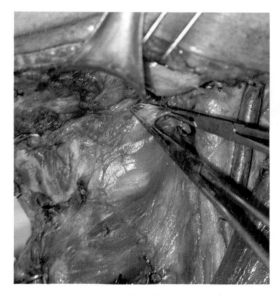

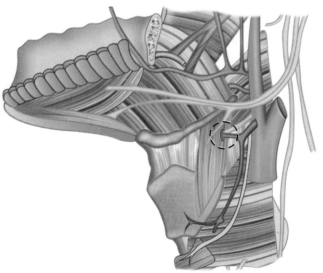

Fig. 8: Dividing the superior laryngeal pedicle, the superior laryngeal artery. A branch of the superior thyroid artery is divided (see indicated by the circle)

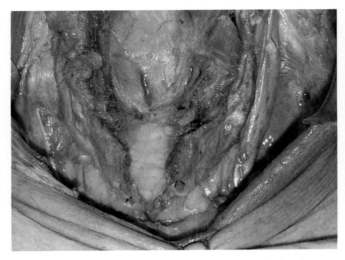

Fig. 9: Dividing the isthmus of the thyroid gland

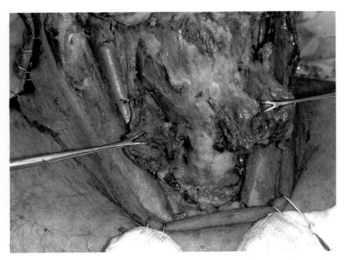

Fig. 10: Dissection of the left thyroid lobe and preservation of the right lobe

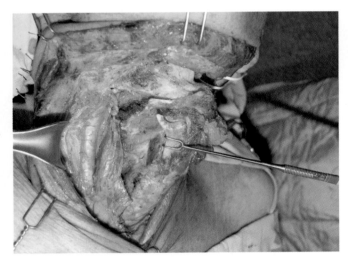

Fig. 11: Rotation of the larynx. The inferior constrictor muscle is detached from the thyroid cartilage ala

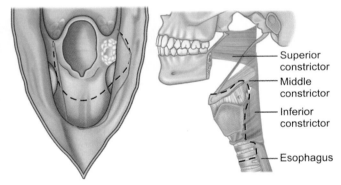

Fig. 12: The borders of the resection

continuity with the whole specimen. The resection of the larynx can now be performed. Figure 12 shows the borders of the resection.

Performing the Tracheal Stoma

When the trachea is exposed at the suprasternal notch, surgery is turned toward performing the tracheal stoma. First, the attachments of the sternocleidomastoid muscle to the medial portion of the clavicles are divided using a monopolar electrocautery. This maneuver will allow performance of a wide and superficial stoma, facilitating treatment of the tracheal stoma and esophageal speech. Next, a circular segment of the skin is excised at the area of the future stoma. This is performed in the midline at the

suprasternal notch. The stoma should be 2–3 cm wide and it varies according to the size of the trachea. Bear in mind that the stoma will shrink during the first year after surgery by a factor of 25%. Therefore, the stoma is usually made larger than anticipated. Attention is turned now to the resection of the trachea. The level of tracheal incision is performed according to the area of the tumor. For glottic or supraglottic tumors, the incision is performed at the lower border of the first tracheal ring, whereas for transglottic or subglottic tumors, resection of the second or even the third tracheal ring is required. The anterior segment of the trachea is incised with a scalpel, and the lumen and endotracheal tube are exposed. A beveled-shaped stoma is performed where the posterior part of the trachea is 0.5 cm higher than its anterior segment (Fig. 13). This will increase the diameter of the stoma and prevent stenosis. The endotracheal tube is removed and a laryngectomy cuffed Laryngoflex® tube is inserted through the skin stoma to the lower stump of the trachea. After the airway is secured, the surgeon should

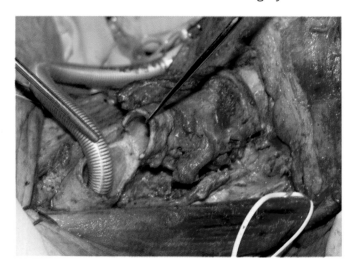

Fig. 13: Division of the trachea. The first tracheal ring is included in the specimen

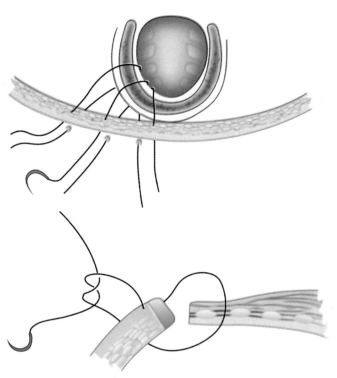

Fig. 14: The trachea is sutured to the skin using half mattress interrupted sutures

inspect the distal stump of the trachea and estimate the subglottic margin of the tumor relative to the inferior border of the glottis. At this stage, the trachea is sutured to the skin using half mattress interrupted sutures (Fig. 14). First sutures are performed at 12, 3, 6, 9 o'clock using half mattress sutures (2-0 nylon). During closure, the skin is advanced over the cartilage by taking larger bites on the skin side than the trachea side. Next, two 4-0 nylon sutures are placed between the previously placed 2-0 sutures. During this procedure, the laryngectomy tube may be removed periodically until the tracheal stoma is completed.

Removal of the Larynx

When the tracheal stoma is completed, surgery is turned for resection of the larynx. The trachea is separated from the esophagus at the "party wall" using an electrocautery. Care is taken not to injure the anterior wall of the esophagus. Now, after full mobilization of the larynx is achieved, attention is turned toward entry of the pharynx. In case of glottic or subglottic tumors, the pharynx is entered at the level of pharyngoepiglottic fold (vallecula) as in Figure 15. On the other hand, in case of a supraglottic tumor and in tumors invading the pyriform sinus, the pharynx is entered from the pyriform sinus at the contralateral side of the tumor. The pharynx is entered using a monopolar electrocautery. After the lumen is entered, dissection is continued with a long Stevens scissors. From this point onwards, circumferential incision of the mucosa is performed under direct vision, verifying safe margins from the tumor. Subsequent removal of the larynx is performed and the specimen is transected in the posterior midline and inspected, confirming complete resection of the tumor with adequate margins as in Figures 16 and 17.

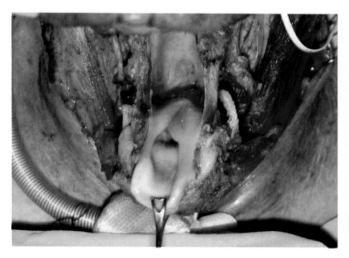

Fig. 15: Entering the pharynx. In this case, the pharynx was entered through the vallecula. After entering the pharynx, the epiglottis is held with a Babcock grasper

Performing of the Tracheoesophageal Puncture

If primary tracheoesophageal puncture (TEP) is indicated, it is performed at this stage. The authors routinely perform TEP in all patients undergoing total laryngectomy excluding

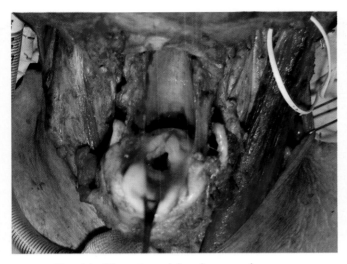

Fig. 16: Dissection of the pharyngeal mucosa

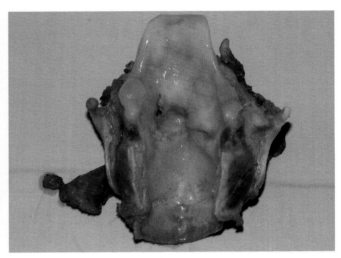

Fig. 17: The laryngectomy specimen.
A left transglottis tumor is shown

patients previously treated with chemoradiation. In these patients, primary TEP is associated with postoperative leak and valve dislodges, and therefore secondary puncture is preferred. A right-angled clamp is delivered through the pharynx to the level of the cervical esophagus, right posterior to the upper lip of the stoma (Fig. 18). The clamp is pushed through the anterior wall of the esophagus toward the membranous trachea. The posterior wall of the trachea is incised with a number 15 blade and its tip is exteriorized in the midline position. Next, a number 12 Foley's catheter is inserted through the puncture using the right-angled clamp. The catheter is then entered through the esophagus to the stomach.

Closure of the Pharyngeal Defect

There are several options to close the mucosa. This includes transverse closure, vertical closure or T-shaped closure (Figs 19A to C). Each of these options has advantages and disadvantages. The authors prefer a vertical closure for three reasons: (i) it is associated with low tension as oppose to the vertical closure; (ii) it is easy to perform and does not involve a bifurcated suture line as oppose to the T-shape closure and; (iii) it results in excellent speech and swallowing result. The closure is performed in two layers using 4-0 vicryl sutures. First, two long sutures are placed at the superior and inferior border of the mucosa and gently retracted to opposite directions, vertically. Next, the mucosa is closed using interrupted sutures beginning at the caudal and cephalad edges of the defect, toward the midline (Fig. 20). Care is taken to assure inversion of the mucosa during closure. The second layer is performed in a similar manner in order to decrease the tension on the first suture line.

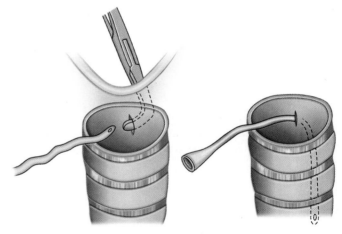

Fig. 18: Performance of the TEP. A right-angled clamp is delivered through the pharynx to the level of the cervical esophagus, right posterior to the upper lip of the stoma. The clamp is pushed through the anterior wall of the esophagus toward the membranous trachea, the trachea is incised with a number 15 blade and its tip is exteriorized in the midline position

Buttressing the Suture Line with Pectoralis Muscle Flap

There is a large variability in the reported rates of post laryngectomy PCF with incidence ranging from 2.6% to 66%. This variability can be largely explained by differences in study period, patient characteristics, surgeon experience and prior therapy. Several studies have specifically examined the utility of PMMF for buttressing the pharyngeal suture line after total laryngectomy. Most authors have reported a significant reduction in the rate of PCF development.

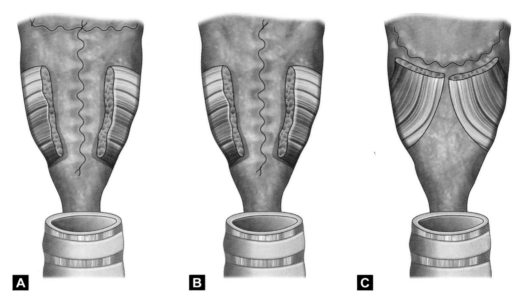

Figs 19A to C: Methods for closure of the pharyngeal mucosa. These include transverse closure (C), Vertical closure (B) and T-shaped closure (A)

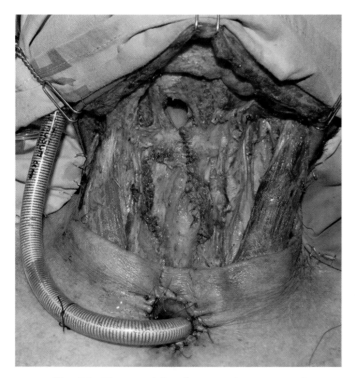

Fig. 20: Closure of the pharyngeal mucosa and suturing of the tracheal stoma

Pectoralis major muscle flap also reduces the need for revision surgery in patients who develop PCF and is indicated in selected group of patients with a higher risk of fistula formation.

Thus, PMMF should not be used as a routine procedure in patients requiring salvage laryngectomy (where the overall rate of PCF is lower than 30%). In view of the increased morbidity, time and cost of adding PMMF to buttress the pharyngeal suture line, it should be used judiciously in patients with prior chemoradiation treatment and those with poor nutritional status. In addition, the size of the surgical defect and the vascularity of the tissues at the pharyngeal suture line are other considerations. Thus, in a selected population of patients at high-risk for PCF, PMMF may be a valuable adjunct for decreasing the risk of complications, morbidity and the potential need for revision surgery.

The muscle is placed over the suture line and between the anterior borders of the sternocleidomastoid muscles laterally, the anterior belly of the digastric muscles superiorly and the suprasternal notch inferiorly (Fig. 21). The wound is copiously irrigated, inspected and hemostasis is performed as indicated. A blood pressure above 120/80 should be confirmed prior to closure for adequate hemostasis. If chyle leak is suspected, a Valsalva maneuver can be performed by keeping a positive ventilation pressure greater than 40 mm Hg for several seconds. Two Jackson-Pratt number 7 drains are placed below and above the PMMF. The platysma is sutured with an absorbable stitches and the skin is closed with 5-0 nylon stitches as in Figures 22 and 23.

In case of advanced tumors with high volume nodal metastases, the larynx and neck dissection specimen can be resected in an en bloc fashion as in Figures 24 and 25.

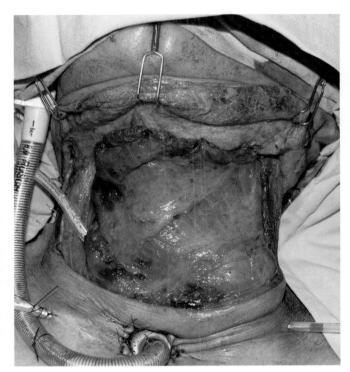

Fig. 21: Buttressing of the suture line with pectoralis major muscle flap

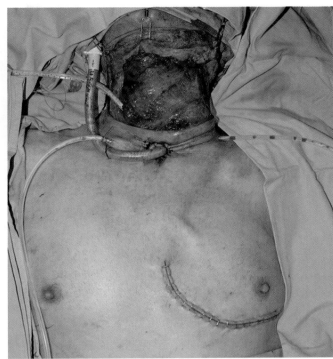

Fig. 22: The donor site of the pectoralis muscle flap

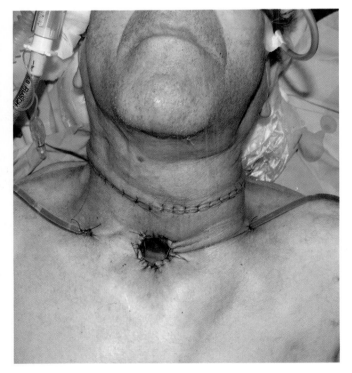

Fig. 23: Closure of the surgical wound

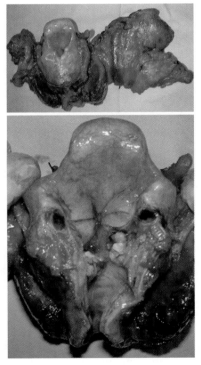

Fig. 24: Laryngectomy with right modified radical neck dissection. T4N2bM0 tumor is shown

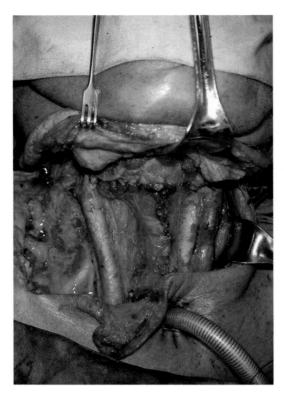

Fig. 25: The surgical field after total laryngectomy left selective neck dissection and right radical neck dissection. In this case, a T closure of the mucosa was performed since the remaining mucosa was insignificant for a vertical closure

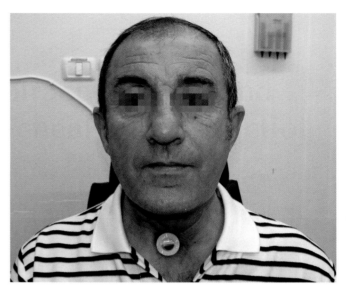

Fig. 26: Postoperative result. The picture was taken 2 months after surgery

POSTOPERATIVE TREATMENT

After the surgery, the patient is extubated and immediately transferred to the post surgery care unit before his transfer to the floor. The wound is kept clean by rinsing it with saline three times a day and covered with antibiotic ointment after each cleansing. High protein, high caloric diet is provided through the catheter placed in the TEP. The drains are removed, either 3 days after the operation or when the fluid is less than 20–30 ml in 24 hours. Prophylactic antibiotic treatment is not indicated in the postoperative period. For pain control, the patients are treated with nonsteroidal anti-inflammatory drugs (diclofenac 75 mg intramuscularly or orally, or rofecoxib 50 mg) once daily and with tramadol (50–100 mg), if the patient asks for them or if the nurses felt it to be necessary.

After 7–10 days, the catheter tube is removed from the TEP and a speech valve is inserted by the speech pathologist. A picture of a patient after total salvage laryngectomy is shown in Figure 26.

HIGHLIGHTS

I. Indications
- Advanced (T4a) squamous cell carcinoma of the larynx
- Recurrent squamous cell carcinoma of the larynx after radiation therapy
- Nonfunctional larynx with significant aspiration and low quality voice
- Poorly differentiated carcinoma of the thyroid with gross laryngotracheal invasion
- Patients who are not suitable for partial laryngectomy.

II. Contraindications
- Tumor invades prevertebral space, encases the carotid artery or invades mediastinal structure
- Presence of distant metastases
- T1-T3 local disease amendable for radiotherapy, chemoradiation or partial laryngectomy
- Selected T4 tumors with minimal thyroid cartilage invasion.

III. Special Preoperative Considerations
- Imaging using CT with contrast
- Imaging with PET-CT in large tumors (T4) for distant metastases work-up
- Previous direct laryngoscope and tissue diagnosis
- Use perioperative antibiotic treatment.

IV. Special Intraoperative Considerations
- Adequate positioning of skin incisions

- Resect the thyroid lobe in the ipsilateral side of the tumor, in tumors invading the subglottis, cricoid or thyroid cartilage.
- Clamp and divide the superior laryngeal pedicle
- Open the pharynx through the vallecula, in case of a glottis tumor, or from the contralateral side of the lesion in case of a supraglottic involvement
- Tumor excision should be performed under direct vision with adequate margins (~1 cm)
- Examine the tumor and its margins after removal of the specimen
- Meticulous mucosal closure reduces the incidence of fistula
- Use the PMMF to buttress the suture line in patients who previously underwent chemoradiation therapy.

V. Special Postoperative Considerations
- Identify complications as early as possible
- Pharyngocutaneous fistula is usually treated conservatively with local pressure
- Early reinstatement of neck and shoulders physiotherapy
- Early restoration of communication means.

VI. Complications
- Bleeding
- Seroma
- Pharyngocutaneous fistula
- Wound infection and dehiscence.

ADDITIONAL READING

1. Ganly I, Patel S, Matsuo J, et al. Postoperative complications of salvage total laryngectomy. Cancer. 2005;103(10):2073-81.
2. Gil Z, Fliss DM. Contemporary management of head and neck cancers. Isr Med 2. Assoc J. 2009;11(5):296-300.
3. Gil Z, Gupta A, Kummer B, et al. The role of pectoralis major muscle flap in salvage total laryngectomy. Arch Otolaryngol Head Neck Surg. 2009;135(10):1019-23.
4. Hanna EY. Laryngeal preservation: what is the best treatment strategy? Curr Oncol Rep. 2004;6(3):167-9.
5. Holsinger FC, Funk E, Roberts DB, et al. Conservation laryngeal surgery versus total laryngectomy for radiation failure in laryngeal cancer. Head Neck. 2006;28(9):779-84.
6. Koch WM. Total laryngectomy with tracheoesophageal conduit. Otolaryngol Clin North Am. 2002;35(5):1081-96.
7. Kraus DH, Pfister DG, Harrison LB, et al. Salvage laryngectomy for unsuccessful larynx preservation therapy. Ann Otol Rhinol Laryngol. 1995;104(12):936-41.
8. Sassler AM, Esclamado RM, Wolf GT. Surgery after organ preservation therapy. Analysis of wound complications. Arch Otolaryngol Head Neck Surg. 1995;121(2):162-5.
9. Weber RS, Berkey BA, Forastiere A, et al. Outcome of salvage total laryngectomy following organ preservation therapy: the Radiation Therapy Oncology Group trial 91-11. Arch Otolaryngol Head Neck Surg. 2003;129(1):44-9.
10. Weingrad DN, Spiro RH. Complications after laryngectomy. Am J Surg. 1983;146(4):517-20.

Chapter **28**

Transfacial Incisions

Ziv Gil, Dan M Fliss

INTRODUCTION

The route of spread of tumors originating in the anterior skull base and paranasal sinuses is determined by the complex anatomy of the craniofacial compartments. These tumors may invade laterally to the orbit and middle fossa, inferiorly to the maxillary antrum and palate, posteriorly to the nasopharynx and pterygopalatine fossa, and superiorly to the cavernous sinus and brain. The recent improvements of endoscopic technology now allow the resection of most benign and malignant neoplasms using minimally invasive techniques. For malignant tumors and for benign tumors with bony involvement, the classical transfacial approaches remain viable surgical techniques. In cases of tumor extension superior or lateral to the paranasal sinuses, transfacial approaches alone cannot provide adequate exposure of the tumor and other supplementary techniques are needed to allow safe resection and reconstruction.

Conventional transfacial approaches involve various skin incisions and osteotomies of the maxillary, frontal and ethmoidal bones. The conventional exposure of the suprastructure of the maxilla involves lateral rhinotomy incision, whereas supra and infrastructure maxillectomy is performed via Weber-Ferguson incisions. Lynch incision may be used to approach the frontal sinus lateral to the supraorbital nerve, where endoscopic resection is unfeasible. Lateral rhinotomy may be combined with a Lynch incision. Dieffenbach incision combined with a lateral rhinotomy incision is used for tumors which extend to the infraorbital rim, lateral orbital wall, zygoma and orbit.

In this chapter, the authors describe the common transfacial incision used alone or in combination for resections at the craniofacial area.

PREOPERATIVE EVALUATION AND ANESTHESIA

All patients scheduled for operation are evaluated preoperatively by a head and neck surgeon and an anesthesiologist. If a free flap is planned, preoperative physical examination by a plastic surgeon is essential. Radiological evaluation of the patients includes axial and coronal computed tomography (CT) and magnetic resonance imaging (MRI) of the head and neck. Broad-spectrum antibiotics are instituted perioperatively. This usually includes a second-generation cephalosporin and metronidazole. All the patients are operated in the supine position.

SURGICAL TECHNIQUE

Figure 1 shows depiction of various transfacial incisions described in this chapter. Summary of the indications for each transfacial approach is given in Table 1.

Lateral Rhinotomy Incision

In cases of malignant tumors, originating in the nasal cavity and maxillary sinus without palatal invasion, the lateral rhinotomy approach is used. Similarly, benign tumors with anterior maxillary wall involvement are also approached with the same incision. This approach allows wide exposure of the maxillary antrum, nasal cavity, ethmoidal sinuses and sphenoid sinus.

The facial incision extends along the lateral border of the nose, approximately 1 cm lateral to the midline. It starts cephalad, medial to the canthus and extends down through the skin crest bordering the nasal ala. It is continued toward

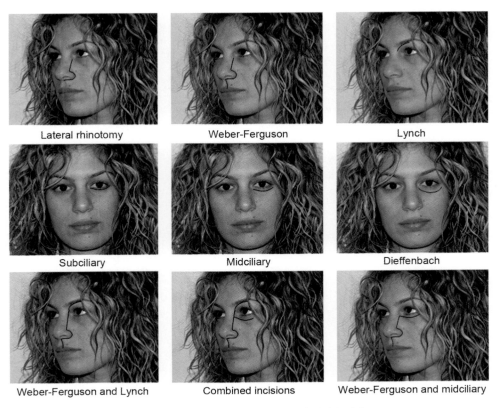

Lateral rhinotomy	Weber-Ferguson	Lynch
Subciliary	Midciliary	Dieffenbach
Weber-Ferguson and Lynch	Combined incisions	Weber-Ferguson and midciliary

Fig. 1: A depiction of various transfacial incisions

the filtrum (Fig. 2). After marking, the skin is injected with lidocaine (0.06%) and epinephrine (1:1,000,000) for hemostasis and hydrodissection purposes. Following the incision with a number 15 blade, the dissection continues with electrocautery. Skin flaps are elevated medially and

Table 1: Summary of the indications for each transfacial approach

Tumor extension	Surgical approach
Nasal cavity Medial maxillary wall Maxillary antrum Anterior and posterior ethmoids Sphenoid sinus	Lateral rhinotomy
Frontal sinus Supraorbital rim Anterior ethmoids	Lynch incision
As in lateral rhinotomy, with infiltration of the hard palate Premaxilla Lateral maxillary wall Maxillary tuberosity	Weber-Ferguson
Infraorbital rim Root of the zygoma Lateral orbital wall	Subciliary Midciliary Dieffenbach

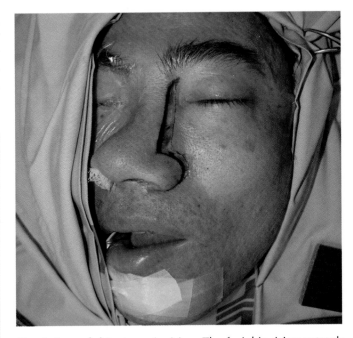

Fig. 2: Lateral rhinotomy incision. The facial incision extends along the lateral border of the nose, approximately 1 cm lateral to the midline. It starts cephalad, medial to the canthus and extends down through the skin crest bordering the nasal ala. It is continued toward the filtrum

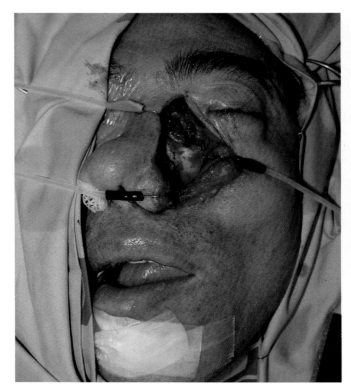

Fig. 3: The limits of the lateral rhinotomy approach. The flaps can be developed to the level of the maxillary tuberosity (laterally), the upper gingival sulcus (inferiorly), the frontal sinus and infraorbital rim (superiorly) and to the nasion and nasal septum (medially)

laterally to the level of the periosteum with the aid of a freer dissector. Care is taken not to injure the infraorbital nerve. If the tumor infiltrates the anterior wall of the maxilla, the skin flaps should be thinner, the fibrofatty tissue and muscles are left on the maxillary bone to be included in the specimen. The flaps can be developed to the level of the maxillary tuberosity (laterally), the upper gingival sulcus (inferiorly), the frontal sinus and infraorbital rim (superiorly) and to the nasion and nasal septum (medially) as in Figure 3. The flaps are held with a 2-0 skin stitches and fish hooks.

Weber-Ferguson Incision

In cases of malignant tumors infiltrating the lateral maxillary wall or palate, total maxillectomy is performed via Weber-Ferguson incision. This incision allows exposure of the superior and inferior aspects of the maxilla and its complete en bloc resection. The facial incision begins as a lateral rhinotomy incision, which is continued toward the filtrum and extended down to the lip in the midline (Figs 4A and B). Inferiorly, the incision continues along the gingivobuccal sulcus extending laterally up to the retromolar area.

After marking, the skin and gingivobuccal sulcus are injected with lidocaine (0.06%) and epinephrine

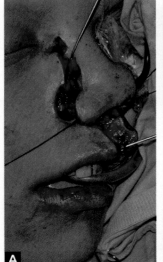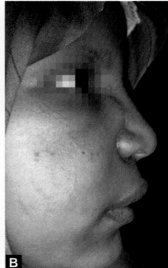

Figs 4A and B: Weber-Ferguson incision. (A) The facial incision begins as a lateral rhinotomy incision, which is continued toward the filtrum and extended down to the lip in the midline; (B) The postoperative result early after surgery

(1:1,000,000) for hemostasis and hydrodissection purposes. Following the incision with a number 15 blade, the dissection continues with electrocautery. Skin flaps are elevated medially and laterally to the level of the periosteum as described above.

A unilateral gingivolabial incision is now made extending up to the lateral buttress of the maxillary. The soft tissue of the cheek is raised from the anterior surface of the maxilla, transecting the infraorbital nerves and vessels if the superior and lateral walls of the maxilla need to be approached. An upper cheek flap is developed laterally and superiorly up to the level of the inferior orbital rim and the maxillary tuberosity (Fig. 5). Inferiorly, it can reach the pterygopalatine fossa.

Lynch Incision

The Lynch incision is used to approach tumors involving the frontal sinus. It can be extended laterally up to the level of the lateral canthus, or inferiorly, to be included in a lateral rhinotomy incision.

The facial incision extends along the lower border of the eyebrow allowing it to be concealed at the hair-skin junction. If the incision is made inside the eyebrow, a thick scar may be noticed giving inferior cosmetic results. The incision is extended down, approximately half a centimeter medial to the medial canthus as in Figures 6A and B.

Following the incision with a number 15 blade, the dissection continues with electrocautery. Skin flaps are elevated in the superior and inferior directions to the level of the periosteum with the aid of a freer dissector. The superior border of the flap is the frontal bone and glabella; its inferior border is the superior orbital rim and roof of the orbit; within its medial border lie the lacrimal fossa with its duct and sac; and the lateral border is the root of the zygoma. Lynch incision can be the extension of a lateral rhinotomy incision as in Figure 7.

Dieffenbach Incision and its Modification

These incisions are used to approach tumors involving the infraorbital rim and zygomatic root. It can be extended medially up to the level of the medial canthus, or inferiorly, to be included in a lateral rhinotomy incision.

The classical Dieffenbach incision extends along the lower border of the eyelid, along a skin crest. The incision extends from the medial canthus to the lateral canthus. Latter modification of this incision is the subciliary incision, which is located just below the cilia of the eyelid or the midciliary incision. The incision is located in the halfway between the Dieffenbach and subciliary incisions as in Figure 8.

Following the incision with a number 15 blade, the dissection continues with electrocautery. Skin flaps are elevated in the superior and inferior directions to the level of the periosteum with the aid of a freer dissector (Fig. 9). The superior border of the flap is infraorbital rim and orbit; its inferior border is the anterior maxillary wall; laterally, it is extended to expose the maxillary tuberosity and root of the zygoma and; medially, it extends to the nasal bone. In elderly population and in previously irradiated patients, the redundant skin and subcutaneous tissue of the lower eyelid tend to swell as the incision may compromise lymphatic

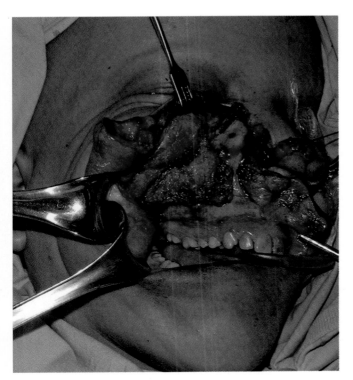

Fig. 5: Extension flaps in Weber-Ferguson approach. The soft tissue of the cheek is raised from the anterior surface of the maxilla, transecting the infraorbital nerves and vessels if the superior and lateral walls of the maxilla need to be approached. An upper cheek flap is developed laterally and superiorly up to the level of the inferior orbital rim and the maxillary tuberosity. Inferiorly, it can reach the pterygopalatine fossa

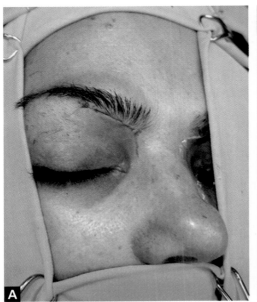
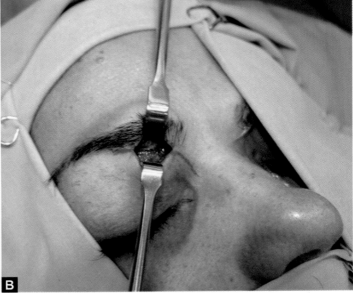

Figs 6A and B: Lynch incision. The facial incision extends along the lower border of the eyebrow allowing it to be concealed at the hair-skin junction. If the incision is made inside the eyebrow, a thick scar may be noticed giving inferior cosmetic results. The incision is extended down, approximately half a centimeter medial to the medial canthus

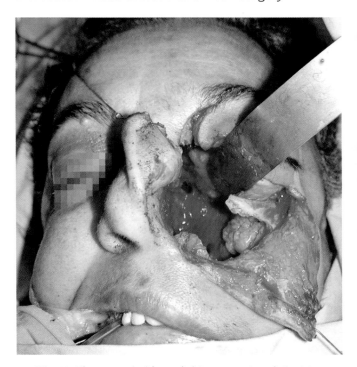

Fig. 7: The extended lateral rhinotomy, Lynch incision

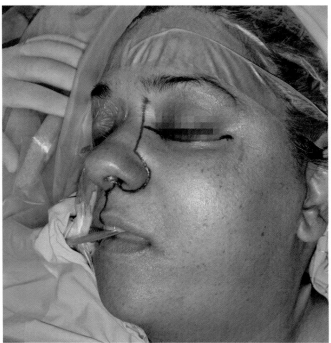

Fig. 8: The subciliary and midciliary incisions. These modifications of the Dieffenbach incision are located just below the cilia of the eyelid or halfway between the Dieffenbach and subciliary incisions

drainage of this area. The skin in this area is closed with subcutaneous continuous number 5-0 prolene stitch to prevent contractions of the thin skin in this area.

HIGHLIGHTS

I. Indications
- Lateral rhinotomy incision
  - Tumor extension
    - Nasal cavity
    - Medial maxillary wall
    - Maxillary antrum
    - Anterior and posterior ethmoids
    - Sphenoid sinus
- Lynch incision
  - Tumor extension
    - Frontal sinus
    - Supraorbital rim
    - Anterior ethmoids
- Weber-Ferguson incision
  - Tumor extension
    - As in lateral rhinotomy, with infiltration of the hard palate
    - Premaxilla
    - Lateral maxillary wall
    - Maxillary tuberosity

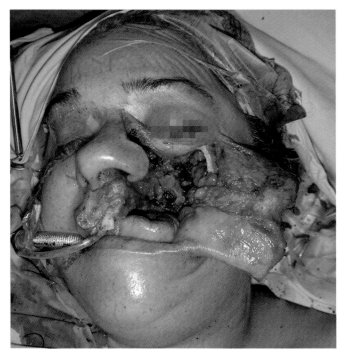

Fig. 9: Extension flaps in extended midciliary incisions. The soft tissue of the cheek is raised from the anterior surface of the maxilla, transecting the infraorbital nerves and vessels if the superior and lateral walls of the maxilla need to be approached. An upper cheek flap is developed laterally and superiorly up to the level of the inferior orbital rim and the maxillary tuberosity. Inferiorly, it can reach the pterygopalatine fossa

- Subciliary incision
  - Tumor extension
    - Infraorbital rim
- Midciliary incision
  - Tumor extension
    - Root of the zygoma
- Dieffenbach incision
  - Tumor extension
    - Lateral orbital wall.

II. Contraindications
- Massive skin infiltration
- Invasion to the base of skull and orbit. Tumors amendable for endonasal surgery

III. Special Preoperative Considerations
- Careful planning of the surgical approach
- Preoperative planning of the reconstruction means.

IV. Special Intraoperative Considerations
- Concealing the facial incision along natural skin crease
- Put the Lynch incision just below the eyebrow
- The vertical part of the lateral rhinotomy incision is placed 0.5 cm medial to the canthus
- Place the lip split portion of the Weber-Ferguson incision in the midline
- The Dieffenbach incision is closed using a subcutaneous fine monocryl suture only.

V. Special Postoperative Considerations
- Daily cleansing of the wound with saline and covering with antibiotic ointment
- Identify wound infection early and treatment with adequate antibiotic coverage.

VI. Complications
- Wound infection
- Skin edema
- Epiphora and stenosis of the lacrimal duct
- Contractures
- Diplopia and telecanthus
- Nerve injury of V1 and V2.

ADDITIONAL READING

1. Cordeiro PG, Santamaria E, Kraus DH, et al. Reconstruction of total maxillectomy defects with preservation of the orbital contents. Plast Reconstr Surg. 1998;102(6):1874-87.
2. Fliss DM, Abergel A, Cavel O, et al. Combined subcranial approaches for excision of complex anterior skull base tumors. Arch Otolaryngol Head Neck Surg. 2007;133(9): 888-96.
3. Gil Z, Fliss DM. Contemporary management of head and neck cancers. Isr Med Assoc J. 2009;11(5):296-300.
4. Shah JP, Gil Z. Current concepts in management of oral cancer—surgery. Oral Oncol. 2009;45(4-5):394-401.
5. Spiro RH, Strong EW, Shah JP. Maxillectomy and its classification. Head Neck. 1997;19(4):309-14.
6. Vural E, Hanna E. Extended lateral rhinotomy incision for total maxillectomy. Otolaryngol Head Neck Surg. 2000;123 (4):512-3.

Chapter 29

Partial Suprastructure Maxillectomy and Partial Infrastructure Maxillectomy

Ziv Gil, Dan M Fliss

Part A: Partial Suprastructure Maxillectomy

INTRODUCTION

Neoplasms of the maxilla and nasal cavity, a rare tumor, accounts for less than 5% of all the head and neck neoplasms. The common primary malignant neoplasms in this area are squamous cell carcinoma, sinonasal undifferentiated carcinoma, adenocarcinoma, minor salivary gland tumors, lacrimal duct neoplasms, esthesioneuroblastoma and melanoma. Rare in the adult population, but more common among children and adolescents are soft tissue sarcomas including rhabdomyosarcoma, Ewing sarcoma and low-grade sarcomas. Secondary tumors of the maxilla usually originate in the skin or skull base and invade the maxillary walls and antrum. Among the benign tumor, the common are inverted papilloma, fibrous dysplasia and juvenile nasopharyngeal angiofibroma. This highly vascular tumor typically originates at the superior margins of the sphenopalatine foramen and occurs predominantly in adolescent males. The chief presenting symptoms of patients with maxillary tumors are prolonged nasal obstruction and recurrent epistaxis. As the tumor grows beyond the maxillary sinus, it may extend into the ethmoid and sphenoid sinuses, the nasopharynx and laterally into the infratemporal fossa. The orbit may be invaded from either direct extension through the lamina papyracea or superior wall of the maxillary sinus, or via the inferior or superior orbital fissures. Superiorly, the tumor may extend into the sphenoid and ethmoid sinuses eroding into the sellae, planum sphenoidale and anterior skull base.

Complete surgical resection has been the preferred treatment for paranasal tumors. With the increasing development of endoscopic modalities in surgical oncology, advanced ablative procedures are being performed endoscopically mainly for management of benign tumors or early stage malignant neoplasms. Future clinical studies are required to evaluate the role of endoscopic surgery for management of early stage malignant tumors arising in the paranasal sinuses. Nevertheless, open partial maxillectomy remains the working horse for most malignant and recurrent benign neoplasms.

In this chapter, the authors will describe the surgical technique of suprastructure maxillectomy. This group of surgeries include medial maxillectomy and partial maxillectomies, not including the hard palate. The classifications of the various maxillectomies described in the literature are shown in Table 1. Since the development of endonasal surgery, medial maxillectomy is rarely performed using an open approach.

PREOPERATIVE EVALUATION AND ANESTHESIA

All patients scheduled for operation are evaluated preoperatively by a head and neck surgeon and an anesthesiologist. If a free flap is planned, preoperative physical examination by a plastic surgeon is essential. Radiological evaluation of the patient includes axial and coronal computed tomography (CT) and magnetic resonance imaging (MRI) of the head and neck (Figs 1A and B). A three-dimensional CT may be used, in selected cases, for planning of the reconstruction procedure. Broad-spectrum antibiotics are instituted perioperatively. This usually includes a second-generation cephalosporin and metronidazole. All the patients are operated in the supine position.

Table 1: The various classifications used to describe the type of maxillectomy

Classification	Resection
Partial suprastructure maxillectomy	1–5 walls sparing the palate
Partial infrastructure maxillectomy	1–5 walls including the palate
Total maxillectomy	All six walls of the maxilla
Extended maxillectomy	All six walls of the maxilla and extra maxillary structure (ethmoid frontal and sphenoid sinuses, orbit, skull base, skin, pterygoid muscles, PPF, ITF)
Medial maxillectomy	Medial maxillary wall
Limited maxillectomy	One wall of the maxilla
Subtotal maxillectomy	2–5 walls of the maxilla
Cordiro classification Type I	One or two maxillary walls not including the palate
Cordiro classification Type II	Palate, upper alveolus, anterior and posterior walls
Cordiro classification Type III	All six walls of the maxilla including the floor of the orbit or exenteration
Cordiro classification Type IV	Orbital exenteration and resection of five maxillary walls sparing the palate

PPF: Pterygopalatine fossa; ITF: Infratemporal fossa

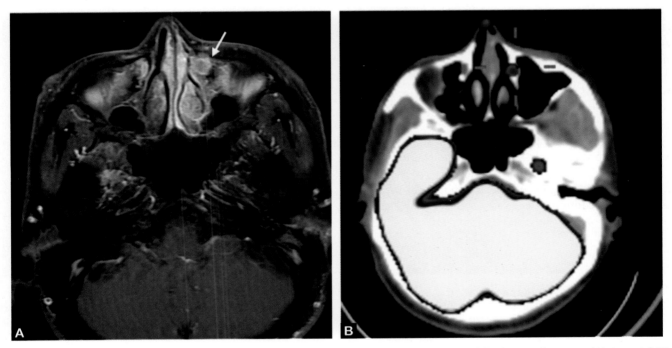

Figs 1A and B: Preoperative imaging of a patient with poorly differentiated carcinoma of the lacrimal system. (A) An axial T1 MRI with gadolinium (left) and; (B) PET-CT image (right) are shown. The white arrow indicates the location of the tumor

SURGICAL TECHNIQUE

The lateral rhinotomy approach is used for most suprastructure maxillectomies in order to gain access to the tumor and its borders. This includes tumors originating in the nasal cavity, ethmoid sinuses, sphenoid sinus and maxillary sinus without palatal invasion. Similarly, benign tumors with anterior maxillary wall involvement may also approach with the same incision.

Skin Incision and Development of Flaps

A temporary tarsorrhaphy is performed before surgery to protect the cornea. The lateral rhinotomy incision extends along the lateral border of the nose, approximately half a cm from dorsum of the nose (Fig. 2). It starts cephalad, medial to the medial canthus and extends down through the skin crest bordering the nasal ala. It is continued toward the filtrum (Fig. 3). After marking, the skin is injected with lidocaine (0.06%) and epinephrine (1:1,000,000) for hemostasis and hydrodissection purposes. Following the incision with a number 15 blade, the dissection continues with electrocautery up to the level of the nasal bone and medial buttress of the maxilla. Skin flaps are elevated medially and

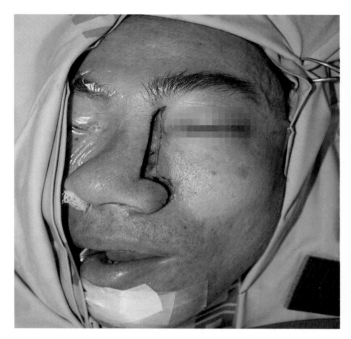

Fig. 3: Skin incision. The patient has a poorly differentiated carcinoma of the lacrimal bone

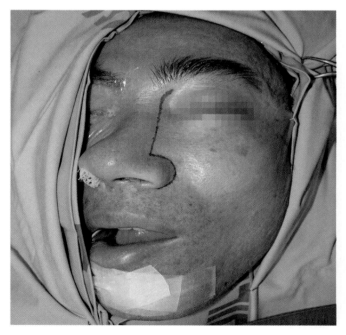

Fig. 2: The lateral rhinotomy incision. The incision extends along the lateral border of the nose, approximately half a centimeter from dorsum of the nose. It starts cephalad, medial to the medial canthus and extends down through the skin crest bordering the nasal ala

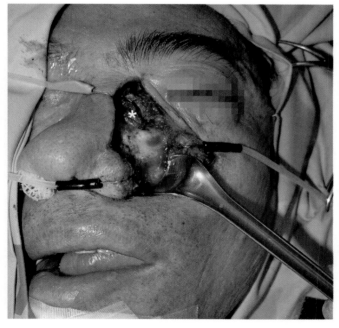

Fig. 4: Development of the subperiosteal flaps. Skin flaps are elevated medially and laterally to the level of the periosteum with the aid of a Freer elevator and electrocautery. Care is taken not to injure the infraorbital nerve at the anterior maxillary wall approximately 1 cm below the infraorbital rim. The flap is elevated superficial to the area of the tumor (*)

laterally to the level of the periosteum with the aid of a freer elevator and electrocautery (Fig. 4). Care is taken not to injure the infraorbital nerve, which will be piercing the anterior maxillary wall approximately 1 cm below the infraorbital rim. The flaps can be developed to the level of the maxillary tuberosity (laterally), the upper gingival (inferiorly), the frontal sinus and infraorbital rim (superiorly) and to the pyriform aperture and nasal septum (medially). The flaps are held with a 2-0 skin stitches and fish hooks.

Osteotomies and Medial Maxillectomy

At this stage, the anterior maxillary wall is widely exposed and the infraorbital nerve is identified and preserved. The bone is inspected carefully in order to identify its integrity and the areas of tumor infiltration. Attention is now turned to perform the maxillectomy. If not invaded by tumor, the anterior maxillary wall is fractured with a fine osteotome to pave the way for the osteotomies. The opening in the bone is widened with a Kerrison Rongeur and the cavity of the maxillary antrum is inspected (Fig. 5). At this stage, a thin suction may be used to evacuate secretions that often encompass parts of the antrum. The osteotomies along the anterior and medial walls of the maxilla are now performed with a motorized reciprocating saw. The lines of the osteotomies are inferior border of the fossa canina, above the dental roots; superiorly, the orbit; laterally, the malar

eminence and; medially the nasal cavity (Fig. 6). In children, the inferior line is higher than usual, since the second line of teeth does not erupt yet. The medial and part of the anterior wall of the maxilla is now retracted anteriorly with a Babcock's grasper and the tumor is freed from its attachments with a Mayo scissors and Freer elevator. If necessary, the rest of the tissue is extirpated with a Kerrison Rongeur. Hemostasis is performed with warm saline. The cavity is inspected and hemostasis is completed with bipolar electrocautery (Fig. 7). In most cases, branches of the sphenopalatine artery can be identified at the posterior wall of the maxilla, lateral and superior to the choana. These are clamped with medium size clip to prevent further bleeding.

Subtotal Suprastructure Maxillectomy

If resection of the lateral and superior walls of the maxilla is indicated, the infraorbital nerve is likely to be involved by the tumor and therefore, it is sound to extirpate along with the specimen. In rare cases, the nerve can be rerouted from its foramen and repositioned laterally and superiorly along with the upper cheek flap. However, this only account for benign tumors without perineural invasion. In all other cases, the nerve is sectioned allowing further development of the flaps superiorly and laterally. The flaps are now developed superiorly toward the orbit and laterally exposing the malar eminence and lateral buttress of the maxilla as in Figures 8A and B.

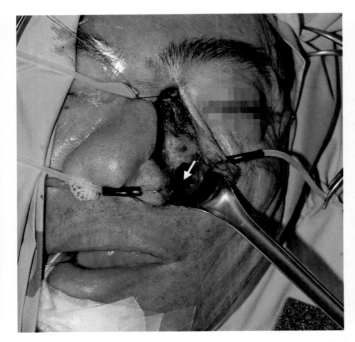

Fig. 5: Opening of the anterior maxillary wall. If not invaded by tumor, the anterior maxillary wall is fractured with a fine osteotome to pave the way for the osteotomies. The opening in the bone (arrow) is widening with a Kerrison Rongeur and the cavity of the maxillary antrum is inspected

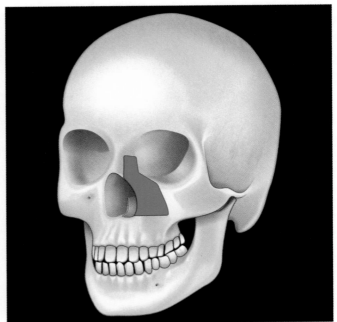

Fig. 6: Osteotomies in medial maxillectomy. The lines of the osteotomies are inferior border of the fossa canina above the dental roots; superiorly, the infraorbital rim; laterally, an oblique line medial to the infraorbital nerve and; medially, the nasal cavity

If resection of the roof and lateral wall of the maxilla are indicated, care is taken to preserve the infraorbital rim and malar eminence if possible. Preservation of these two structures allows maintenance of the contour of the orbit and cheek bone for better cosmesis. Furthermore, resection of the infraorbital rim will imminently lead to enophthalmos and diplopia. Therefore, reconstruction of these bony structures is indicated if violated.

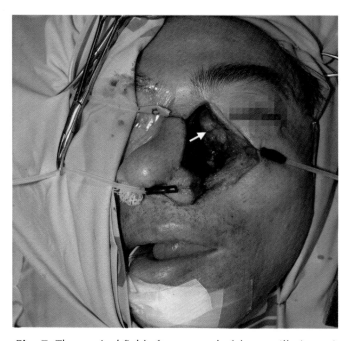

Fig. 7: The surgical field after removal of the maxilla (arrow)

Before continuing with the osteotomy, the inferior and medial walls of the orbit are entered from above the infraorbital rim and along the lamina papyracea. This is performed with a fine, angled freer elevator, superficial to the periorbit. The eye is retracted superiorly and laterally with a flat malleable retractor and the medial canthal ligament is transected. The anterior ethmoidal artery is clipped and the dissection continues posteriorly and laterally exposing the whole portion of the lamina papyracea. With the retractor protecting the orbital content, the lateral, inferior and superior osteotomies are performed with a reciprocating saw as indicated by the location of the tumor. The osteotomies are completed with a medium size osteotome. The specimen is now retracted inferiorly and anteriorly and separated from its surrounding tissue with Mayo scissors and freer elevator.

Care is now taken to resect the lamina papyracea, which forms the superior wall of the maxilla. If the tumor involves the whole portion of the superior maxillary wall, the infraorbital rim and lamina papyracea are included in the superior osteotomy and a suprastructure maxillectomy is achieved in an en bloc fashion as in Figure 9.

The wound is rinsed with warm saline and the internal maxillary artery is identified and clipped at the posterior maxillary wall. Hemostasis in the pterygopalatine fossa (PPF) area is achieved with a bipolar electrocautery and strips of surgicel®.

Reconstruction

Following suprastructure maxillectomy, one reconstruction is needed only after resection of the infraorbital rim. This will require rigid reconstruction, which can be achieved

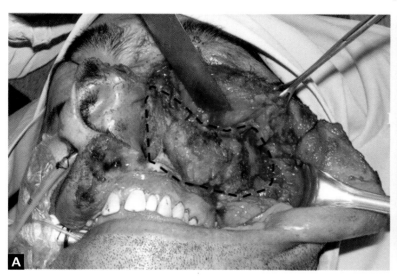

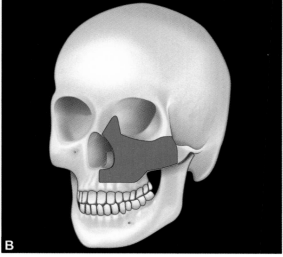

Figs 8A and B: Elevation of the skin flaps after the infraorbital nerve was resected. The flaps are developed superiorly toward the orbit and laterally exposing the malar eminence and lateral buttress of the maxilla. With the retractor protecting the orbital content, the lateral, inferior and superior osteotomies are performed with a reciprocating saw as indicated by the location of the tumor (dashed line)

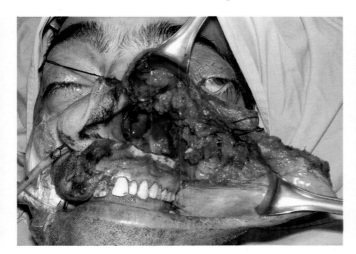

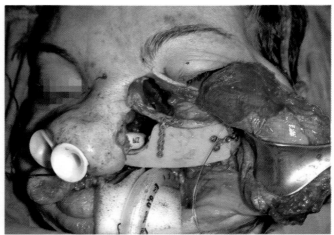

Fig. 9: Partial suprastructure maxillectomy with resection of the infraorbital rim and malar eminence. If the tumor involves the whole portion of the superior maxillary wall, the infraorbital rim and lamina papyracea are included in the superior osteotomy and a suprastructure maxillectomy is achieved in an en bloc fashion

Fig. 10: Reconstruction of the floor of the orbit. The infraorbital rim can be reconstructed with bone graft if postoperative radiotherapy is not indicated

by a malleable titanium mesh or split calvarial bone graft (Fig. 10). Alternative solutions are prefabricated titanium mesh or artificial bone substitutes (medpore®, porex®). Reconstruction of the lamina papyracea is usually not directed.

POSTOPERATIVE TREATMENT

Vaseline gauze is applied to the cavity for hemostasis and the wound is closed in layers with number 4-0 vicryl sutures and number 5-0 nylon stitches. After closing, the wound is covered with a thin film of antibiotic ointment.

After surgery, the patient is extubated and transferred to the floor. The wound is kept clean by rinsing it with saline three times a day during the first 7 days after the operation and covered with antibiotic ointment, after each cleansing. Broad-spectrum antibiotics are continued until the packing is removed. For pain control, the patients are treated with nonsteroidal anti-inflammatory drugs (diclofenac 75 mg intramuscularly or orally, or rofecoxib 50 mg) once daily and with tramadol 50–100 mg if the patient asks for them or if the nurses felt it to be necessary. Daily nasal irrigation with saline is indicated every 2–3 hours during the first year after the operation. Similarly, nasal suctioning should be performed in these patients for 12 months after the surgery or after the adjuvant radiotherapy.

HIGHLIGHTS

I. **Indications**
   - Malignant tumors invading the maxilla without palatal invasion
   - Benign and malignant tumors not suitable for endoscopic resection.

II. **Contraindications**
   - Palatal invasion
   - Involvement of extramaxillary compartment.

III. **Special Preoperative Considerations**
   - Proper preoperative imaging
   - Endoscopic evaluation
   - Ophthalmologic evaluation if orbital invasion is suspected.

IV. **Special Intraoperative Considerations**
   - Proper placement of the lateral rhinotomy skin incision
   - Preserve the infraorbital nerve if possible
   - Preserve the infraorbital rim and malar eminence
   - Clip the internal maxillary artery
   - Protect the eye before resection of the lamina papyracea
   - Appropriate reconstruction of the orbital floor, if indicated.

V. **Special Postoperative Considerations**
   - Antibiotic coverage until the packing is removed
   - Frequent cleansing and suction of nasal secretion are required during the first year after surgery.

VI. Complications
- Wound infection
- Paresthesias of V2
- Bleeding
- Enophthalmos
- Cerebrospinal fluid leak
- Epiphora due to lacrimal duct stenosis
- Diplopia and telecanthus
- Optic nerve injury and blindness.

ADDITIONAL READING

1. Cordeiro PG, Santamaria E. A classification system and algorithm for reconstruction of maxillectomy and midfacial defects. Plast Reconstr Surg. 2000;105(7):2331-46.
2. Fliss DM, Abergel A, Cavel O, et al. Combined subcranial approaches for excision of complex anterior skull base tumors. Arch Otolaryngol Head Neck Surg. 2007;133(9): 888-96.
3. Gil Z, Fliss DM. Contemporary management of head and neck cancers. Isr Med Assoc J. 2009;11(5):296-300.
4. Katz TS, Mendenhall WM, Morris CG, et al. Malignant tumors of the nasal cavity and paranasal sinuses. Head Neck. 2002;24(9):821-9.
5. Kenady DE. Cancer of the paranasal sinuses. Surg Clin North Am. 1986;66(1):119-31.
6. Lavertu P, Roberts JK, Kraus DH, et al. Squamous cell carcinoma of the paranasal sinuses: the Cleveland Clinic experience 1977-1986. Laryngoscope 1989;99:1130-6.
7. Lee CH, Hur DG, Roh HJ, et al. Survival rates of sinonasal squamous cell carcinoma with the new AJCC staging system. Arch Otolaryngol Head Neck Surg. 2007;133(2):131-4.
8. Myers LL, Nussenbaum B, Bradford CR, et al. Paranasal sinus malignancies: an 18-year single institution experience. Laryngoscope. 2002;112(11):1964-9.
9. Sessions RB, Humphreys DH. Technical modifications of the medial maxillectomy. Arch Otolaryngol. 1983;109(9):575-7.
10. Spiro RH, Strong EW, Shah JP. Maxillectomy and its classification. Head Neck. 1997;19(4):309-14.

Part B: Partial Infrastructure Maxillectomy

INTRODUCTION

Infrastructure maxillectomy may include one to five walls of the maxillary bone, but will always include resection of the hard palate. Neoplasms that necessitate infrastructure maxillectomy may be primary tumor of the palate or secondary tumors infiltrating the palate from the paranasal sinuses, buccal mucosa or skin. Being part of the oral cavity, the most common malignancy originating in this area is squamous cell carcinoma. About 5% of the oral cavity carcinomas are primary cancers of the hard palate. Other common malignant neoplasms are of minor salivary origin. These include mucoepidermoid carcinoma, adenoid cystic carcinoma and polymorphous low-grade adenocarcinoma. Melanomas and osteosarcoma or soft tissue sarcomas may rarely involve the palate. Among the benign tumors of this area are pleomorphic adenoma, fibrous dysplasia and ameloblastoma, the most common. Tumors and cysts of dental origin originating in the upper alveolus may also necessitate infrastructure maxillectomy. Secondary tumors of hard palate are mainly squamous cell carcinoma of the paranasal sinuses or skin, minor salivary gland tumors and sarcomas.

The chief presenting symptoms of patients with tumors of the upper alveolus and hard palate are: growing lesion, loose dentition, ill-fitting dentures, palatal and facial numbness, facial swelling and evidence of nasal fistula. Pain is an ominous sign of malignancy, whereas prolonged nasal obstruction and recurrent epistaxis suggest involvement of the nasal cavity and paranasal sinuses. As the tumor grows beyond the hard palate, it may extend superiorly into the paranasal sinuses, posteriorly to oropharynx and laterally to the buccal mucosa and lip.

Complete surgical resection remains the main treatment for malignant tumors of the hard palate and upper alveolus, since they are relatively resistant to radiotherapy and chemotherapy. Exceptions are soft tissue sarcomas in children and adolescence, and lymphomas. As in other cancers of the head and neck, the goals of surgery are not only extirpation of the tumor with free margins, but also adequate reconstruction of the defect to allow good functional and esthetic outcome and better quality of life. Therefore, the reconstruction part of surgery is as important as the resection and should be planned and prepared several days before surgery, as indicated in the last part of this chapter.

In this chapter, the authors will describe the surgical technique of partial infrastructure maxillectomy and its means of reconstruction. This group of surgeries include, partial maxillectomy and subtotal maxillectomy including the superior alveolar ridge with or without the hard palate. The classification of the partial infrastructure maxillectomies are given in Table 2.

Table 2: Infrastructure partial maxillectomies and their classifications*

Main classification (secondary classification)	Resection
Limited maxillectomy (partial maxillectomy)	Hard palate or lateral alveolar ridge, premaxilla
Inferior maxillectomy	Alveolar ridge and hard palate, limited to the floor of the maxilla
Subtotal maxillectomy	Two to five walls of the maxilla, including the floor of the maxilla
Cordiro classification Type I	One or two maxillary walls not including the palate
Cordiro classification Type II	Palate, upper alveolus, anterior and posterior walls

* If bilateral maxillectomy is performed the word "bilateral" is used first, followed by specific description of the procedure on each side

PREOPERATIVE AND PROSTHESIS EVALUATION

Patients scheduled for operation are evaluated preoperatively by a head and neck surgeon and an anesthesiologist. All patients should also undergo clinical examination by an oral and maxillofacial surgeon, and dental prosthesis evaluation. If a free flap is planned, preoperative physical examination by a plastic surgeon is essential. Radiological evaluation of the patients includes axial and coronal CT for demonstration of the bony structures and MRI of the head and neck for soft tissue evaluation. A three-dimensional CT may be used is selected cases for planning of the reconstruction procedure. Laboratory work-up includes complete blood count, coagulation tests and a type and screen.

Dental prosthesis should be prepared ahead of time, as early as possible, during the preoperative work-up. This time is needed for the patient and prosthodontist to discuss the functional and esthetic outcomes of the procedure and to design a temporary obturator that is to be used during surgery and in the immediate postoperative period. This prosthesis allows the holding of packing after the operation for hemostasis and early oral intake.

Since the operation is considered clean-contaminated surgery, broad-spectrum antibiotics are instituted perioperatively. This usually includes a second-generation cephalosporin and metronidazole. All the patients are operated in the supine position. Nasal intubation in the contralateral nostril is usually performed for partial maxillectomies involving the palate and alveolar ridge. If subtotal maxillectomy is indicated, oral endotracheal intubation may be used, with the tube reflected to the contralateral side. Tracheostomy is rarely indicated in these cases.

SURGICAL TECHNIQUE

Surgical Anatomy

The following section is designed to briefly highlight the surgical anatomy of the hard palate and upper alveolar ridge. The maxillary sinuses and nasal cavity are separated from the oral cavity by the floor of the maxillary sinuses, the upper alveolar ridge and the hard palate (Fig. 11). The hard palate is composed of a single anterior primary palate and two pairs of secondary palates posterolaterally. The posterior aspect of the hard palate is formed by the pyramidal process of the palatine bone (posterior nasal spine and maxillary tuberosity). The alveolar ridge is composed of the lateral alveolar ridge on each side and the premaxilla in the middle (between the incisor teeth). The hard palate and alveolar ridge are lined by a stratified squamous epithelium containing hundreds of minor salivary glands. The hard palate has three major foramina transmitting arteries and nerves; a single anterior midline incisive foramen and the two posterolateral greater palatine foramina. The incisive foramen transmits the nasopalatine artery and nerve, and the greater palatine

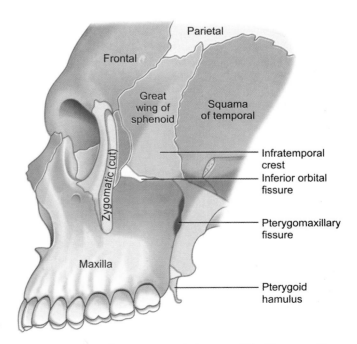

Fig. 11: Surgical anatomy of the maxilla. The maxillary sinuses and nasal cavity are separated from the oral cavity by the floor of the maxillary sinuses, the upper alveolar ridge and the hard palate

foramen conveys the greater and lesser palatine artery and nerve on each side. The blood supply to the hard palate and alveolar ridge is provided by a pair of greater palatine arteries, the nasopalatine artery and branches of the facial artery on each side.

Limited Maxillectomy

Limited maxillectomy also known as partial lateral maxillectomy is performed through the mouth avoiding the need of facial incisions. The approach is used for resection of benign or malignant tumors involving the upper alveolar ridge or hard palate. This is indicated mainly for resection of small tumors originating in the mucosa, teeth or gingival. In case of benign tumors, several millimeters are sufficient to reassure complete tumor resection, whereas in malignant tumors, margins of at least 2 cm are required to prevent close margins (< 0.5 cm at the closed dimension in the final pathological specimen). Positive or close margins are not only poor prognostic factor, but also will always require the implementation of adjuvant radiation therapy.

The procedure starts by marking of the margins of the resection. The lips and buccal mucosa are held with two Richardson retractors. Next, the gingivobuccal sulcus and hard palate are injected with lidocaine (0.06%) and epinephrine (1:1,000,000) for hemostasis purpose. The tumor is shown in Figure 12. A gingivolabial and hard palate incisions are made with monopolar electrocautery to prevent bleeding. As the incision reaches the bony wall of the maxilla, flaps are elevated medially and laterally in the level of the periosteum with the aid of a freer dissector (Fig. 13). In order to preserve the teeth abutting the margins of the specimen, the authors recommend extraction of one tooth

on each side of the specimen. This will allow the surgeon to perform the osteotomy safely and easily in the middle of the tooth socket preserving the contralateral tooth and its root. The osteotomy is performed with an electrical reciprocating sagittal saw, starting from the side of the previously extracted tooth laterally. It continues superiorly along the lateral alveolar ridge and above the roots of the teeth and then down toward the extracted tooth medially. The dissection continues along the medial border of the alveolar ridge and hard palate. Care is taken not to injure the infraorbital nerve, which will be piercing the anterior maxillary wall approximately 1 cm below the infraorbital rim. In some cases, it may be easier to first fracture the anterior wall of the maxillary sinus below the infraorbital nerve with a small osteotome and to introduce the saw through this opening.

The final part of the resection is separation of the specimen posteriorly along the pterygoid plates. This osteotomy is performed last to reduce blood loss, since control of bleeding from the pterygopalatine fossa and internal maxillary artery can be only performed after the specimen is removed. A long retractor is placed laterally in alveolar ridge and a large curved osteotome is placed behind the last molar aiming superomedial to the palate (Fig. 14). The osteotomy starts in a superior direction and as the pterygoids are fractured it continues in a lateral to medial direction above the alveolar ridge. At this stage, the surgeon should expect a brisk bleeding and two suctions should be used to keep the surgical bed bloodless during the last stage

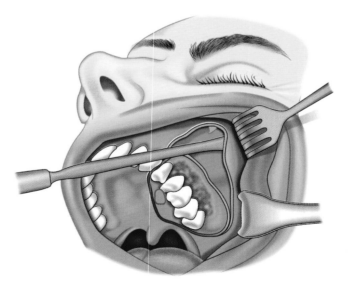

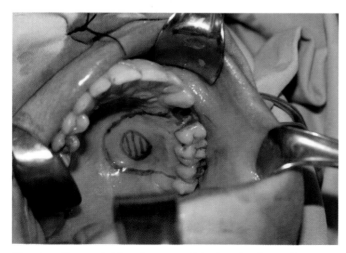

Fig. 12: Pleomorphic adenoma of the hard palate. The tumor and resection margins are shown. In order to preserve the teeth abutting the margins of the specimen, the authors recommend extraction of one tooth on each side of the specimen

Fig. 13: Making of the mucosal incisions along. A gingivolabial and hard palate incisions are made with monopolar electrocautery to prevent bleeding. As the incision reaches the bony wall of the maxilla, small flaps are elevated medially and laterally to the level of the periosteum with the aid of a freer dissector

of the operation. Once the specimen is freed, a curve Mayo scissors and straight osteotome are used to separate the specimen from the sinonasal mucosa, the remnants of the pterygoid muscles and the lateral and posterior walls of the maxillary sinus. After the specimen is removed, hemostasis is performed with the 4 × 4 gauze soaked with 50% hydrogen peroxide diluted with saline. The internal maxillary artery and its branches are clipped and hemostasis is finalized

with a bipolar electrocautery. Bleeding form the area of the pterygopalatine fossa is best controlled with one or two strips of surgicel® or avitene®. The maxillary cavity and specimen are inspected to evaluate proper margins. Frozen section analysis may be used to confirm complete resection during the operation. Figure 15 shows the surgical field after resection. The authors do not recommend the use of split thickness skin graft or artificial grafts to align the maxillary sinus, since it is quickly epithelized several weeks after surgery. The surgical specimen is shown in Figure 16.

The cavity is packed with Xeroform gauze and a dental obturator is used to hold the gauze in place as in Figure 17.

Subtotal Maxillectomy

This procedure is directed for treatment of large tumors, which originate in the upper alveolar ridge and extend to the nasal cavity and maxillary antrum as well as for cancers of the paranasal sinuses, which infiltrate the hard palate. The procedure starts with delineation of the superior border of the resection.

The surgery is performed via a transfacial approach and a Weber-Ferguson incision. This incision allows exposure of the superior and inferior aspects of the maxilla and its complete en bloc resection. The facial incision extends along the lateral border of the nose, approximately half a cm from dorsum of the nose. It starts cephalad, medial to the medial canthus and extends down through the skin crest bordering the nasal ala. It is continued toward the filtrum and extended down to the lip in the midline (Figs 18A and B). Inferiorly, the incision continues along the gingivobuccal sulcus extending laterally up to the retromolar area.

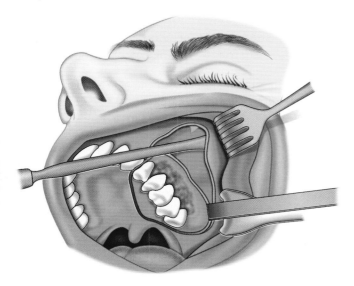

Fig. 14: The posterior osteotomy. The final part of the resection is separation of the specimen posteriorly along the pterygoid plates. A large curved osteotome is placed behind the last molar aiming superomedial to the palate

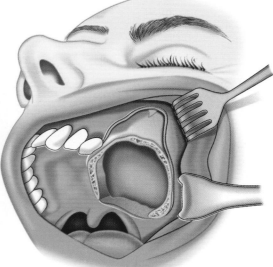

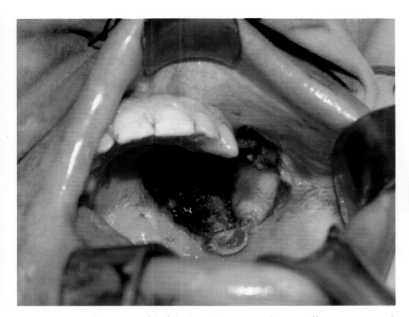

Fig. 15: The surgical field after resection. The maxillary cavity and specimen are inspected to evaluate proper margins

After marking, the skin and gingivobuccal sulcus are injected with lidocaine (0.06%) and epinephrine (1:1,000,000) for hemostasis and hydrodissection purposes. Following the incision with a number 15 blade, the dissection continues with electrocautery. Skin flaps are elevated medially and laterally to the level of the periosteum as described above.

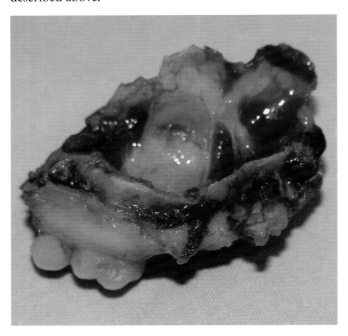

Fig. 16: The surgical specimen

A unilateral gingivolabial incision is now made, extending up to the lateral buttress of the maxillary. The soft tissue of the cheek is raised from the anterior surface of the maxilla, transecting the infraorbital nerves and vessels if the superior and lateral walls of the maxilla are needed to be approached. An upper cheek flap is developed laterally and superiorly up to the level of the inferior orbital rim and the maxillary tuberosity.

At this stage, the anterior maxillary wall is widely exposed and the infraorbital nerve is identified and preserved if possible. The bone is inspected carefully in order to identify its integrity and the areas of tumor infiltration. Attention is now turned to perform the upper osteotomies. If not invaded by tumor, the anterior maxillary wall is fractured with a fine osteotome to pave the way for the performance of the osteotomies. The opening in the bone is widened with a Kerrison Rongeur and the cavity of the maxillary antrum is inspected. At this stage, a thin suction may be used to evacuate secretions that often encompass parts of the antrum. The osteotomies along the anterior and medial walls of the maxilla are now performed with a motorized sagittal reciprocating saw. The lines of the osteotomies are superior to the infraorbital rib and lateral to the zygomatic process of the maxilla. The medial border of the osteotomy is the nasal septum. If indicated, the infraorbital rim and nasal septum can be included in the specimen.

Attention is now turned to the inferior maxillectomy. A gingivolabial and hard palate incisions are made with monopolar electrocautery. As the incision reaches the bony

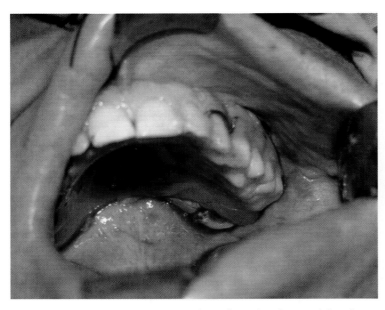

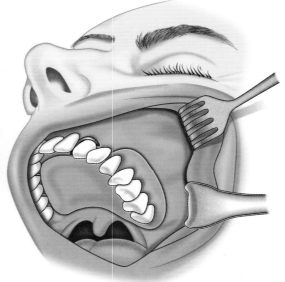

Fig. 17: The palate after fitting of the obturator. The cavity is packed with Xeroform gauze and a dental obturator is used to hold the gauze in place

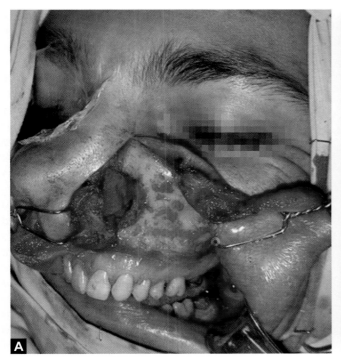

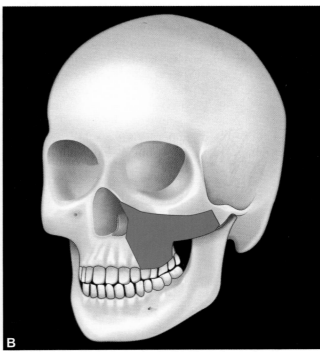

Figs 18A and B: Inferior partial maxillectomy. The surgery involves lateral rhinotomy incision

wall of the maxilla, small flaps are elevated to the level of the periosteum with the aid of a freer dissector. Teeth extractions of one tooth on each side of the specimen are performed if needed, to allow the surgeon to direct the osteotomies into the tooth socket preserving the abutting tooth. The osteotomies are performed laterally and medially down toward the extracted teeth. The osteotomy continues along the medial border of the alveolar ridge and hard palate. The soft palate is dissected from the hard palate with an electrocautery, completing the posterior border of the dissection.

The final part of the resection is separation of the specimen posteriorly along the pterygoid plates. A long retractor is placed laterally in alveolar ridge and a large curved osteotome is placed behind the last molar aiming superomedial to the palate (Fig. 19). This maneuver is aimed to fracture the medial and lateral pterygoid plates separating the specimen from its attachments to the medial and lateral pterygoid muscles. The osteotomy starts in a superior direction and as the pterygoids are fractured, it continues in a lateral to medial direction above the alveolar ridge. Suctions are used to keep the surgical bed bloodless during the last stage of the operation. Once the specimen is freed, a curve Mayo scissors and straight osteotome are used to separate the specimen from the sinonasal mucosa, the remnants of the pterygoid muscles and the lateral and posterior walls of the maxillary sinus. After the specimen is removed,

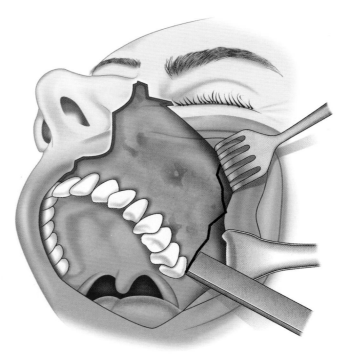

Fig. 19: Separation of the specimen posteriorly along the pterygoid plates. A long retractor is placed lateral alveolar ridge and a large curved osteotome is placed behind the last molar aiming superomedial to the palate

hemostasis is performed with the 4 × 4 gauze soaked with 50% hydrogen peroxide diluted with saline. The internal maxillary artery and its branches are clipped and hemostasis is finalized with a bipolar electrocautery. Bleeding form the area of the pterygopalatine fossa is best controlled with one or two strips of surgicel® or avitene®. The maxillary cavity and specimen are inspected to evaluate proper margins. The wound is rinsed with warm saline and the internal maxillary artery is identified and clipped at the posterior maxillary wall. Figure 20 shows the surgical field after resection. If the resection of the premaxilla is indicated, degloving of the soft tissue of the lower face is performed exposing of the pyriform aperture and the anterior maxillary walls bilaterally. It is then possible to extend the maxillectomy to the lower nasal cavity and laterally.

The cavity is packed with Xeroform gauze and a dental obturator is used to hold the gauze in place (Fig. 20).

A bilateral maxillectomy can be performed in a similar way. In this case, the medial osteotomy is extended to the contralateral side to include the premaxilla.

Reconstruction

Following tumor extirpation, maxillary defects require reconstruction in order to provide a barrier between the nasal cavity and maxillary sinuses, and the oral cavity. Reconstructive failure carries potential, functional and esthetic problems that may hamper oral intake and speech.

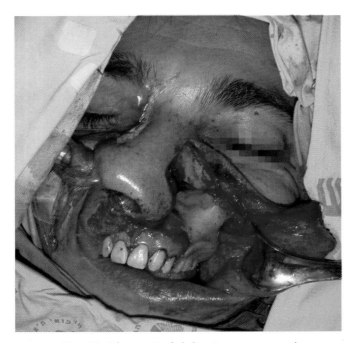

Fig. 20: The surgical defect is reconstructed with an obturatormy

The reconstruction technique is designed according to the location and size of the defect, based on radiological and intraoperative calculations. Temporary obturator is prefabricated before the operation and molded during the procedure after the specimen has been removed. This can be achieved by a prosthodontist with a thermoplastic or self-solidified material, which allow full stenting of the maxillary defect. The obturator is fixed to the remaining teeth by wires that were implanted in the obturator. The temporary prosthesis is replaced by a permanent obturator two weeks after surgery. In many cases, a permanent prosthesis is finally costumed several months after surgery and radiation therapy have completed. The reader is referred to Chapter 7 for further reading regarding dental rehabilitation after ablative surgeries.

Rarely, free flap reconstruction is indicated after subtotal infrastructure maxillectomy. The cases that do require tissue transfer are bilateral maxillectomies and large resections of the premaxilla, including the septum and nasal bones. In these cases, reconstruction is achieved with composite bone flaps including fibula or iliac crest osteofasciomusculocutaneous free flaps and microvascular anastomosis. This type of reconstruction is beyond the scope of this chapter.

POSTOPERATIVE TREATMENT

The incision is closed with inverted absorbable sutures and nylon stitches. After closing, the wound is covered with a thin film of antibiotic ointment. No dressing is used to cover the wound in order to permit easy access to the area of incision for examination and treatment. The wound is kept clean by rinsing it with saline three times a day during the first week after the operation and covered with antibiotic ointment after each cleansing. Broad-spectrum antibiotics are continued until the packing is removed. The nasal packing is removed 5–7 days following the operation. Daily washing of the cavity is recommended after the packing is removed.

Pain Control

Maxillectomies are associated with a considerable level of pain during the early postoperative period. While many analgesic regimens are available [e.g. *pro re nata* (PRN), scheduled dosing, intravenous patient-controlled analgesia], it was shown that a PRN protocol is not adequate for the management of pain following surgery. Intravenous patient-controlled analgesia (PCA) with morphine (1 mg bolus) should be administered, with a 10-minute lockout interval and no basal infusion during the first three postoperative days. This is followed by selective nonsteroidal anti-inflammatory drug [(NSAID) (diclofenac 75 mg intramuscularly or orally, or rofecoxib 50 mg)]. Second-line treatment consists of intramuscular meperidine 1 mg/kg (50–100 mg) repeated every 3–4 hours if required, but not exceeding a maximum of 150 mg as a single dose, or morphine via slow intravenous injection (4–10 mg, titrated according to effect). Tramadol is used as PRN treatment during this period and a single starting dose of 50 mg (20 drops) is prescribed (40 drops, 100 mg/ml). If the desired analgesic effect is not achieved within 30–60 minutes, an additional 20 drops are administered. The total daily dose should not exceed 400 mg of tramadol (equivalent to 160 drops or 4.0 ml). A downward adjustment of the dose and/or prolongation of the interval between doses are carried out for the elderly.

HIGHLIGHTS

I. Indications
- Small tumors involving the lateral alveolar ridge
- Large tumors of the upper alveolar ridge and hard palate
- Tumors involving the hard palate, nasal cavity and maxillary sinuses.

II. Contraindications
- Metastatic disease
- Involvement of extramaxillary compartment (combined approach)
- Carotid involvement
- Intracranial involvement.

III. Special Preoperative Considerations
- Proper preoperative imaging
- Tissue diagnosis
- Endoscopic evaluation
- Evaluation by maxillofacial surgeon and prosthodontist
- Construction of a temporary prosthesis.

IV. Special Intraoperative Considerations
- Proper placement of the lateral skin incision
- Tooth extraction to allow preservation of the remaining tooth
- Preserve the infraorbital rim and malar eminence if possible
- Clip the internal maxillary artery
- Perform the posterior osteotomy (pterygoid plates) last.

V. Special Postoperative Considerations
- Antibiotic coverage until the packing is removed
- Pain management
- Frequent cleansing and suction of nasal secretion are required during the first year after surgery.

VI. Complications
- Paresthesias of V2
- Bleeding
- Enophthalmos
- Epiphora due to lacrimal duct stenosis
- Diplopia and telecanthus
- Optic nerve injury and blindness.

ADDITIONAL READING

11. Cordeiro PG, Santamaria E. A classification system and algorithm for reconstruction of maxillectomy and midfacial defects. Plast Reconstr Surg. 2000;105(7):2331-46.
12. Fliss DM, Abergel A, Cavel O, et al. Combined subcranial approaches for excision of complex anterior skull base tumors. Arch Otolaryngol Head Neck Surg. 2007;133(9): 888-96.
13. Gil Z, Fliss DM. Contemporary management of head and neck cancers. Isr Med Assoc J. 2009;11(5):296-300.
14. Katz TS, Mendenhall WM, Morris CG, et al. Malignant tumors of the nasal cavity and paranasal sinuses. Head Neck. 2002;24(9):821-9.
15. Kenady DE. Cancer of the paranasal sinuses. Surg Clin North Am. 1986;66(1):119-31.
16. Lavertu P, Roberts JK, Kraus DH, et al. Squamous cell carcinoma of the paranasal sinuses: the Cleveland Clinic experience 1977-1986. Laryngoscope 1989;99:1130-6.
17. Lee CH, Hur DG, Roh HJ, et al. Survival rates of sinonasal squamous cell carcinoma with the new AJCC staging system. Arch Otolaryngol Head Neck Surg. 2007;133(2):131-4.
18. Myers LL, Nussenbaum B, Bradford CR, et al. Paranasal sinus malignancies: an 18-year single institution experience. Laryngoscope. 2002;112(11):1964-9.
19. Spiro RH, Strong EW, Shah JP. Maxillectomy and its classification. Head Neck. 1997;19(4):309-14.
20. Truitt TO, Gleich LL, Huntress GP, et al. Surgical management of hard palate malignancies. Otolaryngol Head Neck Surg. 1999;121(5):548-52.

Chapter **30**

Total Maxillectomy

Ziv Gil, Dan M Fliss

INTRODUCTION

Tumors originating in the maxillary sinus are relatively rare. The clinical symptoms in patients with maxillary cancer are frequently nonspecific and include pain, malaise and weight loss. Other symptoms may be directly associated with the location of the primary tumor. Lesions originating in the palate or septum may cause irritation and be visible to the patients. On the other hand, patients with sinonasal tumors suffer from nasal secretions, recurrent epistaxis or nasal obstruction. Whereas most oral cavity tumors are likely to be discovered by the patient or by the dentist upon routine examination, sinonasal tumors are inaccessible to self examination and are routinely diagnosed at an advanced stage. The duration of the symptoms depends on the biological behavior of the disease. In case of a slowly growing tumor of paranasal origin, airway obstruction may develop slowly and the disease which is obscured from the patient and the physician may develop months or years before the diagnosis is established.

Evaluation of patients with suspected maxillary cancer should include complete history and physical evaluation with emphasis on the head and neck. Fiberoptic evaluation of the paranasal sinuses and upper aerodigestive tracts is indicated in all patients, in order to evaluate the tumor extent and potential for resection. In the absence of distant metastases, complete tumor extirpation is the mainstay of treatment for most cancer cases in this area. Exceptions are lymphoma and soft tissue sarcomas of the childhood, which are treated with chemotherapy and radiation.

Total maxillectomy include resection of all six walls of the maxilla. It is used more commonly for large malignant tumors, which infiltrate the hard palate and antrum. Conventional exposure is achieved via a Weber-Ferguson incision with or without subciliary extension as indicated. This approach allows exposure of the medial and lateral buttresses of the maxilla and resection of the superior and inferior extensions of the tumor. Since, cervical lymph nodes are rarely encountered in cases of maxillary carcinomas, neck dissection should only be performed if regional metastases are identified, based on clinical or radiological evaluation.

In this chapter, the authors will describe the surgical technique of total maxillectomy and its means of reconstruction.

PREOPERATIVE AND PROSTHESIS EVALUATION

Patients scheduled for operation are evaluated preoperatively by a head and neck surgeon and an anesthesiologist. All patients should also undergo clinical examination by an oral and maxillofacial surgeon and dental prosthesis evaluation. If a free flap is planned, preoperative physical examination by a plastic surgeon is essential. Radiological evaluation should always include both computed tomography (CT) and magnetic resonance imaging (MRI) of the head, neck and paranasal sinuses for evaluation of bony and soft tissue involvement, respectively. Patients should be evaluated for involvement of cranial nerves, the orbit, skull base and dural or brain infiltration using both CT and MRI. Suspicious neck metastases can be evaluated with CT, MRI or ultrasound. Chest radiograph should be performed for evaluation of lung metastases. Patients can be also evaluated for the presence of metastases using positron emission tomography (PET)-CT. Due to the high yield in staging metastatic disease, utilizing metabolic PET imaging can replace staging techniques employing multiple imaging modalities (i.e. chest X-ray, neck and liver ultrasound, total body CT and bone mapping).

Dental prosthesis should be prepared ahead of time, as early as possible during the preoperative work-up. This time is needed for the patient and prosthodontist to discuss the functional and esthetic outcomes of the procedure and to design a temporary obturator that is to be used during surgery and in the immediate postoperative period. This prosthesis allows the holding of packing after the operation for hemostasis and early oral intake.

Since the operation is considered clean-contaminated surgery, broad-spectrum antibiotics are instituted perioperatively. This usually includes a second-generation cephalosporin and metronidazole. All the patients are operated in the supine position. Since the maxillectomy will include both the oral and nasal cavities, the endotracheal tube will always be at the field of operation. The authors prefer to perform an oral endotracheal intubation with a "South" facing tube, which provides good access for the surgeon needing to work in the nasal passages. Tracheostomy is rarely indicated in these cases.

SURGICAL TECHNIQUE

Surgical Anatomy

The maxilla is composed of six walls: (i) the superior wall, which includes floor of the orbit and the lamina papyracea; (ii) the inferior wall, which includes hard palate and alveolus; (iii) the posterior wall, which includes the pterygoid plates; (iv) the anterior wall, which includes the fossa canina; (v) the medial wall, which includes the inferior, middle and superior conchas and; (vi) the lateral wall, which includes the malar eminence. The posterior aspect of the hard palate is formed by the pyramidal process of the palatine bone. The walls of the maxilla are rather thin and fragile, and they are supported by two robust bony segments; the medial and lateral buttress of the maxilla (Figs 1A and B). The hard palate and alveolar ridge are lined by a stratified squamous epithelium containing hundreds of minor salivary glands. The antrum and medial wall are covered by a thin respiratory epithelium and the external portion of the anterior, superior and lateral walls are lined by periosteum.

Skin Incision and Development of a Superior Cheek Flap

Total maxillectomy is also known as radical maxillectomy. This procedure is directed for treatment of large tumors,

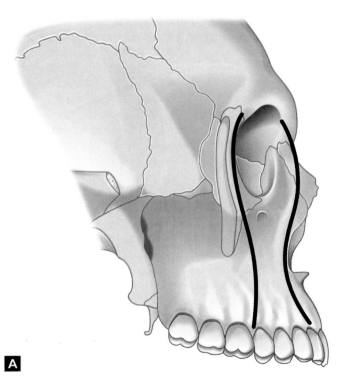

A

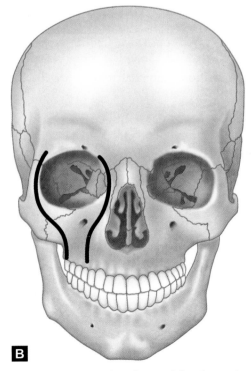

B

Figs 1A and B: Surgical anatomy of the maxilla. The walls of the maxilla are rather thin and fragile, and they are supported by two robust bony segments; the medial and lateral buttress of the maxilla

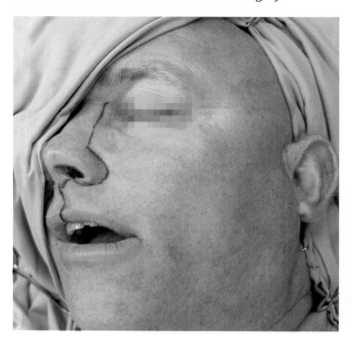

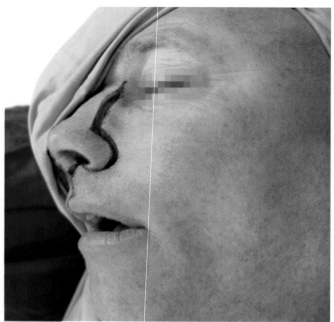

Fig. 2: Weber-Ferguson incision. The facial incision extends along the lateral border of the nose, approximately half a centimeter from dorsum of the nose. It starts cephalad, medial to the medial canthus and extends down through the skin crest bordering the nasal ala. It is continued toward the filtrum and extended down to the lip in the midline

Fig. 3: Skin incision

which originate in the upper alveolar ridge and extend to the nasal cavity and maxillary antrum as well as for cancers of the paranasal sinuses, which infiltrate the hard palate. The surgery is performed through a transfacial approach. In malignant tumors, intraoperative margins of at least 2 cm are required to reassure wide margins free of tumor in the final pathological specimen. Positive or close margins (< 0.5 cm from the tumor front) are not only a poor prognostic factor, but will also require the implementation of adjuvant radiation therapy.

Surgery is performed via a transfacial approach using a Weber-Ferguson incision (Figs 2 and 3). This incision allows exposure of the superior and inferior aspects of the maxilla and its complete en bloc resection. The facial incision extends along the lateral border of the nose, approximately half a centimeter from the dorsum of the nose. It starts cephalad, medial to the medial canthus and extends down through the skin crease bordering the nasal ala. It is continued toward the philtrum and extended down to the lip in the midline. Inferiorly, the incision continues along the gingivobuccal sulcus extending laterally up to the retromolar area.

After marking, the skin, palate and gingivobuccal sulcus is injected with lidocaine (0.06%) and epinephrine (diluted at 1:100,000) for hemostasis and hydrodissection purposes. Following incision of the skin with a number 15 blade, the dissection continues with electrocautery. Skin flaps are

elevated medially and laterally in the level of the periosteum using a freer elevator. The flaps are elevated medially to the nasal bone, pyriform aperture and nasal spine. The septum is inspected to rule out involvement by the tumor. The soft tissue of the cheek is raised from the anterior surface of the maxilla, transecting the infraorbital nerve and vessel. A unilateral gingivolabial incision is now made extending up to the lateral buttress of the maxilla. An upper cheek flap is developed superiorly to the infraorbital rim and the orbit is entered. The orbit is retracted gently with a malleable flat retractor in a superolateral direction and the superior surface of the medial and inferior walls of the orbit are exposed. Care is taken to skeletonize the bone, keeping the integrity of the periorbit. The anterior ethmoidal artery is transected and coagulated on the medial orbital wall. Laterally, the flap is elevated to the level of the malar eminence and up to the root of the zygoma as in Figure 4.

At this stage, the anterior, superior, lateral, medial and inferior walls of the maxillary bone are widely exposed and the bone is inspected carefully in order to identify its integrity and the areas of tumor infiltration. If the tumor infiltrates to anterior wall of the maxilla, the upper cheek flap should be elevated superficial to the subcutaneous tissue and facial muscles. The mucosa of the palate is now incised to the level of the bone and small flaps are developed with a freer elevator making just enough space for the osteotomy to be performed. Next, extraction of one tooth in the area of the planned osteotomy is performed. This allows the surgeon to perform the osteotomy safely and easily in the middle of the tooth socket, preserving the contralateral tooth and its root as in Figure 5.

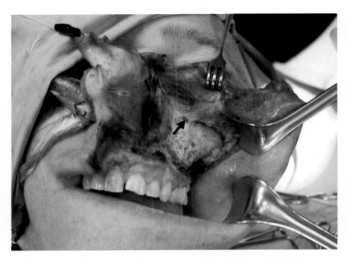

Fig. 4: Development of an upper cheek flap. Skin flaps are elevated medially and laterally to the level of the periosteum with the aid of a freer elevator and electrocautery. Superiorly, the infraorbital rim is exposed and laterally, the flap is elevated lateral to the malar eminence up to the root of the zygoma. The arrow points to the infraorbital nerve

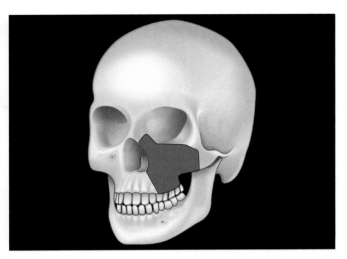

Fig. 5: The upper osteotomies

Attention is now turned to perform the upper osteotomies (Fig. 5). The borders of the osteotomies are superiorly, the orbit; laterally, the zygomatic process of the maxilla and buccal fat pad; medially, the nasal bones and nasal cavity; and inferiorly, the oral cavity. If involved by the tumor, the nasal septum can be included in the specimen.

With the retractor protecting the orbital content and long retractor holding the cheek flap laterally, the superior medial and lateral osteotomies are performed with a reciprocating saw. Care is taken to prevent injury to the optic nerve and rectus muscles. In addition, it is important not to enter the skull base and dura at the pterional area. The osteotomies are completed with a medium size osteotome to prevent inadvertent injury to these structures. If the infraorbital rim is aimed to be preserved, resection of the lamina papyracea is achieved by blunt dissection with a freer elevator and vial forceps, and the thin bone is outfractured in several pieces.

Attention is now turned to the inferior maxillectomy. The osteotomies are performed laterally and medially down toward the extracted teeth. The soft palate is dissected from the hard palate with an electrocautery, completing the posterior border of the dissection. The osteotomies are completed along the hard palate (Fig. 6).

The final part of the resection is separation of the specimen posteriorly along the pterygoid plates. A long retractor is inserted lateral to the alveolar ridge and a large curved osteotome is placed behind the last molar aiming superomedial to the palate. This maneuver is directed to fracture the medial and lateral pterygoid plates, separating the specimen from its attachments to the medial and

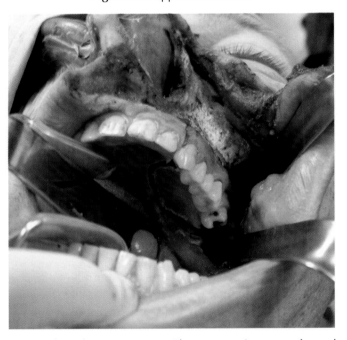

Fig. 6: The inferior osteotomy. The osteotomies are performed laterally and medially down toward the extracted teeth. The soft palate is dissected from the hard palate with an electro-cautery and the palatal osteotomies are completed

lateral pterygoid muscles (Fig. 7). The osteotomy starts in a superior direction and as the pterygoid plates are fractured, it continues in a lateral to medial direction above the alveolar ridge. Since, brisk bleeding is expected during this stage of the operation, suctions are used to keep the surgical bed bloodless during this part. Once the specimen is freed, a curve Mayo scissors and straight osteotome are used to separate the specimen from the sinonasal mucosa, the remnants of the pterygoid muscles, and the lateral and posterior walls of the maxillary sinus. After the specimen is removed

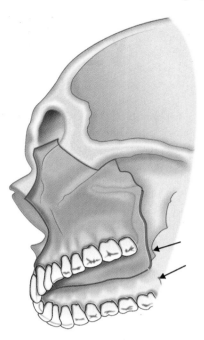

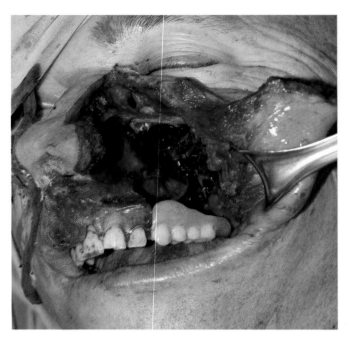

Fig. 7: The posterior osteotomy. A long retractor is inserted lateral to the alveolar ridge and a large curved osteotome is placed behind the last molar aiming superomedial to the palate (arrows). This maneuver is directed to fracture the medial and lateral pterygoid plates separating the specimen from its attachments to the medial and lateral pterygoid muscles. The osteotomy starts in a superior direction and as the pterygoids are fractured, it continues in a lateral to medial direction above the alveolar ridge

Fig. 8: The surgical field after removal of the specimen. The surgical cavity and specimen are inspected to evaluate proper margins. The wound is rinsed with warm saline and the internal maxillary artery is identified and clipped at the posterior maxillary wall

(Fig. 8), hemostasis is performed with a 4 × 4 gauze soaked with 50% hydrogen peroxide diluted with saline. The internal maxillary artery and its branches are clipped and hemostasis is finalized with a bipolar electrocautery. Bleeding from the area of the pterygopalatine fossa is best controlled with one or two strips of Surgicel®. The surgical cavity and specimen are inspected to evaluate proper margins. The wound is rinsed with warm saline and the internal maxillary artery is identified and clipped at the posterior maxillary wall. If the resection of the premaxilla or the contralateral side is indicated, degloving of the soft tissues of the lower face is performed exposing the pyriform aperture and the anterior maxillary walls bilaterally. It is then possible to extend the maxillectomy to the lower nasal cavity and laterally.

The cavity is packed with Xeroform gauze and a dental obturator is used to hold the gauze in place as in Figure 9.

Reconstruction

Following tumor extirpation, maxillary defects require reconstruction in order to provide a barrier between the nasal cavity, maxillary sinuses and the oral cavity. Reconstructive failure carries potential, functional and esthetic problems that may hamper oral intake and speech.

The reconstruction technique is designed according to the location and size of the defect, based on radiological and intraoperative calculations. Temporary obturator is prefabricated before the operation and molded during the procedure after the specimen is removed. This can be achieved by a prosthodontist with a thermoplastic or self solidified material, which allow full stenting of the maxillary defect. The obturator is fixed to the remaining teeth by wires that were implanted in the obturator (Fig. 9). The temporary prosthesis is replaced by a permanent obturator 2 weeks after surgery. In many cases, a permanent prosthesis is finally costumed several months after surgery and radiation therapy has been completed.

Free flap reconstruction may be indicated after total maxillectomy. The cases that definitely require tissue transfer are bilateral maxillectomies and large resections of the premaxilla, including the septum and nasal bones. In these cases, reconstruction is achieved with composite bone flaps including fibula or iliac crest osteofasciomusculocutaneous free flaps and microvascular anastomosis.

Resection of the infraorbital rim or malar eminence and resection of the lamina papyracea may also require free flap reconstruction after total maxillectomy to support the orbital content and for cosmesis. These cases will also require rigid reconstruction, which can be achieved by a malleable titanium mesh or a split calvarial bone graft.

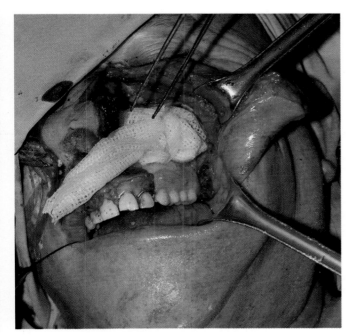

Fig. 9: The cavity is packed with Xeroform® gauze and a dental obturator is used to hold the gauze in place

Reconstruction of the lamina papyracea is directed to prevent prolapse of the orbital content into the maxillary antrum. This is rarely the case, if the medial or inferior portion of the peri orbital walls are resected. However, if both the inferior rim of the orbit is removed it can be reconstructed with titanium mesh coated with fascia.

POSTOPERATIVE TREATMENT

The incision is closed with inverted absorbable sutures and nylon stitches. After closing, the wound is covered with a thin film of antibiotic ointment. No dressing is used to cover the wound in order to permit easy access to the area of incision for examination and treatment. The wound is kept clean by rinsing it with saline 3 times a day during the first week after the operation and covered with antibiotic ointment, after each cleansing. Broad-spectrum antibiotics are continued until the packing is removed. The nasal packing is removed 5 days following the operation. Daily washing of the cavity is recommended after the packing is removed.

Pain Control

Maxillectomies are associated with a considerable level of pain during the early postoperative period. While many analgesic regimens are available [e.g. *pro re nata* (PRN), scheduled dosing, intravenous patient-controlled analgesia (PCR)], it was shown that a PRN protocol is not adequate for the management of pain following surgery. Intravenous-PCA with morphine (1 mg bolus) should be administered, with a 10-minute lockout interval and no basal infusion during the first 3 postoperative days. This is followed by selective nonsteroidal anti-inflammatory drug [(NSAID), for example PO rofecoxib® 50 mg], Second-line treatment consists of intramuscular meperidine 1 mg/kg (50–100 mg) repeated every 3–4 hours if required, but not exceeding a maximum of 150 mg as a single dose or morphine via slow intravenous injection (4–10 mg, titrated according to effect). Tramadol is used as PRN treatment during this period and a single starting dose of 50 mg (20 drops) is prescribed (40 drops, 100 mg/ml). If the desired analgesic effect is not achieved within 30–60 minutes, an additional 20 drops are administered. The total daily dose should not exceed 400 mg of tramadol (equivalent to 160 drops or 4.0 ml). A downward adjustment of the dose and/or prolongation of the interval between doses are carried out for the elderly.

HIGHLIGHTS

I. Indications
- Large tumors of the upper alveolar ridge and hard palate
- Tumors involving the hard palate, nasal cavity and maxillary sinuses.

II. Contraindications
- Metastatic disease
- Involvement of extramaxillary structures or compartments.

III. Special Preoperative Considerations
- Proper preoperative imaging
- Endoscopic evaluation
- Ophthalmologic evaluation if orbital invasion is suspected
- Planning of the reconstruction means
- Evaluation by maxillofacial surgeon and prosthodontist
- Construction of a temporary obturator.

IV. Special Intraoperative Considerations
- Proper placement of the skin incisions
- Preserve the infraorbital rim and malar eminence if possible
- Tooth extraction along the osteotomy site to allow preservation of the remaining teeth
- Meticulous dissection along the lamina papyracea
- Careful dissection along the lateral skull base and cribriform plate
- Clip the internal maxillary artery
- Appropriate reconstruction.

V. Special Postoperative Considerations
- Early identification of complications
- Antibiotic coverage until the packing is removed
- Frequent cleansing and suction of nasal secretion are required during the first year after surgery
- Quick restoration of oral intake.

VI. Complications
- Bleeding
- Enophthalmos
- Epiphora due to lacrimal duct stenosis
- Diplopia and telecanthus
- Optic nerve injury and blindness
- Cerebrospinal fluid leak
- Hematoma
- Skin necrosis
- Wound infection and dehiscence.

ADDITIONAL READING

1. Cordeiro PG, Santamaria E. A classification system and algorithm for reconstruction of maxillectomy and midfacial defects. Plast Reconstr Surg. 2000;105(7):2331-46.
2. Fliss DM, Abergel A, Cavel O, et al. Combined subcranial approaches for excision of complex anterior skull base tumors. Arch Otolaryngol Head Neck Surg. 2007;133(9):888-96.
3. Gil Z, Fliss DM. Contemporary management of head and neck cancers. Isr Med Assoc J. 2009;11(5):296-300.
4. Katz TS, Mendenhall WM, Morris CG, et al. Malignant tumors of the nasal cavity and paranasal sinuses. Head Neck. 2002;24(9):821-9.
5. Kenady DE. Cancer of the paranasal sinuses. Surg Clin North Am. 1986;66(1):119-31.
6. Lavertu P, Roberts JK, Kraus DH, et al. Squamous cell carcinoma of the paranasal sinuses: the Cleveland Clinic experience 1977-1986. Laryngoscope. 1989;99:1130-6.
7. Lee CH, Hur DG, Roh HJ, et al. Survival rates of sinonasal squamous cell carcinoma with the new AJCC staging system. Arch Otolaryngol Head Neck Surg. 2007;133(2):131-4.
8. Myers LL, Nussenbaum B, Bradford CR, et al. Paranasal sinus malignancies: an 18-year single institution experience. Laryngoscope. 2002;112(11):1964-9.
9. Spiro RH, Strong EW, Shah JP. Maxillectomy and its classification. Head Neck. 1997;19(4):309-14.
10. Truitt TO, Gleich LL, Huntress GP, et al. Surgical management of hard palate malignancies. Otolaryngol Head Neck Surg. 1999;121(5):548-52.

Chapter **31**

The Subcranial Approach to the Anterior Skull Base

Ziv Gil, Dan M Fliss

INTRODUCTION

The subcranial approach is a single-stage procedure used in cases of tumors involving the anterior skull base. The concept of a broad subcranial approach to the entire anterior skull base was first introduced by Raveh for cases of traumatic injuries and was later adapted for surgical extirpations of tumors involving this anatomic region. The extent of exposure of the subcranial approach, includes the frontal sinus anteriorly, the clivus posteriorly, the frontal lobe superiorly and the paranasal sinuses inferiorly. Laterally, the boundaries of this approach are both superior orbital walls. The subcranial approach has several major advantages over the traditional craniofacial resection: (i) it affords a broad exposure of the anterior skull base from below rather than through the transfrontal route; (ii) it provides an excellent access to the medial orbital walls and to the sphenoethmoidal, nasal and paranasal cavities; (iii) it allows simultaneous intradural and extradural tumor removal and safe reconstruction of dural defects; (iv) it does not require facial incisions; (v) it is performed with minimal frontal lobe manipulation.

The subcranial approach involves coronal incision and osteotomy of the nasofrontal orbital bone segment, which allows access to the intra- and extracranial compartments of the anterior skull base. Although, the subcranial approach permits complete tumor resection in the majority of cases, there are still situations in which the inferior, lateral or posterior aspects of the tumor are not adequately exposed. These include neoplasms with extensions to the maxillary antrum and palate caudally, to the cavernous sinus posteriorly, to the orbital apex, pterygopalatine fossa (PPF) or infratemporal fossa (ITF) laterally and

involvement of the nasopharynx and inferior aspect of the clivus inferoposteriorly. In addition, the endonasal approach has now replaced the subcranial approach in most cases of benign and malignant tumors of the anterior and middle skull base.

In this chapter, the authors will describe the surgical procedure of the subcranial approach, which is used in their institution for extirpations of tumors involving the anterior skull base and paranasal sinuses.

PREOPERATIVE EVALUATION AND ANESTHESIA

All patients scheduled for operation are evaluated preoperatively by a head and neck surgeon, a neurosurgeon and an anesthesiologist. Patients younger than 18 years are also examined by a pediatrician. If a free flap is planned, preoperative physical examination by a plastic surgeon is essential. Radiological evaluation of the patients includes axial and coronal computed tomography (CT), and magnetic resonance imaging (MRI) of the head and neck. Neuroangiography evaluations may also be performed in cases of highly vascular tumors invading the skull base or the cavernous sinus. Figures 1 and 2 show typical preoperative CT and MRI scan of patients with tumors involving the anterior skull base.

Patients who underwent prior skull base or craniofacial procedures for extirpation of malignant tumors are also evaluated using a positron emission tomography-CT hybrid (PET-CT) using the Discovery LS PET/CT system (GE Medical) prior to the operative procedure. The PET part of PET-CT is performed twice, using a 2-D and a 3-D

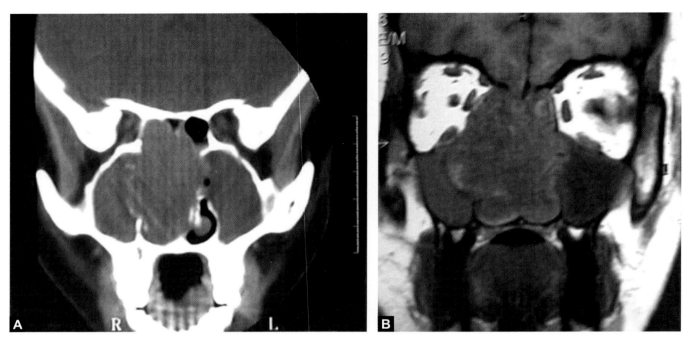

Figs 1A and B: A preoperative coronal CT (A) and MRI (B) of a 16-year-old girl with esthesioneuroblastoma invading the anterior skull base nasal cavity and right maxillary sinus

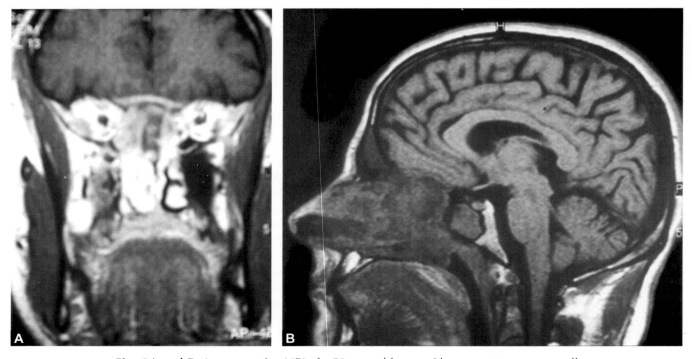

Figs 2A and B: A preoperative MRI of a 53-year-old man with recurrent squamous cell carcinoma invading the anterior skull base, nasal cavity and frontal sinus

acquisition protocols for comparison purposes. The authors reported an upstaging of 20% of the patients (10 of 50) using this novel method. Electromyographic monitoring of the cranial nerves and neuronavigation (BrainLab® interface) may be also used in selected cases.

The authors recommend to routinely shampooing the head with chlorhexidine (Septal Scrub®) the night before the operation. Broad-spectrum antibiotics are instituted perioperatively. All the patients are operated in the supine position without shaving the hair at the surgical site. No tracheostomy is performed. A lumbar spine catheter is inserted for a period of 3–5 days for cerebrospinal fluid (CSF) drainage to facilitate frontal lobe retraction and to reduce the risk of postoperative CSF leak.

SURGICAL TECHNIQUE

After the induction of anesthesia, the patient's hair is shampooed vigorously with 4% w/v chlorhexidine (Septal Scrub®) parted with a sterile comb along the proposed incision line and tied in clumps by rubber bands. The operative field is then scrubbed with surgical sponges containing chlorhexidine solution (0.05% w/v) and draped with sterile towels that are clipped in place with surgical staples.

The skin is incised above the hairline and a bicoronal flap is created in a supraperiosteal plane. A flap is elevated anteriorly beyond the supraorbital ridges and laterally superficial to the temporalis fascia (Fig. 3A). The pericranial flap is elevated up to the periorbits and the supraorbital nerves and vessels are carefully separated from the supraorbital notch. The lateral and medial walls of the orbits are then exposed (Fig. 3B), and the anterior ethmoidal arteries are clipped or coagulated. The pericranium is elevated above the nasal bones and the flap is rotated forward and held over the face throughout the rest of the procedure (Fig. 3B). Titanium micro or mini plates are applied to the frontal bones and removed before performing the osteotomies, to ensure the exact repositioning of the bony segments at the end of the operation. An osteotomy of the anterior or the anterior and posterior frontal sinus walls together with the proximal nasal bony frame, part of the superior and medial wall of the orbit and a segment of the superoposterior nasal septum is then performed. For type A osteotomy, the anterior frontal sinus wall as well as the proximal nasal frame are osteotomized and removed in one block (Fig. 4A). If a type B osteotomy is planned, burr holes are made and the posterior frontal sinus wall is resected after the dura has been detached from the frontal, orbital and ethmoid roofs (Fig. 4B). A part of the distal nasal bone is preserved in order to support the nasal valve. In cases of lateral invasion of a tumor, the osteotomy

lines can be extended to include the lateral segments of the orbital roofs. After the frontonaso-orbital bone segment is osteotomized, it is stored in saline until the reconstructive procedure. A bilateral ethmoidectomy and a sphenoidotomy are then performed. This approach enables the exposure and assessment of the tumor in its circumference. The tumor is extirpated at this stage and the dura or brain parenchyma is also resected when involved by tumor. Frozen sections may be taken during surgery in order to assess the tumor's margins. One side of the cribriform plate and olfactory filaments can be preserved whenever possible.

Reconstruction Following Subcranial Surgery

Following tumor extirpation, cranial base defects require reconstruction in order to provide a secure barrier between the intracranial content and the paranasal cavity. Reconstructive failure carries potential life-threatening complications (e.g. CSF leakage and meningitis) that may delay the initiation of adjuvant therapy.

Reconstruction of the anterior skull base is technically challenging and may be further complicated by several factors. Firstly, there is a paucity of local tissue that is available for transfer into the defect. Secondly, previous radiation treatment significantly reduces tissue perfusion that delays normal wound healing. Finally, many of these patients have undergone multiple surgeries prior to the index operation, thus increasing its complexity and secondary to scar tissue formation, decreasing tissue perfusion.

The reconstruction technique is designed according to the size and location of the cranial defect based on radiological and intraoperative calculations. Primary closure of the dura is performed whenever possible. In cases of extensive skull base defects, a second surgical team simultaneously harvests a large fascia lata sheath (20 × 10 cm). The size of the fascia used for reconstruction is tailored according to the dimension of the dural and skull base defects. First, the dura is repaired with fascia lata patch with the goal of watertight closure (Fig. 5A, yellow arrow). The fascia is tacked under the edges of the dura and carefully sutured in place. The dural repair is then covered with a second layer of fascia that is applied against the entire undersurface of the ethmoid roof, the sella and the sphenoidal area (Fig. 5A). Fibrin glue is used in order to provide additional protection against CSF leak. Never put the fibrin glue between the two layers of fascia lata, since the two layers adhere better when there is no additional material between them. The frontal sinus is cranialized in order to prevent mucocele formation. After removing all the mucosa from its undersurface, the earlier osteotomized segment is repositioned in its original anatomical place. Wrapping of

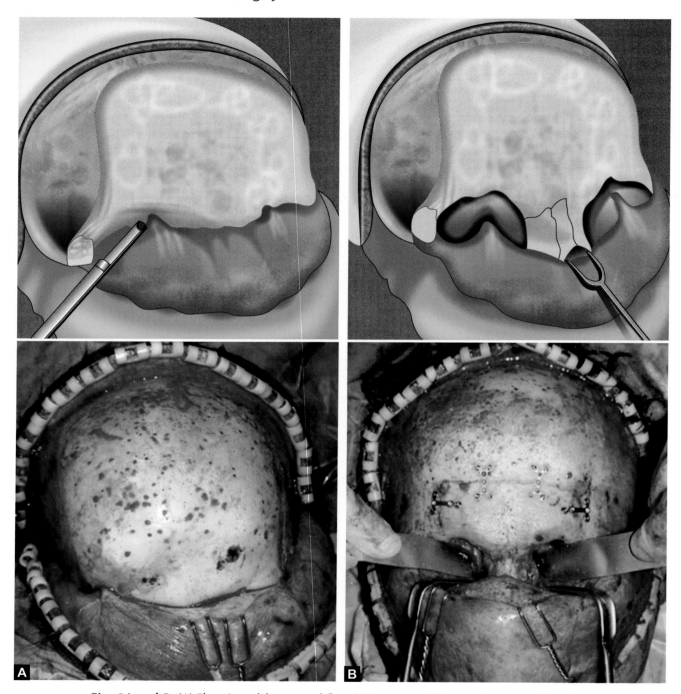

Figs 3A and B: (A) Elevation of the coronal flap; (B) Exposure of the superior part of the orbits

the bone segment (Fig. 5B) is accomplished by a double sided covering of the bone segment with the pericranial flap. This vascularized tissue is guided underneath the bony segment to cover the intranasal surface and then it is externalized over the entire frontal area. The bone segment and its overlying pericranial flap are fixed with the prebent titanium plates (Fig. 5B). A medial compression method is used to reduce the telecanthus. In this method, two threads are guided through the medial canthal ligament and driven underneath the frontonaso-orbital segment. The threads are tightened and fixed to the contralateral frontal titanium plates in order to enable medial compression and alignment

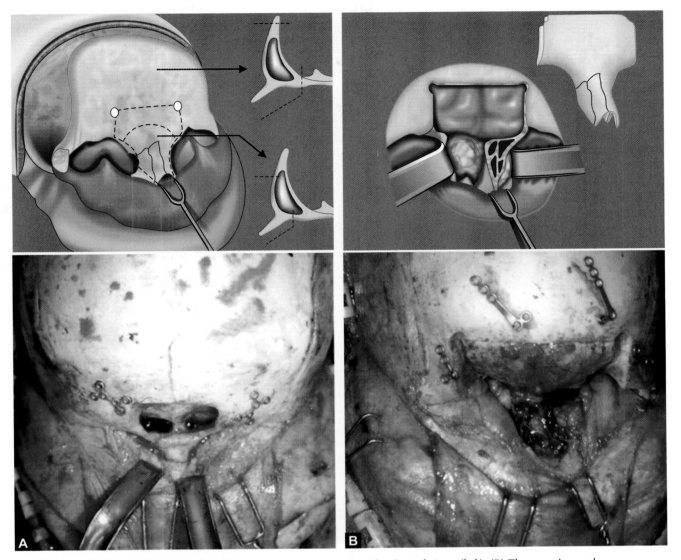

Figs 4A and B: (A) Osteotomy of the anterior wall of the frontal sinus (left); (B) The anterior and posterior frontal sinus walls (right). The tumor is seen in the nasal cavity

thereby avoiding the telecanthus altogether. Vaseline gauze is applied to the reconstructed skull base to provide additional support against dural pulsation.

Vacuum drains are left in place and the incision is closed with inverted absorbable sutures and skin staples. After closing, the wound is covered with a thin film of antibiotic ointment. No dressing is used to cover the wound in order to permit easy access to the area of incision for examination and treatment.

POSTOPERATIVE TREATMENT

After surgery, the patients are extubated and immediately transferred to the critical care unit for 24 hours. The patients should routinely undergo CT scan after the operation to rule out bleeding or tension pneumocephalus. The wound is kept clean by rinsing it with saline three times a day during the first 10 days after the operation and covered with antibiotic ointment after each cleansing. It is advised to the patient to

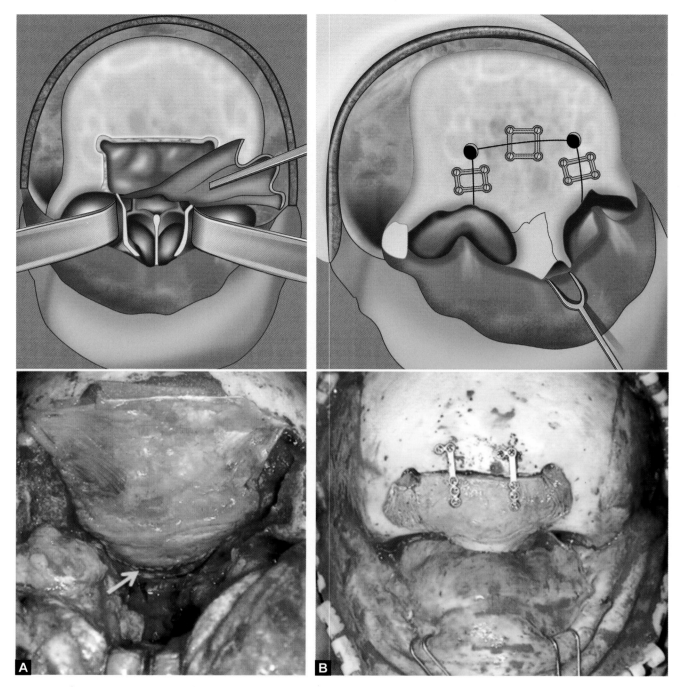

Figs 5A and B: Reconstruction of the dura following tumor resection. (A) Primary reconstruction of the dura is performed with a fascia lata sheath (yellow arrow). This is covered by a second layer of fascia lata; (B) Wrapping of the frontal bone segment is performed to reduce osteonecrosis

wash his hair with Chlorhexidine once daily. The drains are removed either, 3 days after the operation or when the fluid is less than 20 ml in 24 hours. Broad-spectrum antibiotics are instituted preoperatively and continued until the packing is removed. For pain control, the patients are treated with nonsteroidal anti-inflammatory drugs (diclofenac 75 mg intramuscularly or orally, or rofecoxib 50 mg) once daily and with tramadol (50–100 mg) if the patient asks for them or if the

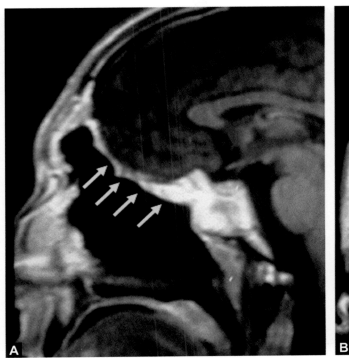 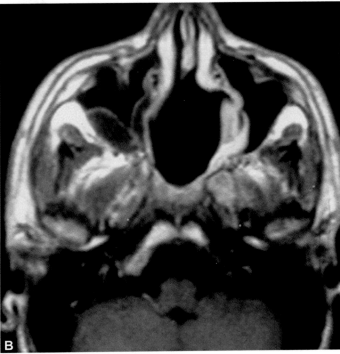

Figs 6A and B: Postoperative MRI of the patient (in Figure 2) performed 12 months after surgery. On the sagittal view, the arrows indicate the fascia lata flap

nurses felt it to be necessary. Stool softeners are administered to reduce the chance of Valsalva induced increase intracranial pressure. The lumbar drain is kept to drain 10cc/hour CSF and is removed 3–5 days after the operation and the nasal packing is removed 7 days following the operation. Daily washing of the head is recommended after the patient is mobile. Figures 6A and B show the postoperative MRI of the patient shown in figure 2. The fascia lata is delineated by the yellow arrows.

HIGHLIGHTS

I. Indications
- Tumors involving the anterior base of skull base not amendable for endoscopic surgery
- The tumor extend to the anterior maxillary wall, frontal sinus, sphenoid sinus or skin.

II. Contraindications
- Tumors amendable for minimally invasive (endoscopic) surgery.
- Metastatic disease
- Massive brain involvement
- Palatal involvement
- Cavernous sinus involvement in malignant tumors.

III. Special Preoperative Considerations
- The subcranial approach is a multidisciplinary team effort
- Use broad-spectrum prophylactic antibiotic treatment to reduce infections
- Insert a lumbar drain after administering anesthesia to facilitate frontal lobe retraction and to reduce the risk of postoperative cerebrospinal fluid leak.
- Do not shave the head to improve patient's satisfaction.

IV. Special Intraoperative Considerations
- Preserve the distal one third of the nasal bone
- Preserve the pericranium for further use
- Protect the supraorbital nerve during flap elevation
- Use a small craniotomy as possible to minimize osteonecrosis.
- Assure a tight dural seal in order to prevent cerebrospinal fluid leak. Never put bio glue between the two layers of fascia lata to facilitate adherence
- Proper repair of the telecanthus reduces the risk for diplopia.

V. Special Postoperative Considerations
- Immediate extubation is required to allow continuous neurological monitoring

- Never ventilate a patient with a positive pressure after extubation in order to avoid life-threatening tension pneumocephalus.
- Admit the patient to an intensive care unit for 24 hours after surgery
- Continue cerebrospinal drainage and close monitoring for 3–5 days
- Frequent cleansing and suction of nasal secretion are required during the first year after surgery.

VI. Complications
- Meningitis
- Cerebrospinal fluid leak
- Tension pneumocephalus
- Wound infection
- Osteonecrosis and fistula of the naso-fronto-orbital segment
- Diplopia and telecanthus.

ADDITIONAL READING

1. Fliss DM, Gil Z, Spektor S, et al. Skull base reconstruction after anterior subcranial tumor resection. Neurosurg Focus. 2002;12(5):e10.
2. Fliss DM, Zucker G, Cohen A, et al. Early outcome and complications of the extended subcranial approach to the anterior skull base. Laryngoscope. 1999;109(1):153-60.
3. Gil Z, Abergel A, Spektor S, et al. Quality of life following surgery for anterior skull base tumors. Arch Otolaryngol Head Neck Surg. 2003;129(12):1303-9.
4. Gil Z, Constantini S, Spektor S, et al. Skull base approaches in the pediatric population. Head Neck. 2005;27(8):682-9.
5. Gil Z, Fliss DM. Pericranial wrapping of the frontal bone after anterior skull base tumor resection. Plast Reconstr Surg. 2005;116(2):395-9.
6. Raveh J, Laedrach K, Speiser M, et al. The subcranial approach for fronto-orbital and anteroposterior skull base tumor. Arch Otolaryngol Head Neck Surg. 1993;119(4):385-93.

Chapter 32

Parotidectomy

Ziv Gil, Dan M Fliss

INTRODUCTION

The salivary gland system contains the parotid glands, the submandibular glands, the sublingual gland and hundreds of minor salivary glands located below the mucosa of the upper aerodigestive tracts. The parotid is the largest gland of the salivary system and it is located superficial to the mandibular ramus and extends posteriority to the retromandibular fossa, anteriority to the masseter muscle, superiorly to the preauricular area and inferiorly below the mandible. The glandular secretions of the parotid gland are drained by an intralobular and interlobular collecting duct system and conducted to the oral cavity via the Stensen's duct (Fig. 1). The gland is pierced by the facial nerve, which separates the gland to superficial and deep lobes, with a relative volume of 80% and 20%, respectively. The facial nerve exits the base of skull through the stylomastoid foramen, located in the mastoid part of the temporal bone. The nerve exits the foramen lateral to the styloid process and forms the main trunk (*pes enserinus*), which then divides into two main branches: (i) the zygomaticotemporal and; (ii) cervicofacial trunks. The two main branches are divided into five main branches: (i) the temporal; (ii) zygomatic; (iii) buccal; (iv) marginal mandibular and; (v) cervical branches.

The parotid gland is the most common origin for tumors of the salivary gland system. Tumors originating in the parotid glands are usually presented as a single, slow growing subcutaneous mass. Although most of these tumors grow from the superficial lobe toward the skin, tumors can grow medially toward the parapharyngeal space and present as an oropharyngeal, submucosal mass. Symptoms of pain or facial nerve paralysis as well as enlarged cervical lymph nodes are suggestive of malignancy.

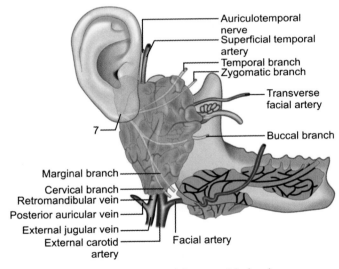

Fig. 1: Anatomy of the parotid gland

Approximately 80% of the tumors arising in the parotid gland are benign. Approximately 80% of benign tumors that arise in the parotid gland are pleomorphic adenoma (PA, mixed tumor) and the rest include Warthin's tumor, oncocytoma, monomorphic adenoma and benign cysts. Most of the adenomas arise between the age of 30 years and 50 years, and are slightly more common in women, whereas Warthin's tumor is more common in the elderly population, among smokers and in men. Malignant tumors of the parotid gland are found in 20% of the patients. The common malignant tumors are mucoepidermoid carcinoma, adenoid cystic carcinoma, adenocarcinoma, acinic cell carcinoma, carcinoma ex-pleomorphic adenoma (malignant mixed tumor) and lymphoma. Most squamous cell carcinomas of the parotid gland are secondary to skin metastases from the scalp and forehead. Tumors, which may present as multicenter and bilateral lesions are Warthin's tumor and acinic cell carcinoma.

Every lesion in the parotid gland requires further evaluation and most are treated with surgery. Two exceptions are lymphoma and an asymptomatic Warthin's tumor in the elderly patient. Pleomorphic adenoma, the most common tumor of the parotid glands, is normally a well-circumscribed, encapsulated tumor. However, these tumors may have small protrusions known as pseudopodia that extend beyond the central tumor mass. The tumor is composed of a mixture of glandular epithelium and myoepithelial cells within a mesenchyme-like background. The epithelium often forms ducts and cystic structures or may occur as islands or sheets of cells.

Recurrent pleomorphic adenoma may follow surgical resection of both the conventional or giant variants, but even after superficial or total parotidectomy, recurrence rates of up to 2.5% have been reported. Even though many hypotheses for recurrences of parotid gland pleomorphic adenoma have been advanced, including cellular, biological and genetic factors, to date only obvious or underestimated tumor spillage or incomplete excision are accepted contributors to recurrent disease. For malignant tumors, both stage and grade of the primary tumor are established prognostic factors of survival. The pattern of spread of parotid cancers includes direct extension to the skin, bones or muscles, spreading through cervical lymph nodes or nerve invasion. Adenoid cystic carcinoma is known for its high rate of neural invasion and lung metastases.

In this chapter, the technique practiced by the authors for surgical removal of the parotid gland with preservation of the facial nerve will be described in details. This technique allows complete extirpation of the tumor with wide margins and preservation of the facial nerve function. The surgical technique for removal of deep lobe parotid tumors is also described.

PREOPERATIVE EVALUATION

Radiological evaluation is required prior to surgery, since it can influence decision-making regarding the treatment. Imaging usually includes computed tomography (CT) with contrast or ultrasound. This allows evaluation of the tumor site and size, presence of additional lesions, nodal metastases and tumor infiltration to vessels, muscles, nerves, cartilages and bony tissue. Fine needle aspiration (FNA) may be used for tissue diagnosis prior to surgery. This is mainly important for differentiation between benign and malignant disease and

more importantly for the diagnosis of parotid lymphoma, which requires a nonsurgical treatment. The accuracy of FNA in case of a parotid gland tumor is approximately 90%. Ultrasound of the neck may be used as an adjunct for fine needle aspiration in small tumors.

All patients are evaluated by a head and neck surgeon. In case of a suspected malignant tumor, which may require facial nerve resection, also necessitate evaluation by a reconstructive surgeon for facial nerve grafting.

The authors do not recommend routine administration of prophylactic antibiotics in clean operations. First-generation cephalosporins and metronidazole are routinely used if the operation includes dissection in the oral cavity. Surgery is performed under general anesthesia without muscle relaxation. This allows the surgeon monitoring of the facial nerve function during dissection with electrocautery. Intraoperative monitoring of the facial nerve is performed in selected cases, including recurrent tumors or previous radiation treatment.

SURGICAL TECHNIQUE

Skin Incision

The patient is placed on the operating room table in a supine position. The head is stabilized with a soft donut holder and the whole operating table is then elevated in an angle with the head up in order to minimize bleeding. The surgical access is planned through a modified Blair incision (Figs 2A and B). Marking of the incision is preferably performed with the neck slightly flexed in order to identify the lines of relaxed skin tension. The incision normally extends from the tragus, encircles the lobule and then drops down posterior to the helix along the nuchal hair line. In young patients, the incision is performed on the free edge of the tragus, however, in elderly persons it is better concealed along a preauricular vertical skin crest. For large tumors or for those located in an accessory parotid, the incision can be extended 2–3 cm below the ramus of the mandible along a transverse skin crest in the lower neck. If neck dissection is indicated, the incision is extended medially up to the level of the cricoid cartilage. After incision marking, a donut is placed to support the head, which is rotated toward the contralateral side. The patient is then prepped and draped in a standard surgical fashion. A Betadine® 5% sterile ophthalmic prep solution containing 5% povidone-iodine (0.5% available iodine) is used for prepping of the periocular region (lids, brow and cheek). A transparent adhesive drape sheath (Steri-Drape™) is placed on the face to allow intraoperative monitoring of facial movements during surgery. If indicated, facial nerve monitoring electrodes are inserted prior to

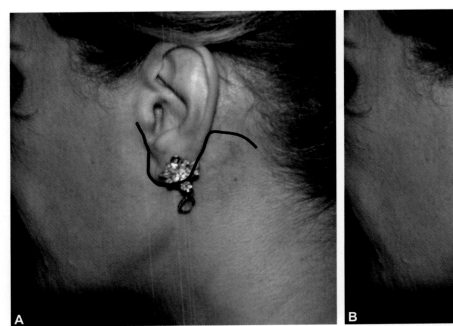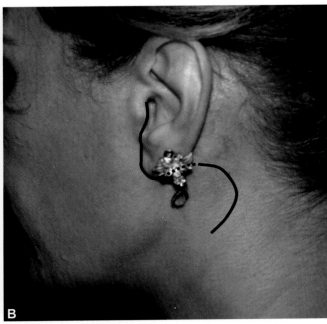

Figs 2A and B: Planning of the skin incision. (A) The incision normally extends from the tragus, encircles the lobule and then drops down posterior to the helix along the nuchal hair line. In young patients, the incision is performed on the free edge of the tragus, however, in elderly persons it is better concealed along a preauricular vertical skin crest; (B) For large tumors or for those located in an accessory parotid, the incision can be extended 2–3 cm below the ramus of the mandible along a transverse skin crest in the lower neck

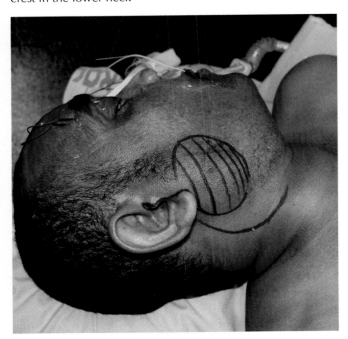

Fig. 3: Positioning of the facial nerve monitoring electrodes. If indicated, facial nerve monitoring electrodes are inserted prior to draping for monitoring the function of the orbicularis oculi (blue electrodes) and orbicularis oris muscles (yellow electrodes). The neck incision and tumor area are marked on the patient

draping for monitoring of the function of the orbicularis oculi and orbicularis oris muscles as in Figure 3.

Skin Incision and Elevation of the Flap

After marking, the skin is injected with lidocaine (0.06%) and epinephrine (1:1,000,000) to reduce the amount of pain after surgery and for hemostasis. The skin is incised with a number 15 blade and subsequent dissection of the subcutaneous tissue is carried out with an electrocautery at the lowest effective setting. The flaps are elevated superficial to the capsule of the parotid gland, which is composed of the superficial musculoaponeurotic system (SMAS). Keeping the flap superficial to the SMAS and deep to the subcutaneous fatty tissue, lowers the risk of skin perforation and tumor spillage and diminishes the rate of Frey's syndrome (Fig 4). The flap is elevated anteriorly to the edge of the tumor, while the subcutaneous fat is retained on the skin flap. Care is taken to prevent injury to the distal branches of the facial nerve as they exit the gland. Lower in the neck, subplatysmal flaps are elevated superiorly, 2 cm below the ramus of the mandible. While elevating a small posterior flap, care is taken to prevent injury to the anterior wall of the cartilaginous part of the external auditory canal. Next, the anterior border of the sternocleidomastoid muscle is exposed over the mastoid bone and the tail of the parotid gland is separated from the muscle. This is achieved by placing several Babcock's graspers

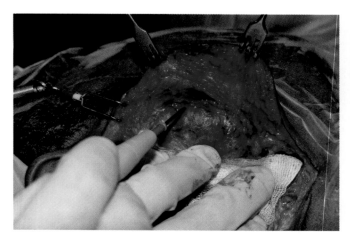

Fig. 4: Skin incision and elevated skin flaps. The skin is incised with a number 15 blade and subsequent dissection of the subcutaneous tissue and the platysma is carried out with an electrocautery at the lowest effective setting. The anterior flap is elevated 1–2 cm anteriorly to the edge of the tumor

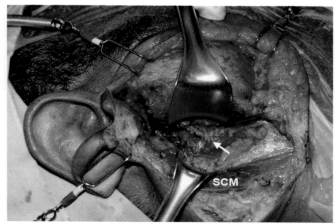

Fig. 5: Exposure of the posterior belly of the digastric muscle. The muscle crosses the angle formed by the sternocleido-mastoid muscle and the ramus of the mandible in the middle. The white arrow indicates the posterior belly of the digastric muscle. SCM: Sternocleidomastoid muscle

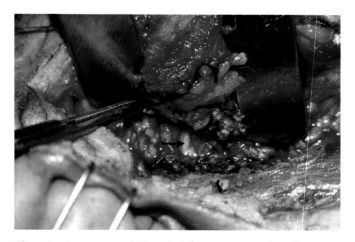

Fig. 6: Exposure of the facial nerve. As the dissection continues toward the facial nerve, one or two Army-Navy angled retractors are placed at the tympanomastoid fissure, retracting the posterior edge of the gland anteriorly. The nerve is indicated by the arrow

on the tail of the parotid, retracting the gland anteriorly. Care is taken to try and preserve the branches of the greater auricular nerve. If the nerves enter the superficial edge of the parotid, it needs to be resected.

Identifying the Facial Nerve

In order to allow safe and accurate identification of the facial nerve, the operation should be performed, while minimizing bleeding and while monitoring of the facial muscle movements. A bipolar electrocautery is used to minimize thermal trauma to the nerve. The next step of the dissection is identifying the posterior belly of the

digastric muscle (Fig. 5). The muscle is easily identified at its attachment to the mastoid bone. Early exposure of the posterior belly of the digastric muscle is a key point for identification of the main trunk of the facial nerve, which lies deep to the muscle. The operation continues using a fine hemostat along the posterior border of the tragus, at the tympanomastoid fissure. Meticulous dissection is performed releasing the cartilaginous anterior wall of the external auditory canal from the parotid capsule. Bipolar electrocautery is used for hemostasis during dissection of the fibrous tissue. As the dissection continues toward the facial nerve, one or two Army-Navy angled retractors are placed at the tympanomastoid fissure, retracting the posterior edge of the gland anteriorly (Fig. 6). The main trunk of the facial nerve is identified according to the following anatomical landmarks: (i) the mastoid process; (ii) the anteroinferior surface of the cartilaginous wall of the external auditory canal and; (iii) the posterior belly of the digastric muscle (Fig. 7). The main trunk lies at a point where all the three landmarks meet. Occasionally, the small branch of the stylomandibular artery is identified superficial to the nerve. This artery should be carefully ligated and divided in order to keep a bloodless surgical field.

Dissection along the Facial Nerve

After the main trunk of the facial nerve is identified, the dissection is continued superficial to the nerve with a fine hemostat and bipolar electrocautery. First, the main two branches of the nerve: (i) the cervicofacial and; (ii) zygomaticotemporal are exposed and the glandular tissue is reflected superficially (Fig. 8). The dissection is performed in a plane superficial to the epineurium of the facial nerve

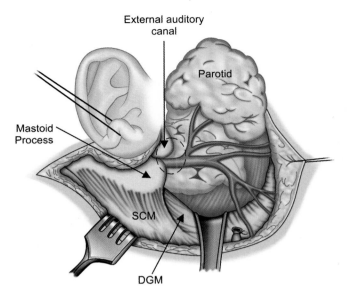

Fig. 7: Anatomic landmarks of the facial nerve. The main trunk of the facial nerve is identified according to the anatomical landmarks; the mastoid process, the anteroinferior surface of the cartilaginous wall of the external auditory canal and the posterior belly of the digastric muscle (DGM). The main trunk lies at a point where all the three landmarks meet (circle). SCM: Sternocleidomastoid muscle

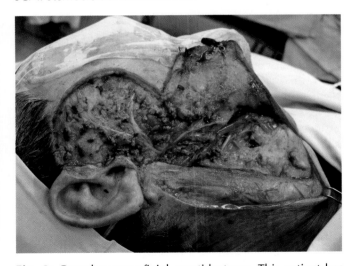

Fig. 9: Complete superficial parotidectomy. This patient has squamous cell carcinoma of the skin overlying the parotid gland. Surgery included composite resection of the skin, superficial parotidectomy and selective neck dissection

branches allowing accurate identification of the nerve branches and complete extirpation of the glandular tissue superficial to the nerve. The dissection is continued along the distal branches of the nerve starting with its superior divisions. The hemostat is directed superficially along the nerve and held open, while the bipolar is used for hemostasis. A number 15 blade is used to divide the glandular tissue.

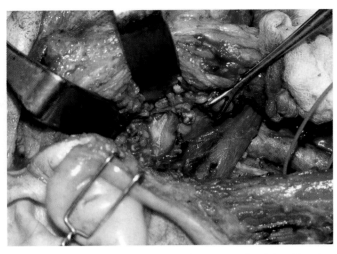

Fig. 8: Dissection along the facial nerve. After identification of the facial nerve trunk, its two main branches—the cervicofacial and zygomaticotemporal branches are exposed

The Stensen's duct may be identified adjacent to the buccal branches of the nerve. If identified, the duct is divided and tied. The dissection continues along the lower branches of the facial nerve in a similar fashion.

After the parotid tissue is dissected free of the upper and lower branches of the nerve, the operation continues anterior to the neoplasm along the anterior edge of the gland and the specimen is fully extirpated from its surrounding tissue.

A complete removal of the superficial lobe is most probably indicated only in case of large tumors, malignant neoplasm or during revision surgery for multifocal pleomorphic adenoma (Figs 9 and 10). Otherwise, the dissection should achieve wide surgical margins with glandular tissue free of tumor circumferentially to the tumor.

In cases of malignant neoplasms, such as high-grade mucoepidermoid carcinoma or adenoid cystic carcinoma, the surgeon may not be able to dissect the tumor off the nerve due to perineural invasion of the carcinoma. In these cases, the nerve should be excised en bloc with the tumor and reconstruction should be performed with a greater auricular or sural nerve graft. The greater auricular nerve should not be used when in close proximity to the tumor.

Excision of a Deep Lobe Parotid Tumor

A pleomorphic adenoma of the deep lobe may be encountered in minority of cases. The dissection is performed using a similar technique as described previously for tumor located in the superficial lobe. However, the surgeon may leave the superficial lobe attached to its anterior border allowing exposure of the area deep to the facial nerve (Fig. 11). Next, the nerve is meticulously freed circumferentially. This may be achieved by elevating the nerve on a vessel loop or nerve

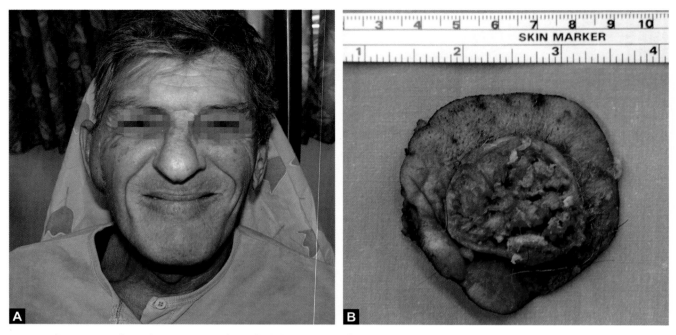

Figs 10A and B: The postsurgical result. (A) A picture taken 2 weeks after surgery showing the reconstruction with an anterolateral thigh free flap. The facial nerve function is normal; (B) The surgical specimen

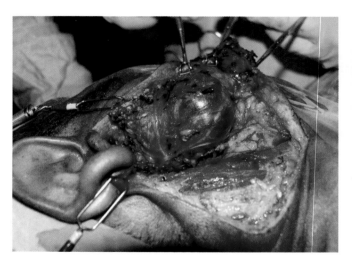

Fig. 11: Excision of a deep lobe parotid gland tumor. A superficial parotidectomy is performed and the deep lobe parotid tumor is exposed deep to the facial nerve

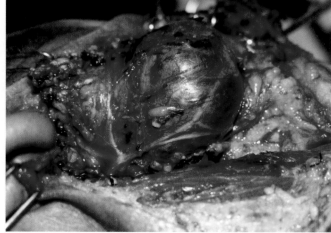

Fig. 12: Mobilization of the tumor from the deep lobe. The nerve is meticulously freed circumferentially. This may be achieved by elevating the nerve on a vessel loop or nerve hook. Freeing the nerve from its deep attachments will allow mobilization of the deep lobe in between its upper and lower branches

hook. Freeing the nerve from its deep attachments will allow mobilization of the deep lobe in between its upper and lower branches (Fig. 12). The dissection is finalized by separating the tumor from the fibrofatty tissue at the lateral border of the parapharyngeal space (Fig. 13). The surgical field after removal of the tumor is shown in Figure 14.

The wound is copiously irrigated, inspected and hemostasis is performed as indicated. A blood pressure above 120/80 should be confirmed prior to closure for an adequate hemostasis. A Jackson-Pratt number 7 drain is left at the surgical bed. The superficial lobe is flipped back over the facial nerve and sutured in place with a number 4-0 vicryl suture (Figs 15A and B). The platysma and SMAS are sutured with absorbable stitches and the skin is closed with 5-0 nylon stitches.

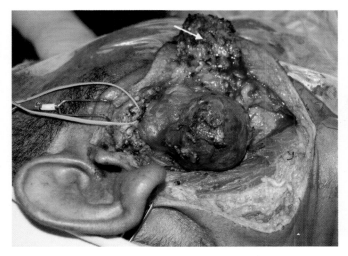

Fig. 13: Delivery of the tumor between the facial nerve branches. The dissection is finalized by separating the tumor from the fibrofatty tissue at the lateral border of the para-pharyngeal space. The arrow indicates the superficial lobe that was flipped over anteriorly

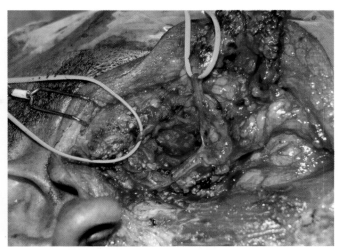

Fig. 14: The surgical field after removal of the deep lobe parotid gland tumor

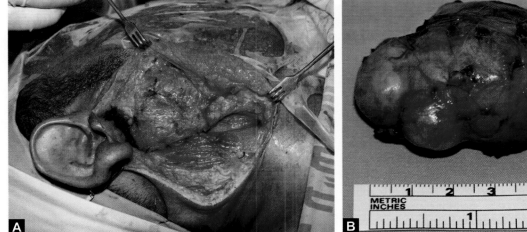

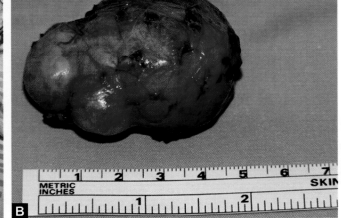

Figs 15A and B: Closure of the surgical wound. The superficial lobe is flipped back over the facial nerve and sutured in place with a number 4-0 vicryl suture. On the right the specimen, which is a deep lobe pleomorphic adenoma is resected completely without disruption of the capsule

Retrograde Dissection of the Facial Nerve

Rarely, retrograde dissection of the facial nerve branches is indicated. This technique should be utilized, when the common technique for identification of the main facial nerve trunk fails. Indications for retrograde facial nerve dissection include: (i) inability to identify the main nerve trunk; (ii) fibrosis due to prior surgery; (iii) tumor located superficial to the main trunk and; (iv) tumors that are adherent to the mastoid process. The dissection starts by identifying the marginal mandibular branch of the facial nerve, which has a relatively fewer anatomical variations relative to the other branches. The marginal mandibular branch can be usually identified superficial to the submandibular gland, at the angle of the mandible and superficial to the facial vein and artery. The dissection continues from anterior to posterior along the nerve branch. The nerve becomes wider as the retrograde dissection progresses. After identifying the main branches, the dissection continues as described earlier.

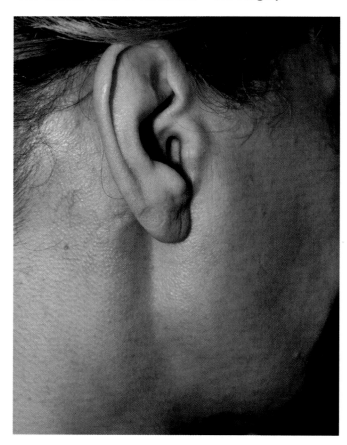

Fig. 16: A postoperative picture
taken six months after surgery

POSTOPERATIVE TREATMENT

After the surgery, the patient is extubated and immediately transferred to the post surgery care unit before the transfer to the floor. The wound is kept clean by rinsing it with saline three times a day and covered with antibiotic ointment after each cleansing. The drains are removed either 3 days after the operation or when the fluid is less than 20 ml in 24 hours. Prophylactic antibiotic treatment is not indicated in the postoperative period. A postoperative picture taken 6 months after surgery (Fig. 16) shows an excellent cosmetic result.

HIGHLIGHTS

I. Indications
- Benign or malignant tumors of the superficial lobe of the parotid gland
- Benign neoplasms of the deep lobe of the parotid gland
- Chronic inflammation, chronic sialadenitis and sialolithiasis of the parotid gland resistant to conservative therapy.

II. Contraindications
- Malignant neoplasms with facial nerve involvement
- Lymphoma of the parotid gland.

III. Special Preoperative Considerations
- Imaging using CT with contrast
- Use of intraoperative facial nerve monitoring when indicated
- Complete blood count and coagulation function test.

IV. Special Intraoperative Considerations
- Operation is performed without relaxation for cranial nerve monitoring
- Preserve the greater auricular nerve if possible
- Identify the posterior belly of the digastric early during the operation
- Identify the facial nerve using the posterior belly of the digastric muscle, the external auditory canal and the mastoid process.
- The authors do not recommend to rely on the tragal pointer as the sole anatomical landmark of the nerve
- Dissection should be performed superficial to the epineurium of the facial nerve
- Avoid stretching of the facial nerve during retraction
- Use bipolar electrocautery during the dissection
- Never cut through the glandular tissue without knowing the location of the facial nerve and its branches.
- Always monitor the movement of the facial muscles during dissection
- Careful hemostasis and clean surgical field lowers the risk of nerve injury
- Proper surgical technique and careful hemostasis during and after surgery diminish the risk of bleeding
- Avoid flap necrosis in elderly patients or after radiation therapy by proper planning of the skin incision and elevation of the flap in a correct plane
- Avoid capsular rapture during surgery
- Avoid enucleation of a parotid tumor
- The facial nerve is located more superficial and caudal, in infants and children
- A nerve stimulator may be used as an adjunct to assist identification of the nerve.

V. Special Postoperative Considerations
- Identify complications as early as possible
- Bleeding in this area can lead to hematoma and infection. Open and evacuate the wound in the operating room when growing hematoma is identified.
- Salivary leak is usually treated conservatively with local pressure.

VI. Complications
- Bleeding
- Seroma
- Frey's syndrome
- Wound infection
- Fistula
- Temporary facial nerve palsy
- Permanent facial nerve paralysis
- Anesthesia in the periauricular area.
  - Direct consequence of surgery rather than a complication.

ADDITIONAL READING

1. Arriaga MA, Myers EN. The surgical management of chronic parotitis. Laryngoscope. 1990;100(12):1270-5.
2. Carew JF, Spiro RH, Singh B, et al. Treatment of recurrent pleomorphic adenomas of the parotid gland. Otolaryngol Head Neck Surg. 1999;121(5):539-42.
3. Frankenthaler RA, Luna MA, Lee SS, et al. Prognostic variables in parotid gland cancer. Arch Otolaryngol Head Neck Surg. 1991;117(11):1251-6.
4. Lai SY, Weinstein GS, Chalian AA, et al. Parotidectomy in the treatment of aggressive cutaneous malignancies. Arch Otolaryngol Head Neck Surg. 2002;128(5):521-6.
5. Murrah VA, Batsakis JG. Salivary duct carcinoma. Ann Otol Rhinol Laryngol. 1994;103(3):244-7.
6. Osborne RF, Shaw T, Zandifar H, et al. Elective parotidectomy in the management of advanced auricular malignancies. Laryngoscope. 2008;118(12):2139-45.
7. Spiro JD, Spiro RH. Cancer of the parotid gland: role of 7th nerve preservation. World J Surg. 2003;27(7):863-7.
8. Spiro RH. Diagnosis and pitfalls in the treatment of parotid tumors. Semin Surg Oncol. 1991;7(1):20-4.

Chapter **33**

Selective Neck Dissection of Levels I–IV

Ziv Gil, Dan M Fliss

INTRODUCTION

In head and neck cancers, the type, grade, site and stage of the primary tumor determine the risk of cervical metastases and therefore, the form of treatment. In oral tongue squamous cell carcinoma, the risk of neck metastasis is also significantly associated with the depth of tumor invasion. The patterns of spread of cancer to cervical lymph nodes can be predicted based on the anatomical location of the primary tumor. Therefore, in the absence of a clinical evidence of neck disease, the pathological features of the primary tumor along with its site of origin and clinical T stage are used to stratify the risk of positive neck metastases and therefore, the need for a neck dissection. When the risk for positive neck lymph nodes exceeds 15–25%, elective neck dissection is indicated not only for treatment, but also as a staging procedure for evaluation of the need for an adjuvant therapy. Exact knowledge of the anatomy of the neck and its adjacent structures and, the risk and location of common cervical metastases, are essential for the operative treatment of head and neck cancer. A selective neck dissection, directed to the basins at risk for lymphatic spread is commonly used for this purpose. For example, resection of levels I–IV is performed for oral cavity cancers and of levels II–IV is performed for cancers of the larynx and hypopharynx (Fig. 1). Due to the rich lymphatic system of the supraglottis and the frequent involvement of multiple subsites, supraglottic tumors will necessitate bilateral neck dissection. Similarly, tongue and glottic tumors that cross the midline will also necessitate neck dissection bilaterally. Advances in the anatomical elucidation of the neck, understanding the biological behavior of tumors and improvement in surgical methods have contributed to the emergence of the selective neck dissection technique resulting in excellent survival and functional outcomes.

Although, a selective neck dissection is generally performed in patients without clinical evidence of neck metastases, there is emerging data that the same operation can be also performed on patients with positive lymph nodes that are anatomically amenable, provided an adequate surgical margin can be safely obtained. These mainly include patients with a single positive lymph node less than 3 cm in size (N1 neck stage). Radical neck dissection is reserved for patients with clinical or radiological evidence of neck disease, when complete tumor removal is unattainable without sacrificing of cranial nerves, the internal jugular vein and the sternocleidomastoid muscle. These may often include those patients with group of lymph nodes greater than 6 cm in size and with macroscopic evidence of extracapsular extension. For patients with multiple nodes but with no evidence of extracapsular extension (neck stage of N2), comprehensive neck dissection with preservation of the sternocleidomastoid muscle, internal jugular vein and spinal accessory nerve is often used.

In this chapter, the technique practiced by the authors for surgical removal of the lymphatic tissue of neck levels I, II, III and IV, which is frequently used in patients with oral cavity squamous cell carcinoma, without clinical evidence of positive neck nodes will be described in details. This technique allows complete extirpation of the neck lymphatic system, preservation of the cranial nerves and sternocleidomastoid muscle. The surgical technique for removal of levels II, III and IV, which is usually practiced in thyroid and larynx carcinomas, is identical sparing level I. In contrast to oral cavity and larynx squamous cell carcinomas, for differentiated thyroid carcinoma, neck dissection of levels II–IV is only utilized when there is clinical evidence of positive lymph nodes.

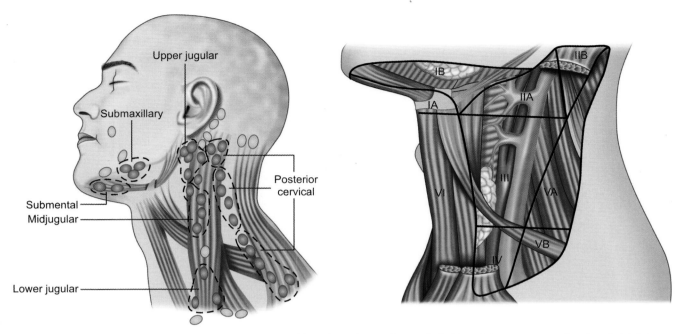

Fig. 1: The levels of the neck. The distribution of lymph nodes in the neck (left) and the corresponding levels (right)

PREOPERATIVE EVALUATION AND ANESTHESIA

All patients scheduled for operation are evaluated preoperatively by a head and neck surgeon and an anesthesiologist. Radiological evaluation of the neck is mandatory for clinical staging prior to surgery. Neck imaging usually includes computed tomography (CT) with contrast. This allows evaluation of nodal metastases and tumor infiltration to vessels, muscles, nerves, cartilages and bony tissue. Ultrasound of the neck may be used as an adjunct for fine needle aspiration. The radiological staging of the patients with advance stage (stage III–IV) is completed by using a positron emission tomography-CT hybrid (PET-CT) that is used for assessing the presence of regional and distal metastases. Imaging should be used at all times prior to surgery since it can influence decision-making regarding the treatment. All patients should also undergo routine blood tests including complete blood count and coagulation function tests.

The authors do not recommend routine administration of prophylactic antibiotics in clean operations. First-generation cephalosporins and metronidazole are routinely used if the operation includes dissection in the oral cavity or larynx. Surgery is performed under general anesthesia without muscle relaxation. This allows the surgeon monitoring of the spinal accessory, hypoglossal, phrenic and marginal mandibular nerves, and brachial plexus during dissection

with electrocautery. Intraoperative monitoring of the facial nerve is performed in selected cases, when the dissection includes the parotid gland.

SURGICAL TECHNIQUE

Skin Incision

The patient is placed on the operating room table in a supine position. The head is stabilized with a soft donut holder and the whole operating table is then elevated in an angle with the head up in order to minimize bleeding. The surgical access is planned through a transverse neck incision (Fig. 2). Marking of the incision is preferably performed with the neck slightly flexed in order to identify the lines of relaxed skin tension. The incision normally extends from the mastoid tip to the cricoid arch, 2–3 fingers below the ramus of the mandible along a transverse skin crest in the lower neck. In cases of thyroid surgery, the normal thyroidectomy incision can be extended laterally along a skin crest up to the posterior border of the sternocleidomastoid muscle. Eliminating the horizontal component of the skin incision in this case allows access to levels II–VI and a better cosmetic outcome than the traditional hockey stick incision. After incision marking, a roll is placed under the shoulders to hyperextend the neck and the head is rotated toward the contralateral side.

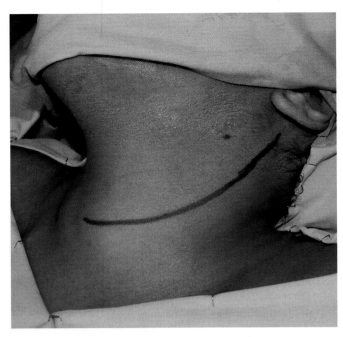

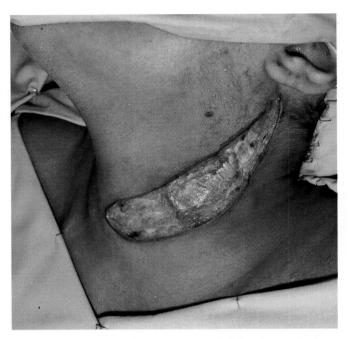

Fig. 2: Planning of the neck incision. Marking of the incision is preferably performed with the neck slightly flexed in order to identify the lines of relaxed skin tension. The incision normally extends from the mastoid tip to the cricoid arch, 2–3 fingers below the ramus of the mandible along a transverse skin crest in the lower neck. The levels of the neck are shown on the right

Fig. 3: Skin incision. After injection with lidocaine and adrenaline, the skin is incised with a number 15 blade and subsequent dissection of the subcutaneous tissue and the platysma is carried out with an electrocautery at the lowest effective setting

This position moves the lymphatic content of the neck anteromedial and cephalad, and facilitates dissection of levels II–IV. The patient is then prepped and draped in a standard surgical fashion.

Skin Incision and Elevation of Subplatysmal Flaps

The skin is incised with a number 15 blade and subsequent dissection of the subcutaneous tissue and the platysma is carried out with an electrocautery at the lowest effective setting (Fig. 3). Subplatysmal flaps are elevated superiorly, 1 cm below the ramus of the mandible and inferiorly to the sternum (Fig. 4). This plane separates the superficial cervical fascia from the superficial layer of the deep cervical fascia. Care is taken to prevent injury to the marginal mandibular branch of the facial nerve. The nerve runs within the fascia superior to the submandibular gland. Injury to the nerve is prevented by elevation of the flap immediately below the platysma leaving the superficial layer of the deep cervical fascia on the submandibular gland. If dissection of the pre- and postvascular lymph nodes is indicated, the flap is elevated to the level of the mandible exposing the facial artery

and vein. The routine removal of the pre- and postvascular lymph nodes in the neck dissection is not included. There are two main indications for extirpation of these nodes: (i) skin or lip cancers for which the lymph nodes around the facial artery may be the primary echelon and; (ii) clinical or radiological evidence of positive nodes at this level. The flaps are retracted and held using skin hooks.

Dissection along the Sternocleidomastoid Muscle

The superficial layer of the deep cervical fascia that unwraps the sternocleidomastoid muscle should be stripped from the muscle. This dissection is usually started by placing hemostats on the fascia at the anterior border of the muscle retracting the tissue medially (Fig. 5). The dissection is started at the posterior border of the muscle, along the entire length of the muscle in a lateral to medial plane. The dissection is made with electrocautery and small vessels interconnecting the superficial and deep borders of the muscle are electrocautered with a bipolar or clamped and divided. When the dissection reaches the external jugular vein, the vein is clamped at its superior border and preserved. This vein may be used later for free flap anastomosis if this is indicated. The branches of the great auricular nerve is preserved if possible, however

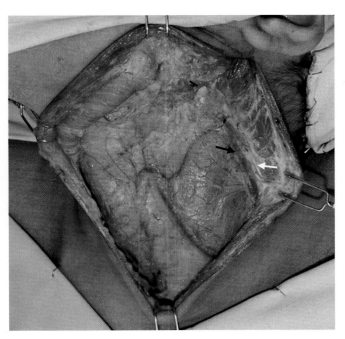

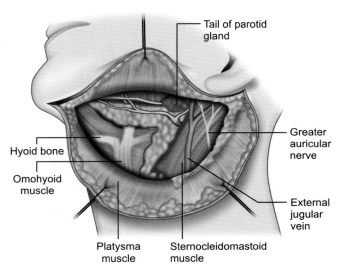

Tail of parotid gland

Greater auricular nerve

External jugular vein

Hyoid bone

Omohyoid muscle

Platysma muscle

Sternocleidomastoid muscle

Fig. 4: Elevation of superior and inferior platysmal flaps. Subplatysmal flaps are elevated superiorly 1 cm below the ramus of the mandible and inferiorly to the sternum. The greater auricular nerve (white arrow) and external jugular vein (black arrow) are indicated

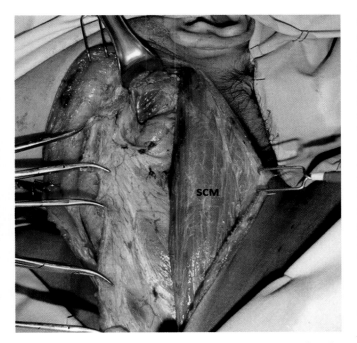

SCM

Fig. 5: Dissection along the sternocleidomastoid muscle. The dissection is started at the posterior border of the sternocleidomastoid muscle (SCM) along the entire length of the muscle in a lateral to medial plane

division of the nerve may be indicated to release the sternocleidomastoid muscle at its superior border. As the deep aspect of the muscle is approached, care is taken to avoid injury to the spinal accessory nerve that enters the muscle at the junction of its upper and middle-third and lateral to its medial border (Fig. 6). The dissection now continues deep to the muscles from medial to lateral along its entire length. The dissection continues laterally up to the posterior border of the muscle completely releasing the muscle from its fascia. At this point, the omohyoid muscle is elevated with a Adson clamp and divided at the junction of its anterior and posterior belly with electrocautery (Fig. 7). Alternatively, if there is no evidence of nodal metastases in level IV, the muscle can be separated from its surrounding tissue and retracted with a Richardson retractor in an inferolateral direction, exposing the supraclavicular area.

Dissection along the Spinal Accessory Nerve

After the sternocleidomastoid muscle is exposed and stripped from its surrounding tissue, the spinal accessory nerve is identified at its upper-third. The next step is exposure of the posterior belly of the digastric muscle. The muscle crosses the angle formed by the sternocleidomastoid muscle and the ramus of the mandible in the middle (Fig. 8). Exposure of

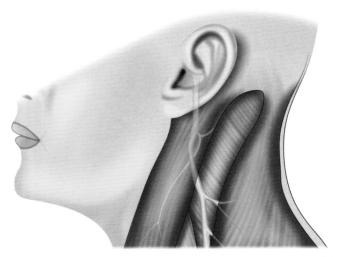

Fig. 6: The spinal accessory nerve. The spinal accessory nerve that enters the muscle at the junction of its upper and middle-third and lateral to its medial border

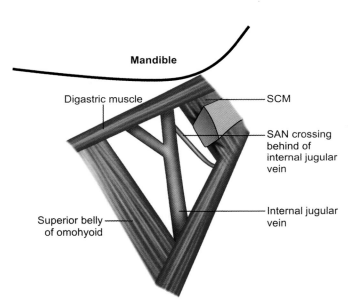

Fig. 8: The posterior belly of the digastric muscle. The muscle crosses the angle formed by the sternocleidomastoid muscle (SCM) and the ramus of the mandible in the middle.
SAN: Spinal accessory nerve

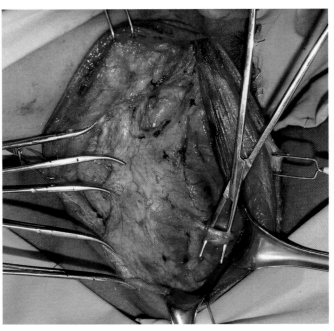

Fig. 7: Dividing the omohyoid muscle. The omohyoid muscle is elevated with a Adson clamp and divided at the junction of its anterior and posterior belly with electrocautery

the posterior belly of the digastric muscle begins by retraction of the sternocleidomastoid muscle with a Richardson retractor laterally and of the ramus of the mandible with an Army-Navy retractor cephalad. The next step is separation of the tissue superficial to the digastric muscle with a Adson clamp and electrocautery. The spinal accessory nerve, which

runs between the upper third of the sternocleidomastoid muscle and the posterior belly of the digastric muscle in now exposed. A Adson clamp is used to elevate the lymphatic tissue away from the nerve and the tissue is cauterized and divided with a bipolar and a scalpel, releasing the tethered nerve (Fig. 9). Using this technique, the nerve is completely exposed from its entry to the sternocleidomastoid muscle inferiorly to the posterior belly of the digastric muscle. Care is taken not to injure the internal jugular vein, which lies immediately deep to the superior portion of the nerve. The nerve is then elevated on a vessel loop and separated circumferentially from its surrounding tissue (Fig. 10). Frequently, a small artery runs parallel to the nerve. This artery should be preserved in order to maintain the vascular supply to the nerve.

Once the nerve is freed, dissection is continued posterior and cephalad to the nerve in level IIb, also known as the submuscular recess. Here, the tissue which lies on the splenius capitis and lavatory scapula muscles and between the posterior belly of the digastric muscle and the posterior border of the superior third of the sternocleidomastoid muscle is extirpated. Dissection is performed with electrocautery from lateral to medial without injuring the spinal accessory nerve. Within this area, frequently lie branches of the occipital and sternocleidomastoid arteries, which are cauterized with a bipolar. The dissection continues

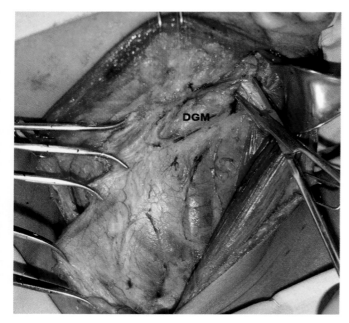

Fig. 9: Exposure of the spinal accessory nerve. The spinal accessory nerve runs between the upper third of the sterno-cleidomastoid muscle and the posterior belly of the digastric muscle within the lymphatic tissue. A Adson clamp is used to elevate the lymphatic tissue away from the nerve and the tissue is cauterized and divided with a bipolar and a scalpel, releasing the tethered nerve.
DGM: Digastric muscle

in a superior to inferomedial direction with electrocautery. As the dissection reaches the nerve, bipolar cauterization and sharp dissection are used in order to reduce injury to spinal accessory nerve. At this point, the lymphatic content of level IIb is passed beneath the spinal accessory in order to keep it in continuity with the whole specimen as in Figure 10.

Dissection along the Transverse Cervical Plexus and Brachial Plexus

After separating of the tissue overlying the spinal accessory nerve, the dissection continues between the posterior border of the sternocleidomastoid muscle and the internal jugular vein. At this level, lie the sensory branches of the transverse cervical plexus (Fig. 11). The fatty tissue overlying the internal jugular vein is now grabbed with 3–4 Babcock's graspers and retracted medially. The specimen can be now freed from the cervical roots (Fig. 12). While the dissection continues medially, the anterior scalene muscle is exposed. As the dissection reaches the supraclavicular area, the fatty tissue that overlies the brachial plexus is gently divided and tied. The brachial plexus can now be easily identified at the root of the neck between the anterior and middle scalene muscles. Again, care is taken to stay superficial to the fascia overlying the scalene muscles to prevent the rare, but most devastating complication of brachial plexus or phrenic nerve injury. A dissection at the supraclavicular area (level IV) should be performed carefully in order to preserve the transverse

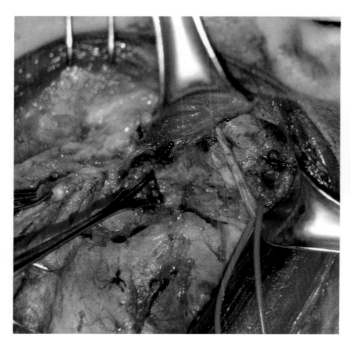

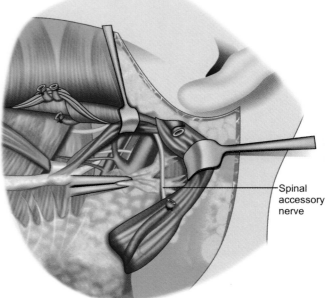

Spinal accessory nerve

Fig. 10: Dissection of level IIb. The tissue, which lies on the splenius capitis and lavatory scapula muscles, and between the posterior belly of the digastric muscle and the posterior border of the superior third of the sternocleidomastoid muscle, is extirpated

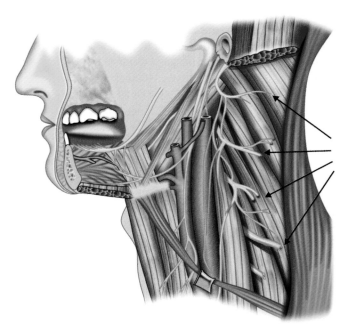

Fig. 11: The cervical plexus and its relation to the great vessels and muscles of the neck. Arrows indicate the cervical roots

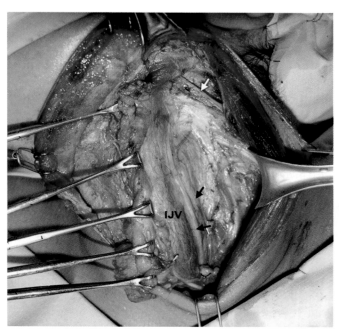

Fig. 12: Dissection along the transverse cervical plexus and brachial plexus. The fatty tissue overlying the internal jugular vein (IJV) is grabbed with 5–4 Babcock's graspers and retracted medially and the specimen is freed from the cervical roots. While the dissection continues medially, the anterior scalene muscle is exposed. The spinal accessory nerve (white arrow), common carotid artery (upper black arrow) and vagus nerve (lower black arrow) are indicated

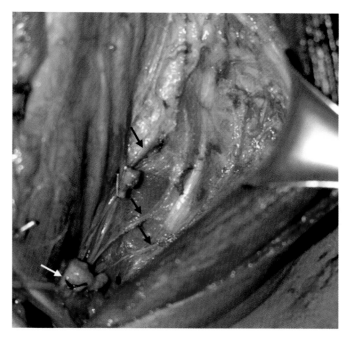

Fig. 13: The supraclavicular area. The fatty tissue at the supra-clavicular area is tied to prevent chylous leak (white arrow). In addition, care is taken to preserve the deep branches of the cervical nerves that contribute to the spinal accessory nerve (2nd, 3rd and 4th) and phrenic nerve (3rd, 4th and 5th) (black arrows)

cervical artery, supraclavicular artery and thyrocervical trunk. The fatty tissue at the supraclavicular area is tied to prevent chylous leak shown as white arrow in Figure 13. In addition, care is taken to preserve the deep branches of the cervical nerves that contribute to the spinal accessory nerve (2nd, 3rd and 4th) and phrenic nerve (3rd, 4th and 5th) as in Figure 13. Again, this is accomplished by staying superficial to the fascia overlying the scalene muscles. The fascia is only violated if invaded by tumor. The dissection now continues toward the common carotid artery.

Dissection along the Common Carotid Artery and Internal Jugular Vein

As the dissection continues from lateral to medial, the carotid sheath is exposed. Here, dissection with a fine Adson clamp is preferred to prevent accidental injury to the vagus nerve or to the adventitia of the carotid artery. This method is preferred in previously irradiated neck or in revision surgery. A sharp dissection with a number 15 knife can be performed instead. The carotid sheath is exposed but not violated and the dissection is continued anterior to the artery in order to preserve the sympathetic trunk, which lies deep to the artery. The Babcock's clamps are now repositioned to allow adequate traction (from lateral to medial) of the tissue overlying the carotid sheath and internal jugular vein. Here, the operation is always performed with a sharp dissection allowing complete removal of the fascia investing the internal jugular vein (Fig. 14). This is achieved by moving the scalpel along the entire length of the vein in a cephalad to caudal direction and vice versa. A gauze sponge may be used here to keep the tension of the specimen. As the vein is freed from the specimen, the thin branches of the vein are carefully divided and tied with a 4-0 silk suture. Next, the larger branches of the facial and middle thyroid veins are identified, clamped, divided and ligated in a similar way. The area in the lower part of the vein may contain large lymphatic vessels; the thoracic duct on the left and the right lymphatic duct, if a right neck dissection is performed. Regardless if identified or not, the tissue that accompanies the vessels is clamped with small titanium clips or tied with number 3-0 silk suture.

The surgeon should be aware that within the area of level IV, the jugular vein may be rotated and folded on itself and accidental injury with the blade should be avoided. Bleeding as a result of injury to the wall of the internal jugular vein can be easily controlled by suturing of the cut with a number 6-0 interrupted sutures. On the cephalad portion of the internal jugular vein, the dissection is continued inferior to the posterior belly of the digastric muscle. Here, it is advised to use meticulous dissection with a thin hemostat in order to prevent injury to the internal jugular vein deep to the muscle or to its lingual branch. In case of clinical evidence of positive nodes in level II, the digastric belly can be retracted cephalad exposing the most distal part of the vein at the base of skull. This maneuver may also prevent accidental injury to a folded vein. Injury in this area may be difficult to control and hemostasis may require tying of the vein. Rarely, the dissection in this area can be challenging, if a large metastatic lymph node with extracapsular extension if involved. If the surgeon is concerned of vein injury or of leaving cancerous tissue in this area, the dissection may be continued from another direction. For example, dissection of level I may be continued from medial to lateral according to the need of surgery and the location of the tumor leaving upper level II for the very last part of the procedure.

As the internal jugular vein is completely freed from its fascia, the dissection is continued medially toward the carotid sheath and the specimen is completely freed from the great vessels of the neck.

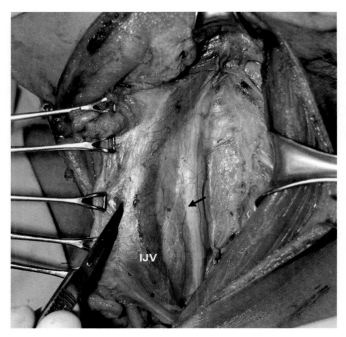

Fig. 14: Dissection along the common carotid artery and internal jugular vein. The Babcock's clamps are now repositioned to allow adequate traction (from lateral to medial) of the tissue overlying the carotid sheath and internal jugular vein (IJV). Here, the operation is always performed with a sharp dissection allowing complete removal of the fascia investing the internal jugular vein

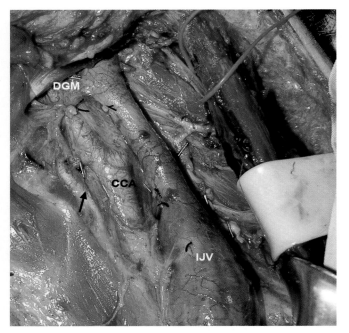

Fig. 15: Dissection along the strap muscles. The dissection continues at the medial border of the dissection along the sternohyoid and sternothyroid muscles. The superior thyroid artery (black arrow) is preserved by staying superficial to the strap muscles.
DGM: Digastrics muscle; IJV: Internal jugular vein; CCA: Common carotid artery

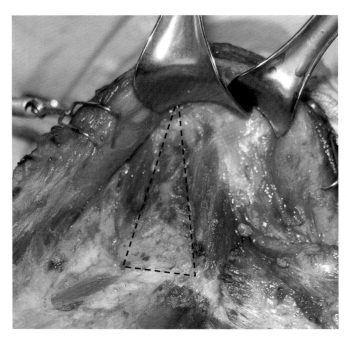

Fig. 16: Dissection of the submental triangle. This dissection includes all the fatty tissue between the anterior belly of the digastrics muscle in the contralateral and ipsilateral side of the dissection

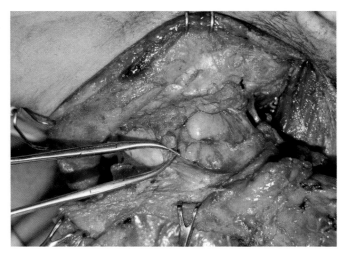

Fig. 17: Ligation of the facial artery and vein

Dissection along the Strap Muscles

The specimen is now retracted superiorly and the branches of the ansa cervicalis nerve are divided and kept on the specimen along with the anterior belly of the omohyoid muscle. The dissection continues at the medial border of the dissection along the sternohyoid and sternothyroid muscles. The superior thyroid artery and external branch of the superior thyroid artery are preserved by staying superficial to the strap muscles (Fig. 15). The dissection is continued from lateral to medial and from inferior to superior toward the hyoid bone and the digastric muscle. The anterior branches of the ansa hypoglossi may be used here to trace the hypoglossal nerve, which lies inferior to the posterior belly of the digastric muscle, anterior to the distal portion of the internal jugular vein and superficial to the internal and external branches of the carotid artery. Care is now taken to the last part of the operation, extirpation of level I.

Dissection of the Submandibular and Submental Lymph Nodes

The borders of level I are: (i) the ramus of the mandible and its symphysis superiorly; (ii) the digastric muscle inferiorly and posteriorly; (iii) the hyoid bone in the midline and inferiorly and; (iv) the anterior belly of the contralateral digastric muscle medially (Fig. 1). The deep border of the

dissection is the mylohyoid muscle. First the lymphatic tissue of the submental triangle is dissected (level Ia). The dissection here starts by delineating the superior, lateral and medial borders of the dissection. The specimen is retracted inferiorly and the anterior bellies of the digastric muscles on the ipsilateral and contralateral sides are identified (Fig. 16). The dissection continues below the symphysis of the mandible from superior to inferior. As the mylohyoid muscle is exposed, the submental vessels are ligated with a bipolar.

Next, the tissue between the digastric muscle and the ramus of the mandible is extirpated (level Ib) along with the whole specimen. The dissection starts by delineating the superior border for the dissection parallel to the lower part of the ramus of the mandible. In order to preserve the marginal mandibular branch of the facial nerve, it is advisable to first identify the facial vein, which lies superficial to the submandibular gland. The vein is clamped, divided and ligated, and distal portion is reflected superiorly, protecting the nerve (Fig. 17). The nerve lies superficial to the facial artery and vein (Fig. 18). After the facial artery and vein are ligated, their distal stump is reflected up protecting the nerve.

The dissection is now safely continued below the distal stump of the vein. As the dissection continues superficial to the submandibular gland, the facial artery is identified and divided releasing the gland. The specimen is now retracted with a Babcock's clamp caudally and the mylohyoid muscle is exposed. The muscle is gently retracted medially with an angled retractor exposing the lingual nerve and the submandibular ganglion (Fig. 19). Before the clamping the tissue inferior to the lingual nerve, the submandibular gland is rotated superiorly exposing the medial portion of the hypoglossal nerve. Only now, when both the lingual

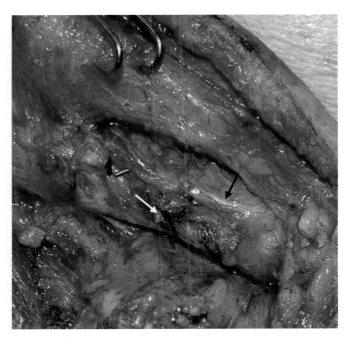 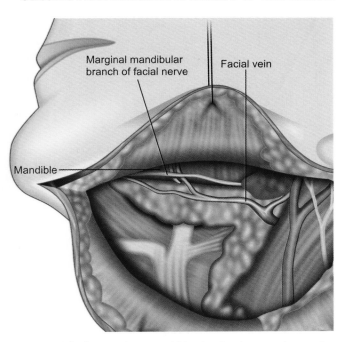

Fig. 18: The marginal mandibular branch of the facial nerve. The nerve (black arrow) runs within the fascia superior to the submandibular gland. Injury to the nerve is prevented by elevation of the flap immediately below the platysma leaving the superficial layer of the deep cervical fascia on the submandibular gland. The nerve lies superficial to the facial artery and vein. After the facial artery and vein are ligated (white arrow), their distal stump is reflected up protecting the nerve

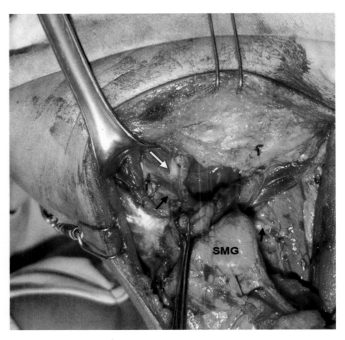 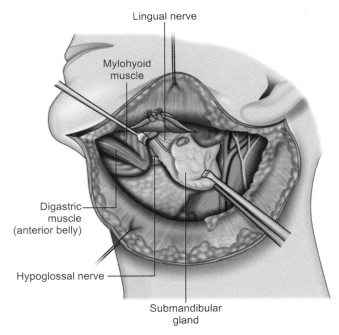

Fig. 19: Dissection of level IIb. The submandibular gland (SMG) is reflected inferiorly. The lingual nerve (white arrow) and hypoglossal nerve (black arrows) are identified before ligation of the submandibular ganglion and Wharton's duct

and hypoglossal nerves are identified superior to the medial portion of the digastric muscle, a clamp is placed below the lingual nerve and its neighboring vessels are divided and ligated (Fig. 20). Next, the submandibular duct and its surrounding tissue is clamped and divided inferior to the lingual nerve. The dissection of the submandibular triangle

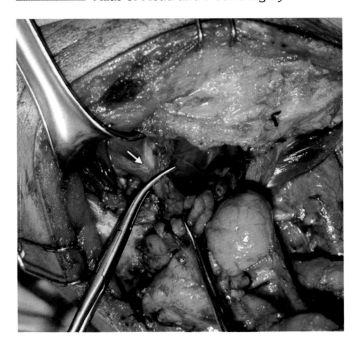

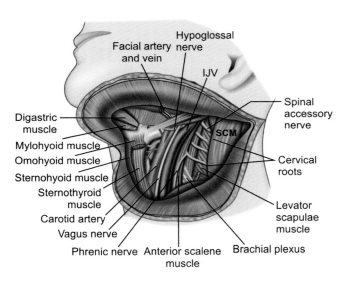

Fig. 20: Dividing of the tissue below the lingual nerve. Only when both the lingual (white arrow) and hypoglossal nerves are identified superior to the medial portion of the digastric muscle, a clamp is placed below the lingual nerve (submandibular ganglion) and its neighboring vessels are divided and ligated

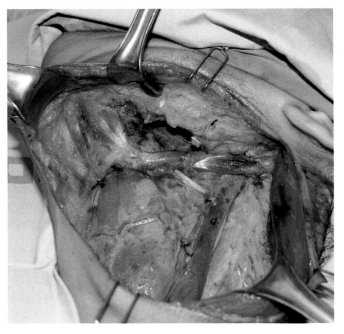

Fig. 21: The surgical field after completion of the neck dissection.
IJV: Internal jugular vein; SCM: Sternocleidomastoid muscle

is completed by division of the facial artery on the second time above the digastric muscle (Fig. 21).

The specimen is oriented and each level is submitted separately to the pathology lab for analysis (Fig. 22). The wound is copiously irrigated, inspected and hemostasis is performed as indicated. A blood pressure above 120/80

should be confirmed prior to closure for adequate hemostasis. If a chyle leak is suspected, a Valsalva maneuver can be performed by keeping positive ventilation. A Jackson-Pratt number 7 drain is left at the surgical bed, the platysma is sutured with absorbable stitches and the skin is closed with 5-0 nylon stitches or with clips.

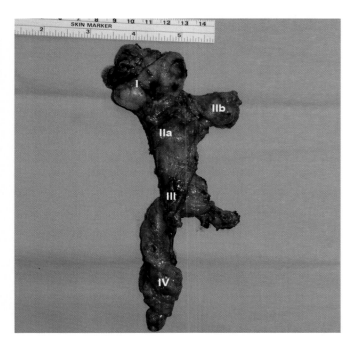

Fig. 22: The surgical specimen. The levels of the neck are indicated. After the neck dissection is completed, the specimen is oriented and each level is submitted separately to the pathology laboratory for analysis

POSTOPERATIVE TREATMENT

After the surgery, the patient is extubated and immediately transferred to the post surgery care unit before his transfer to the floor. The wound is kept clean by rinsing it with saline three times a day and covered with antibiotic ointment after each cleansing. The drains are removed either, 3 days after the operation or when the fluid is less than 20–30 ml in 24 hours. Prophylactic antibiotic treatment is not indicated in the postoperative period. For pain control, the patients are treated with nonsteroidal anti-inflammatory drugs (diclofenac 75 mg intramuscularly or orally, or rofecoxib 50 mg) once daily and with tramadol (50–100 mg) if the patient asks for them or if the nurses felt it to be necessary. If free flap is also performed, selective COX-2 inhibitors should be avoided.

HIGHLIGHTS

I. Indications
- Squamous cell carcinoma of the oral cavity with no clinical or radiological evidence of lymph node metastases.
- Head and neck squamous cell carcinoma with clinical or radiological evidence of small lymph node metastasis (clinical stage of N1).
- Clinical evidence of nodal disease in well-differentiated thyroid cancers (levels II–IV)
- Larynx cancer with or without evidence of cervical metastases (levels II–IV).

II. Contraindications
- Clinical evidence of multiple or large positive lymph nodes (clinical stage of N2 or N3)
- Positive lymph nodes in level V
- Involvement of the internal jugular vein or spinal accessory nerve
- Tumor invades the prevertebral fascia, encases carotid artery or involves mediastinal structures.

III. Special Preoperative Considerations
- Imaging using CT with contrast
- Imaging with PET-CT
- Complete blood count and coagulation function tests.

IV. Special Intraoperative Considerations
- Operation is performed without relaxation for cranial nerve monitoring
- Preserve the external jugular vein if free flap reconstruction is indicated
- Identify the spinal accessory nerve in the upper third of the sternocleidomastoid
- Identify the posterior belly of the digastric before freeing the accessory nerve from its surrounding tissue.
- Preserve the spinal branches, which contribute to the accessory nerve
- Dissection should be performed superficial to the fascia overlying the scalene muscles to prevent phrenic nerve injury.
- Careful dissection along the carotid artery diminishes the risk of vascular injury and vagus nerve paralysis
- Sharp dissection along the internal jugular vein allows complete removal of the fascia overlying the great vessels.
- Meticulous dissection of the supraclavicular area and the use of silk ties to prevent chylous leak.
- Prevent injury to the internal jugular vein near the skull base by meticulous dissection with a hemostat
- Utilize the facial vein as a guide to prevent injury to the marginal mandibular branch of the facial nerve
- Identify both the lingual and hypoglossal nerves before dividing the submandibular ganglion
- Proper surgical technique and careful hemostasis during and after surgery diminish the risk of bleeding.
- Valsalva maneuver may be used to identify occult chyle leak at the root of the neck.

V. Special Postoperative Considerations
- Identify complications as early as possible

- Bleeding in this area can lead to an imminent airway obstruction. Open and evacuate the wound at the bedside if airway obstruction occurs.
- Chyle leak is usually treated conservatively with modified diet and local pressure.
- Early reinstatement of neck and shoulders physiotherapy.

VI. Complications
- Bleeding
- Seroma
- Chylous leak
- Wound infection
- Cranial nerve paralysis (spinal accessory and shoulder dysfunction, hypoglossal, lingual, marginal mandibular branch of the facial nerve, vagus, phrenic, brachial plexus, sympathetic trunk)
- Anesthesia in the periocular area (a direct consequence of surgery rather than a complication)
- Jugular vein thrombosis in perioperative radiotherapy treatment.

ADDITIONAL READING

1. Andersen PE, Warren F, Spiro J, et al. Results of selective neck dissection in management of the node-positive neck. Arch Otolaryngol Head Neck Surg. 2002;128(10):1180-4.

2. Byers RM, Clayman GL, McGill D, et al. Selective neck dissections for squamous carcinoma of the upper aerodigestive tract: patterns of regional failure. Head Neck. 1999;21(6):499-505.

3. Byers RM, Weber RS, Andrews T, et al. Frequency and therapeutic implications of "skip metastases" in the neck from squamous carcinoma of the oral tongue. Head Neck. 1997;19(1):14-9.

4. Carvalho AL, Kowalski LP, Borges JA, et al. Ipsilateral neck cancer recurrences after elective supraomohyoid neck dissection. Arch Otolaryngol Head Neck Surg. 2000;126(3):410-2.

5. Ferlito A, Rinaldo A, Silver CE, et al. Elective and therapeutic selective neck dissection. Oral Oncol. 2006;42(1):14-25. Epub 2005 Jun 23.

6. Gil Z, Carlson DL, Boyle JO, et al. Lymph node density is a significant predictor of outcome in patients with oral cancer. Cancer. 2009 ;115(24):5700-10.

7. Kupferman ME, Patterson M, Mandel SJ, et al. Patterns of lateral neck metastasis in papillary thyroid carcinoma. Arch Otolaryngol Head Neck Surg. 2004;130(7):857-60.

8. Pellitteri PK, Ferlito A, Rinaldo A, et al. Planned neck dissection following chemoradiotherapy for advanced head and neck cancer: is it necessary for all? Head Neck. 2006;28(2):166-75.

9. Puri SK, Fan CY, Hanna E. Significance of extracapsular lymph node metastases in patients with head and neck squamous cell carcinoma. Curr Opin Otolaryngol Head Neck Surg. 2003;11(2):119-23.

Chapter **34**

Comprehensive Neck Dissection of Levels II–V

Ziv Gil, Dan M Fliss

INTRODUCTION

Head and neck cancers include tumors originating in the skin, oral cavity, oropharynx, hypopharynx, larynx, nasopharynx, paranasal sinuses and thyroid. Demographic and geographic factors as well as exposure to different carcinogens (e.g. nicotine, alcohol or viruses) contribute to the differential incidence of these tumors. Tumors originating at different sites also vary by pathophysiology, biological behavior and sensitivity to radiotherapy and chemotherapy. Such factors play an important role in tailoring appropriate treatment for these patients.

The most common malignant tumors of the head and neck include squamous cell carcinomas (SCC), salivary gland and thyroid carcinomas. Management of head and neck cancers should be planned according to the tumor's characteristics, patient factors and the expertise of the medical team. The main goals of therapy are ablation of cancer while minimizing morbidity, preservation of function and improvement of patient's quality of life. When the risk for positive neck lymph nodes exceeds 15%, elective neck dissection is indicated, while palpable neck disease necessitates in most cases comprehensive clearance of all of the lymphatic basins in the neck.

In this chapter, the technique practiced by the authors for surgical removal of the lymphatic tissue of neck levels II, III, IV, V, which is frequently used in patients with thyroid cancers, scalp or skin cancers with clinical evidence of positive neck nodes in any of these levels will be described in details. This technique allows complete extirpation of the neck lymphatic system, preservation of the cranial nerves, large vessels and sternocleidomastoid muscle.

TAILORING OF SURGERY

The general principle of the surgery is extirpation of the lymphatic basins of the primary tumor, while preserving the accessory nerve, internal jugular vein and the sternocleidomastoid muscle. These include the submandibular, submental, jugulodigastric, midjugular, lower jugular, posterior neck and retroauricular nodes. Figure 1 shows a depiction with the location of the nodes to be resected. Radical or modified radical neck dissection is reserved for cases in which complete tumor removal is unattainable without scarifying any or all of these structures.

The type, grade, site and stage of the primary tumor determine the risk of cervical metastases and therefore, the form of treatment. The patterns of spread of cancer to cervical lymph nodes are predictable based on the anatomical location of the primary tumor. Therefore, in the absence of a clinical evidence of neck disease, the pathological features of the primary tumor along with its site of origin and clinical T stage are used to stratify the risk of positive neck metastases and therefore, the need for a neck dissection. When the risk for positive neck lymph nodes exceeds 15–25%, elective neck dissection is indicated. A selective neck dissection of levels II–V is usually indicated for thyroid cancers with clinical evidence of neck metastases. Other indications are advance skin squamous cell carcinoma in the postauricular area, malignant melanoma with positive sentinel lymph node or presence of nodal metastases in levels II–V. Carcinomas of the oropharynx, nasopharynx, larynx and hypopharynx are usually treated with primary radiotherapy with or without chemotherapy even in the presence of neck disease. Selective neck dissection of levels II–V is reserved for patients who fail the nonsurgical treatment.

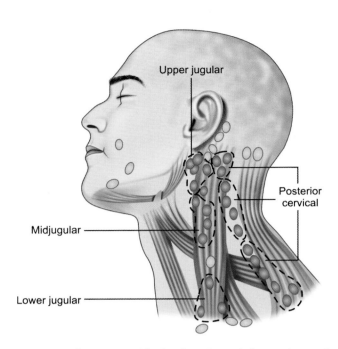

Fig. 1: A depiction with the location of the nodes to be resected. These include the jugulodigastric, midjugular, lower jugular, posterior neck and retroauricular nodes

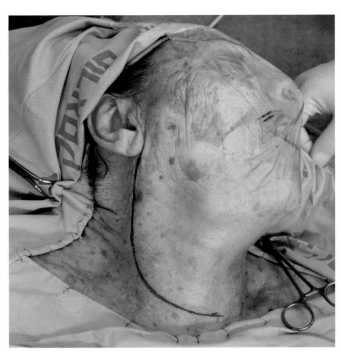

Fig. 2: Planning of the neck incision. A patient with T4N2bM0 poorly differentiated carcinoma of the parotid gland. The surgical access is planned through a hockey stick neck incision, which is extended in its upper-part posterior to a standard parotidectomy incision

PREOPERATIVE EVALUATION AND ANESTHESIA

Physical examination and preoperative imaging are required for clinical staging and treatment planning. The nasopharynx, hypopharynx and larynx are evaluated with a flexible endoscope, while the floor of mouth and base of tongue are better assessed using a manual exam. Radiologic evaluation of patients should include computed tomography (CT) scan of the head and neck, while well-differentiated thyroid cancers are better evaluated using ultrasound. For tongue cancers, magnetic resonance imaging (MRI) may offer better assessment of local invasion. Positron emission tomography (PET) or integrated PET-CT system offer a good assessment of locoregional and distant metastases. Pathological diagnosis prior to surgery is essential to verify suspicious neck nodes. It can be easily achieved by ultrasound guided fine needle aspiration. All patients scheduled for operation are evaluated preoperatively by a head and neck surgeon and by an anesthesiologist.

Routine administration of prophylactic antibiotics in clean operations is not recommended. To allow continuous monitoring of the cranial nerves, surgery is performed under general anesthesia without muscle relaxation.

SURGICAL TECHNIQUE

Skin Incision

The patient is placed on the operating room table in a supine position. The head is stabilized with a soft donut holder and the whole operating table is then elevated in an angle with the head up in order to minimize bleeding. The surgical access is planned through a hockey stick neck incision (Fig. 2). The incision normally extends from the nuchal line to 2 cm above the clavicle, at the level of the posterior border of the sternocleidomastoid muscle. Preferably it is placed along a transverse skin crest in the lower neck. Marking of the incision is preferably performed with the neck slightly flexed in order to identify the lines of relaxed skin tension. Alternatives, which are rarely used, include a standard Y incision with low or high bifurcation or a double Y incision (Martin's incision). However, our experience is that if placed correctly, a single incision allows convenient resection of all lymphatic tissue and better cosmetic results, especially in previously irradiated patients, which may have compromise blood supply to the flaps. In cases of thyroid surgery, it is advisable to extend the normal thyroidectomy incision further laterally along a skin crest lateral to the posterior border of the sternocleidomastoid muscle. In this technique, concealing the incision in a normal skin crest, eliminates the horizontal component of the incision and gives a better cosmetic result. After incision marking, a roll is placed under the shoulders to hyperextend the neck and the head is rotated toward the contralateral side. This position moves the lymphatic content of the neck anteriomedial and cephalad, and facilitates the dissection. The patient is then prepped and draped in a standard surgical fashion.

Skin Incision and Elevation of Subplatysmal Flaps

The skin is incised with a number 15 blade and subsequent dissection of the subcutaneous tissue and the platysma is carried out with an electrocautery at the lowest effective setting. Subplatysmal flaps are elevated superiorly, 2 cm below the ramus of the mandible medially. Posteriorly, the flap is elevated up to the occipital area and caudally up to the anterior border of the trapezius muscle (Figs 3A and B). In the presence of metastatic disease in this area, the flap may be extended posteriorly toward the nuchal line. The platysma does not reach the posterior triangle of the neck and therefore, the thickness of the flap should be kept approximately half a centimeter in this area. A too thick flap will encompass the

lymphatic tissue that need to be extirpated, whereas a thin flap may lead to skin necrosis, especially in elderly or previously irradiated patients. Anteriorly, the flap is elevated to the level of the strap muscles and inferiorly, over the clavicle. While elevating the posterior flap, care is taken to prevent injury to the spinal accessory nerve, which lies superficially within the fatty tissue of the posterior neck. Injury to the nerve is prevented by its early identification in the mid-posterior triangle. The nerves can be identified in two fingers distance above the bifurcation of the greater auricular nerve (Erb's point). When identified, the spinal accessory nerve is exposed using a fine hemostat and preserved throughout its course along the posterior triangle (Fig. 4). The nerve is gently retracted with a vessel loop and meticulously freed from its surrounding tissue and bipolar cautery. The flaps are then retracted and held using skin hooks.

Dissection Posterior to the Sternocleidomastoid Muscle

The dissection continues posteriorly, superficial to the trapezius muscle. The entire fibrofatty tissue of the neck from the suboccipital area to the supraclavicular fossa is now dissected in a posterior to medial direction starting above the

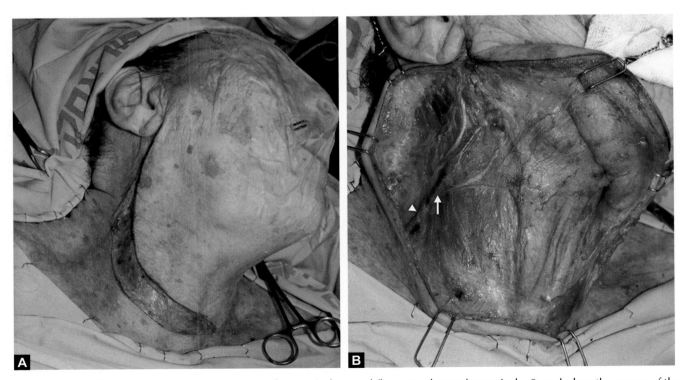

Figs 3A and B: Elevation of superior and inferior flaps. Subplatysmal flaps are elevated superiorly, 2 cm below the ramus of the mandible medially. Posteriorly, the flap is elevated up to the occipital area and caudally up to the anterior border of the trapezius muscle. The platysma does not reach the posterior triangle of the neck and therefore, the thickness of the flap should be kept approximately half a centimeter in this area. The white arrow indicates Erb's point, a site at the lateral root of the cervical plexus, where six types of nerves meet. The white arrowhead indicates the external jugular vein

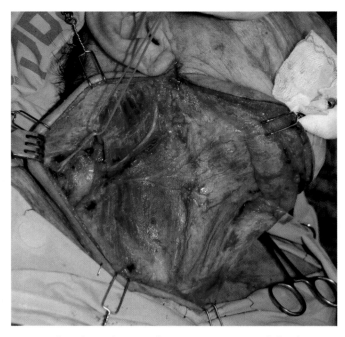

Fig. 4: Identifying the spinal accessory nerve. While elevating the posterior flap, care is taken to prevent injury to the spinal accessory nerve, which lies superficially within the fatty tissue of the posterior neck. The nerves can be identified in two fingers distance above the bifurcation of the greater auricular nerve (Erb's point). Here, the nerve is elevated on a vessel loop (blue)

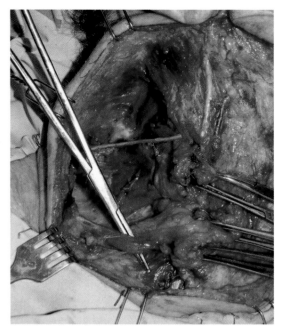

Fig. 5: Dissection above and below the spinal accessory nerve. The entire fibrofatty tissue of the neck from the suboccipital area to the supraclavicular fossa is now dissected in a posterior to medial direction starting above the nerve and continuing below it. Above the clavicle, the posterior belly of the omohyoid muscle is identified and divided

nerve and continuing below it (Fig. 5). While dissection of the level Va is predominantly performed with a monopolar cautery, a blunt dissection with a hemostat is performed in level Vb. This is done mainly to prevent inadvertent injury to the brachial plexus and transverse cervical artery, which lies within the fibrofatty tissue of the supraclavicular area. Note that the surgery does not include dissection inferior to the clavicle, as bleeding and nerve injury may occur in this area. The external jugular vein is divided lower in the neck and included in the specimen. As the dissection continues, the fibrofatty tissue is retracted medially with Babcock's graspers revealing the fascia overlying the splenius capitis, lavatory scapula and scalene muscles (Fig. 6). During this dissection, the peripheral cutaneous branches of the cervical plexus are divided and ligated. This is important since within each of these branches lay an artery that may cause significant bleeding after the operation. Care is taken not to injure the cervical branches that supply the spinal accessory nerve (2nd, 3rd and 4th) and those supplying the phrenic nerve (3rd, 4th and 5th). At this point, brachial plexus and its fascia can be identified between the anterior and middle scalene muscles and the phrenic nerve on the surface of the anterior scalene muscle. The posterior belly of the omohyoid muscle is identified and transected to be included in the specimen.

The dissection continues until the posterior border of the sternocleidomastoid muscle and the dissection is now continued anteriorly.

Dissection Along Sternocleidomastoid Muscle

To include both the posterior and anterior triangles in the same specimen, it requires a combined approach from posterior to anterior of the sternocleidomastoid muscle and vice versa. Therefore, attention is now turned to dissection along the sternocleidomastoid muscle. The superficial layer of the deep cervical fascia that unwrap the sternocleidomastoid muscle should be stripped from the muscle. This dissection is usually started by placing the hemostats on the fascia at the anterior border of the muscle, retracting the tissue medially (Fig. 7). The dissection is started at the posterior border of the muscle along the entire length of the muscle in a lateral to medial plane. The dissection is made with an electrocautery and small vessels interconnecting the superficial and deep borders of the muscle are electrocautered with a bipolar or clamped and divided. When the dissection reaches the external jugular vein, the vein is clamped at its superior border if not performed previously. As the deep aspect of the muscle is approached, care is taken to avoid injury to the proximal part of the spinal accessory nerve that enters

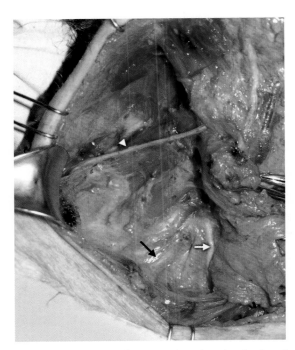

Fig. 6: Dissection along the posterior triangle. As the dissection continues, the fibrofatty tissue is retracted medially with Babcock's graspers revealing the fascia overlying the splenius capitis, lavatory scapula and scalene muscles. During this dissection, the peripheral cutaneous branches of the cervical plexus are divided and ligated. The spinal accessory nerve (white arrowhead), brachial plexus (black arrow) and phrenic nerve (white arrow) are indicated

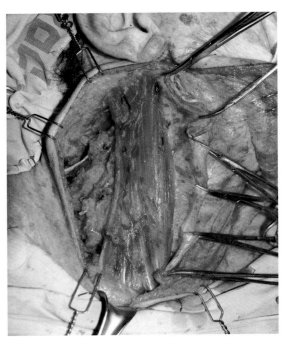

Fig. 7: Dissection along the sternocleidomastoid muscle. The dissection is started at the posterior border of the muscle along the entire length of the muscle in a lateral to medial plane. Hemostats are placed anterior to the muscle and the fascia overlying the sternocleidomastoid muscle is stripped over the muscle

the muscle at the junction of its upper and middle-third and lateral to its medial border (Fig. 8). The dissection now continues deep to the muscles from anterior to posterior along its entire length. The dissection continues laterally up to the posterior border of the muscle completely releasing the muscle from its fascia. Attention is now turned to free the proximal part of the spinal accessory nerve.

Releasing the Entire Length of the Spinal Accessory Nerve

After the sternocleidomastoid muscle is exposed and stripped from its surrounding tissue the spinal accessory nerve is identified at its upper-third. The next step is exposure of the posterior belly of the digastric muscle. The muscle crosses the angle formed by the sternocleidomastoid muscle and the ramus of the mandible in the middle. Exposure of the posterior belly of the digastric muscle begins by retraction of the sternocleidomastoid muscle with a Richardson retractor laterally and the ramus of the mandible with an Army-Navy retractor cephalad. The next step is separation of the tissue superficial to the digastric muscle with a Adson clamp and electrocautery. The spinal accessory nerve, which runs

between the upper third of the sternocleidomastoid muscle and deep to the posterior belly of the digastric muscle in now exposed. A Adson clamp is used to elevate the lymphatic tissue away from the nerve and the tissue is cauterized and divided with a bipolar and a scalpel releasing the tethered nerve (Fig. 9). Using this technique, the nerve is completely exposed from its entry to the sternocleidomastoid muscle inferiorly to the posterior belly of the digastric muscle. Care is taken not to injure the internal jugular vein, which lies immediately deep to the superior portion of the nerve. The nerve is then elevated on a vessel loop and separated circumferentially from its surrounding tissue. Frequently a small artery runs parallel to the nerve. This artery should be preserved in order to maintain the vascular supply to the nerve.

Once the nerve is freed, dissection is continued posterior and cephalad to the nerve in level IIb, also known as the submuscular recess. Here the tissue, which lies on the splenius capitis and lavatory scapula muscles, deep to the superior third of the sternocleidomastoid muscle is extirpated. Dissection is performed with an electrocautery from lateral to medial without injuring the spinal accessory nerve. Within this area frequently lie branches of the occipital and sternocleidomastoid arteries, which are cauterized

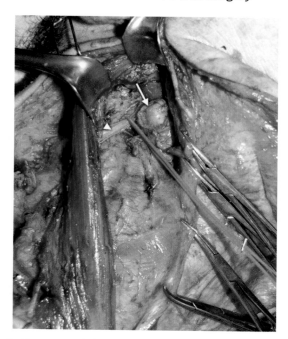

Fig. 8: Exposure of the proximal portion of the spinal accessory nerve. As the deep aspect of the muscle is approached, care is taken to avoid injury to the spinal accessory nerve that enters the muscle at the junction of its upper and middle-third and lateral to its medial border. The arrowhead indicates the spinal accessory muscle and the white arrow indicates a neighboring metastatic lymph node

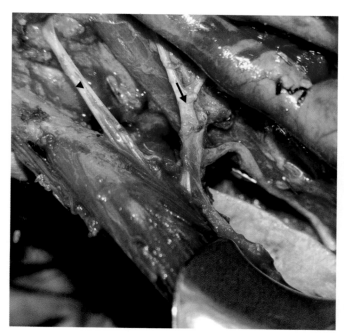

Fig. 9: Separating the spinal accessory nerve from the specimen. The spinal accessory nerve runs between the upper third of the sternocleidomastoid muscle and the posterior belly of the digastric muscle within the lymphatic tissue. A Adson clamp is used to elevate the lymphatic tissue away from the nerve and the tissue is cauterized and divided with a bipolar and a scalpel releasing the tethered nerve. Both the spinal (arrow) and cranial (arrowhead) nerve branches of the nerve should be preserved

with a bipolar. The dissection continues in a superior to inferomedial direction with electrocautery. As the dissection reaches the nerve, bipolar cauterization and sharp dissection are used in order to reduce injury to spinal accessory nerve. At this point, the lymphatic content of level IIb is passed beneath the spinal accessory in order to keep it in continuity with the whole specimen.

At this point, the sternocleidomastoid is retracted in a superoposterior direction and the spinal accessory nerve is exposed piercing the middle portion of the muscle. The nerve can be now completely dissected and separated from the muscle using Adson clamp and biolar cautery. The preserved nerve is now completely released from the specimen and from the muscle. The sternocleidomastoid is now pooled superiorly with a Richardson retractor and the previously dissected content of level V is passed below the muscle in continuity with the whole specimen.

Dissection along the Common Carotid Artery and Internal Jugular Vein

After the specimen is delivered forward underneath the sternocleidomastoid muscle and the spinal accessory nerve, the dissection continues toward the great vessels. The muscle is retracted posteriorly and the fatty tissue overlying the

internal jugular vein is now grabbed with 3–4 Babcock's graspers and retracted medially. The specimen can be now freed from the cervical roots. While the dissection continues medially, the anterior scalene muscle is exposed. The deep layer of the deep cervical fascia is routinely left on the scalene muscle in order to protect the phrenic nerve, which runs parallel to the muscle. Care is also taken to preserve the deep branches of the cervical nerves that contribute to the spinal accessory nerve and phrenic nerve.

The dissection now continues toward the common carotid artery. Here, dissection with a fine Adson clamp is preferred to prevent accidental injury to the vagus nerve or to the adventitia of the carotid artery. This method is preferred in previously irradiated neck or in revision surgery. A sharp dissection with a number 15 knife can be performed instead. The carotid sheath is exposed but not violated and the dissection is continued anterior to the artery in order to preserve the sympathetic trunk, which lies deep to the artery. The Babcock's clamps are now repositioned to allow adequate traction (from lateral to medial) of the tissue overlying the carotid sheath and internal jugular vein. Here, the operation is always performed with a sharp dissection allowing complete removal of the fascia investing

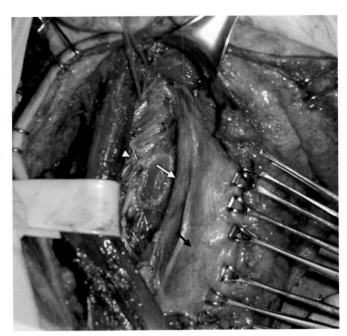

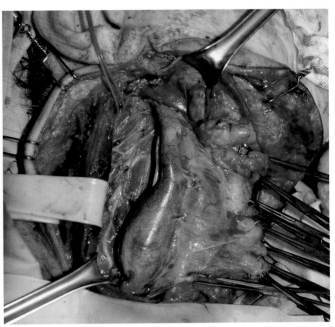

Fig. 10: Dissection along the common carotid artery and internal jugular vein. The Babcock's clamps are now repositioned to allow adequate traction (from lateral to medial) of the tissue overlying the carotid sheath and internal jugular vein. Here, the operation is always performed with a sharp dissection allowing complete removal of the fascia investing the internal jugular vein. The common carotid artery (white arrow), internal jugular vein (black arrow) and the stumps of the cervical roots (white arrowhead) are indicated

Fig. 11: Dissection along the internal jugular vein. The Babcock's clamps are now repositioned to allow adequate traction (from lateral to medial) of the tissue overlying the internal jugular vein. Here, the operation is always performed with a sharp dissection allowing complete removal of the fascia investing the internal jugular vein

the internal jugular vein (Figs 10 and 11). This is achieved by moving the scalpel along the entire length of the vein in a cephalad to caudal direction and vice versa. A gauze sponge may be used here to keep the tension of the specimen. As the vein is freed from the specimen, the thin branches of the vein are carefully divided and tied with a 4-0 silk suture. Next, the larger branches of the facial and middle thyroid veins are identified, clamped, divided and ligated in a similar way. The area in the lower part of the vein may contain large lymphatic vessels; the thoracic duct on the left and the right lymphatic duct, if a right neck dissection is performed. Regardless, if identified or not, the tissue that accompanies the vessels is clamped with small titanium clips or tied with number 3-0 silk suture.

On the cephalad portion of the internal jugular vein, the dissection is continued inferior to the posterior belly of the digastric muscle. Here, it is advised to use meticulous dissection with a thin hemostat in order to prevent injury to the internal jugular vein deep to the muscle or to its lingual branch. In case of clinical evidence of positive nodes in level II, the digastric belly can be retracted cephalad exposing the most distal part of the vein at the base of skull. This

maneuver may also prevent accidental injury to a folded vein. Injury in this area may be difficult to control and hemostasis may require tying of the vein. Rarely, the dissection in this area can be challenging, if a large metastatic lymph node with extracapsular extension is involved. As the internal jugular vein is completely freed form its fascia, the dissection is continued medially toward the carotid sheath and the specimen is completely freed from the great vessels of the neck.

Dissection along the Strap Muscles

This is the last part of the operation. The specimen is now retracted superiorly and the branches of the ansa cervicalis nerve are divided and kept on the specimen along with the anterior belly of the omohyoid muscle. The dissection continues at the medial border of the dissection along the sternohyoid and sternothyroid muscles. The superior thyroid artery and external branch of the superior laryngeal artery are preserved by staying superficial to the strap muscles (Fig. 12). The dissection is continued from lateral to medial and from inferior to superior toward the hyoid bone and the digastric muscle. The anterior branches of the ansa hypoglossi may be used here to trace the hypoglossal nerve, which lies inferior to the posterior belly of the digastric muscle, anterior to the distal portion of the internal jugular vein and superficial

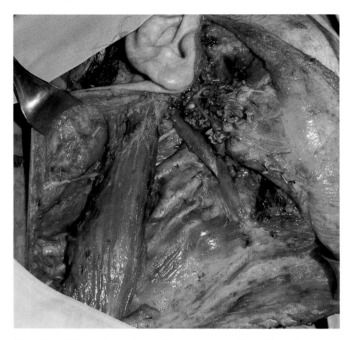

Fig. 12: Dissection along the strap muscles. The dissection continues at the medial border of the dissection along the sternohyoid and sternothyroid muscles. In this case, the neck dissection also involves superficial parotidectomy and dissection of the submandibular triangle

to the internal and external branches of the carotid artery. As the strap muscles are exposed, the omohyoid muscle is freed from the hyoid bone and the selective neck dissection is completed by including the lymphatic tissue anterior and posterior to the sternocleidomastoid muscle in the whole specimen.

The specimen is oriented and each level is submitted separately to the pathology laboratory for analysis. The wound is copiously irrigated, inspected and hemostasis is performed as indicated. A blood pressure above 120/80 should be confirmed prior to closure for an adequate hemostasis. If a chyle leak is suspected, a Valsalva maneuver can be performed by keeping a positive ventilation pressure for several seconds. Two Jackson-Pratt number 7 drains are left at the surgical bed; one to drain the posterior triangle and the second is placed along the great vessels and the digastric muscle. The platysma is sutured with absorbable stitches and the skin is closed with 5-0 nylon stitches or with clips.

POSTOPERATIVE TREATMENT

After the surgery, the patient is extubated and immediately transferred to the post surgery care unit before his transfer to the floor. In some cases, it may be advisable to connect the

drains to low pressure suction for 24 hours in order to ensure continuous negative pressure and adherence of the flaps. The wound is kept clean by rinsing it with saline three times a day and covered with antibiotic ointment after each cleansing. The drains are removed either, 3 days after the operation or when the fluid is less than 20–30 ml in 24 hours. Prophylactic antibiotic treatment is not indicated in the postoperative period. For pain control, the patients are treated with nonsteroidal anti-inflammatory drugs (diclofenac 75 mg intramuscularly or orally, or rofecoxib 50 mg) once daily and with tramadol (50–100 mg) if the patient asks for them or if the nurses felt it to be necessary.

HIGHLIGHTS

I. **Indications**
   - Advance skin squamous cell carcinoma in the postauricular area with no clinical of radiological evidence of lymph node metastases.
   - Malignant melanoma with positive sentinel lymph node
   - Thyroid cancers with clinical evidence of neck metastases in level V
   - Patients with oropharynx, nasopharynx, larynx or hypopharynx squamous cell carcinoma who failed nonsurgical treatment
   - Any head and neck carcinoma with clinical or radiological evidence of lymph node metastasis in level II–V, not amendable for chemoradiation
   - Neck metastases from postauricular skin cancers and resection of occipital nodes.

II. **Contraindications**
   - Involvement of the internal jugular vein or spinal accessory nerve
   - Tumor invades the prevertebral fascia, encases carotid artery or involves mediastinal structures
   - Metastatic disease (not including differentiated thyroid cancer and adenoid cystic carcinoma).

III. **Special Preoperative Considerations**
   - Imaging using CT with contrast
   - Imaging with PET-CT in large tumors (T4) for distant metastases work-up
   - Complete blood count and coagulation function tests, blood type and cross.

IV. **Special Intraoperative Considerations**
   - Operation is performed without relaxation for cranial nerve monitoring
   - Early identification of the spinal accessory nerve in the posterior triangle

- Preserve the spinal branches, which contribute to the accessory and phrenic nerves
- Dissection should be performed superficial to the fascia overlying the scalene muscles to prevent injury to the phrenic nerve and brachial plexus.
- Sharp dissection along the internal jugular vein allows complete removal of the fascia overlying the great vessels.
- Meticulous dissection of the supraclavicular area and the use of silver clips prevent chyle leak
- Proper surgical technique and careful hemostasis during and after surgery diminish the risk of bleeding
- Valsalva maneuver may be used to identify occult chyle leak at the root of the neck.

V. **Special Postoperative Considerations**
- Identify complications as early as possible
- Bleeding in this area can lead to an imminent airway obstruction. Open and evacuate the wound at the bedside if airway obstruction occurs.
- Chyle leak is usually treated conservatively with modified diet and local pressure
- Early reinstatement of neck and shoulders physiotherapy.

VI. **Complications**
- Bleeding
- Seroma
- Chyle leak
- Wound infection

- Cranial nerve paralysis (spinal accessory and shoulder dysfunction, hypoglossal, lingual, marginal mandibular branch of the facial nerve, vagus, phrenic, brachial plexus, sympathetic trunk).
- Paresis of the spinal accessory nerve is almost always a temporary consequence of surgery
- Anesthesia in the perioricular area (a direct consequence of surgery rather than a complication)
- Jugular vein thrombosis in perioperative radiotherapy treatment.

ADDITIONAL READING

1. Byers RM. Treatment of the neck in melanoma. Otolaryngol Clin North Am. 1998;31(5):833-9.
2. Lentsch EJ, Myers JN. Melanoma of the head and neck: current concepts in diagnosis and management. Laryngoscope. 2001;111(7):1209-22.
3. Patel RS, Clark JR, Gao K, et al. Effectiveness of selective neck dissection in the treatment of the clinically positive neck. Head Neck. 2008;30(9):1231-6.
4. Patel SG, Coit DG, Shaha AR, et al. Sentinel lymph node biopsy for cutaneous head and neck melanomas. Arch Otolaryngol Head Neck Surg. 2002;128(3):285-91.
5. Shah JP, Kraus DH, Dubner S, et al. Patterns of regional lymph node metastases from cutaneous melanomas of the head and neck. Am J Surg. 1991;162(4):320-3.
6. Vauterin TJ, Veness MJ, Morgan GJ, et al. Patterns of lymph node spread of cutaneous squamous cell carcinoma of the head and neck. Head Neck. 2006;28(9):785-91.

Chapter 35

Selective Neck Dissection of Levels VI and VII

Ziv Gil, Dan M Fliss

INTRODUCTION

The incidence of thyroid carcinomas has increased in the last decade, mostly due to widespread use of imaging modalities in modern medicine, without significant impact on the survival. Nevertheless, surgery remained a routine procedure for management of carcinomas originating in the thyroid gland with neck metastases. The most common malignant tumor originating in the thyroid gland is papillary carcinoma, followed by follicular, medullary and anaplastic carcinomas. While anaplastic cancers are considered usually inoperable, differentiated thyroid carcinomas (papillary and follicular) often require treatment of the primary tumor and clearance of nodal metastases if clinical evidence of positive lymph nodes is evident. The primary echelon for malignant tumors of the thyroid are the para and pretracheal lymph nodes, also known as level VI and VII of the neck (Fig. 1). Management of head and neck cancers should be planned according to the tumor's characteristics, patient factors and the expertise of the medical team. In medullary thyroid cancer, dissection of para and pretracheal regions may be performed without evidence of locoregional metastases, whereas differentiated thyroid cancers are usually performed as a therapeutic procedure (positive nodes). Palpable neck disease or radiological evidence of nodal metastases will necessitate, in most cases, selective neck dissection of the lateral neck along with central compartment cleanup.

The goal of neck dissection of levels VI and VII is to assure complete removal of the disease, preservation of the parathyroid glands and preventing injury to the recurrent laryngeal nerves. In order to perform a safe and efficient surgery, the surgeon should be familiar with the anatomy of the thyroid gland and the various anatomical locations of the vital structures along the course of the gland. Improper

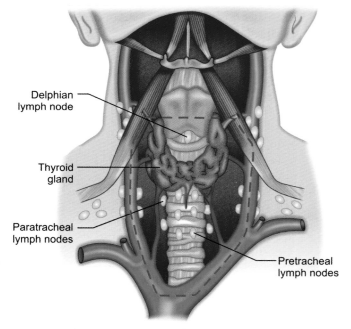

Fig. 1: A depiction with the location of the nodes to be resected. The central lymphatic compartment of the neck is contained laterally between the common carotid arteries. Level VI is limited superiorly by the hyoid bone and inferiorly by the upper border of the manubrium of the sternum. Level VII extends from the inferior border of level VI to the upper border of the aortic arch. The red line delineates the area of the central compartment neck dissection

surgical technique may imminently cause unnecessary disabilities to the patient including hypocalcemia and vocal cord paralysis, which may lead to significant morbidity.

In this chapter, the technique practiced by the authors for surgical removal of the lymphatic tissue of neck levels VI and VII, which is frequently used in patients with thyroid cancers with clinical evidence of positive neck nodes in any of these levels will be described in details. This technique may be also used for advanced hypopharyngeal and laryngeal carcinomas, when radiotherapy is contraindicated or as salvage procedures. The surgical technique for removal of levels II–VII, which is usually practiced when comprehensive clearance of all neck nodes is indicated, is similar to the technique described in this chapter, adding selective dissection of the lateral neck compartments as described in Chapters 33 and 34.

PREOPERATIVE EVALUATION AND ANESTHESIA

Physical examination and preoperative imaging are required for clinical staging and treatment planning. The neck is palpated and the glottis is evaluated with a flexible endoscope or a mirror. Radiologic evaluation of patients with poorly differentiated carcinomas include computed tomography (CT) scan of the neck and mediastinum with contrast, while well-differentiated thyroid cancers are better evaluated using ultrasound. Integrated positron emission tomography (PET) and CT offers a good assessment of locoregional and distant metastases in squamous cell carcinomas or in poorly differentiated thyroid cancer. Pathological diagnosis prior to surgery is essential to verify suspicious neck nodes. It can be easily achieved by ultrasound guided fine needle aspiration. All patients scheduled for operation are evaluated preoperatively by a head and neck surgeon and by an anesthesiologist.

The authors do not recommend routine administration of prophylactic antibiotics since these are clean operations. First-generation cephalosporins may be used if the sterility of the surgery is compromised. Unless contraindicated, placement of number six, 5–7 tracheal tubes is recommended to prevent trauma to the vocal cords. Surgery is performed under general anesthesia with muscle relaxation. In cases of aggressive thyroid cancers, insertion of an endoesophageal tube is recommended to facilitate identification of the esophagus during surgery. Intraoperative monitoring of the recurrent laryngeal nerve is performed in selected cases. These include revision surgery, recurrent thyroid cancer, unilateral vocal cord paralysis and surgery after previous external beam radiation therapy.

SURGICAL ANATOMY

The central lymphatic compartment of the neck is contained laterally between the common carotid arteries. Level VI is limited superiorly by the hyoid bone and inferiorly by the upper border of the manubrium of the sternum. Level VII extends from the inferior border of level VI to the upper border of the aortic arch. Figure 1 shows a depiction with the location of the nodes to be resected. Within this compartment lies the thyroid and parathyroid glands with their blood supply, the superior and recurrent laryngeal nerve. Neighboring structures are the thyroid cartilage, cricoid, trachea, hypopharynx and cervical esophagus. The upper mediastinum contains the innominate artery, brachiocephalic vein and thymus.

SURGICAL TECHNIQUE

Skin Incision

The patient is placed on the operating room table in a supine position. The head is stabilized with a soft donut holder and the whole operating table is then elevated in an angle with the head up in order to minimize bleeding.

The surgical access is planned through a horizontal neck incision (Fig. 2). Marking of the incision is preferably performed with the neck slightly flexed in order to identify the lines of relaxed skin tension. The incision extends to the anterior borders of the sternocleidomastoid muscles on each side, 2 cm above the clavicles. If lateral neck dissection is also indicated, the incision is extended laterally up to the anterior border of the trapezius along the same skin crest, eliminating the need for vertical extension.

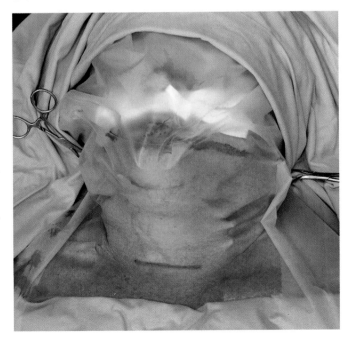

Fig. 2: Planning of the neck incision. The incision extends 2 cm lateral to the anterior borders of the sternocleidomastoid muscles on each side and 2 cm above the clavicles

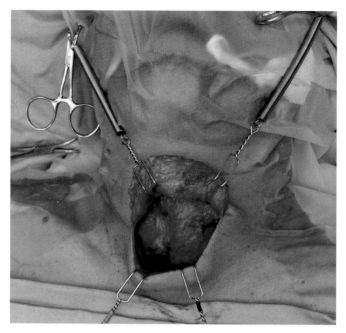

Fig. 3: Elevation of superior and inferior flaps. Subplatysmal flaps are elevated superiorly above the hyoid bone down to the level of the sternum

After incision marking, a roll is placed under their shoulders to hyperextend the neck. The patient is then prepped and draped in a standard surgical fashion. A transparent plastic cover is used to drape the head (from the level of mandible, upward) to allow the anesthesiology and surgical teams continuous monitoring of the tube connectors (Fig. 2). This also prevents unnecessary traumatization of the skin by stapling or stitching.

Skin Incision and Elevation of Subplatysmal Flaps

After marking, the skin is injected with lidocaine (0.06%) and epinephrine (1:1,000,000) to reduce the amount of pain after surgery and for hemostasis. The skin is incised with a number 15 blade and subsequent dissection of the subcutaneous tissue and the platysma is carried out with a monopolar electrocautery at the lowest effective setting. Subplatysmal flaps are elevated superiorly above the hyoid bone down to the level of the sternum (Fig. 3). This plane separates the superficial cervical fascia from the superficial layer of the deep cervical fascia. Care is taken to prevent injury to the anterior jugular veins, which are left on the superficial layer of the deep cervical fascia. The flaps are retracted and held using skin hooks. If total thyroidectomy is indicated, it is now performed using the technique described in chapter 38 of this book. Otherwise, a central compartment neck dissection is performed as described below.

Dissection along the Tracheoesophageal Groove and Preservation of the Recurrent Laryngeal Nerve

The technique described here is practiced for thyroid cancers. If total thyroidectomy is performed in the same operation, the recurrent laryngeal nerve and parathyroid glands are identified and preserved during surgery (Fig. 4). Once a total thyroidectomy is completed, attention is turned to the selective neck dissection of level VI. Otherwise, the nerve should be identified early in the operation in the tracheoesophageal groove and the inferior parathyroid glands are likely to be sacrificed. The surgeon should be aware of the different variations in the location of the recurrent laryngeal nerve. On the left side, the nerve crosses anterior to the aortic arch, loops under it and ascend in a relatively constant position along the tracheoesophageal groove. On the other hand, the course of the right nerve is less predicted, since it crosses anterior to the subclavian artery and ascend posterior to the artery and relatively more laterally than in the left side. When identified, the nerve should be untethered from the surrounding tissue and reflected away from the specimen. All dissections along the nerve should be performed only with a fine clamp and any retraction of the nerve with hook or vessel loop should be avoided to prevent neuropraxia and temporary vocal cord paralysis. Dissection with monopolar electrocautery near the nerve may cause neuropraxia and temporary vocal cord paralysis due to thermal trauma and therefore should be avoided.

Dissection along the Common Carotid Artery

After the recurrent laryngeal nerve is identified and preserved, the dissection continues along the carotid sheath. If bilateral neck dissection is indicated, the right side of the neck is approached first. The fibrofatty tissue that overlies the common carotid artery is stripped from the vessel using dissection with fine Adson clamp. This is performed when the surgeon stands cephalad to the patient, in a superior to inferior direction (Fig. 5). As the dissection continues inferiorly, the innominate artery (i.e. brachiocephalic trunk) is exposed. The dissection continues medially along the artery and the inferior thyroid vessels are clamped, divided and ligated. In this area, the remnants of the thymic tissue are reflected superiorly along with the whole specimen using Babcock's graspers. It is important to clamp and tie all the tissue positioned in the upper mediastinum area to prevent retraction of vessels into the mediastinum, which are difficult to control and may lead to inadvertent injury to the recurrent laryngeal nerves. The nerve can be now identified passing deep to the innominate artery and coursing superior to it in a lateral to medial direction. The dissection along the recurrent laryngeal nerve is now completed and its entire portion is reflected away from the specimen. Care is now

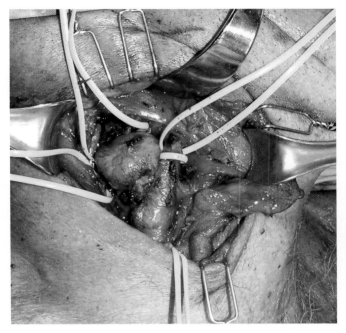

Fig. 6: Dissection along the carotid bifurcation. The dissection starts by ligation of the common feeder of the tumor coming from the bifurcation of the carotid. This vessel along with some other small branches coming from the external carotid artery are ligated or clipped. The next step is meticulous dissection of the carotid body tumor from the main vessels

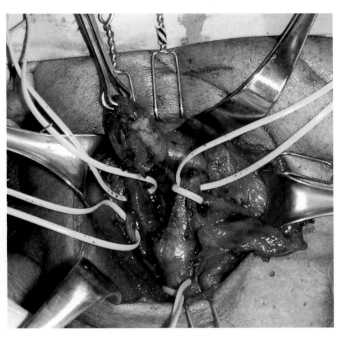

Fig. 7: Dissection along the internal carotid artery. The next step is to meticulously dissect the tumor off the internal and external branches of the carotid artery

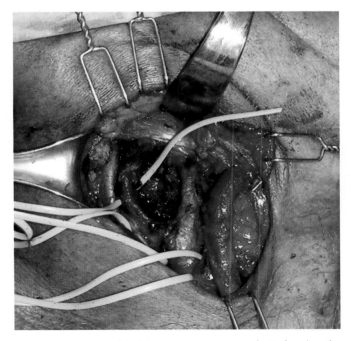

Fig. 8: The surgical field after tumor removal. Only after the neighboring cranial nerves are identified and the great vessels are controlled, the tumor can be resected

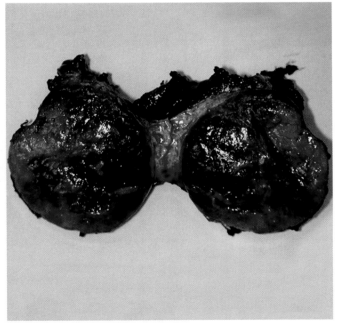

Fig. 9: The surgical specimen

each cleansing. The drain is removed either, 3 days after the operation or when the fluid is less than 20–30 ml in 24 hours. Prophylactic antibiotic treatment is not indicated in the postoperative period. For pain control, the patients are treated with nonsteroidal anti-inflammatory drugs (diclofenac 75 mg intramuscularly or orally, or rofecoxib 50 mg) once daily and with tramadol (50–100 mg) if the patient asks for them or if the nurses felt it to be necessary.

HIGHLIGHTS

I. **Indications**
   - Clinical and radiological evidence of carotid body tumor
   - Recurrent carotid body tumors.

II. **Contraindications**
   - Evidence of distant metastases
   - Tumor that invades the skull base or involves mediastinal structures are excised by combined approaches.
   - Simultaneous resection of bilateral carotid body tumors should be avoided. If indicated, these tumors should be excised in a stepwise procedure.
   - Stable small carotid body tumor in elderly or high-risk patients can be followed radiologically with MRI.

III. **Special Preoperative Considerations**
   - Imaging using CT and MRI with contrast
   - Complete blood count and coagulation function tests
   - Embolization for large tumors is optional
   - Consultation with vascular surgery team when indicated.

IV. **Special Intraoperative Considerations**
   - Operation is performed without relaxation for cranial nerve monitoring.
   - Identify the carotid artery and its branches, and use vessel loops for proximal and distal control of bleeding.
   - Identify the spinal accessory nerve, vagus nerve and hypoglossal nerve early during the operation to prevent accidental injury

   - Identify the superior laryngeal nerve posterior and medial to the tumor to avoid its injury
   - Ligate the large vessels feeding the tumor.
   - Proper surgical technique and careful hemostasis during surgery diminish the risk of bleeding.

V. **Special Postoperative Considerations**
   - Identify complications as early as possible
   - Bleeding in this area can lead to an imminent airway obstruction. Open and evacuate the wound at the bedside if airway obstruction occurs.

VI. **Complications**
   - Bleeding
   - Seroma
   - Wound infection
   - Superior laryngeal nerve injury (the most common nerve injury)
   - Other cranial nerve paralysis (spinal accessory and shoulder dysfunction, hypoglossal, lingual, marginal mandibular branch of the facial nerve, vagus, sympathetic trunk)
   - Anesthesia in the periocular area (a direct consequence of surgery rather than a complication)
   - First bite syndrome
   - In cases of bilateral tumor excision, patients may experience labile blood pressure postoperatively, which is difficult to control medically. These patients should be admitted to the intensive care unit for observation.

ADDITIONAL READING

1. Heath D. The human carotid body in health and disease. J Pathol. 1991;164(1):1-8.
2. Knight TT, Gonzalez JA, Rary JM, et al. Current concepts for the surgical management of carotid body tumor. Am J Surg. 2006;191(1):104-10.
3. Liapis C, Gougoulakis A, Karydakis V, et al. Changing trends in management of carotid body tumors. Am Surg. 1995;61(11):989-93.
4. Shamblin WR, ReMine WH, Sheps SG, et al. Carotid body tumor (chemodectoma). Clinicopathologic analysis of ninety cases. Am J Surg. 1971;122(6):732-9.

Chapter 37

Surgical Management of Parapharyngeal Space Tumors

Ziv Gil, Dan M Fliss

INTRODUCTION

The parapharyngeal space (PPS) is a deep space in the neck, in the shape of an inverted teepee. Its base attaches the skull base and the apex reaches the level of the hyoid bone. Its medial side is delineated by the naso- and oropharynx, its anterolateral side by the masticator space, its posterolateral side by the deep lobe of the parotid gland and its posteromedial side by the retropharyngeal space (Figs 1A and B). Less than 1% of all the head and neck neoplasms that originate involve the PPS. These tumors can be either primary or secondary tumors, which infiltrate or metastasize to the PPS. Most of the tumors involving the PPS are benign (80%) with those originating from the parotid glands comprise half of them. The rest are of schwannomas, paragangliomas or enlarged lymph nodes. These tumors may be undetected for a long period of time, after which they usually present as an asymptomatic mass displacing oropharyngeal structures medially. Other symptoms of PPS tumors include change in voice, trismus, mass in the upper neck, cranial nerve deficits, serous otitis media due to Eustachian tube obstruction and obstructive sleep apnea. The complex anatomy of the PPS accounts for the diversity of surgical approaches for removal of tumor in this anatomical area. The standard approaches to the PPS include the transcervical approach, the transparotid-transcervical approach and the transcervical-transmandibular approach. For large tumors, which involve the infratemporal fossa, the transcervical-infratemporal fossa approach is commonly used. The surgical approach is tailored according to the anatomical extent of the tumor, its histologic type (benign or malignant) and the patient's medical history (previous surgeries or radiation treatment).

This chapter describes the preoperative evaluation and surgical approaches used for removal of tumors of the PPS. These techniques allow wide exposure and complete extirpation of the tumor, while preserving the cranial nerves in this area.

PREOPERATIVE EVALUATION AND ANESTHESIA

Imaging

Imaging should be used at all times prior to surgery since it can influence decision-making regarding the treatment. A contrast computerized tomography (CT) scan and a basic magnetic resonance imaging (MRI) study with fat suppression should be utilized in patients with PPS for preoperative evaluation and decision-making regarding the treatment. A T2-weighted MRI study with fat suppression is usually added (Figs 2A and B). Anterior displacement of the carotid artery and the internal jugular vein (poststyloid tumors) is suggestive for paraganglioma and schwannoma. Visualization of a vascular flow void on MRI study is usually sufficient for diagnosis of paraganglioma, but magnetic resonance angiography (MRA) may be added for supportive evidence for vascular tumors. A dynamic MRI can be also utilized for uncertain cases. In this test, a bolus injection of a standard dose of gadolinium is injected and a short T1-weighted study is directed at the region of interest and sequentially repeated for about 2 minutes. The time curve of the signal intensity is then generated on a workstation and compared to that of a blood vessel when possible. A sharp and

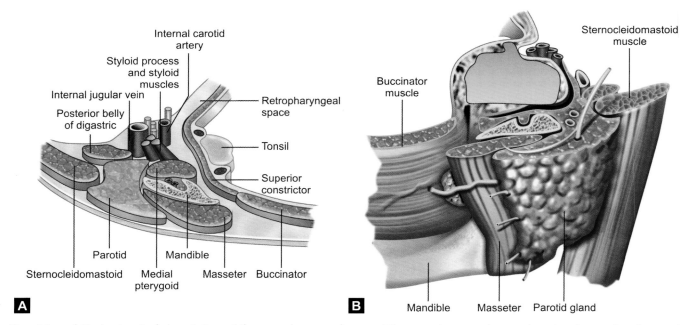

Figs 1A and B: Anatomical description of the parapharyngeal space. The parapharyngeal space has the shape of an inverted teepee. Its base attaches the skull base and the apex reaches the level of the hyoid bone. Its medial side is delineated by the naso- and oropharynx, its anterolateral side by the masticator space, its posterolateral side by the deep lobe of the parotid gland and its posteromedial side by the retropharyngeal space

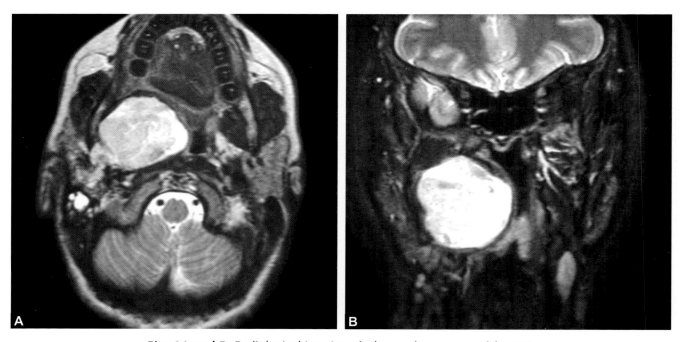

Figs 2A and B: Radiological imaging of a large schwannoma of the PPS.
A T2-weighted MRI image showing a parapharyngeal space tumor

early rise of signal intensity that is followed by a rapid drop (also called washout), similar in shape and magnitude to that seen in the blood vessels is characteristic of vascular lesions. Prestyloid tumors are most frequently of salivary gland origin. These can be secondary tumors, which originate in the deep lobe of the parotid gland or primary minor salivary gland tumors in the PPS. Computed tomography (CT) or MRI are used to demonstrate a preserved fat plane between the deep parotid lobe and the tumor, which is indicative of a separate tumor of the PPS, most commonly originating from extraparotid minor salivary glands. The lack of visualization of this plane may indicate a tumor originating in the deep lobe of the parotid gland or a large tumor that is either compressing this plane or rarely, invading it. If a malignant tumor is suspected, the radiological staging of the patient is completed by using a positron emission tomography-CT hybrid (PET-CT) that is used for assessing the presence of regional and distal metastases.

Tissue Diagnosis

The utility of fine needle aspiration (FNA) biopsy is questionable in tumors of the PPS for several reasons: (i) It is difficult to reach via ultrasound and frequently will require CT guided FNA, which is technically challenged; (ii) It can potentially cause bleeding and airway obstruction in case of vascular tumors; (iii) It cannot distinguish between malignant or benign paragangliomas and has low specificities in tumors, which harbor islands of carcinoma in large pleomorphic adenoma. Finally, imaging is usually sufficient to guide the surgical treatment. For these reasons, the authors do not recommend routine FNA for PPS tumors. In any case, considering the risk of vascular injury as well as the complexity of future resection after adherence of the tumor to the pharyngeal mucosa, a peroral biopsy of PPS tumor should not be performed. Peroral FNA may be used in selected cases, especially in those which are suspected to be malignant, especially of lymphomas and metastatic lesions for which nonsurgical treatment is indicated.

Patients with suspected paragangliomas will require preoperative embolization a few days prior to the operation. Surgery is performed under general anesthesia without muscle relaxation. This allows the surgeon monitoring of the spinal accessory, hypoglossal, vagus, phrenic and marginal mandibular nerves during dissection with electrocautery. Intraoperative monitoring of the facial nerve is performed in selected cases, when the dissection includes the parotid gland, mainly transcervical-transparotid approaches.

SURGICAL TECHNIQUE

Various surgical approaches for the resection of PPS tumors are used (Figs 3A to D). Table 1 shows the various indications for each one of the approaches described herein.

The Transcervical Approach for Resection of PPS Tumor

The transcervical is the optimal approach for removal of tumors of the PPS that originate in the pre or postvascular compartment. These usually include schwannomas, para-gangliomas and pleomorphic adenoma of the PPS; both of which account for most tumors in this area as in Figures 3A to D.

The patient is placed on the operating room table in a supine position. The head is stabilized with a soft donut holder and the whole operating table is then elevated in an angle with the head up in order to minimize bleeding. The surgical access is planned through a modified Blair incision (Fig. 4). Marking of the incision is preferably performed with the neck slightly flexed in order to identify the lines of relaxed skin tension. The incision normally extends from the mastoid tip to the cricoid arch, 2–3 fingers below the ramus of the mandible along a transverse skin crest in the lower neck. After incision marking, a roll is placed under the shoulders to hyperextend the neck and the head is rotated toward the contralateral side.

Skin Incision and Elevation of Subplatysmal Flaps

The skin is incised with a number 15 blade and subsequent dissection of the subcutaneous tissue and the platysma is carried out with an electrocautery at the lowest effective setting. Subplatysmal flaps are elevated superiorly exposing the internal jugular vein (Fig. 5). This plane separates the superficial cervical fascia from the superficial layer of the deep cervical fascia. Care is taken to prevent injury to the marginal mandibular branch of the facial nerve. The nerve runs within the fascia superior to the submandibular gland. Injury to

Table 1: The various approaches to the parapharyngeal space tumors and their indications

Radiological Description	Likely Diagnosis	Surgical Approach
Prevascular tumors	Benign salivary gland tumor	Transcervical
Postvascular tumors	Schwannoma, paraganglioma	Transcervical
Deep lobe parotid tumors with PPS extension	Benign salivary gland tumor	Transcervical-transparotid
Large malignant tumors with skull base involvement	Malignant salivary gland tumors, sarcomas	Transmandibular
Large tumors with infratemporal fossa involvement	Schwannoma, paraganglioma, salivary gland tumors, sarcomas	Transcervical-infratemporal fossa

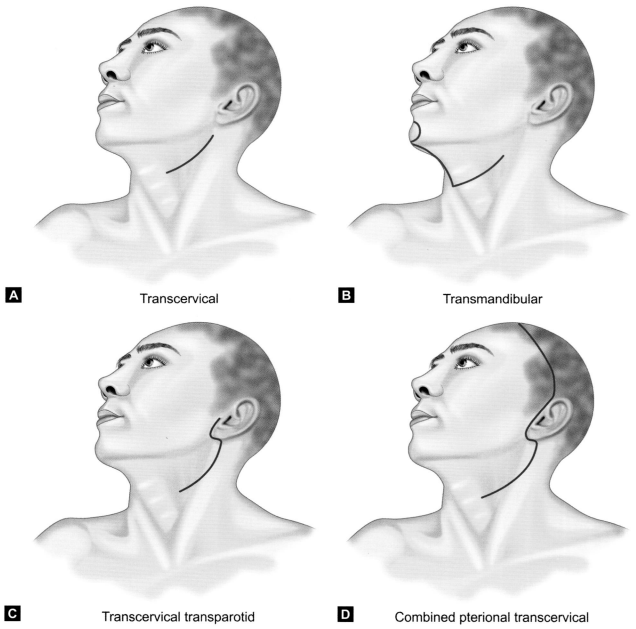

A   Transcervical

B   Transmandibular

C   Transcervical transparotid

D   Combined pterional transcervical

Figs 3A to D: The various incisions according to the different approaches to the parapharyngeal space

the nerve is prevented by elevation of the flap immediately below the platysma leaving the superficial layer of the deep cervical fascia on the submandibular gland.

Exposure of the Sternocleidomastoid and Digastric Muscle

The dissection now continues along the superficial layer of the deep cervical fascia that unwrap the sternocleidomastoid muscle. The authors usually start this dissection by placing

hemostats on the fascia at the anterior border of the muscle, retracting the tissue medially. The dissection is started at the anterior border of the muscle along its entire length in a lateral to medial plane. The dissection is made with an electrocautery and small vessels interconnecting the superficial and deep borders of the muscle are electrocautered with a bipolar or clamped and divided (Fig. 6). The branches of the great auricular nerve is preserved if possible, however division of the nerve may be indicated to release the

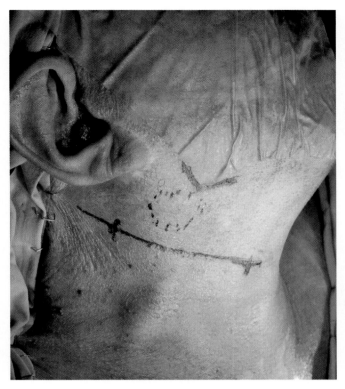

Fig. 4: Planning of the skin incision. A transcervical approach to a parapharyngeal space schwannoma

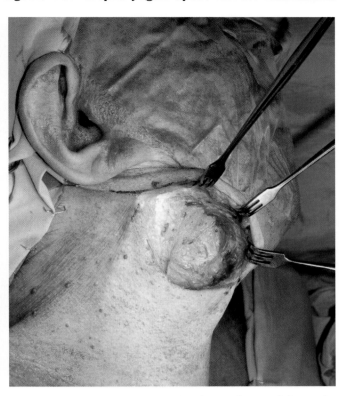

Fig. 5: Elevation of superior and inferior platysmal flaps. The skin is incised with a number 15 blade and subsequent dissection of the subcutaneous tissue and the platysma is carried out with an electrocautery at the lowest effective setting. Subplatysmal flaps are elevated superiorly, 1 cm below the ramus of the mandible and inferiorly to the sternum

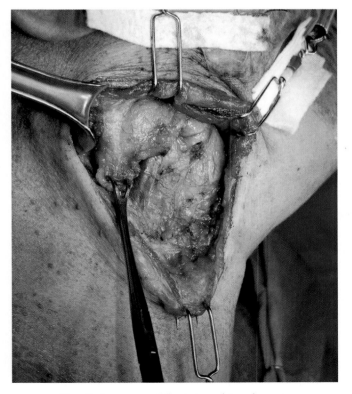

Fig. 6: Exposure of the internal jugular vein

sternocleidomastoid muscle at its superior border. As the deep aspect of the muscle is approached, care is taken to avoid injury to the spinal accessory nerve that enters the muscle at the junction of its upper and middle-third, and lateral to its medial border (Fig. 7). The dissection now continues deep to the muscles from medial to lateral.

After the sternocleidomastoid muscle, the cranial nerves and large vessels of the neck are exposed to prevent accidental injury during tumor resection. After exposing the spinal accessory nerve, the posterior belly of the digastric muscle is identified (Fig. 7). The muscle crosses the angle formed by the sternocleidomastoid muscle and the ramus of the mandible in the middle. Exposure of the posterior belly of the digastric muscle begins by retraction of the sternocleidomastoid muscle with a Richardson retractor laterally and of the ramus of the mandible with an Army-Navy retractor cephalad.

The next step is identifying the internal jugular vein, common carotid artery and its branches. The dissection continues medially toward the common carotid artery. As the dissection continues from lateral to medial, the carotid

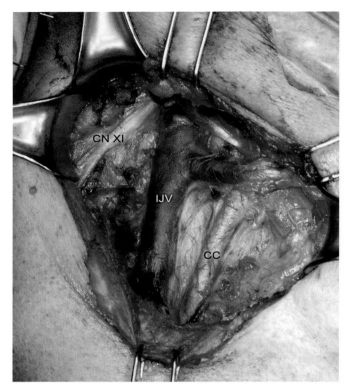

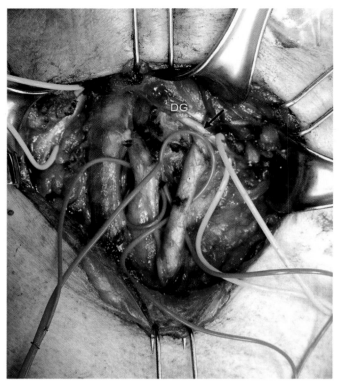

Fig. 7: Exposure of the spinal accessory nerve and great vessels. As the deep aspect of the muscle is approached, care is taken to avoid injury to the spinal accessory nerve that enters the muscle at the junction of its upper and middle-third and lateral to its medial border. The sternocleidomastoid is retracted posteriorly, the spinal accessory nerve (CN XI), internal jugular vein (IJV) and common carotid artery (CC) are identified

Fig. 8: The hypoglossal nerve, posterior belly of the digastric and the stylohyoid muscles are identified. The hypoglossal nerve (arrow) is identified and preserved. If the tumor grossly extends toward the skull base, the posterior belly of the digastric muscle (DG) can be transected exposing the most distal part of the tumor; the base of skull

sheath is exposed (Fig. 8). Here, the authors prefer dissection with a fine Adson clamp to prevent accidental injury to the vagus nerve or to the adventitia of the carotid artery. This method is preferred in previously irradiated neck or in revision surgery. The carotid sheath is exposed but not violated and the dissection is continued anterior to the artery in order to preserve the sympathetic trunk, which lies deep to the artery. Babcock's clamps are used to allow adequate traction (from lateral to medial) of the tissue overlying the carotid sheath and internal jugular vein. As the internal jugular vein is exposed, the dissection is continued cephalad up to the posterior belly of the digastric muscle. During this dissection, the internal and external branches of the carotid artery are identified. The vagus nerve, which runs along the carotid artery is identified and preserved. Vessel loops are placed around the internal and external branches of the carotid artery to enable proximal control of these vessels in case of arterial bleeding. Vessel loops are used to mark the cranial nerves and great vessels in the field and to allow their retraction.

As the dissection is continued toward the digastric muscle, the hypoglossal nerve should be identified (shown by the arrow in Figure 8). The nerve lies inferior to the posterior belly of the digastric muscle anterior to the distal portion of the internal jugular vein and superficial to the internal and external branches of the carotid artery. The anterior branches of the ansa hypoglossi may also be used here to trace the nerve.

The tumor is now identified and its association with the cranial nerves should be explored (Fig. 9). The tumor is now separated from the surrounding tissue. Here, it is advised to use meticulous dissection with a thin hemostat in order to prevent injury to the great vessels and cranial nerves. If the tumor grossly extends toward the skull base, the posterior belly of the digastric muscle can be retracted cephalad or transected exposing the most distal part of the tumor; the base of skull. The stylohyoid muscle and stylomandibular ligament may be also divided to allow wide approach to the PPS from below. This maneuver may also prevent accidental injury to the internal jugular vein at the jugular foramen.

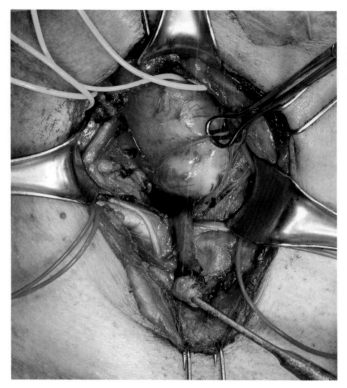

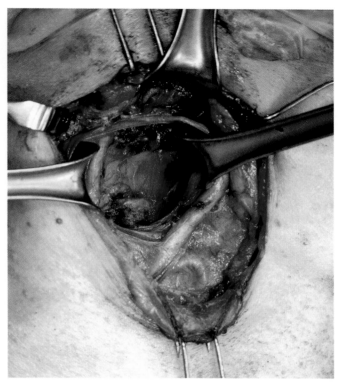

Fig. 9: Exposure of the tumor. The digastric muscle is retracted superiorly, the carotid artery is retracted anteriorly and the sternocleidomastoid muscle is retracted posteriorly. The fascia overlying the tumor is dissected and the tumor is exposed. A finger dissection is used to deliver the tumor inferiorly from the PPS

Fig. 10: The surgical field after tumor removal. The specimen is retracted with a Babcock's clamp caudally and the mylohyoid muscle is exposed. The muscle is gently retracted medially with an angled Army-Navy retractor, exposing the lingual nerve and the submandibular ganglion. Only, when both the lingual and hypoglossal nerves are identified superior to the medial portion of the digastric muscle, a clamp is placed below the lingual nerve and its neighboring vessels are divided and ligated

Injury in this area may be difficult to control and hemostasis may require tying of the vein. In large PPS tumors, which extend to the neck, removal of the submandibular gland can improve exposure and facilitate finger dissection in the PPS.

As the specimen is completely freed from its surrounding tissue, the proximal and distal margins are clamped and tied with a number 3-0 silk suture and the tumor is removed as in Figures 10 and 11.

Figures 12A to D show another case of PPS schwannoma, excised via a transcervical approach. The specimen is oriented and submitted separately to the pathology laboratory for analysis. The wound is copiously irrigated, inspected and hemostasis is performed as indicated. A blood pressure above 120/80 should be confirmed prior to closure for an adequate hemostasis. If a chyle leak is suspected, a Valsalva maneuver can be performed by keeping a positive ventilation pressure greater than 15 mm Hg for several seconds. A Jackson-Pratt number 7 drain is left at the surgical bed, the platysma is sutured with absorbable stitches and the skin is closed with 5-0 nylon stitches or with clips.

The Transcervical-Transparotid Approach for Resection of Deep Lobe Parotid Tumor in the PPS

This approach is suitable for tumors of the PPS originating in the deep lobe of the parotid gland. The most common tumor in this area is pleomorphic adenoma (Figs 13A and B). A routine superficial parotidectomy is performed with dissection of all facial branches as distally as possible to allow maximal mobilization of the branches. The various branches are then sharply dissected away from the deep lobe of the parotid (Fig. 14). A routine transcervical exposure of the PPS is gained via the cervical part of the Blair incision. After the facial nerve has been dissected away from the tumor, a Richardson retractor is used to elevate the posterior belly of the digastric muscle superiorly exposing the tumor in the PPS (Fig. 15). The submandibular gland is excised or retracted anteriorly and the digastric muscle is divided (Fig. 16). The thin fibrous tissue in this area is divided and the tumor is

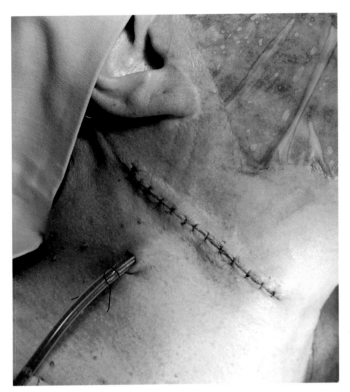

Fig. 11: Skin closure

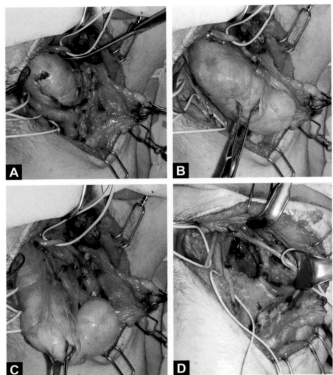

Figs 12A to D: A transcervical approach to PPS schwannoma. The tumor was exposed via a transcervical approach. The hypoglossal vagus and spinal accessory nerves are marked with yellow vessel loops

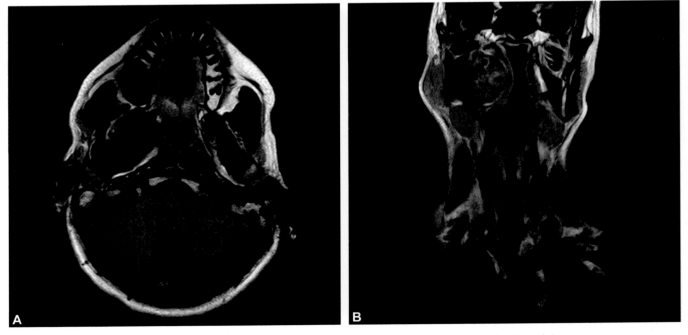

Figs 13A and B: Preoperative imaging of a PPS tumor originating in the deep lobe of the parotid gland. (A) An axial T1 MRI; and (B) Coronal MRI

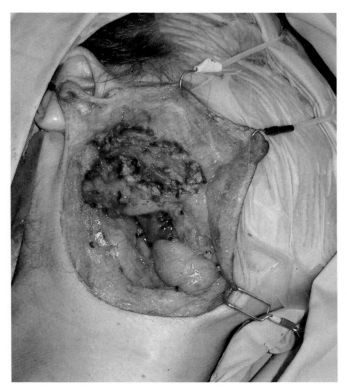

Fig. 14: Transcervical-transparotid approach. In this case of a deep lobe pleomorphic adenoma, a routine superficial parotidectomy is performed with dissection of the facial branches as distally as possible to allow maximal mobilization of the gland

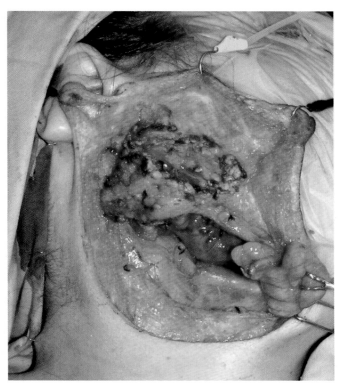

Fig. 15: The submandibular gland is retracted medially exposing the PPS

removed with blunt dissection that is possible once exposure of the PPS is maximal (Fig. 17). The finger dissection in this area should be performed with care to prevent accidental disintegration and spillage of the tumor and its content (Fig. 18). The loose areolar tissue that surrounds the tumor is divided and separated with scissors to enable delivery of the tumor through the neck as in Figure 19.

The Transmandibular Approach

This approach is suitable for patients with extremely large tumor, malignant neoplasms, previously operated and irradiated patients, and for highly vascular lesions as in Figure 20.

The surgical access is planned through a lip-split incision extended to a horizontal neck incision toward the ipsilateral side of the tumor. The lip incision is performed in the midline circumferencing the chin toward the side of the tumor, extended caudally up to the level of the cricoid cartilage. This incision is then extended laterally to a formal collar neck incision up to the level of the mastoid bone. After marking of the incision, the patient is prepped and draped in a standard surgical fashion.

Subplatysmal flaps are elevated superiorly, 1 cm below the ramus of the mandible and inferiorly to the clavicle. Care is taken to prevent injury to the marginal mandibular branch of the facial nerve. After elevation of the flaps, the fascia overlying the sternocleidomastoid muscle is incised and the common carotid artery and its branches are identified. The internal jugular vein is also exposed and ligated if indicated. The case presented in Figure 21 demonstrates a recurrent pleomorphic adenoma encasing the internal and external carotid arteries. The tumor is meticulously dissected off the great vessels. The hypoglossal nerve is identified and preserved at this stage (shown by the arrow in Figure 21). After the lip and skin of the chin are split at the midline, the incision is extended to the level of the outer cortex of the mandible. The incision is extended to the gingivolabial sulcus, preserving half a centimeter of the oral mucosa on the mandible for later suturing of the incision. The soft tissue overlying the mandible is elevated bilaterally, deep to the periosteum approximately 2–3 cm on each side of the planned osteotomy. Care is taken to preserve the mental nerve, which enters the mental foramen. Before performing the osteotomy, two titanium miniplates are prebanded and fixed to the mandible. One is fixed to the anterior face of the cortex and the second to the inferior border of the mandible. This two-point fixation minimizes free movement of the mandible. Attention is now

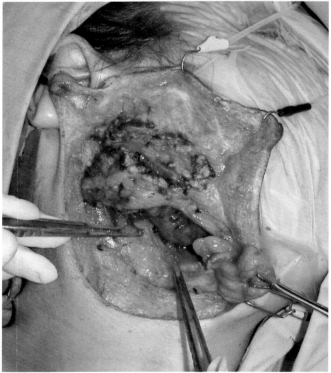

Fig. 16: Dividing the digastric muscle. The tendon of the digastric muscle is divided in order to gain access to the PPS

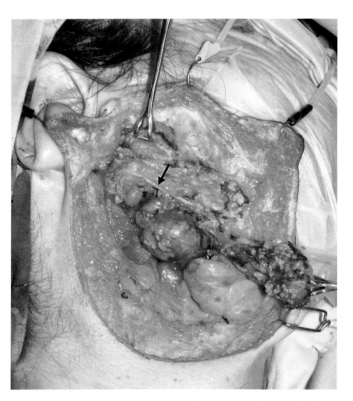

Fig. 17: Exposure of the tumor. The marginal mandibular branch of the facial nerve (arrow) is shown

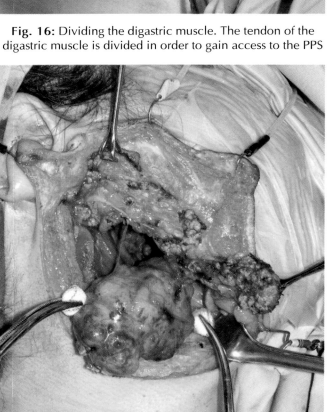

Fig. 18: Delivery of the tumor. A finger dissection is used to deliver the tumor out from the PPS

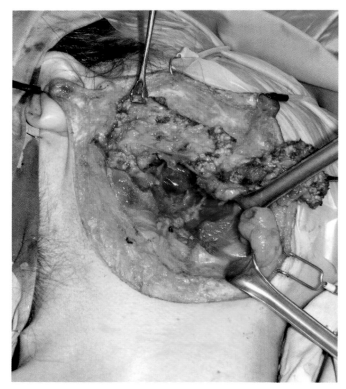

Fig. 19: The surgical field after removal of the tumor

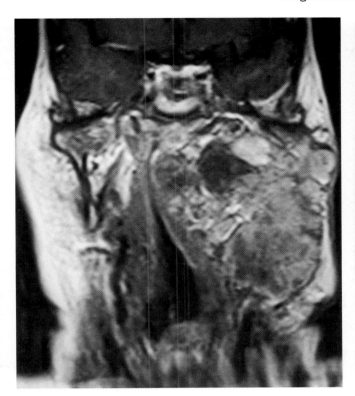

Fig. 20: Transmandibular approach. An MRI showing a large parapharyngeal recurrent pleomorphic adenoma

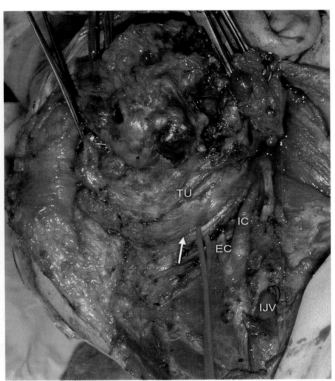

Fig. 21: The tumor encasing the carotid artery. The surgery starts with exposure and control of the carotid artery and its branches. The internal jugular vein is ligated. The structures shown are: internal carotid artery (IC); external carotid artery (EC); common carotid artery (CC); internal jugular vein (IJV); hypoglossal nerve (arrow) and; tumor (TU)

turned to the osteotomy. As a general rule, the osteotomy is performed in a paramedian position in the ipsilateral side of the tumor. Paramidline mandibulotomy is preferred to lateral or medial mandibulotomy. The mandibulotomy is performed in an angled direction. The angled osteotomy is presumed to provide better stability. Osteotomy is performed with a reciprocal, sagittal mechanical saw with a thin blade to minimize bone loss. Once the mandible is split, the ramus in the ipsilateral side is swung laterally. The gingivolabial incision is extended toward the anterior pillar of the tonsil allowing further exposure of the parapharyngeal space. Division of the mylohyoid muscle is required to allow lateral retraction of the mandible. After achieving adequate exposure of the oral and base of tongue, attention is turned to resect the tumor. Excision of the tumor is achieved in a monoblock fashion (Figs 22 and 23). Reconstruction is performed with an anterolateral thigh free flap as in Figures 24A and B.

Reconstructive Considerations

A primary closure of the surgical defect should be routinely used when possible. When the facial nerve is sacrificed, a reconstruction procedure is required. In these cases, an

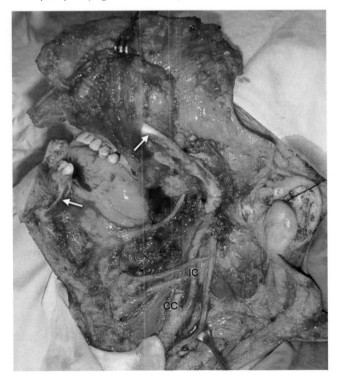

Fig. 22: The surgical field after tumor removal. The common carotid (CC), internal carotid (IC) and mandibular osteotomies (arrows) are indicated

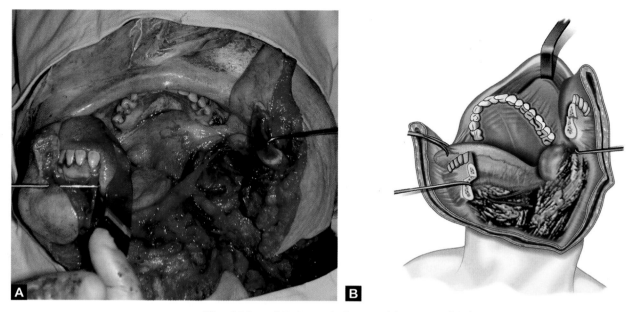

Figs 23A and B: Lateral picture of the surgical field

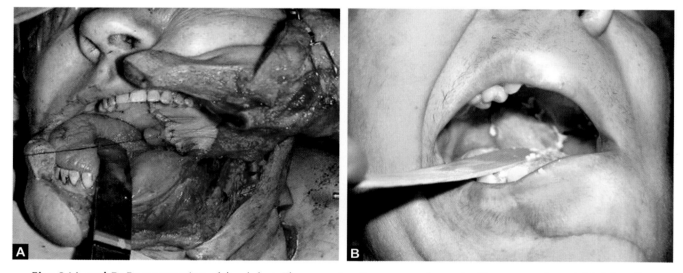

Figs 24A and B: Reconstruction of the defect. The reconstruction was performed with an anterolateral thigh free flap

interposition greater auricular nerve graft is used during the same procedure. High-risk patients, with a low life expectancy, did not undergo reconstruction of the facial nerve. Larger defects require regional flaps (temporalis muscle flap) or free flaps (radial forearm or anterolateral thigh free flaps).

POSTOPERATIVE TREATMENT

If mandibular split is not performed, these surgeries rarely require airway protection or tracheostomy. After

the operation, the patient is extubated and immediately transferred to the post surgery care unit before his transfer to the floor. The wound is kept clean by rinsing it with saline three times a day and covered with antibiotic ointment after each cleansing. The drains are removed either, 3 days after the operation or when the fluid is less than 20–30 ml in 24 hours. Prophylactic antibiotic treatment is not indicated in the postoperative period. For pain control, the patients are treated with nonsteroidal anti-inflammatory drugs (diclofenac 75 mg intramuscularly or orally, or rofecoxib 50 mg) once daily and with tramadol (5–100 mg) if the patient asks for them or if the nurses felt it to be necessary. If free flap is also performed, selective COX-2 inhibitors should be avoided.

HIGHLIGHTS

I. Indications
- Isolated salivary gland tumors, schwannomas and paragangliomas of the PPS
- Deep lobe parotid tumors invading the PPS
- Large PPS tumors with infratemporal fossa involvement
- Malignant tumor of the PPS.

II. Contraindications
- Lymphoma
- Carcinomas of oropharyngeal or nasopharyngeal origin emendable for chemoradiation therapy
- Evidence of distant metastases
- Tumor invades the prevertebral fascia, encases carotid artery or involves mediastinal structures
- Stable small paragangliomas can be followed radiologically with MRI.

III. Special Preoperative Considerations
- Imaging using CT and MRI with contrast
- Imaging with PET-CT in malignant tumors for distant metastases work-up
- Embolization for vascular tumors
- Neurosurgical and reconstructive consultation when indicated.

IV. Special Intraoperative Considerations
- Operation is performed without relaxation for cranial nerve monitoring
- Identify the carotid artery and its branches and use vessel loops for control of bleeding
- Identify the spinal accessory nerve, vagus nerve and hypoglossal nerve early during the operation to prevent accidental injury
- Divide the posterior belly of the digastric, stylohyoid muscle and stylomandibular ligament to allow exposure of the PPS
- Remove the submandibular gland and the styloid process if indicated to facilitate exposure of the PPS

- Careful finger dissection should be performed in the PPS to prevent tumor spillage
- Proper surgical technique and careful hemostasis during and after surgery diminish the risk of bleeding.

V. Special Postoperative Considerations
- Identify complications as early as possible
- Bleeding in this area can lead to an imminent airway obstruction. Open and evacuate the wound at the bedside if airway obstruction occurs
- Early reinstatement of temporomandibular joint and jaw physiotherapy should be used to prevent trismus.

VI. Complications
- Bleeding
- Seroma
- Wound infection
- Cranial nerve paralysis (spinal accessory and shoulder dysfunction, hypoglossal, lingual, marginal mandibular branch of the facial nerve, vagus, phrenic, brachial plexus, sympathetic trunk)
- Anesthesia in the periauricular area (a direct consequence of surgery rather than a complication)
- Jugular vein thrombosis in perioperative radiotherapy treatment
- First bite syndrome
- Frey's syndrome (in transparotid approach).

ADDITIONAL READING

1. Carrau RL, Myers EN, Johnson JT. Management of tumors arising in the parapharyngeal space. Laryngoscope. 1990;100(6):583-9.
2. Cohen SM, Burkey BB, Netterville JL. Surgical management of parapharyngeal space masses. Head Neck. 2005;27(8):669-75.
3. Khafif A, Segev Y, Kaplan DM, et al. Surgical management of parapharyngeal space tumors: a 10-year review. Otolaryngol Head Neck Surg. 2005;132(3):401-6.
4. Olsen KD. Tumors and surgery of the parapharyngeal space. Laryngoscope. 1994;104(5 Pt 2 Suppl 63):1-28.
5. Shahinian H, Dornier C, Fisch U. Parapharyngeal space tumors: the infratemporal fossa approach. Skull Base Surg. 1995;5(2):73-81.

Chapter 38

Hemi and Total Thyroidectomy

Ziv Gil, Dan M Fliss

INTRODUCTION

Surgery has become a routine procedure for management of neoplasms arising in the thyroid gland. The main objective of thyroid surgery is ablation of one or both of the thyroid lobes (Table 1). In case of thyroid cancer, complete removal of the tumor with adjacent thyroid tissue is indicated. Decision regarding hemi or total thyroidectomy is made according to tumor and patient's factors. The first includes histology, tumor size, extrathyroidal extension, differentiation and presence of locoregional or distant metastases (Table 2). Patient's factors include age, sex, family history and previous exposure to radiation. Multifocal disease and presence of solid nodules in the contralateral lobe is also considered as an indication for total thyroidectomy. The second goal of thyroid surgery is preservation of the parathyroid glands and their blood supply. Meticulous and proper surgical technique allows maintenance of normal calcium homeostasis without the need of supplements. The third goal of surgery is to prevent injury to the superior and recurrent laryngeal nerves. Preservation of the recurrent laryngeal nerve should be pursued in all cases of well differentiated thyroid cancers, if the vocal cords are functional. In case of a paralyzed vocal cord or in poorly differentiated thyroid cancers, sacrificing of one recurrent laryngeal nerve may be required. In order to perform a safe and efficient thyroid surgery, the surgeon should be familiar with the anatomy of the thyroid gland and the variations of the anatomical locations of the vital structures along the course of the gland, which will facilitate safe and efficient surgery. Improper technique may imminently lead to unnecessary complications, which may include hypocalcemia, vocal cord paralysis and superior laryngeal nerve palsy that can cause significant morbidity to patients.

Table 1: Goals of thyroid surgery

1. Ablation of one or both of the thyroid lobes
2. Preservation of the parathyroid glands and their blood supply
3. Prevent injury to the superior and recurrent laryngeal nerves

Table 2: Risk factors for recurrent disease in patients with thyroid cancer

Low-risk Factors	High-risk Factors
Patient factors	Patient factors
Age < 45	Age > 45
Female	Male
	Exposure to radiation
	Family history
Tumor Factors	*Tumor Factors*
Low-grade	High-grade
Size < 1.5 cm	Size > 1.5 cm
Single nodule	Multifocal disease
Unilateral nodule	Bilateral nodules
	Extrathyroid extension
	Nodal metastases
	Distant metastases

In this chapter, the technique practiced by the authors for surgical ablation of the thyroid gland will be described in details. This technique allows complete resection of the thyroid tissue, preservation of all parathyroid glands along with their blood supply, the recurrent and the superior laryngeal nerve.

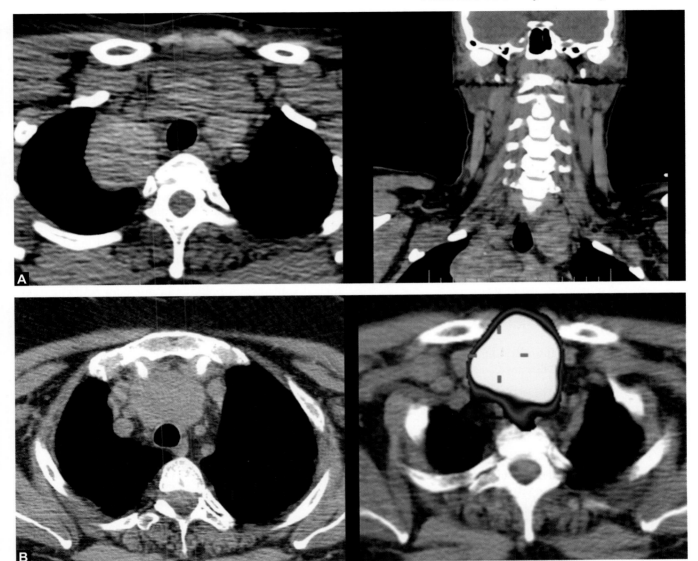

Figs 1A and B: (A) Preoperative CT scan of a patient with a large retrosternal goiter; (B) Preoperative coronal CT and PET-CT of a 52-year-old woman with papillary carcinoma invading the upper mediastinum

PREOPERATIVE EVALUATION AND ANESTHESIA

All patients scheduled for operation are evaluated preoperatively by a head and neck surgeon and an anesthesiologist. Patients younger than 18 years are also examined by a pediatrician. Radiological evaluation of the patient includes ultrasound of the neck. In case of giant or retrosternal goiters, axial and coronal computed tomography (CT) without contrast is indicated. Clinical suspicion of aggressive thyroid cancers with tracheal, vascular or esophageal involvement may necessitate CT with contrast or magnetic resonance imaging (MRI) of the neck to assess infiltration of the tumor to neighboring structures. Flexible tracheoscopy and esophagoscopy may be also used in these cases to examine intraluminal invasion. Figure 1A shows preoperative CT scan of a patient with a large retrosternal goiter.

Patients with complaints of hoarseness, stridor or dysphagia, and clinical findings of hemoptysis, vocal cord palsy and recent fast growth of the tumor should alert the surgeon toward diagnosis of poorly differentiated cancer. These patients may also be evaluated using a positron emission tomography-CT hybrid (PET-CT) prior to the operative procedure. A PET-CT scan of a patient with an aggressive papillary carcinoma of the thyroid gland involving the upper mediastinum is shown in Figure 1B.

It is recommended to routinely perform ultrasound guided fine needle aspiration (FNA) in all patients scheduled for thyroid surgery. Immunohistochemical staining of the cytologic sampling of calcitonin as well as calcitonin plasma levels should be performed in medullary carcinoma, if suspected during the anamnesis. All patients should undergo routine blood tests including thyroid function assessment, plasma calcium levels, complete blood count and coagulation function tests.

The authors do not recommend routine administration of prophylactic antibiotics since these are clean operations. First-generation cephalosporins may be used if the sterility of the surgery is compromised. Unless contraindicated, placement of number six, 5 - 7 tracheal tubes is recommended to prevent trauma to the vocal cords. Surgery is performed under general anesthesia with muscle relaxation. Intraoperative monitoring of the recurrent laryngeal nerves is performed in selected cases. These include revision surgery, recurrent thyroid cancer, unilateral vocal cord paralysis and surgery after previous external beam radiation therapy.

SURGICAL TECHNIQUE

Skin Incision

The patient is placed on the operating room table in a supine position. The head is stabilized with a soft donut holder and the whole operating table is then elevated in an angle with the head up in order to minimize bleeding.

The surgical access is planned through a horizontal neck incision (Fig. 2). Marking of the incision is preferably performed with the neck slightly flexed in order to identify the lines of relaxed skin tension. The incision is normally extended between the anterior borders of the sternocleidomastoid muscles, 2 cm above the clavicles. There are two options to gain access to the superior poles of the thyroid in patients with long neck: (i) higher incisions or; (ii) longer incision. The most important factor for positioning of the skin incision is to hide it along a transverse skin crest in the lower neck. From the authors' experience, correct placement of the incision is more important than its size. Female patients with large breasts, require higher incision than usual to prevent drop of the incision below the clavicles. Such incisions located over the manubrium tend to widen during time, become hypertrophic and cause poor cosmetic result. The length of a normal skin incision for thyroid surgery is normally 4 cm and the incision can be extended laterally for cervical access to large goiters. After incision marking, a roll is placed under the shoulders to hyperextend the neck. This positioning moves the thyroid gland anterior and cephalad.

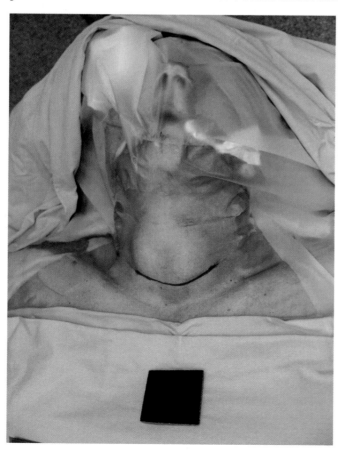
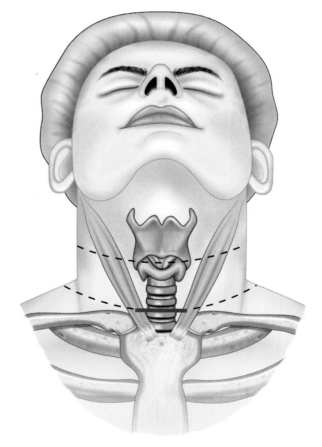

Fig. 2: Positioning and skin incision planning

The surgeon should be aware of the possibility that extension of the neck may pull the endotracheal tube out 2–4 cm from its original location. In such cases, repositioning of the tube caudally may be required. The patient is then prepped and draped in a standard surgical fashion. A transparent plastic cover is used to drape the head (from the level of mandible, upward) to allow the anesthesiology and surgical teams to continuously monitor the tube connectors (Fig. 2). This also prevents unnecessary traumatization of the skin by stapling or stitching.

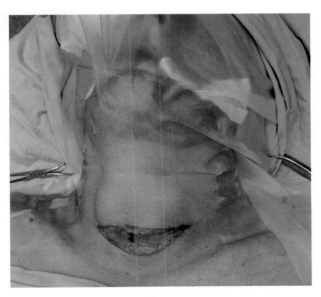

Fig. 3: Skin incision

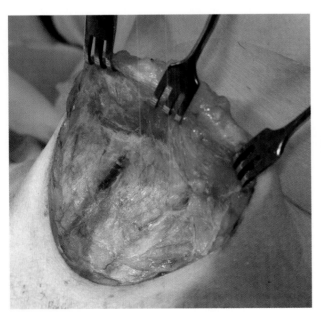

Skin Incision and Elevation of Subplatysmal Flaps

After marking, the skin is injected with lidocaine (0.06%) and epinephrine (1:1,000,000) to reduce the amount of pain after surgery and for hemostasis. The skin is incised with a number 15 blade and subsequent dissection of the subcutaneous tissue and the platysma is carried out with an electrocautery at the lowest effective setting (Fig. 3). Subplatysmal flaps are elevated superiorly, 1 cm above the thyroid notch and inferiorly to the sternum (Figs 4 and 5). This plane separates the superficial cervical fascia from the superficial layer of the deep cervical fascia (Fig. 6). Care is taken to prevent injury to the anterior jugular veins, which are left on the superficial layer of the deep cervical fascia. The flaps are retracted and held using skin hooks.

Exposure of the Thyroid Gland

The superficial layer of the deep cervical fascia is then elevated with forceps and divided along the midline avascular layer, between the infrahyoid strap muscles (Fig. 7). Small vessels interconnecting the anterior jugular veins are electrocautered with a bipolar or clamped and divided. Care is taken to avoid injury to the thyroid gland vessels that are located immediately below this layer. The dissection continues deep to the sternohyoid muscles. The fascia between the strap muscles is divided with electrocautery dissection and the isthmus is exposed as in Figure 7.

In case of small thyroid gland, an adequate exposure is accomplished without dividing the sternothyroid muscles. In case of large thyroid gland or if thyroid carcinoma is suspected, the sternohyoid muscle is separated from the

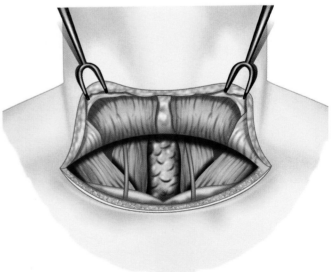

Fig. 4: Elevation of the superior subplatysmal flap

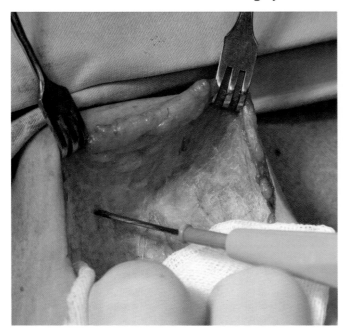

Fig. 5: Elevation of the inferior subplatysmal flap

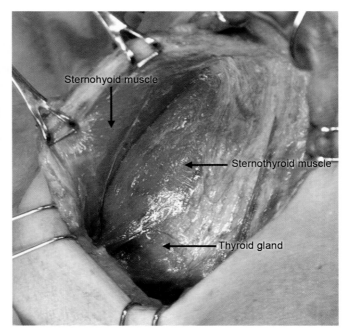

Fig. 6: Separation of the deep and superficial strap muscles

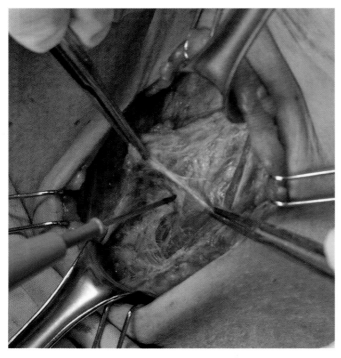

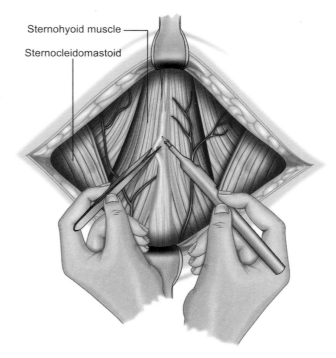

Fig. 7: Midline separation of the sternohyoid muscles

sternothyroid muscle using electrocautery dissection and the sternothyroid muscle is then divided in its upper pole (Fig. 8). This facilitates exposure of the superior thyroid artery. If extrathyroidal extension of the tumors is expected, the muscle is divided both superiorly and inferiorly, and the section of the muscle that abuts the tumor is left on the thyroid capsule in order to assure its removal in continuity with the tumor. Exposing first the side with the underlying pathology is usually preferred. The lobe is examined and palpated before dissection commences.

Dissection along the Superior Pole

Exposure of the superior pole of the thyroid lobe begins by retraction of the strap muscle with a Richardson retractor laterally and with a right angle retractor cephalad. This maneuver facilitates exposure of the tip of the superior pole (Fig. 9). The next step is separation of the superior stump of the sternohyoid muscle from the thyroid. This is performed with electrocautery or bipolar. Now the surgery continues by separating the superior pole from its superomedial attachment to the fascia investing the cricothyroid muscles. This technique is crucial in order to delineate the superior thyroid pole from medial to lateral releasing the tethered pole. Within this area frequently lie tiny vessels interconnecting the superior pole with the fascia investing the cricothyroid muscles. These vessels should be carefully ligated close to the gland in order to prevent unintended injury to the superior laryngeal nerve (SLN) and to facilitate exposure of the superior pole as in Figure 9.

At this stage, the vessels supplying the superior pole are divided (Fig. 10). Mass ligature of the superior pedicle at this stage is ill-advised due to several reasons: (i) the extent of the superior thyroid pole is variable and its upper part can be easily left behind after thyroidectomy causing superfluous uptake during postsurgical radioactive iodine scanning; (ii) the superior laryngeal nerve (SLN) accompanies the superior thyroid vessels and may be injured during bulky ligation of the pedicle; (iii) high ligation of the superior thyroid artery may compromise blood supply to the superior parathyroid glands causing postoperative hypocalcemia; (iv) the superior parathyroid gland is occasionally located posteriorly to the superior pole and may be resected with the specimen and; (v) massive ligation of the superior thyroid pedicle may cause retraction of the vessels cephalad causing bleeding, which may be difficult to control. High and bulky ligation of the superior pole may cause inadvert injury

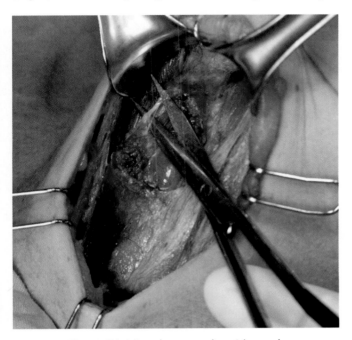

Fig. 8: Dividing the sternothyroid muscle

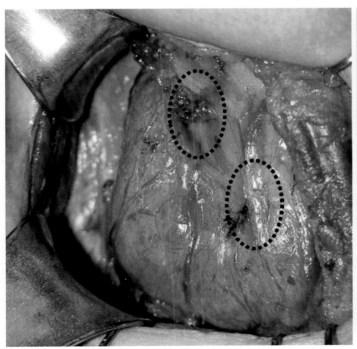

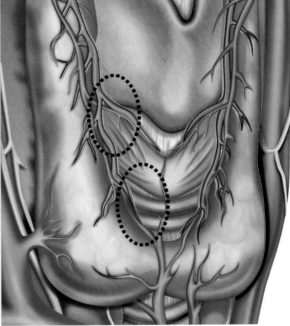

Fig. 9: Exposure of the thyroid lobe . Encircled are tiny vessels interconnecting the superior thyroid pole with the fascia investing the cricothyroid muscles

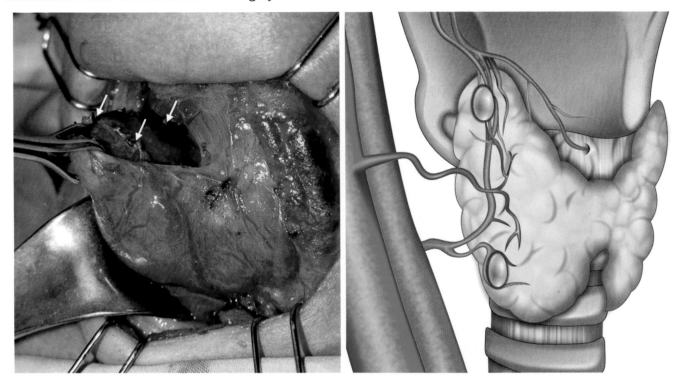

Fig. 10: Dividing the vessels supplying the superior pole. Arrows indicate the ligated blood vessels of the superior pole

to the SLN (Fig. 11). Therefore, it is advisable to ligate the individual branches of the superior thyroid artery and vein. As the dissection continues along its posterior border, the pole gradually drops down caudally away from the SLN and some remaining small posterior vessels can be cauterized safely with a bipolar.

Exposure of the Inferior Pole

After separating of the superior thyroid lobe, the sternohyoid muscle is dissected caudally with electrocautery exposing its inferior pole. At this stage, it is recommended to delineate the inferior border of the thyroid lobe along its border with the trachea. This is performed by gentle dissection with a clamp (Fig. 12). This simple maneuver allows: (i) the identification of the lower border of the gland; (ii) the identification of the inferior thyroid vessels and; (iii) the identification of the trachea. The fascia overlying the inferior pole and its small vessels should be identified and divided carefully in order to prevent injury to the recurrent laryngeal nerve, which may be displaced medially by the tumor.

Subcapsular Dissection of the Thyroid Gland

After separation of the inferior and superior poles of the thyroid lobe, a subcapsular dissection is performed. This technique is recommended in order to prevent devascularization of the parathyroid glands. The gland is rotated medially and retracted gently with two pediatric Babcock

forceps or with small gauze. At this point, the surgery continues with a "subcapsular" dissection along the visceral fascia in a cranial to caudal direction. This fascia is consistent of multiple thin layers of connective tissue that encapsulate the thyroid gland and its superficial thyroid vasculature. The parathyroid glands receive their blood supply from branches of the inferior thyroid artery and less frequently also from the superior thyroid artery. The parathyroid glands and their vascular supplies are invested in these thin layers. The fascia is striped from the underlying thyroid by spreading of a micro clamp and by cauterizing the small vessels with bipolar cautery. While the visceral fascia is reflected laterally, the terminal branches of the inferior thyroid artery are ligated distal to the parathyroid glands and the thyroid "capsule" is peeled away along with the parathyroid glands. This technique allows identification and preservation of the upper and lower parathyroid glands along with their blood supply, which are contained in this adventitial layer. The superior and inferior parathyroid glands can be distinguished from the underlying thyroid tissue by their yellowish brown color (café ole), its fatty consistency and its teardrop shape. Rarely, the surgeon may harvest a small part of a suspected parathyroid gland for fast pathological examination during surgery to confirm its diagnosis. Unintentional devascularization of the parathyroid glands will lead to change in the color of the parathyroids from light to dark brown within few minutes. If a parathyroid gland is detached from its blood

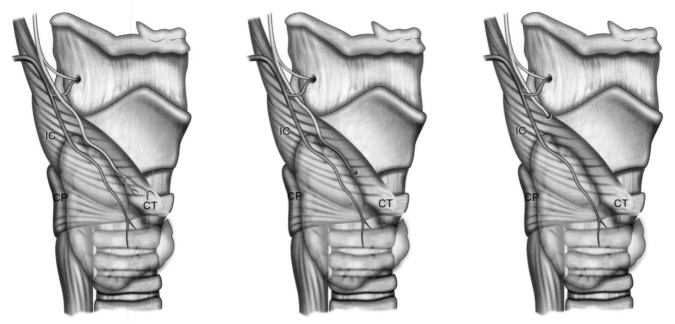

Fig. 11: Anatomical variants of the external branch of the superior laryngeal nerve. In the first variant, the external branch of the superior laryngeal nerve descend superficially to the inferior constrictor muscle running next to the superior thyroid vessels before innervating the cricothyroid muscles. In the second variant, the external branch of the superior laryngeal nerve pierces the inferior constrictor muscle, approximately 1 cm above the cricothyroid membrane. In the third variant, the external branch of the superior laryngeal nerve runs deep to the inferior constrictor muscle which literally protects the nerve from unintended injury. IC: Inferior constrictor; CP: Cricopharyngeus muscle; CT: Cricoid cartilage

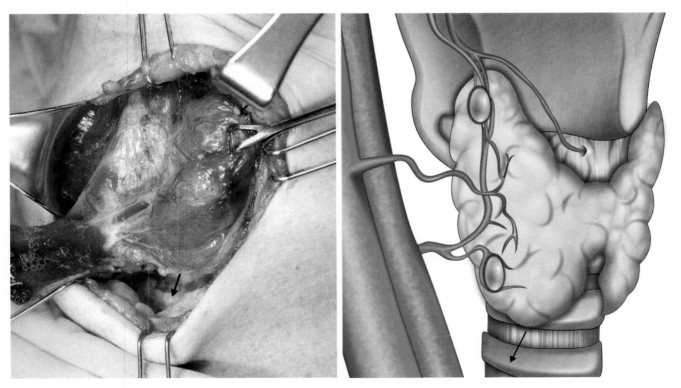

Fig. 12: Exposure of the lower border of the thyroid gland and division of the inferior thyroid vessels. The arrows indicate the trachea

supply, reimplantation of the gland is recommended after confirming its diagnosis using frozen section. Parathyroid gland reimplantation is performed by mincing the devascularized gland into 1 mm cubes and placing it into a small pocket in the middle portion of the sternocleidomastoid muscle. The area of reimplantation is marked with small titanium clips, in case future surgery is indicated.

Dissection along the Tracheoesophageal Groove and Preservation of the Recurrent Laryngeal Nerve

The subcapsular dissection is meticulously continued from medial to lateral and the tissue overlying the surface of the gland is reflected inferiorly and laterally. Small vessels interconnecting the thyroid gland and the visceral fascia are divided with a bipolar electrocautery. These vessels should be divided one by one in order to prevent accidental injury to the recurrent laryngeal nerve. The middle thyroid vein is identified, clamped and ligated immediately on the capsule of the gland.

It has been formerly contemplated that the next step in thyroid surgery should be identification of the recurrent laryngeal nerve. However, identifying the nerve at this point has several pitfalls. First, it almost and always will cause bleeding from injured vessels along the course of the nerve, which will further complicate its identification. Second, it may inadvertently cause injury to the recurrent laryngeal nerve, either directly with the spreading clamp or as a result of attempts of hemostasis of the bleeding near the nerve with clamping or with electrocautery. Finally, it may cause injury to the inferior thyroid vessels and unintentional devascularization of the parathyroid glands. The technique proposed here takes into consideration the different anatomical variations of the recurrent laryngeal nerve (RLN) as depicted in Figure 13. Other variations in the location of the RLN are related to the side of the operated neck. On the left side, the RLN crosses anterior to the aortic arch, loops under it and ascends in a relatively constant position along the tracheoesophageal groove. On the other hand, the course of the right RLN is less predicted, since it crosses anterior to the subclavian artery and ascend posterior to the artery and relatively more laterally than on the left side.

As the subcapsular dissection continues, the gland from the trachea below the middle thyroid vein is separated. This dissection at this stage should include only preidentified tissue including see-through fibrous tissue or vessels in order to prevent injury to the RLN. This maneuver will free the lobe from its attachment to the trachea allowing reflection of the lobe medially, away from the nerve. Usually, the nerve is exposed lateral or below the tubercle of Zuckerkandl (Fig. 14). When identified, the nerve should be untethered

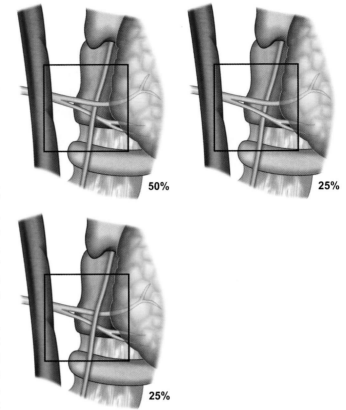

Fig. 13: Anatomical variations of the recurrent laryngeal nerve and its relationships with the middle thyroid vein, the thyroid gland, the Zuckerkandl tubercle, the trachea and the esophagus. The recurrent laryngeal nerve may come into view at this point, lateral to the Zuckerkandl tubercle and superficial to the lateral border of the trachea. In more than half of the cases, the RLN is located along the tracheoesophageal groove, posterior to Berry's ligament (i.e. the posterior suspensory ligament). In the rest of the cases, the RLN may ascend along the paratracheal region, it may pierce the ligament of Berry or lie below the thyroid parenchyma

from the gland and reflected away. If the nerve is found below the lateral border of the thyroid, the gland should be separated from the underlying nerve with a fine clamp. The thyroid is elevated above the nerve and meticulously transected and ligated. All dissections along the nerve should be performed only with a fine clamp and any retraction of the nerve with hook or vessel loop should be avoided to prevent neuropraxia and temporary vocal cord paralysis. It is suggested that blood vessels in this location should be ligated with 4-0 silk sutures to prevent subsequent hemorrhage that may result in an inadvertent injury to the RLN during hemostasis. Electrocautery of bleeding vessels near the nerve

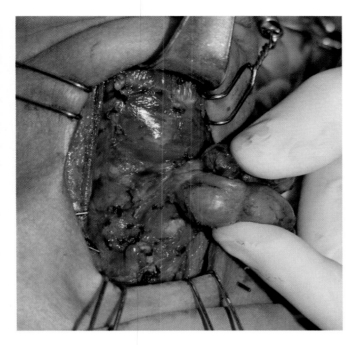

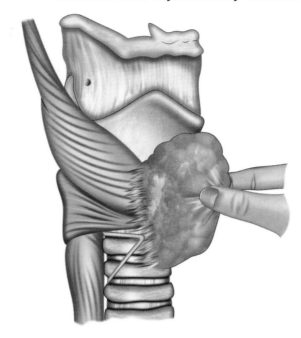

Fig. 14: Exposure of the recurrent laryngeal nerve. This maneuver will free the lobe from its attachment to the trachea, allowing reflection of the lobe medially, away from the nerve

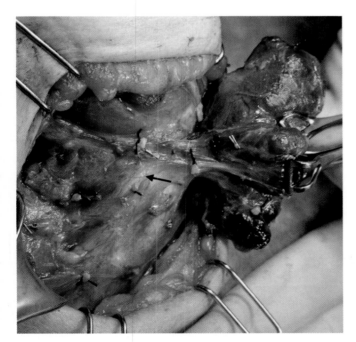

Fig. 15: Dissection along the Berry's ligament. The arrow indicates the recurrent laryngeal nerve

may cause neuropraxia and temporary vocal cord paralysis due to thermal trauma to the fragile nerve bundles.

After displacement of the nerve away from the thyroid gland, the dissection continues along the posterolateral portion of the gland toward the ligament of Berry (Fig. 15). Ligation of any vascular structure in this area should be performed only after identification and preservation of the RLN and all of its branches. At this area the thyroid gland may be tethered by the ligament of Berry to the trachea. This dense fibrotic structure attaches the gland to the first and second tracheal rings. After identification and preservation of the RLN, dissection of the ligament of Berry is carried keeping the nerve in view at all times.

Rarely, the tumor may be adherent to the perineurium or may infiltrate deep to the perineural space. If the recurrent laryngeal nerve is paralyzed preoperatively and intraoperative exploration shows neural invasion by cancer, the nerve should be sacrificed. In cases of neural invasion of differentiated thyroid cancers and normal nerve function, effort should be made to meticulously dissect the tumor from the perineurium rather than from resecting the nerve. In these cases, adjuvant therapy with radioactive iodine may be applied for tumor control. On the other hand, undifferentiated thyroid cancers are likely not to react to radioactive iodine therapy and in these cases the nerve may be sacrificed in order to assure complete tumor resection. Nonetheless, before sacrificing a functional nerve, it is important first to confirm that the contralateral nerve is free of tumor and can be safely preserved during thyroidectomy.

The inferior thyroid arteries and veins are divided and ligated close to the thyroid gland to assure preservation of the blood supply to the parathyroid glands. Dissection along Berry's ligament is continued with electrocautery or with sharp dissection and the thyroid lobe is completely mobilized except for the attachment of the isthmus to the contralateral lobe. A clamp is placed lateral to the isthmus, separating it from the opposite lobe, cut and ligated with continuous vicryl sutures for hemostasis. If total thyroidectomy is indicated, division of the two lobes is not required and the whole thyroid gland is resected in an en bloc fashion. Small amount of oozing along the course of the RLN is best managed with Surgicel® or Avitene® absorbable hemostats. In 10% of the patients, a thyroidea ima artery may be present below the gland, anterior to the trachea. This artery emerges directly from the aorta or occasionally from the brachiocephalic trunk to supply the inferior pole of the gland and should be ligated at the level of the thyroid capsule.

Attention is then turned to dissection of the pyramidal lobe (Fig. 16), which is found in more than 50% of the individuals. The pyramidal lobe can be branched off from the left or right thyroid lobe, or from the isthmus. The lobe is stripped from the underlying cricothyroid muscles using electrocautery from a superior to inferior direction and resected along with the rest of the thyroid gland. The thyroidectomy specimen is then oriented with a silk stitch marking the left or right thyroid lobes (Figs 17 to 19) and submitted to the pathology laboratory for analysis.

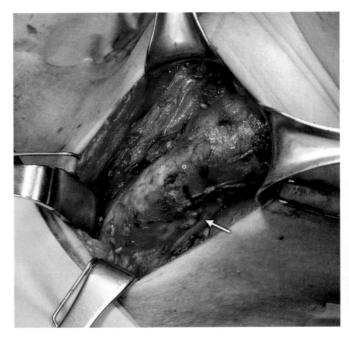

Fig. 17: The surgical field after total thyroidectomy. The arrow indicates the recurrent laryngeal nerve

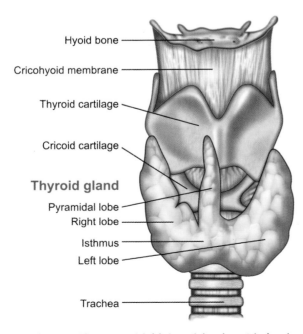

Fig. 16: The pyramidal lobe of the thyroid gland

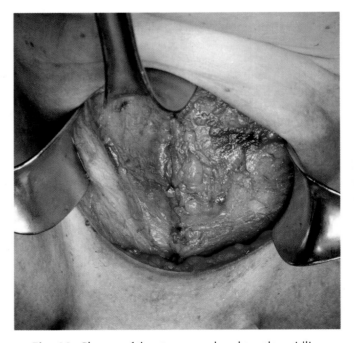

Fig. 18: Closure of the strap muscles along the midline

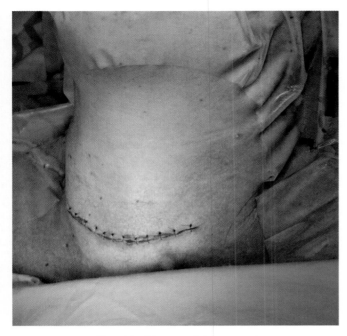

Fig. 19: Closure of the wound

POSTOPERATIVE TREATMENT

After surgery, the patients are extubated and immediately transferred to the critical care unit for 24 hours. The patients routinely undergo CT scan after the operation to rule out bleeding or tension pneumocephalus. The wound is kept clean by rinsing it with hydrogen peroxide three times a day during the first 10 days after the operation and covered with antibiotic ointment after each cleansing. The drains are removed either, 3 days after the operation or when the fluid was less than 20 ml in 24 hours. Broad-spectrum antibiotics are instituted preoperatively and continued until the packing is removed. For pain control, the patients are treated with nonsteroidal anti-inflammatory drugs (diclofenac 75 mg intramuscularly or orally, or rofecoxib 50 mg) once daily and with tramadol (50–100 mg) if the patient asks for them or if the nurses felt it to be necessary.

HIGHLIGHTS

I. Indications
- Significantly enlarged thyroid gland
- Suspected thyroid cancer
- Differentiated or undifferentiated thyroid carcinomas
- Medullary thyroid carcinoma
- Graves disease refractory to nonsurgical treatment.

II. Contraindications
- Tumor invades the prevertebral fascia, encases carotid artery, or involves mediastinal structures.
- Anaplastic thyroid carcinoma.

III. Complications
- Bleeding
- Seroma
- Wound infection
- Recurrent laryngeal nerve paralysis leading to hoarseness and aspirations
- Temporary hypocalcemia
- Permanent hypocalcemia
- Bilateral recurrent laryngeal nerve paralysis, requiring tracheostomy.

IV. Special Preoperative Considerations
- Imaging using ultrasound
- Ultrasound guided fine needle aspiration
- Thyroid function tests and calcium level
- Evaluation of neck nodes by ultrasound.

V. Special Intraoperative Considerations
- Dividing the sternothyroid muscle higher as possible
- Ligation of the blood vessels medial to the superior pole
- Ligation of the blood vessels of the superior pole close to the thyroid gland
- Identifying of the trachea in the midline
- Subcapsular dissection and preservation of the parathyroid glands and their blood supply
- Identify the recurrent laryngeal nerve at its closest location to the thyroid gland
- Proper surgical technique and careful hemostasis during and after surgery diminish the risk of bleeding.

VI. Special Postoperative Considerations
- Identify complications early as possible.
- Bleeding in this area can lead to an imminent airway obstruction. Open and evacuate the wound at the bedside if airway obstruction occurs.
- Identify and treat hypocalcemia promptly.

ADDITIONAL READING

1. Farrag TY, Agrawal N, Sheth S, et al. Algorithm for safe and effective reoperative thyroid bed surgery for recurrent/persistent papillary thyroid carcinoma. Head Neck. 2007;29 (12):1069-74.
2. Fliss DM, Zucker G, Cohen A, et al. Early outcome and complications of the extended subcranial approach to the anterior skull base. Laryngoscope. 1999;109(1):153-60.

3. Gil Z, Abergel A, Leider-Trejo L, et al. A comprehensive algorithm for anterior skull base reconstruction after oncological resections. Skull Base. 2007;17(1):25-37.

4. Gil Z, Abergel A, Spektor S, et al. Quality of life following surgery for anterior skull base tumors. Arch Otolaryngol Head Neck Surg. 2003;129(12):1303-9.

5. Gil Z, Constantini S, Spektor S, et al. Skull base approaches in the pediatric population. Head Neck. 2005;27(8): 682-9.

6. Gil Z, Fliss DM. Contemporary management of head and neck cancers. Isr Med Assoc J. 2009;11(5):296-300.

7. Gil Z, Fliss DM. Pericranial wrapping of the frontal bone after anterior skull base tumor resection. Plast Reconstr Surg. 2005(2);116(2):395-8.

8. Gil Z, Patel SG. Surgery for thyroid cancer. Surg Oncol Clin N Am. 2008;17(1):93-120, viii.

9. McCaffrey JC. Aerodigestive tract invasion by well-differentiated thyroid carcinoma: diagnosis, management, prognosis, and biology. Laryngoscope. 2006;116(1):1-11.

10. Myers EN, Pantangco IP. Intratracheal thyroid. Laryngoscope. 1975;85(11 pt 1):1833-40.

11. Newman E, Shaha AR. Substernal goiter. J Surg Oncol. 1995;60(3):207-12. Review.

12. Pagedar NA, Freeman JL. Identification of the external branch of the superior laryngeal nerve during thyroidectomy. Arch Otolaryngol Head Neck Surg. 2009;135(4):360-2.

13. Randolph GW, Kamani D. The importance of preoperative laryngoscopy in patients undergoing thyroidectomy: voice, vocal cord function, and the preoperative detection of invasive thyroid malignancy. Surgery. 2006;139(3):357-62.

14. Raveh J, Laedrach K, Speiser M, et al. The subcranial approach for fronto-orbital and anteroposterior skull-base tumor. Arch Otolaryngol Head Neck Surg. 1993;119(4):385-93.

15. Shaha AR, Shah JP, Loree TR. Low-risk differentiated thyroid cancer: the need for selective treatment. Ann Surg Oncol. 1997;4(4):328-33.

16. Shemen LJ, Strong EW. Complications after total thyroidectomy. Otolaryngol Head Neck Surg. 1989;101(4):472-5.

Chapter 39

Mandibular Split Approaches to Cancers of the Oral Cavity

Ziv Gil, Dan M Fliss

INTRODUCTION

During the last decade the management of oral cavity squamous cell carcinoma (OSCC) changed dramatically, mostly due to reconstruction means and the use of adjuvant treatment modalities. Management of OSCC should be tailored according to characteristics of the tumor and, patient and surgeon preferences. The main goals of therapy are: (i) ablation of cancer while minimizing morbidity; (ii) preservation or restoration of function and; (iii) improvement of the patient's quality of life. These goals are achieved by a multidisciplinary team including specialists in head and neck surgery, reconstructive surgery, radiation oncology, medical oncology, dental surgery, prosthetics, pathology and rehabilitation medicine. Adjunctive teams including speech and swallowing, psychiatry or addiction services may also participate in the management of these patients as indicated.

Tumors originating in the oral cavity require surgical ablation. As a rule, early stage (stage I and II) OSCC should be managed with a single modality, while advanced tumors are managed with a multimodality therapy. Therefore, advanced stage OSCC will require adjuvant treatment, which includes radiation therapy with or without chemotherapy. The overall objective of all surgical oncology procedures is to excise all tumor extensions with sufficient surgical margins. Tumors originating in the oral cavity, which are accessible and relatively nonsensitive to radiation, are managed surgically. Patients with distant metastases are considered nonsurgical candidates with the exception of adenoid cystic carcinoma. The tumor should be resected if possible in an en bloc fashion in order to decrease the possibility of tumor spillage, to allow resection of the adjoining lymphatic system and to ensure the presence of negative margins. A 2 cm margin can be achieved in most cases of oral cavity carcinomas.

Patients with OSCC, has a 3% risk per year of developing a second primary tumor even after complete tumor ablation. Prevention (smoking and alcohol cessation) and early detection should be a principal objective of postoperative patient care. Follow-up of patients with OSCC is aimed at early detection of primary tumor recurrence, locoregional or distant metastases, or of a second primary tumor. Routine head and neck examination and yearly chest X-ray imaging are part of the management of these patients after surgery. Computed tomography (CT), magnetic resonance imaging (MRI) and positron emission tomography (PET-CT) imaging can be used for early detection of recurrence in this population.

In this chapter, the technique practiced by the authors for resection of large oral cavity tumors, which require mandibular split, will be described in details. This technique allows complete resection of the tumor and requires reconstruction with a free flap tissue transfer.

PREOPERATIVE EVALUATION AND ANESTHESIA

All patients scheduled for operation are evaluated preoperatively by a head and neck surgeon, an anesthesiologist, an oral and maxillofacial surgeon and a plastic surgeon. Patients younger than 18 years are also examined by a pediatrician. Radiological evaluation of the patients includes computed tomography (CT) with contrast, magnetic

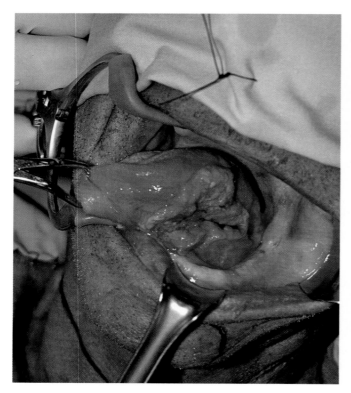

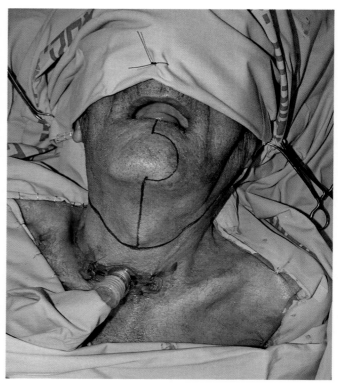

Fig. 1: Anterior oral tongue squamous cell carcinoma, clinically T3N1M0 stage IV. The tumor invades the floor of mouth but not the mandible. The tumor crosses the midline and the depth of invasion is greater than 10 mm

Fig. 2: Positioning and skin incision planning. Tracheostomy is performed at the beginning of the operation

resonance imaging (MRI) and positron emission tomography (PET-CT). Figure 1 shows an invasive T3 OSCC of tongue of a patient with a tumor infiltrating the oral tongue, base of tongue and floor of mouth. Flexible endoscopy is used in these cases to examine the larynx, hypopharynx and cervical esophagus. All patients should undergo routine blood tests including complete blood count and coagulation function tests.

Most patients with advanced disease will require adjuvant treatment. Therefore, it is suggested to evaluate the need for teeth extraction before the operation. In addition, placement of percutaneous endoscopic gastrostomy (PEG) or jejunostomy (PEJ) is indicated if adjuvant chemoradiation is expected and if low oral patency is expected.

SURGICAL TECHNIQUE

Composite Subtotal Glossectomy via Paramedian Mandibulotomy

Since this is a clean contaminated operation, prophylactic antibiotic treatment with first generation cephalosporin

and metronidazole is indicated. Surgery is performed under general anesthesia with muscle relaxation. After endotracheal or nasal intubation, a tracheostomy is performed. The tracheostomy tube is usually inserted as low as possible in the neck to separate it from the neck flaps.

Skin Incision

The patient is placed on the operating room table in a supine position. The head is stabilized with a soft donut holder and the whole operating table is then elevated in an angle with the head up in order to minimize bleeding.

The surgical access is planned through a lip-split incision, extended to a horizontal neck incision toward the ipsilateral side of the tumor (Fig. 2). The incision will allow raising of a lower cheek flap, exposure of the mandibulotomy site and neck dissection. The author is referred to Chapter 33 for description of the neck dissection. Marking of the incision is preferably performed with the neck slightly flexed in order to identify the lines of relaxed skin tension. The lip incision is performed in the midline, circumferencing the chin toward the side of the tumor, extended caudally up to the level of the cricoid cartilage. This incision is then extended laterally to a formal collar neck incision up to the level of the mastoid bone. After marking of the incision, the patient is prepped and draped in a standard surgical fashion.

Elevation of Subplatysmal Flaps

The skin is incised with a number 15 blade and subsequent dissection of the subcutaneous tissue and the platysma is carried out with an electrocautery at the lowest effective setting. Subplatysmal flaps are elevated superiorly, 1 cm below the ramus of the mandible and inferiorly to the clavicle. This plane separates the superficial cervical fascia from the superficial layer of the deep cervical fascia. Care is taken to prevent injury to the marginal mandibular branch of the facial nerve. The nerve runs within the fascia superior to the submandibular gland. Injury to the nerve is prevented by elevation of the flap immediately below the platysma leaving the superficial layer of the deep cervical fascia on the submandibular gland. If dissection of the pre- and postvascular lymph nodes is indicated, the flap is elevated to the level of the mandible, exposing the facial artery and vein. Routine removal of the pre- and postvascular lymph nodes is not included in the neck dissection. There are three main indications for extirpation of these nodes: (i) skin or lip cancers for which the lymph nodes around the facial artery may be the primary echelon; (ii) tumors of the floor of mouth or mandible abutting the pre- and postvascular nodes and; (iii) clinical or radiological evidence of positive nodes at this level. The flaps are retracted and held using skin hooks (Fig. 3). The lower flaps should remain separate from the tracheostomy incision in order to prevent contamination of the surgical area by tracheal secretions.

Mandibulotomy

After the lip and skin of the chin are split at the midline, the incision is extended to the level of the outer cortex of the mandible. The soft tissue overlying the mandible is elevated bilaterally, deep to the periosteum approximately 2–3 cm on each side of the planned osteotomy (Fig. 4). In the presented case, the mandible was stripped from the gingival mucosa to ensure 2 cm margins from the tumor. The osteotomy site is marked with a pen in a paramedian position. If possible, care is taken to preserve the mental nerve, which enters the mental foramen (Figs 5 and 6). Before performing the osteotomy, two titanium miniplates are prebanded and fixed to the mandible. One is fixed to the anterior face of the cortex and the second

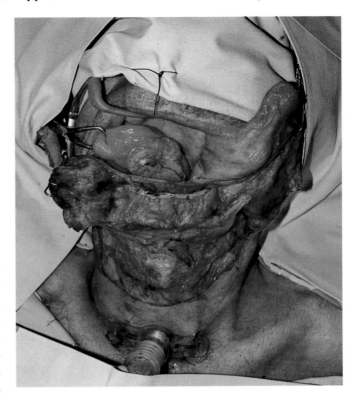

Fig. 3: Skin incision and elevation of the subplatysmal flaps and lower cheek flap. An upper and lower platysmal flaps are elevated. A lip-split incision is performed and a lower cheek flap is developed. The mandible is exposed and the mucosa overlying the mandible is included in the specimen along with the floor of mouth. In this edentulous patient, there is no mandibular involvement

to the inferior border of the mandible (Fig. 7). This two-point fixation minimizes free movement of the mandible. Attention is now turned to the osteotomy. As a general rule, the osteotomy is performed in a paramedian position in the ipsilateral side of the tumor. Paramidline mandibulotomy is preferred to lateral or medial mandibulotomy for several reasons: (i) the osteotomy is performed through a wider space between the lateral incisor and canine; (ii) it preserves dentition and; (iii) the genioglossus and geniohyoid muscles. Lateral mandibulotomy has several disadvantages, including unequal pull of the muscles, which increases movement of the segments during mastication, denervation of the teeth medial to the osteotomy and devascularization of the distal segment of the mandible. For these reasons and since the osteotomy is within the lateral portal of the radiation beam, lateral osteotomy is associated with high-risk of osteoradionecrosis.

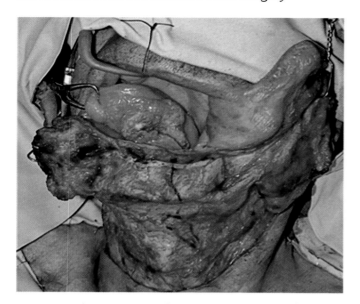

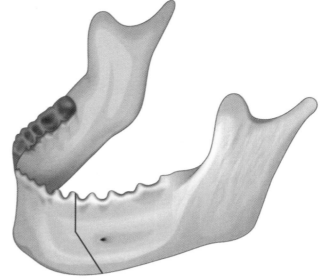

Fig. 4: Exposure and marking of the osteotomy site. The mandibulotomy is performed in an angled direction to allow maximum fixation

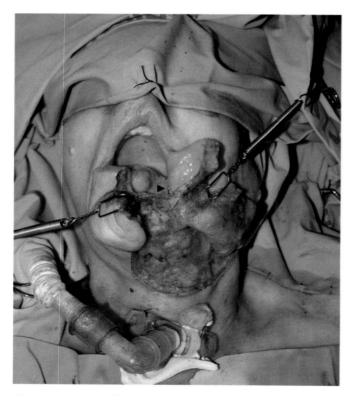

Fig. 5: Exposure of the mandibulotomy site. A sleeve of buccal mucosa is left on the mandible to facilitate watertight closure of the oral cavity (arrowhead)

The mandibulotomy can be performed in a straight line, in a step ladder fashion or in an angled direction. The angled osteotomy is presumed to provide better stability (Figs 8 and 9). Osteotomy is performed with a reciprocal sagittal mechanical saw with a thin blade to minimize bone loss. Once the mandible is split, the ramus in the ipsilateral side is swung laterally (Fig. 10). The gingivolabial incision is extended toward the anterior pillar of the tonsil, allowing further exposure of the base of tongue (Fig. 11). Division of the mylohyoid muscle is required to allow lateral retraction of the mandible. After achieving adequate exposure of the oral and base of tongue, attention is turned to resect the tumor. Two centimeter margins from the tumor are required to achieve complete tumor resection (Fig. 12). During the resection, brisk bleeding is expected from the lingual artery and its branches, which are controlled with number 4-0 silk sutures and bipolar electrocautery. Excision of the tumor is achieved in a monoblock fashion along with the floor of mouth and lymph nodes of the neck (Figs 13 and 14). After removal of the tumor, the margins are sent for frozen section evaluation. The surgical specimen is shown in Figure 15. Reconstruction is performed with a fascia lata sling flap for supporting of the floor of mouth (Fig. 16). An anterolateral thigh free flap is used for reconstruction of the tongue and floor of mouth as in Figure 17.

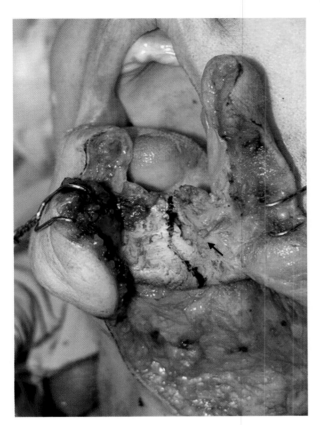

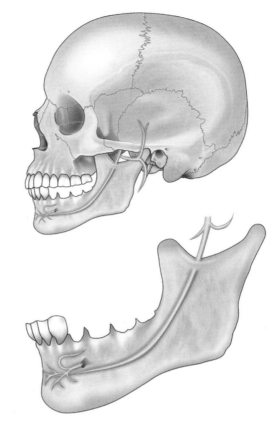

Fig. 6: Marking of the osteotomy site. An angled osteotomy is performed to allow maximum fixation in two dimensions. The mental nerve at its entrance to the mental foramen is shown (arrow)

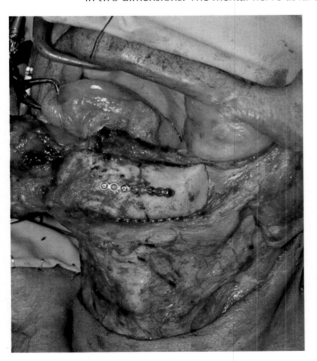

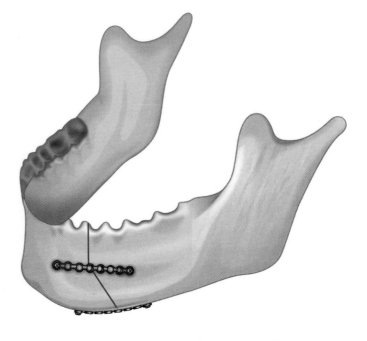

Fig. 7: Fixation of the titanium miniplates prior to the osteotomy. Titanium miniplates are placed in two different dimensions; anterior and inferior to the mandible, to allow maximal fixation in two dimensions

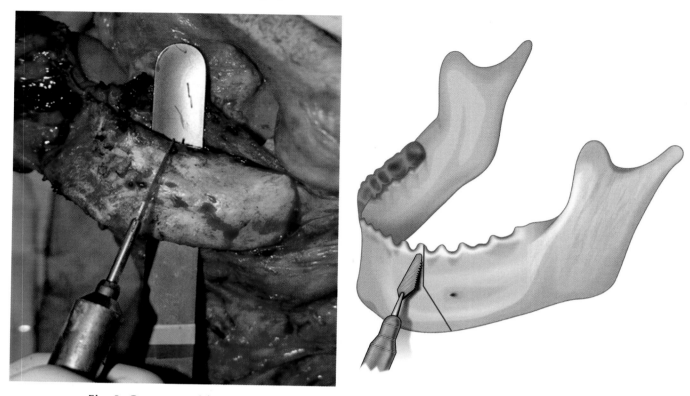

Fig. 8: Osteotomy of the mandible. An angled paramedian osteotomy is the procedure of choice

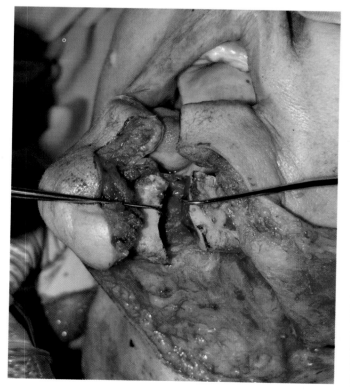

Fig. 9: A paramedian mandibulotomy

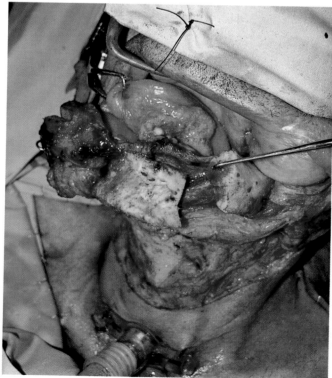

Fig. 10: Separation of the mandible

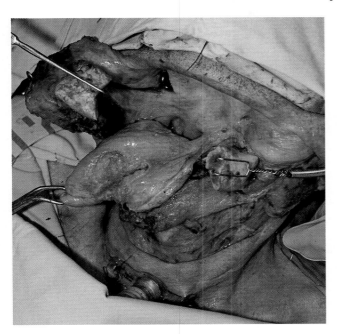

Fig. 11: Exposure of the tumor

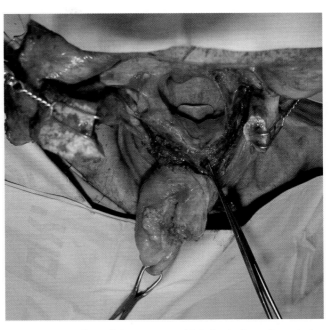

Fig. 12: Resection of the tumor, which includes subtotal glossectomy and resection of the base of tongue, floor of mouth, hyoid bone, left tonsillar fossa, mylohyoid muscle and the extrinsic muscles of the tongue. The epiglottis and hypopharynx mark the inferior margin of the resection

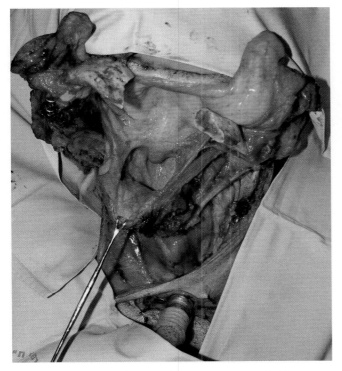

Fig. 13: The surgical area after tumor removal. The upper limit of the resection is the palate. The posterior margin of the resection is the base of tongue

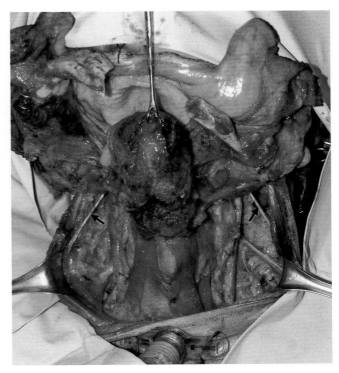

Fig. 14: The caudal margin of the resection is the thyroid cartilage. A bilateral selective neck dissection including levels I–IV is also performed. Arrows indicate the spinal accessory nerves

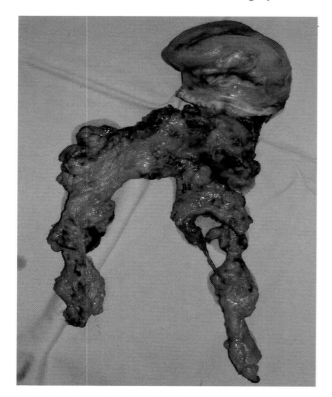

Fig. 15: The surgical specimen. The composite resection includes the tongue, base of tongue on the left, floor of mouth, extrinsic muscles of the tongue and floor of mouth and bilateral neck dissection. The tumor is resected en bloc with the lymphatic tissue of the neck

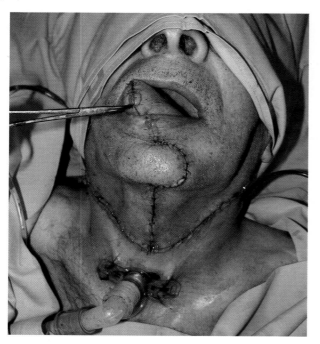

Fig. 17: The defect is reconstructed with an anterolateral thigh free flap

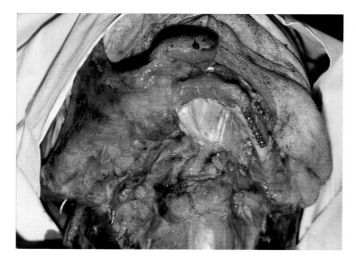

Fig. 16: The floor of mouth is supported with a fascia lata sheath

Composite Resection of a Recurrent OSCC via Paramedian Mandibulotomy

The next case shows resection of a recurrent floor of mouth OSCC tumor. The clinical T1NoMo tumor, recurred in the deep extrinsic muscles of the tongue. The composite resection is performed via paramedian mandibulotomy. Figure 18 shows the planning of the incision. In this case, the mental nerve is preserved. Marking of the osteotomy site and preplating is performed before the osteotomy (Fig. 19). Following the mandibulotomy, the area of the tumor in the extrinsic muscles of the tongue is exposed (Fig. 20). The surgical site after tumor resection is shown in Figure 21.

Reconstruction

The reconstruction technique is designed according to the size and location of the defect based on radiological and intraoperative calculations. There are three options for reconstruction after partial glossectomy: (i) primary closure; (ii) reconstruction with a rotational pectoralis major flap and; (iii) free flap reconstruction. The first option is performed when the defect is small, a rare situation in this type of operation. The second type of reconstruction is performed for large defects in patients who cannot tolerate long operation. Free flap reconstruction is performed in most patients for reconstruction of function when the surgical defect is sizeable. Anterolateral thigh musculocutaneous flap or radial forearm flap are often used for this purpose (Fig. 17).

The specimen is oriented and submitted to the pathology laboratory for analysis. The wound is copiously irrigated, inspected and hemostasis is performed as indicated. A blood pressure above 120/80 should be confirmed prior to closure

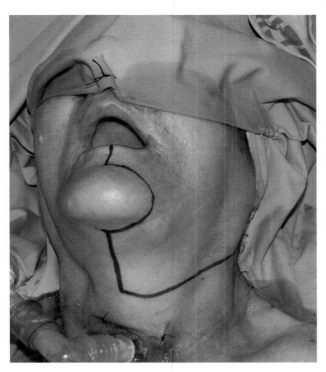

Fig. 18: Planning of the skin incision in a patient with recurrent oral cavity squamous cell carcinoma . This rT1N0M0 tumor recurred in the area of the extrinsic muscles of the tongue

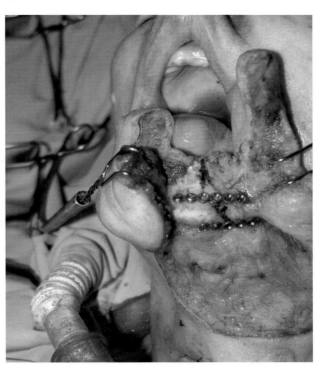

Fig. 19: Plating is performed with titanium miniplates before the osteotomy. The plates are positioned anterior and inferior to the mandible to assure maximal three-dimensional fixation

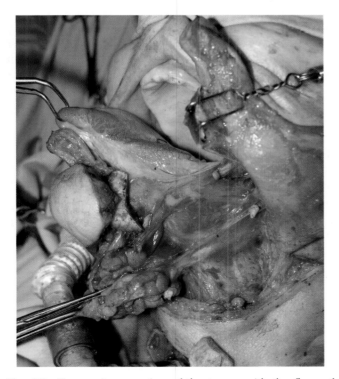

Fig. 20: Composite resection of the tumor with the floor of mouth, suprahyoid muscles and sublingual and submandibular glands

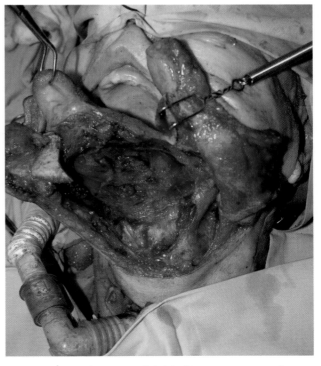

Fig. 21: The surgical field after tumor removal

for adequate hemostasis. A Jackson-Pratt number 7 drain is left at the surgical bed. The prebanded titanium plates are used to fixate the mandible. The mucosa and subcutaneous tissue are approximated and sutured with number 4-0 vicryl suture. The platysma is sutured with absorbable stitches and the skin is closed with 5-0 nylon stitches or with clips.

HIGHLIGHTS

I. **Indications**
   - Large oral tongue tumors
   - Tumor of the base of tongue
   - Tumors of the floor of mouth that do not involve the mandible.

II. **Contraindications**
   - Oropharynx or base of tongue squamous cell carcinoma amendable for chemoradiation treatment
   - Tumor involving the internal or common carotid
   - Tumors involving the prevertebral fascia
   - Metastatic disease.

III. **Special Preoperative Considerations**
   - Routine imaging including CT and MRI
   - Prior evaluation by a maxillofacial surgeons for need of teeth extraction
   - Prophylactic antibiotic treatment
   - Placement of percutaneous endoscopic gastrostomy in selected patients
   - Prior planning of the reconstruction means.

IV. **Special Intraoperative Considerations**
   - Nasal intubation in case of trismus
   - Always perform temporary tracheostomy
   - Place the skin incision along a transverse skin crest in the lower neck
   - Paramedian mandibulotomy
   - Prevent injury to the marginal mandibular branch of the facial nerve
   - Preserve the mental nerve
   - Fix the titanium miniplates before the osteotomy to allow accurate repositioning of the bone
   - Leave a sleeve of mucosa over the lower alveolar ridge to facilitate mucosal closure

   - Perform angled osteotomy of the mandible to provide better stability
   - Frozen sections are used for intraoperative evaluation of surgical margins
   - Adequate reconstruction for restoration of structure and function.

V. **Special Postoperative Considerations**
   - Early detection of complications
   - Nasogastric tube feeding
   - Oral cleansing
   - Removal of the tracheostomy tube when the airway is patent.

VI. **Complications**
   - Bleeding
   - Malunion of the mandible
   - Wound infection
   - Nerve injury
   - Wound dehiscence
   - Fistula.

ADDITIONAL READING

1. Gourin CG, Johnson JT. A contemporary review of indications for primary surgical care of patients with squamous cell carcinoma of the head and neck. Laryngoscope. 2009;119(11): 2124-34.
2. McGregor AD, MacDonald DG. Patterns of spread of squamous cell carcinoma to the ramus of the mandible. Head Neck. 1993;15(5):440-4.
3. Neligan PC, Gullane PJ, Gilbert RW. Functional reconstruction of the oral cavity. World J Surg. 2003;27 (7): 856-62.
4. Patel RS, Dirven R, Clark JR, et al. The prognostic impact of extent of bone invasion and extent of bone resection in oral carcinoma. Laryngoscope. 2008;118(5):780-5.
5. Shaha AR. Mandibulotomy and mandibulectomy in difficult tumors of the base of the tongue and oropharynx. Semin Surg Oncol. 1991;7(1):25-30. Review.
6. Shah JP, Gil Z. Current concepts in management of oral cancer—surgery. Oral Oncol. 2009;45(4-5):394-401. Epub 2008 Jul 31.

Chapter 40

Medialization Laryngoplasty

Jacob T Cohen

INTRODUCTION

Medialization laryngoscopy is considered as being the procedure of choice for the management of a paralyzed vocal fold. It can be performed alone or in combination with arytenoid adduction. The first vocal fold medialization was developed by Brunings in 1911. He medialized the paralytic vocal fold by injecting paraffin inside the body of the vocal fold. Later, Payr described an external approach for medialization using an anterior thyroid lamina cartilage flap that collapsed inwards, resulting in medialization of the vocal fold. Neither of these two approaches gained much popularity. Almost forty years later, Meurman described an external medialization procedure using autologous rib cartilage grafts placed between the thyroid ala and the inner perichondrium. This procedure resulted in a high incidence of complications, probably as a result of perichondrial and mucosal perforations.

Numerous modifications of these external approaches have since been reported in the literature, with Isshiki being the first to introduce the concept of alloplastic implant material for medialization using an external approach with a Silastic implant. Isshiki is credited with the ultimate success and popularity of this technique, which he classified as a type I thyroplasty. This procedure offers the advantages of being performed under local anesthesia with minimal or no discomfort to the patient. The patient's position is anatomic thus allowing better assessment of voice during the procedure; it is potentially reversible and structural integrity of the vocal fold is preserved because the prosthesis is placed

lateral to the inner perichondrium of the thyroid lamina. Its disadvantages include the fact that it is an open procedure, which is technically more difficult to perform than injection medialization techniques and the closure of the posterior glottis is limited.

More recently, Gore-Tex (polytetrafluoroethylene) strips have been used to maintain vocal fold medialization. The biocompatibility of Gore-Tex has been demonstrated for more than four decades of clinical use in vascular, cardiac and reconstructive surgery. The material was developed in the late 1960s by W L Gore and Associates. This semiporous material allows minimal amount of tissue in-growth without significant surrounding inflammation. It has the advantage of a very low extrusion rate while retaining the ability for easy removal, when necessary.

The advantages of an external approach to modify vocal fold tension and position without altering the structural components (i.e. the mucosal fold and underlying muscle body) have expanded the role of laryngeal framework surgery. Isshiki and Koufman have reported their continuing successful experience with medialization and tensioning procedures for the management of vocal fold bowing and dysphonia resulting from sulcus vocalis and soft tissue deficits. Medialization laryngoplasty is the current popular choice for management of vocal fold paralysis, vocal fold bowing resulting from aging or cricothyroid joint fixation, sulcus vocalis and soft tissue defects resulting from excision of pathologic tissue.

PREOPERATIVE EVALUATION AND ANESTHESIA

All patients scheduled for medialization laryngoplasty are evaluated preoperatively by a laryngologist, a speech and language pathologist and an anesthesiologist. The surgical candidates who are younger than 18 years of age are also examined by a pediatrician. Laryngeal function impairments are determined by using subjective criteria based on patient's clinical symptoms, such as breathiness, aspiration and exertion intolerance, and more objective criteria that include perceptual assessment and performance of phonatory tasks consisting of mean and maximum phonation time, acoustic analysis (i.e. spectrographic analysis, measurement of fundamental frequency, perturbation of frequency and amplitude, signal/noise ratio).

Electromyography (EMG) is the only current available test for evaluating the integrity of the laryngeal motor unit in the presence of vocal fold motion impairment. Laryngeal EMG is useful for prognosis by determining the presence of denervation or reinnervation potentials. Medialization thyroplasty should be considered soon after denervation has been documented by EMG and in the presence of aspiration or severe dysphonia. If there is visual or EMG evidence of recovery, medialization by injection of a resorbable material, such as Cymetra, can be considered as a temporizing procedure. Despite normal voluntary electric activity, vocal fold immobility may be present as a result of laryngeal synkinesis, joint ankylosis or posterior web formation.

All patients who are planned for medialization laryngoplasty must undergo a videostroboscopic examination, which is still the most useful means of preoperative and postoperative evaluation of all patients undergoing laryngeal procedures, providing visual assessment of glottal closure and status of the mucosal wave.

Medialization laryngoplasty is performed under local anesthesia with intravenous sedation in an operating room setting in order to deal with potential airway problems. Intravenous 20 mg dexamethasone is given preoperatively to minimize edema and prophylactic intravenous antibiotic is administered as well. Local anesthesia is injected in the skin incision site and then subcutaneously to the deeper layers overlying the thyroid cartilage via an injection of 1% lidocaine hydrochloride with 1:100,000 epinephrine, to a volume of 10–15 ml (Fig. 1).

SURGICAL TECHNIQUE

With the patient in the supine position, the nasal passages are decongested and anesthetized using 4 cc of 5% cocaine solution. A flexible fiberoptic laryngoscope is then inserted through the nose up to the level at which the vocal cords can be observed. The endoscope is suspended above the patient and is attached to a video camera connected to a monitor so that the glottis can be viewed throughout the operation. The patient is prepared for a sterile procedure and a horizontal incision is outlined over the middle aspect of the thyroid lamina. A 5 cm incision is made through the skin down to the subplatysmal plane. Superior and inferior subplatysmal flaps are elevated, exposing the thyroid notch superiorly and the inferior borders of the cricoid cartilage (Fig. 2). The strap muscles are split in the midline and retracted laterally off the thyroid lamina leaving the outer perichondrium intact (Fig. 3). A single large skin hook is implanted in the anterior-superior aspect of the contralateral ala and retracted laterally providing exposure of the ipsilateral lamina. A small curved inferiorly based perichondrium flap is elevated down to the lower edge of the thyroid ala. Using an 18G needle, a small

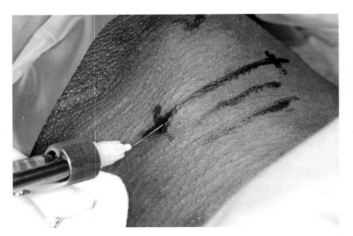

Fig. 1: Local anesthesia is injected in the skin incision site and then subcutaneously to the deeper layers overlying the thyroid cartilage

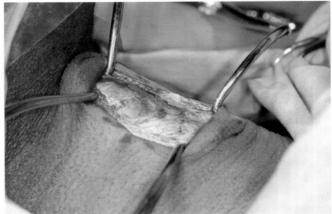

Fig. 2: A 5 cm incision is made through the skin down to the subplatysmal plane. Superior and inferior subplatysmal flaps are elevated, exposing the thyroid notch superiorly and the inferior borders of the cricoid cartilage

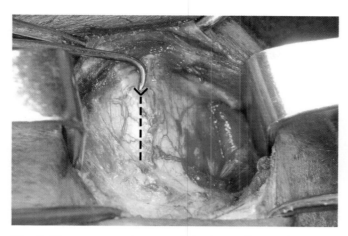

Fig. 3: The strap muscles are split in the midline and retracted laterally off the thyroid lamina leaving the outer perichondrium intact. The thyroid notch and midline are highlighted with black lines

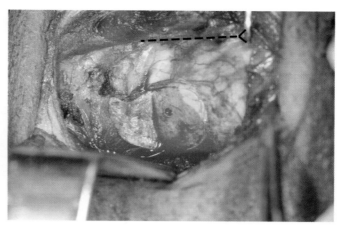

Fig. 4: A small curved inferiorly based perichondrium flap is elevated down to the lower edge of the thyroid ala. Using an 18G needle, a small hole is created 3 or 4 mm above the lower edge of the thyroid cartilage and 1 cm posterior to the midline. The thyroid notch and midline are highlighted with black lines

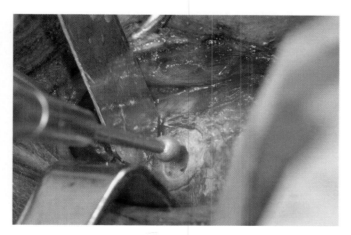

Fig. 5: A 6–8 mm window is created through the thyroid ala using a 5 mm diamond burr

Undermining is extended 4–5 mm both posteriorly and inferiorly, and 2–3 mm anteriorly (Figs 6A and B). A 3–4 mm wide strip of Gore-Tex is cut, soaked in an antibiotic solution and then progressively packed between the thyroid cartilage and the perichondrium in the pocket (Fig. 7). While the patch is being inserted, the patient is instructed to pronounce several sustained vowels (a/e), as well as a few words until the best voice quality has been achieved. The position and the size of the implant are also determined by video monitoring. The patch is then secured inside the hole of the thyroid lamina (Fig. 8) and the window is closed by suturing the external perichondrium and prelaryngeal muscles (Fig. 9). A suction drain is placed for 24 hours. The subcutaneous tissue is sutured by 4-0 absorbable suture and the skin is sutured with interrupted 5-0 nylon sutures (Fig. 10).

hole is created 3 or 4 mm above the lower edge of the thyroid cartilage and 1 cm posterior to the midline (Fig. 4). Once the needle passes through the cartilage, it is withdrawn and a small 27G needle is inserted through the hole. The video monitor provides confirmation of the correct needle placement in relation to the glottis. If the position of the hole appears to be too low or too high, a second hole is created until the position is considered to be satisfactory and a 6–8 mm window is created through the thyroid ala using a 5 mm diamond burr (Fig. 5).

Drilling is stopped when the inner perichondrium becomes visible. A small dissector (such as dental elevator) is introduced and a pocket is formed beneath the window.

POSTOPERATIVE TREATMENT

After surgery, the wound is kept clean by rinsing it with hydrogen peroxide three times a day and covered with antibiotic ointment during the first 7 postoperative days. Oral antibiotics are continued for 6 days after the procedure. The suction drain is removed after 24 hours and the patient is discharged 48 hours after surgery. Patients are re-examined and sutures are removed 7 days postoperatively. Follow-up examinations are scheduled at 1 month and then again after 3 months. All patients undergo a videostroboscopic examination during the postoperative evaluation in order to assess glottal closure and mucosal wave status.

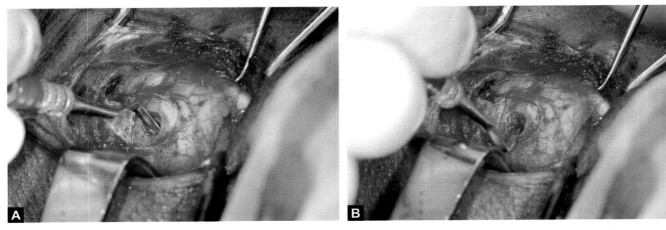

Figs 6A and B: A small dissector (such as dental elevator) is introduced and a pocket is formed beneath the window. Undermining is extended 4–5 mm both posteriorly and inferiorly, and 2–3 mm anteriorly

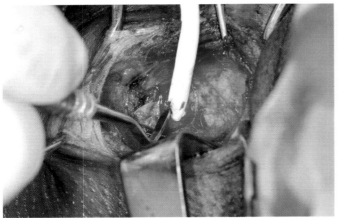

Fig. 7: A 3–4 mm wide strip of Gore-Tex is cut, soaked in an antibiotic solution and then progressively packed between the thyroid cartilage and the perichondrium in the pocket

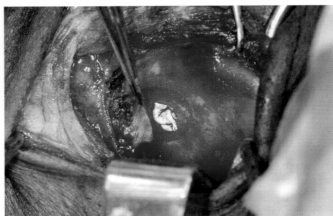

Fig. 8: The patch is then secured inside the hole of the thyroid lamina

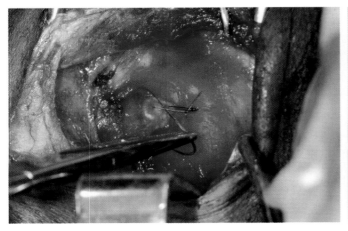

Fig. 9: The window is closed by suturing the external perichondrium and prelaryngeal muscles

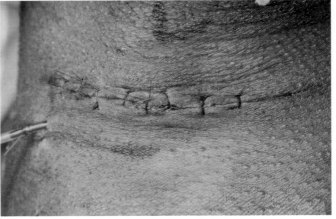

Fig. 10: A suction drain is placed for 24 hours and the skin is sutured with interrupted 5-0 nylon sutures

HIGHLIGHTS

I. Indications
- Vocal fold paralysis
- Vocal fold paresis
- Vocal fold/folds bowing
- Vocal fold soft tissue deficit
- Arytenoid fixation
- Sulcus vocalis.

II. Contraindications
- Post radiotherapy thyroid cartilage chondronecrosis
- Post hemilaryngectomy
- Violation of the laryngeal mucosa during the procedure
- Post type IV cordectomy
- Airway obstruction.

III. Special Preoperative Considerations
- Prophylactic antibiotics
- Good video stroboscopic evaluation.

IV. Special Intraoperative Considerations
- Positioning of the fiberoptic laryngoscope for good visualization of the larynx during surgery, is the single most important factor for success.
- The perichondrium must be kept intact
- Position of the cartilage window is the key for surgical success
- Do not extend the pocket superiorly toward the ventricle.

V. Special Postoperative Considerations
- Prophylactic antibiotics
- No voice rest is needed.

VI. Complications
- Wound infection
- Implant migration
- Neck hematoma/seroma.

ADDITIONAL READING

1. Cohen JT, Bates DD, Postma GN. Revision Gore-Tex medialization laryngoplasty. Otolaryngol Head Neck Surg. 2004;131 (3):236-40.
2. Isshiki N, Okamura H, Ishikawa T. Thyroplasty type I (lateral compression) for dysphonia due to vocal cord paralysis or atrophy. Acta Otolaryngol. 1975;80(5-6):465-73.
3. Koufman JA. Laryngoplasty for vocal cord medialization: an alternative to Teflon. Laryngoscope. 1986;96(7): 726-31.
4. Koufman JA. Surgical correction of dysphonia due to bowing of the vocal cords. Ann Otol Rhinol Laryngol. 1989;98(1 Pt 1): 41-5.
5. Zeitels SM, Mauri M, Dailey SH. Medialization laryngoplasty with Gore-Tex for voice restoration secondary to glottal incompetence: indications and observations. Ann Otol Rhinol Laryngol. 2003;112(2):180-4.

Chapter 41

Minimally Invasive Video-Assisted Thyroidectomy

Paolo Miccoli, Gabriele Materazzi, Piero Berti

INTRODUCTION

The first endoscopic procedures proposed to reduce the invasiveness of surgery in the neck were the endoscopic and video-assisted parathyroidectomies. It was quite evident that parathyroid adenomas were ideal candidates for a minimal access surgery, as these tumors are mostly benign and characterized by their limited size. Later on, the same accesses proved suitable for removing small thyroid nodules and new approaches were soon proposed, in some cases also modifying the old ones. At present, some controversies still exist about what should be considered a real minimally invasive operation for thyroid. Although, the concern raised by some about the possible adverse effect of CO_2 insufflation in the neck was probably over evaluated, the procedure of minimally invasive video-assisted thyroidectomy (MIVAT) setup by the authors in 1998, was characterized by the use of an external retraction avoiding any gas inflation, which is not necessary to create an adequate operative space in the neck. This approach to the thyroid has been used in Department of Surgery, University of Pisa, for the last 8 years on more than 2,500 patients with results that can successfully rival those of standard open surgery also in terms of operative time. Of course, this is not an operation, which might be proposed for any patient. Its main limit is represented by the necessity of a severe selection of the patients undergoing surgery. Only 10–30% of the cases, according to different authors, fulfill the inclusion criteria for a MIVAT.

PREOPERATIVE EVALUATION AND ANESTHESIA

The inclusion criteria and the main contraindications are summarized in Table 1. The most relevant limit is represented by the size of both the nodule and the gland as measured by means of an accurate ultrasonographic study performed preoperatively. In endemic goiter countries, indeed, the gland volume can be relevantly independent from the nodule volume and this aspect might be responsible for the necessity of converting the procedure. Ultrasonography can also be useful to exclude the presence of a thyroiditis, which might make the dissection troublesome. In case, if ultrasonography only gives the suspicion of thyroiditis, autoantibodies should be measured in the serum. In any case, when a correct

Table 1: Inclusion criteria and contraindications for MIVAT

Indications	Contraindications
Thyroid volume lower than 25 ml	Large goiters
Nodule diameter lower than 3 cm	Thyroiditis
Multinodular goiter	Locally advanced carcinoma
Low risk papillary carcinoma (< 2 cm)	Metastatic lymph nodes central and lateral compartment
Graves disease	Coagulative disorders

diagnosis is performed preoperatively, thyroiditis must be considered as a contraindication.

One of the most controversial aspects in terms of indications is the opportunity of treating malignancies. No doubt "low-risk" papillary carcinomas constitute an ideal indication for MIVAT, but a good selection has to take into account the exact profile of possible lymph node involvement in the neck. In fact, although the completeness of a total thyroidectomy achievable with video-assisted procedures is beyond debate, the greatest caution should be taken when approaching a disease involving either metastatic lymph nodes or an extracapsular invasion of the gland. In these cases, an endoscopic approach might be inadequate to obtain a full clearance of the nodes or the complete removal of the neoplastic tissue (infiltration of the trachea or the esophagus). Again, an accurate echographic study is of paramount importance in order to select the right cases undergoing video-assisted surgery.

The operation is generally performed with patient under general anesthesia, but local anesthesia (deep bilateral cervical block) can also be used.

All patients should be rendered euthyroid before surgery. Preoperative preparation of patients with thyrotoxicosis is particularly critical to avoid operative or postoperative thyroid storm. The planned procedure should be discussed with the patient and informed consent must be obtained, particularly focusing on the evenience of converting to an open traditional cervicotomy in case of locally advanced cancer because of difficult endoscopic dissection due to thyroiditis and intraoperative bleeding.

Routine preoperative laryngoscopy is strongly recommended in all patients undergoing thyroid surgery in order to identify preoperatively asymptomatic vocal cord hypomotility or palsy.

SURGICAL TECHNIQUE

Operating Room Set-Up

Patient

- Supine position without neck hyperextension
- Conventional neck preparation and draping
- A sterile drape covering the skin.

Team

- The surgeon is on the right side of the table (Fig. 1).
- The first assistant is on the left side of the table (opposite to the surgeon).
- The second assistant is at the head of the table.
- The third assistant is on the left side of the table.
- The scrub nurse is behind the surgeon on the right side of the table.

Instrumentation

Minimally Invasive Video-Assisted Thyroidectomy Kit

- Minimally invasive video-assisted thyroidectomy kit is shown in Figure 2.
- Forward oblique telescope 30° (diameter 5 mm, length 30 cm)
- Suction dissector with cut-off hole with stylet (blunt, length 21 cm)
- Ear forceps (very thin, serrated, working length 12.5 cm)
- Conventional tissue retractor (Army-Navy type)
- Small tissue retractor (double-ended, length 12 cm)
- Clip applier for vascular clips
- Straight scissors (length 12.5 cm)
- Ultrasound generator
- Single screen (double screen can be useful, but is not mandatory)
- Electrocautery (monopolar)

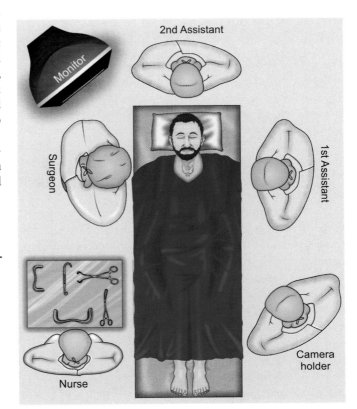

Fig. 1: Operating room set-up team. The surgeon is on the right side of the table; the first assistant is on the left side of the table (opposite the surgeon); the second assistant is at the head of the table; the third assistant is on the left side of the table; the scrub nurse is behind the surgeon on the right side of the table

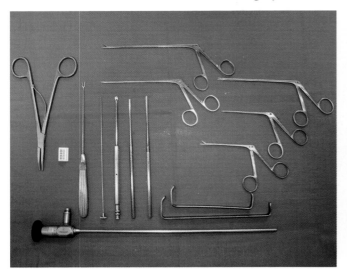

Fig. 2: Instrumentation for minimally invasive video-assisted thyroidectomy

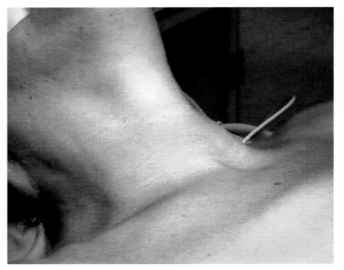

Fig. 3: Minimally invasive video-assisted thyroidectomy position of the patient on the operating table. The neck is not extended

Operative Technique

Preparation of the Operative Space

The patient is positioned in supine position with his neck not extended. Hyperextension must be avoided because it would reduce the operative space (Fig. 3). The skin is protected by means of a sterile film (Tegaderm®). A 1.5 cm horizontal skin incision is performed 2 cm above the sternal notch in the central cervical area. Subcutaneous fat and platysma are carefully dissected so as to avoid any minimum bleeding. During this step, the surgeon should use the electrocautery with its blade protected with a thin film of sterile drape leaving just the tip, to coagulate, in order to avoid damage to the skin or the superficial planes. Two small retractors are used to expose the midline, which has to be incised for 2–3 cm on an absolutely bloodless plane as in Figures 4A and B.

The blunt dissection of the thyroid lobe from the strap muscles is completely carried out through the skin incision by gentle retraction and by using tiny spatulas. When the thyroid lobe is almost completely dissected from the strap muscles, larger and deeper retractors (Army-Navy type) can be inserted and this will maintain the operative space during all the endoscopic parts of the procedure (Fig. 5). Then, a 30° (5 mm or 7 mm) endoscope is introduced through the skin incision. From this moment on, the procedure is entirely endoscopic until the extraction of the lobe of the gland. Preparation of the thyrotracheal groove is completed under endoscopic vision by using small (2 mm in diameter) instruments like spatulas, forceps, spatula-sucker, scissors, etc.

Ligature of the Main Thyroid Vessels

Avoiding the electrocautery (neither bipolar nor monopolar) is particularly important at this point of time when both laryngeal nerves are not yet exposed. Harmonic® device is utilized for almost all the vascular structures, but if the vessel to be coagulated is running particularly close to the inferior laryngeal nerve, then hemostasis is achieved by means of small vascular clips applied by a disposable or reusable clip applier.

The first vessel to be ligated is the middle vein when present, or the small veins between jugular vein and thyroid capsule. This step allows a better preparation of the thyrotracheal groove where the recurrent nerve can be later searched.

During this step, the endoscope has to be held inside the camera with the 30° tip pointing downwards and in an orthogonal axis with the thyroid lobe and trachea.

A further step is represented by the exposure of the upper pedicle, which must be carefully prepared, until an optimal visualization of the different branches is achieved. During this step, the endoscope should be rotated through 180° angle, with the 30° tip pointing upward and held in a parallel direction with the thyroid lobe and trachea, in order to better visualize the upper portion of the operative camera where the superior thyroid vein and artery are running.

The upper pedicle is then prepared by retracting downward and medially the thyroid lobe by means of the retractor and the assistant spatula. The correct position of the retractors (both the first one on the strap muscles and the second one on the upper part of the thyroid lobe) is

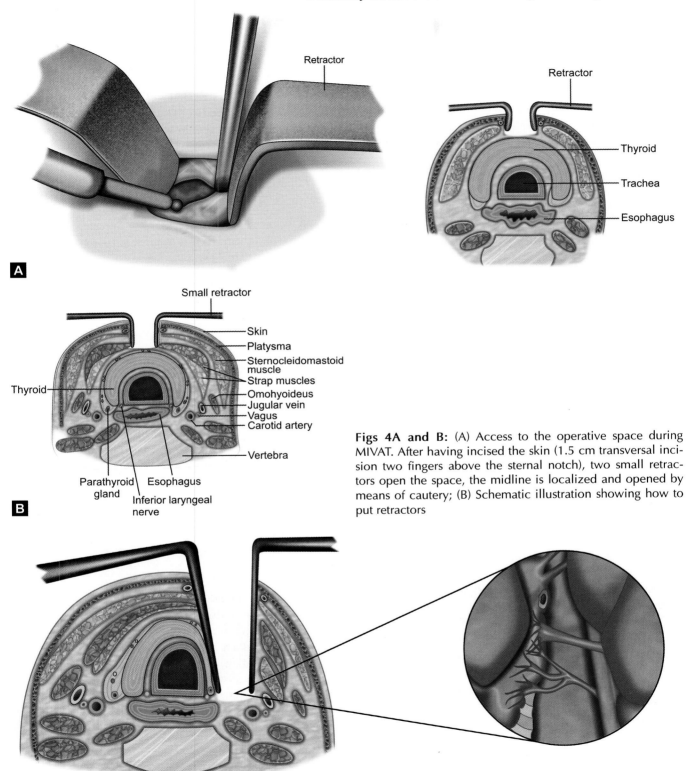

Figs 4A and B: (A) Access to the operative space during MIVAT. After having incised the skin (1.5 cm transversal incision two fingers above the sternal notch), two small retractors open the space, the midline is localized and opened by means of cautery; (B) Schematic illustration showing how to put retractors

Fig. 5: Access to the operative space during MIVAT. When the thyroid lobe is almost completely dissected from the strap muscles, larger and deeper retractors (Army-Navy type) can be inserted and this will maintain the operative space during all the endoscopic part of the procedure

very important during this step in order to obtain the best visualization of the vessels. A further spatula can be used to pull the vessels laterally. This will allow the external branch of the superior laryngeal nerve to be easily identified during most procedures (Fig. 6). Its injury can be avoided by keeping the inactive blade of Harmonic® in the posterior position so as to not transmit the heat to this delicate structure. At this point of time, section of the upper pedicle can be obtained by harmonic scalpel en bloc or selectively, depending on the diameter of the single vessels and/or the anatomical situation as in Figures 7 and 8.

Inferior Laryngeal Nerve and Parathyroid Glands Identification and Dissection

After retracting medially and lifting up the thyroid lobe, the fascia can be opened by a gentle spatula retraction. During this step, the endoscope should be repositioned in an orthogonal axis with the thyroid lobe and trachea pointing downward with an angle of 30°. The recurrent laryngeal nerve appears generally, at this point of time, lying in the thyrotracheal groove posterior to the Zuckerkandl tuberculum (posterior lobe), which constitutes an important landmark in this phase. This way the recurrent nerve and the parathyroid glands are dissected and freed from the thyroid as in Figure 9.

Dissection of the entire nerve from the mediastinum to its entrance into the larynx is not mandatory and might result in wastage of time during the endoscopic phase. It is correct and

very safe to identify the laryngeal nerve and free it from the thyroid capsule as much as possible. It is important to stress that the complete dissection of the nerve can be more easily obtained during the further step, under direct vision, when the thyroid lobe has already been extracted. Also, both the parathyroid glands are generally easily visualized during the endoscopic step, thanks to the camera magnification. Their vascular supply is preserved by selective section of the branches of the inferior thyroid artery. During dissection, when dealing with large vessels or small vessels close to the nerve, hemostasis can be achieved by 3 mm titanium vascular clips.

Extraction of the Lobe and Resection

At this point of time, the lobe is completely freed. The endoscope and the retractors can be removed and the upper portion of the gland can be rotated and pulled out using conventional forceps. A gentle traction over the lobe allows the complete exteriorization of the gland. The operation is now conducted as in open surgery under direct vision. The lobe is freed from the trachea by ligating the small vessels and dissecting the Berry's ligament. At this point of time, it is very important to check the laryngeal nerve once again to avoid its injury before the final step. The isthmus is then dissected from the trachea and divided. After completely exposing the trachea, the lobe is finally removed.

Drainage is not necessary. The midline is then approached by a single stitch, platysma is closed by a subcuticular suture

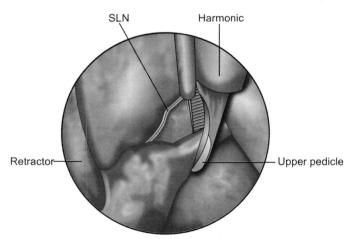

Fig. 6: Endoscopic vision. Dissection of the upper pedicle (left side) during MIVAT. The upper pedicle is prepared by retracting downward and medially the thyroid lobe by means of the retractor and the assistant spatula. The correct position of the retractors (both the first one on the strap muscles and the second one on the upper part of the thyroid lobe) is very important during this step, in order to obtain the best visualization of the vessels. A further spatula can be used to pull the vessels laterally. This will allow the external branch of the superior laryngeal nerve (SLN) to be easily identified

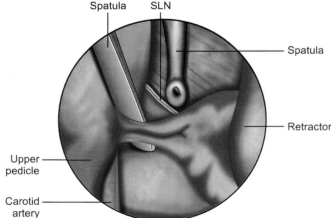

Fig. 7: MIVAT endoscopic vision. Section of the upper pedicle (right side) during MIVAT. Section of the upper pedicle can be obtained by harmonic scalpel "en bloc" or selectively, depending on the diameter of the single vessels and/or the anatomical situation. External branch of the superior laryngeal nerve (SLN) injury can be avoided by keeping the inactive blade of Harmonic® in the posterior position so as to not transmit the heat to this delicate structure

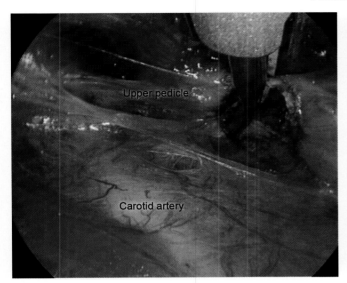

Fig. 8: Endoscopic vision. Section of the upper pedicle by harmonic scalpel. Carotid artery is well visible and under control

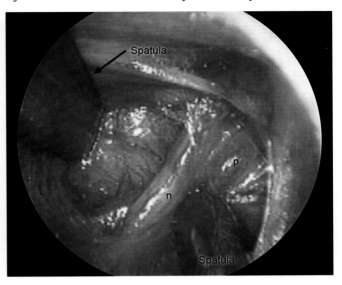

Fig. 9: MIVAT endoscopic vision. Dissection of the inferior laryngeal nerve. The recurrent laryngeal nerve (n) appears lying in the thyrotracheal groove. Parathyroid gland (p) is also well visible

and a cyanoacrylate sealant is used for the skin. If total thyroidectomy is a planned operation, the same procedure is to be performed on the opposite side after the first lobe has been removed.

POSTOPERATIVE TREATMENT

Postoperative Care

After surgery, patients undergoing MIVAT require strict observation during the first 5–10 hours in the ward. Dysphonia, airway obstruction and neck swelling must be carefully checked. No drain is left. So, careful surveillance of postoperative hematomas is required during the immediate postoperative period. Postoperative bleeding risk is very low and dramatically decreases after 5 hours.

In case of postoperative hematoma, if compressive symptoms and airway obstruction are present, reintervention and immediate hematoma evacuation is strongly required.

Patients can start oral intake since the evening on the operative day and can be discharged the day after. On the first and second postoperative day, serum calcium must be checked in order to control hypoparathyroidism by substitutive therapy as described in Table 2.

Wound care is not really necessary after MIVAT because of the glue covering the skin and postoperative pain can be controlled by means of both intravenous (IV) and oral analgesics.

Voice impairments and subjective or objective dysphonia require immediate postoperative vocal cord check by an

Table 2: Management of postoperative hypocalcemia

Management of hypocalcemia following thyroidectomy on the first postoperative day	
Acute symptomatic	Calcium gluconate IV
Asymptomatic calcium ≤7.5* mg/dl	Calcium (3 g) + vitamin D (0.5 μg) per os daily
Asymptomatic calcium, 7.5–7.9 mg/dl	Calcium (1.5 g) per os daily

*Normal range: 8–10 mg/dl

ENT doctor. In case of normal postoperative course, vocal cord check can be delayed after three months.

HIGHLIGHTS

I.   **Indications**
   • "Low-risk" papillary carcinomas with exact profile of possible lymph node involvement.
II. **Contraindications**
   • Thyroiditis.
III. **Special Preoperative Considerations**
   • Ultrasonographic study
   • Echographic study
   • Routine laryngoscopy
   • Euthyroid before surgery.
IV. **Special Intraoperative Considerations**
   • Hyperextension must be avoided to reduce the operative space
   • Avoid damage to the skin or the superficial planes

- Avoid injury to external branch of the superior laryngeal nerve by keeping the inactive blade of Harmonic® in the posterior position
- While dealing with large vessels or small vessels close to the nerve, hemostasis can be achieved by 3 mm titanium vascular clips.

IV. **Special Postoperative Considerations**
   - Strict observation during the first 5–10 hours
   - MIVAP patients are checked for dysphonia, airway obstruction and neck swelling
   - Surveillance of postoperative hematomas
   - Serum calcium must be checked
   - Pain controlled by means of both IV or oral analgesics
   - Vocal cord check by an ENT doctor.

V. **Complications**
   - Dysphonia
   - Voice impairments
   - Airway obstruction
   - Neck swelling.

ADDITIONAL READING

1. Barczyński M, Konturek A, Cichoń S. Minimally invasive video-assisted thyroidectomy (MIVAT) with and without use of harmonic scalpel-a randomized study. Langenbecks Arch Surg. 2008;393(5):647-54. Epub 2008 Jul 4.
2. Del Rio P, Berti M, Sommaruga L, et al. Pain after minimally invasive video-assisted and after minimally invasive open thyroidectomy—results of a prospective outcome study. Langenbecks Arch Surg. 2008;393(3):271-3. Epub 2007 Oct 2.
3. Lombardi CP, Raffaelli M, D'alatri L, et al. Video-assisted thyroidectomy significantly reduces the risk of early post-thyroidectomy voice and swallowing symptoms. World J Surg. 2008;32(5):693-700.
4. Miccoli P, Berti P, Ambrosini CE. Perspectives and lessons learned after a decade of minimally invasive video-assisted thyroidectomy. ORL J Otorhinolaryngol Relat Spec. 2008;70(5):282-6. Epub 2008 Oct 30.
5. Miccoli P, Elisei R, Materazzi G, et al. Minimally Invasive video-assisted thyroidectomy for papillary carcinoma: a prospective study about its completeness. Surgery. 2002;132(6):1070-4.
6. Miccoli P, Materazzi G. Minimally invasive video-assisted thyroidectomy (MIVAT). Surg Clin North Am. 2004;84:735-41.
7. Miccoli P, Minuto MN, Ugolini C, et al. Minimally invasive video-assisted thyroidectomy for benign thyroid disease: an evidence-based review. World J Surg. 2008;32(7):1333-40.
8. Miccoli P, Pinchera A, Materazzi G, et al. Surgical treatment of low- and intermediate-risk papillary thyroid cancer with minimally invasive video-assisted thyroidectomy. J Clin Endocrinol Metab. 2009;94(5):1618-22. Epub 2009 Feb 17.
9. Sgourakis G, Sotiropoulos GC, Neuhäuser M, et al. Comparison between minimally invasive video-assisted thyroidectomy and conventional thyroidectomy: is there any evidence-based information? Thyroid. 2008;18(7):721-7.
10. Terris DJ, Angelos P, Steward DL, et al. Minimally invasive video-assisted thyroidectomy: a multi-institutional North American experience. Arch Otolaryngol Head Neck Surg. 2008;134(1):81-4.

Chapter 42

Minimally Invasive Video-Assisted Parathyroidectomy

Paolo Miccoli, Gabriele Materazzi, Piero Berti

INTRODUCTION

The first endoscopic procedure in the cervical area was performed by M Gagner, who operated on a patient presenting with a primary hyperparathyroidism (PHPT) caused by a hyperplasia of four glands. Primary hyperparathyroidism seemed immediately to be an ideal disease to be approached endoscopically for several reasons: (i) the tumor giving rise to the hyperfunction is almost always benign; (ii) it rarely exceeds 2–3 cm size; (iii) there is no need for any surgical reconstruction after the small mass removal. In 1997, authors ideated and developed minimally invasive video-assisted parathyroidectomy (MIVAP) in Pisa. At present, it might be assumed that MIVAP is considered as a valid option for most of the cases of PHPT and is widely performed in several centers as the first option. In spite of the initial caution though, the introduction of new technologies and instrumentation very much facilitated these procedures shortening significantly, the operative time and enlarging the indications.

PREOPERATIVE EVALUATION AND ANESTHESIA

Minimally invasive video-assisted parathyroidectomy is generally carried out under general anesthesia, although locoregional anesthesia, such as, bilateral cervical block with sedation may be used in selected patients.

An extensive preoperative biological evaluation is necessary to confirm the diagnosis of primary hyperparathyroidism. Once the diagnosis is established, a correct preoperative localization of the lesion is generally considered mandatory before performing MIVAP or any other minimally invasive approach to primary hyperparathyroidism. Localization can be based either on an ultrasound examination or on a double phase ^{99m}Tc-labeled sestamibi scan. In many cases, both imaging studies have already been performed before the patient being referred to the surgeon. The authors prefer an ultrasound examination using a linear transducer (8–13 MHz) with color Doppler capability. In authors' experience, ultrasound has two important advantages over scintigraphy. It is much more accurate in revealing anatomical details; in defining the size and position of the adenoma, and its relationships with vascular structures. The sensitivity of ultrasonography is comparable to scintigraphy. Lesions greater than 3 cm in diameter must be carefully evaluated. Large adenomas are sometimes difficult to remove endoscopically.

No doubt, this is a surgery mostly indicated only for sporadic disease characterized by the presence of a single, well localized adenoma harbored in a virgin neck. This should imply a positive imaging that should be concordant for both ultrasonography and sestamibi scintiscan.

Some contraindications are shown in Table 1.

SURGICAL TECHNIQUE

Operating Room Set-Up

Patient

- Supine position without neck hyperextension
- Conventional neck preparation and draping
- A sterile drape covering the skin.

Table 1: Contraindications for minimally invasive video-assisted parathyroidectomy

Relative Contraindications	Absolute Contraindications
Adenomas >3 cm*	Large goiters
Lack of preoperative localization†	Recurrent disease
Neck surgery on the opposite side of the suspected adenoma§	Extensive previous neck surgery
Previous neck irradiation or small thyroid nodules¶	MEN** and familial PHPT
	Parathyroid carcinoma

*Depending upon their shape, even larger adenomas can be removed
†A bilateral exploration can be performed through a central incision
§A lateral access can be used
¶Concurrent thyroidectomy is possible
**Multiple endocrine neoplasia

Team

- The surgeon is on the right side of the table.
- The first assistant is on the left side of the table (opposite to the surgeon).
- The second assistant is at the head of the table.
- The third assistant is on the left side of the table.
- The scrub nurse is behind the surgeon on the right side of the table.

Instrumentation

Minimally Invasive Video-Assisted Parathyroidectomy Kit

- Forward oblique telescope 30° (diameter 5 mm, length 30 cm)
- Suction dissector with cut-off hole with stylet (blunt, length 21 cm)
- Ear forceps (very thin, serrated, working length 12.5 cm)
- Conventional tissue retractor (Army-Navy type)
- Small tissue retractor (double-ended, length 12 cm)
- Clip applier for vascular clips
- Straight scissors (length 12.5 cm)
- Single screen (double screen can be useful, but is not mandatory).
- Electrocautery (monopolar)

Technique

The access to the operative field is same as described in minimally invasive video-assisted thyroidectomy (MIVAT). A 1.5 cm central, unique incision is performed two fingers above the sterna notch (Fig. 1). In case of redo surgery, a lateral access instead of the standard midline access is possible. This avoids entering fibrous tissue where

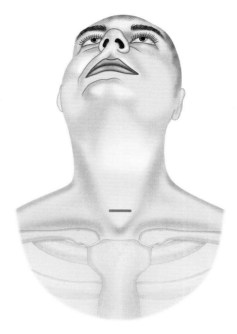

Fig. 1: Minimally invasive video-assisted parathyroidectomy is performed through a central unique incision 1.5 cm long, two fingers above the sternal notch

recognition of anatomical planes and structures, such as, the recurrent nerve may be difficult. The incision is made just medially to the sternocleidomastoid muscle and the same blunt dissection is performed until the thyroid space is well exposed.

The exploration first starts on the side in which the adenoma is supposed to be on the basis of the preoperative imaging, but bilateral exploration can be achieved through the central incision. The endoscopic magnification allows very easy identification of the relevant neck structures like the recurrent laryngeal nerve. Once the adenoma is located, it is dissected without disrupting the capsule performing a cautious blunt dissection by spatulas (Fig. 2). The pedicle of the gland, which is well visible under optical magnification (Figs 3A and B), is then clipped; the use of small disposable vascular clips is strongly suggested (2 mm) because of the relatively small operative field. Washing and cleaning of the operative field can be simply achieved in absence of trocars. Water can be injected directly with a syringe; its aspiration is facilitated by the use of the spatula-shaped aspirator. Smoke and fluids can be sucked without introducing extra instruments into the incision.

The adenoma is then retrieved through the skin incision. No drainage is necessary, but the author strongly advocates,

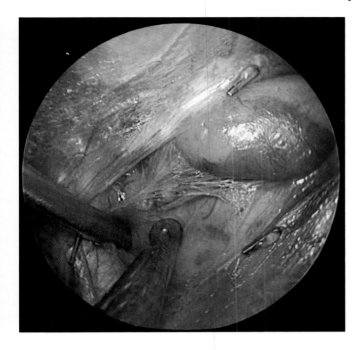

Fig. 2: Endoscopic view of the operative field. The adenoma is visualized and dissected without disrupting the capsule by spatulas

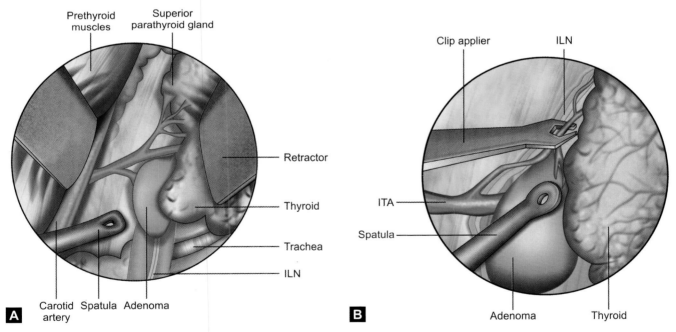

Figs 3A and B: The vascular pedicle of the parathyroid adenoma is cut between vascular clips
ITA: Inferior thyroid artery; ILN: Inferior laryngeal nerve

not closing the midline tightly for better evaluation of early bleedings. Skin is generally closed only by means of a skin sealant (Dermabond®) after a subcuticular running suture has been performed in order to approach the two edges of the incision as in Figure 4.

Quick intraoperative intact parathyroid hormone assay (qPTH) is utilized during the procedure. The completeness of the surgical resection of all hyperfunctioning parathyroid tissue is confirmed by a decrease of more than 50% in qPTH values compared to the highest pre-excision level.

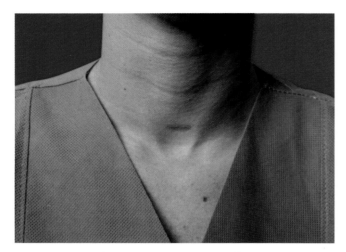

Fig. 4: Skin incision after minimally invasive video-assisted parathyroidectomy, final result

Measurements are obtained when anesthesia is induced, when the adenoma is visualized, and 5–10 minutes after the adenoma is removed.

POSTOPERATIVE TREATMENT

After surgery, patients undergoing MIVAP require observation during the first 5–10 hours in the ward. Dysphonia, airway obstruction and neck swelling must be carefully checked. No drain is left. So, careful surveillance of postoperative hematomas is required during the immediate postoperative period.

Patients can start oral intake, since the evening on the operative day and can be discharged the day after. On the first and second postoperative day, serum calcium must be checked in order to control hypoparathyroidism by substitutive therapy as described in Table 2 of MIVAT.

Voice impairments and subjective or objective dysphonia require immediate postoperative vocal cord check by an ENT doctor. In case of normal postoperative course, vocal cord check can be delayed after three months.

Table 2: Management of postoperative hypocalcemia

Management of hypocalcemia following thyroidectomy on the first postoperative day	
Acute symptomatic	Calcium gluconate IV
Asymptomatic calcium ≤7.5* mg/dl	Calcium (3 g) + vitamin D (0.5 μg) per os daily
Asymptomatic calcium, 7.5–7.9 mg/dl	Calcium (1.5 g) per os daily

*Normal range: 8–10 mg/dl

HIGHLIGHTS

I. Indications
- Sporadic disease characterized by the presence of a single, well localized adenoma harbored in a virgin neck.

II. Contraindications
- Adenomas greater than 3 cm
- Lack of preoperative localization
- Neck surgery on the opposite side of the suspected adenoma
- Previous neck irradiation or small thyroid nodules
- Large goiters
- Recurrent disease
- Extensive previous neck surgery
- MEN and familial PHPT
- Parathyroid carcinoma.

III. Preoperative Considerations
- Ultrasound examination
- Scintigraphy.

IV. Special Intraoperative Considerations
- Thyroid space is exposed by making medial incision to the sternocleidomastoid muscle by making blunt dissection
- Adenoma is dissected without disrupting the capsule
- Quick intraoperative intact parathyroid hormone assay is utilized.

V. Special Postoperative Considerations
- MIVAP patients are checked for dysphonia, airway obstruction, neck swelling
- Surveillance of postoperative hematomas
- Serum calcium must be checked
- Vocal cord check by an ENT doctor.

VI. Complications
- Dysphonia
- Voice impairments
- Airway obstruction
- Neck swelling.

ADDITIONAL READING

1. Barczyński M, Cichoń S, Konturek A, et al. Minimally invasive video-assisted parathyroidectomy versus open minimally invasive parathyroidectomy for a solitary parathyroid adenoma: a prospective, randomized, blinded trial. World J Surg. 2006;30(5):721-31.
2. Berti P, Materazzi G, Picone A, et al. Limits and drawbacks of video-assisted parathyroidectomy. Br J Surg. 2003;90(6): 743-7.
3. Lombardi CP, Raffaelli M, Traini E, et al. Video-assisted minimally invasive parathyroidectomy: benefits and long-term results. World J Surg. 2009;33(11):2266-81.

4. Miccoli P, Bendinelli C, Berti P, et al. Video-assisted versus conventional parathyroidectomy in primary hyperparathyroidism: a prospective randomized study. Surgery. 1999; 126(6):1117-22.

5. Miccoli P, Berti P, Materazzi G, et al. Endoscopic bilateral neck exploration versus quick intraoperative parathyroid hormone assay (qPTH) during endoscopic parathyroidectomy: A prospective randomized trial. Surg Endosc. 2008;22(2):398-400.

6. Miccoli P, Cecchini G, Conte M, et al. Minimally invasive, video-assisted parathyroid surgery for primary hyperparathyroidism. J Endocrinol Invest. 1997;20(7):429-30.

7. Vignali E, Picone A, Materazzi G, et al. A quick intraoperative parathyroid hormone assay in the surgical management of patients with primary hyperparathyroidism: a study of 206 consecutive cases. European Journal of Endocrinology. 2002;146(6):783-8.

Chapter 43

Floor of the Mouth Resection

Giuseppe Spriano, Giovanni Cristalli, Valentina Terenzi, Paolo Marchesi, Valentina Manciocco

INTRODUCTION

The standard treatment of the tumor of the floor of the mouth (FOM) is surgery. The type of surgical resection in patients with carcinoma of the FOM is related to the size and depth of the tumor, its relationship with the mandible and the presence or absence of cervical lymph node metastasis.

Single transoral resection, possibly associated with free skin graft reconstruction is the treatment of choice in case of small tumors (T1/2) without deep infiltration, providing low morbidity (deep invasion of more than 3 mm is considered as a risk for metastatic disease in neck).

Marginal mandibulectomy is best suited for tumors encroaching on, adherent to or superficially invading the mandibular cortex, where it is possible to get adequate 3-D margin regardless of the dentition or history of previous radiotherapy. Segmental jaw resection is reserved for tumors extensively invading the mandibular medullary cavity, when the mandible channel is infiltrated (lymphatic infiltration of V3) or when the mandible is thin and atrophic, and marginal resection would not leave an adequate rim of bone.

The resection of the primary tumor and metastatic lymph nodes is considered by most authors, the classic surgical approach to cancer. The "pull-through" operation is the gold standard treatment in case of tumor invading the floor of the mouth. The operation consists of the tumor excision from submandibular route avoiding the resection of the mandibular arch.

Otherwise, in case of tumors involving the posterior FOM, to achieve an adequate exposure and adequate locoregional control, a conservative transmandibular approach with a lip-splitting incision should be performed.

In case of T4a tumors with massive adjacent tissue involvement, a radical resection with segmental mandibulectomy en bloc with neck dissection(s) is mandatory.

TREATMENT PLANNING

Treatment depends on tumor characteristics and patient-related factors as illustrated in Table 1.

PREOPERATIVE ASSESSMENT

Preoperative examination includes anamnesis and physical examination. It is important to evaluate the patient's general condition to plan an adequate surgical treatment (possibility to perform the surgical resection under local anesthesia, in case of small lesion in patients with bad general conditions).

In case of extensive tumors with risk of bleeding or when there are contraindications to orotracheal intubation, it is useful to perform a tracheotomy under local anesthesia.

Table 1: Tumor factors and patient-related factors

Tumor Factors	Patient Factors
Site and subsite of origin	General medical condition
T and N stage	Performance status
Mandibular invasion	Occupation
Grading	Lifestyle (smoking/drinking)
Depth of infiltration	Socioeconomic considerations
Previous treatment (surgery/radiotherapy)	

Diagnostic assessment consist of local inspection and imaging that helps to plan adequate resection type, principally evaluating the proximity and the relationship between tumor and mandible (the final decision on mandibulectomy could be taken intraoperatively) and the tumor extension to adjacent sites. It is important to evaluate the site and the extent of the surgical defect for planning an appropriate reconstruction.

To assess tumor stage, radiological investigations required are:

- Neck ultrasound to investigate cervical node involvement.
- Head and neck computed tomography (CT) scan (Fig. 1). and/or magnetic resonance imaging (MRI) to evaluate tumor extension (Fig. 2), possible bone invasion and cervical node involvement.
- Orthopantomogram (Fig. 3) to plan marginal or segmental mandibulotomy, if required, to investigate general status of dentature and to check how tall is the mandible.
- Thorax spiral CT scan to investigate the presence of lung metastasis or secondary tumor.

SURGICAL TECHNIQUES

Transoral Excision

Indications

T1-2, N0 tumors with limited deep infiltration (depth less than 3 mm).

Contraindication

Clinically node positive (cN+) tumors.

Complications

- Dehiscence of the oral suture
- Infections
- Bleeding
- Tongue anchylosis.

Patient is supine on the operatory table and a folder blanket is placed under the shoulders to extend the neck (if tracheotomy has to be performed). General endotracheal anesthesia is induced. Antibiotic is administered intraoperatively (ampicillin and clavulanic acid 2.2 g). In case of tumor involving the posterior FOM or when partial glossectomy is required, temporary tracheotomy is recommended. If the tumor extends to the oropharynx (base of the tongue), tracheotomy conducted by local anesthesia is preferred. The patient is then prepared and draped including, the site to harvest the Thiersch graft (inguinal cutis can be used). An oral mouth gag (Molt or Denhart 12–14 cm) is placed in the oral cavity.

The line of incision is marked by dots using pick-shaped electrocautery tip. The margin of resection must extend at least 1 cm from the normal tissue. Sublingual gland represents the deep margin of resection. Lingual artery can be identified in the neck and ligated to reduce bleeding. The lingual nerve can be identified and preserved, if there is no suspicion of infiltration. If Wharton's duct involvement is

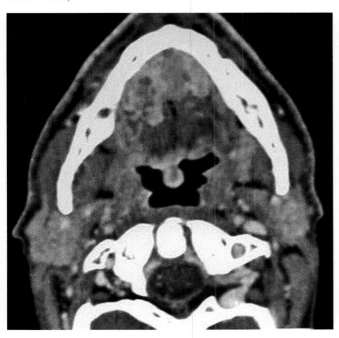

Fig. 1: Computed tomography scan shows the involvement of mylohyoid plane bilaterally

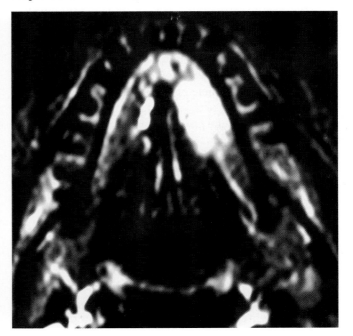

Fig. 2: Magnetic resonance imaging demonstrating cancer of floor of the mouth close to the mandible not invading cortical bone

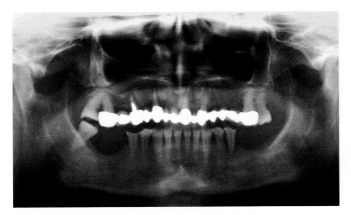

Fig. 3: Preoperative orthopantomogram to evaluate mandibular high according to Cawood-Howell 1988

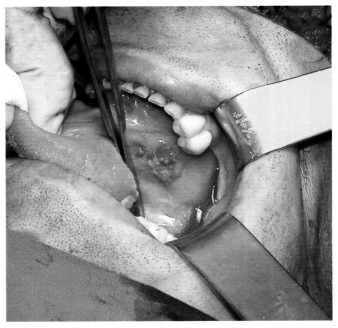

Fig. 4: Squamous cell carcinoma of the anterolateral floor of the mouth pT2N2bM0

present, it is necessary to marsupialize the duct and not to cover it with the skin graft.

If a marginal mandibulectomy is planned and a mandibular subperiosteal plane is clearly identified, it is possible to perform the osteotomy using a drill or a straight osteotome. Attention has to be paid to regularize osteotomy margins using a drill. Local flap can be harvested and positioned to cover the defect.

Margins are checked by frozen section. If they show infiltration (R1) or margins appear close or with dysplasia, a wired excision is required.

Suture can be achieved directly and if this is not possible, a free skin graft may be harvested and positioned in place using a 3-0 or 4-0 absorbable stiches. In superficial tumors an intensive follow up can be used avoiding an elective neck dissection.

Postoperative Treatment

Nasogastric tube feeding is maintained usually for 4–5 days. Tracheostomy is closed 3–4 days after surgery. Antibiotic therapy is administered for 7 days after surgery (the use of ampicillin and clavulanic acid is recommended at the dose of 2.2 g × 2 intravenously. for the first 2 days and 1 g × 2 per os for the remaining 5 days).

Pull-Through

This procedure consists of "en bloc" excision of the tumor and neck dissection(s) through a combined transcervical and transoral approach preserving mandibular continuity.

Indications

- T3–T4a tumors independently to N stage (in case of T4 tumors, no massive bone infiltration has to be present so that a marginal mandibulectomy can be performed)
- T1-T2 tumors (Fig. 4) with deep invasion (more than 3 mm) or cN+.

Contraindications

- Bulky tumors
- Infiltration of mandible (in which segmental mandibulectomy is required).

Complications

- Orocervical salivary fistula
- Bleeding
- Infection
- Complications related to neck dissection
- Tongue anchylosis.

Surgical Technique

The position of the patient is the same as previously described. Tracheotomy is mandatory and is performed at the beginning of the operation. Preparation using bacteriostatic solutions (Betadine) should extend from a line joining the tragus to the ala of the nose, down to the nipples. Depending on the type of reconstruction, specific surgical field has to be prepared.

The first step is neck dissection: selective in N0 cases, radical or modified radical in N1-3. Skin incision (two or three limbs) depends on dissection type. In case of bilateral neck dissection, a visor flap can be harvested. Platysmal flap is dissected until inferior margins of the mandible. Neck dissection is performed, it is possible to ligate the lingual artery to avoid bleeding if hemiglossectomy is planned, and taking care to preserve vessels in case of microsurgical

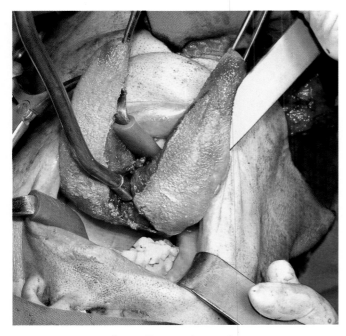

Fig. 5: Transoral resection

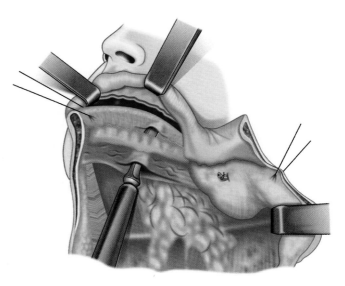

Fig. 6: Subperiosteal detachment of floor of the mouth to the inner face of the mandible (for iconographic reasons, the lip has been interrupted by the artist)

reconstruction. The flap is elevated in the inner subperiosteal plane so that the oral cavity is entered.

Intraoral step: The line of resection must be at least 1 cm from the safety margins and is dotted before by electrocautery as described for transoral resection. The incision proceeds anteriorly, laterally and circumferentially until a mandibular subperiosteal plane is clearly identified. Posteriorly, the mucosa of lingual fold is incised avoiding the step of sectioning the muscle plane (Fig. 5).

If possible, it is better to preserve the anterior digastric muscles. Following a subperiosteal plane (Fig. 6), the mandibular insertions of mylohyoid muscle and the geniohyoid muscle are sectioned. At this point, it is possible to connect the intraoral and extraoral incision and to pull the anterior FOM in continuity with the neck dissection down through the mandibular arch (Figs 7 and 8). Dissection proceeds by sectioning the geniohyoid, mylohyoid muscles and the digastric muscles laterally, beyond the insertion of masseter muscle and inferiorly over the hyoid bone (Figs 9A and B). The tumor is now removed "en bloc" with neck dissection as in Figure 10. Reconstruction using a flap is always necessary.

Postoperative Management

The patient is kept on nasogastric feeding tube till soft tissue healing allows feeding restoration. It usually occurs in 10 days period. In order to identify an orocervical fistula, a methylene blue diluted solution can be administered orally so that it can be detected in the neck drainage (within 24 hours) or through a cervical dehiscence. Tracheotomy is closed on 3rd–4th day or when there is no reasonable risk of surgical revision. Chewing of solid food should be postponed until approximately the sixth postoperative week. To avoid infection, in addition to penicillin and clavulanic acid, adjunctive intravenous metronidazole (500 mg × 2) can be administered.

Blood pressure must be monitored after free flap. Skin paddle of the flap is monitored by the nurse every 1 hour and at the same time, the vacuum of the suction drains must be evaluated.

Conservative Transmandibular Resection

Indications

Tumors with posterior extension to tongue base, lateral oropharynx.

Contraindications

• Associated disease of the mandible (osteoradionecrosis post-radiation, previous bisphosphonate therapy)
• Mandibular infiltration (cT4a bone).

Complications

• Orocervical salivary fistula
• Bleeding
• Infection
• Complications related to neck dissection
• Tongue anchylosis
• Malocclusion
• Teeth lesions
• Pseudarthrosis.

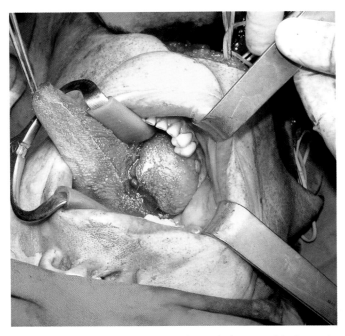

Fig. 7: The tumor is tractioned through the mandibular arch from the neck (pull-through operation)

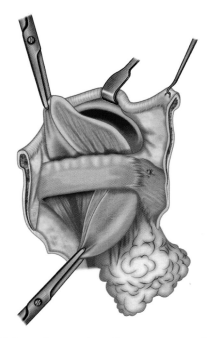

Fig. 8: Pull-through resection allows to respect the continuity between the tumor bed and the neck dissection (for iconographic reasons, the lip has been interrupted by the artist)

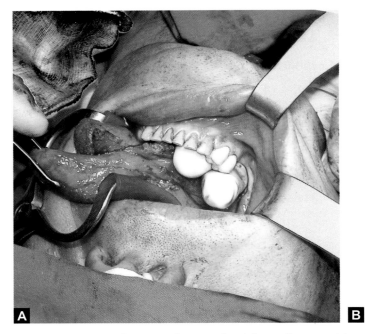

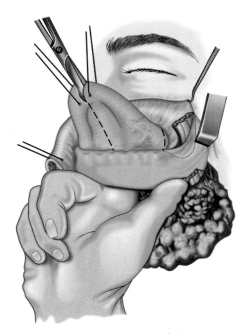

Figs 9A and B: Detachment of oral floor allows a wide transit between the oral cavity and neck by preserving mandibular arch (for iconographic reasons, in Fig. 9B, the lip has been interrupted by the artist)

Surgical Technique

Skin incision depends on the type of neck dissection as described for pull-through operation and is continued superiorly from the mid-submental crease using a straight midline chin incision that extends through the lip and into the depth of the labial alveolar sulcus. It is advisable to preserve an adequate cuff of alveolar mucosa to facilitate incisional closure. The mucosal incision is then extended

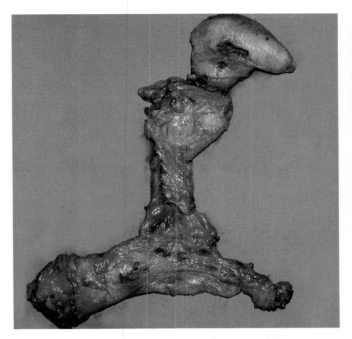

Fig. 10: Surgical specimen shows "en bloc" resection of tumor and neck dissection

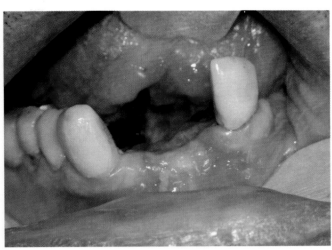

Fig. 11: Squamous cell carcinoma of the anterior floor of the mouth pT4aN2cM0 C

within the labial alveolar sulcus to the region of the mandible corresponding to the site of mandibular osteotomy. Usually the lip splitting is on the midline while the mandible is cut paramediallly and anteriorly to the exit of the mandibular nerve to avoid overlapping of the two cutting lines. Once neck dissection has been performed, the periosteum is elevated in the region of placing the mandibular plate (preplating) before making the osteotomy. The incision must be extended over the alveolar ridge into the lingual sulcus. Mental nerve must be preserved. Periosteum of the inner face of the mandible is detached to insert a malleable retractor to protect soft tissues during the osteotomy. The osteotomy is performed avoiding excessive loss of bone by a slim sagittal saw or a Gigli saw through an oblique line conducted between the second incisor and the canine. Dissection is continued through the submucosal tissues and mylohyoid muscle to swing the mandible laterally. The hypoglossal nerve is preserved, when possible, while the lingual nerve is usually sectioned.

Mandibular contention is then obtained using two titanium miniplates and monocortical 7–11 mm screws. Closure of lingual soft tissues is performed in multiple layers using a microvascular free flap, such as, lateral thigh or forearm flap. Moreover, a pectoralis major pedicled flap can be used.

Anterior/Lateral Composite Resection
Segmental Resection

The aim of the operation is to resect the mandible, the FOM and neck nodes en block.

Indications

T4 tumors (Fig. 11) with extension to mandible, tongue and soft tissues.

Contraindications

- Bad general conditions
- Metastatic disease.

Complications

- Orocervical fistula
- Bleeding
- Infection
- Complications related to neck dissection
- Tongue anchylosis
- Malocclusion
- Teeth lesions
- Pseudarthrosis.

Surgical Technique

Patient preparation is the same as described for transmandibular conservative resection. Tracheotomy is performed even under local anesthesia, if endotracheal intubation is not possible (risk of bleeding, trismus, bulky mass). Dental extraction may be performed at the beginning of the procedure or at the time of tumor excision. According to the type of neck dissection, a two or three limbs skin incision is performed or a visor flap is harvested. If possible, the surgeon making the visor flap has to preserve one mandibular nerve. The section of both mandibular nerve allows a wide exposition of the mandibular arch and of the neck without scars on lips and chin. In other cases (lateral and posterior extension), it is better to use a labial split incision and a cheek flap to expose the mandibular arch. In this way, even if the esthetic results are less satisfying, it may be possible to preserve one of the two mandibular nerve and the reconstructive time is easier. A modification of this approach is necessary, when the cancer infiltrates the floor of the mouth and the mandible up to the skin of the chin. In this case, the infiltrated skin of the chin is excised en bloc with the mandible. The first step is neck dissection.

Mandibulotomy

Mandibular arch is exposed by sectioning tissues of alveolar ridge preserving the periosteum of the outer side of mandible. Facial vein and artery are preserved as recipient vessels for microvascular anastomosis. Marginal branch of facial nerve is identified and preserved (if possible). The periosteum is incised inferior to the attachment of the masseter muscle, which is then elevated from the angle of mandible depending on the extent of the cancer lateral to the mandible.

By electrocautery, the resection continues along the oral floor to the ventral surface of the tongue leaving safety margins of 2 cm. The neck incision is then connected with the intraoral incision. Care must be taken not to compromise the resection margins. In case of approach by visor flap, two Penrose drains must be passed around the flap and used for traction.

A reconstruction plate is shaped and positioned by screws. The anterior position of the mandibular osteotomy is then marked on the mandible.

Osteotomy is planned according to the extension of tumor with at least 2 cm safety margins. Line of osteotomy is generally straight. The osteotomy can be facilitated by removal of a tooth from the line of planned excision. During osteotomy, care should be taken to ensure that adequate bone is left around any remaining dentition. Most of these patients have poor dentition and all the remaining teeth, if compromised must be removed before the reconstruction time. Lateral retraction of mandibular segment is limited by the presence of an intact temporomandibular joint.

Depending on the extent of the cancer, this may be performed either below the notch of the mandible or through the notch with section of the coronoid process and portion of tendon of the temporalis muscle, by disarticulation of the mandible from the glenoid fossa or vertically with preservation of the angle and posterior aspect of the ramus. The latter chance requires mandibular channel intraoperative frozen section to look for lymphatic infiltration.

When both osteotomies have been completed, the mucosal incision can be easily made around the tumor in the oral cavity. The deep tissues are en bloc dissected according to the lesion extension with safe margins.

By sectioning the mylohyoid muscles and geniohyoid muscles of both sides and respecting the continuity with neck dissection, the tumor removal is completed.

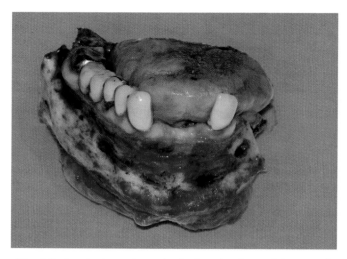

Fig. 12: Surgical specimen including the floor of the mouth and segmental mandibulectomy

At this time, it is possible to separate the specimen (Fig. 12) from the hyoid bone attachment by sectioning inferiorly the geniohyoid muscle and hyoglossus muscle.

Frozen section may be taken and may be accurately registered and labeled. Bone margins cannot be evaluated intraoperatively.

Special Preoperative Considerations

- Evaluate the denture state of the patient, eventually planning teeth extraction, if necessary
- Insert the nasogastric feeding tube after the anesthesia
- Use prophylactic antibiotic treatment to reduce infection.

Special Intraoperative Considerations

- If partial glossectomy is done, the suture can be performed between the mucosal margins and the tongue intrinsic muscles to avoid tongue anchylosis covering the deep plane of resection.
- In case of marginal mandibulectomy (Figs 13 to 16), it is important to preserve at least 10 mm of inferior border of mandible that accounts for almost 50% of the cross sectional area of the mandible, since this usually provides enough structural integrity to withstand the loading forces related to mastication.
- In case of conservative mandibulotomy, a simple transverse osteotomy minimizes bone loss and is the simpler and more rapid method of avoiding stair stepped osteotomy.

Special Postoperative Considerations

- Do not start oral feeding before suture stabilization
- It is important to clean the oral cavity.

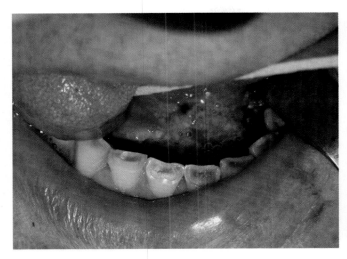

Fig. 13: Squamous cell carcinoma of the anterior floor of the mouth pT2N0M0 (proximal to the mandible)

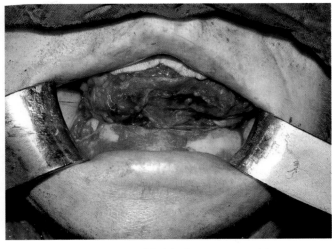

Fig. 14: Surgical field after tumor excision with marginal mandibulectomy

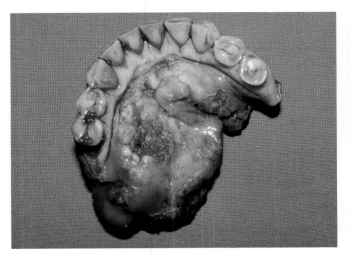

Fig. 15: Surgical specimen

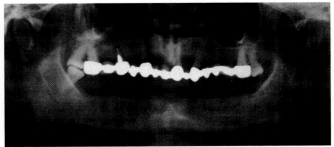

Fig. 16: Postoperative panorex X-ray

RECONSTRUCTION

It depends on the surgical defect. In case of isolated soft tissue defect, reconstruction can be achieved by fasciocutaneous free flap (Figs 17 and 18), such as, radial forearm or anterolateral thigh free flap. When total glossectomy is performed, a more bulky free flap can be harvested. If a free flap is not recommended, a pectoralis major pedicled flap can be harvested.

Reconstruction (Figs 19 to 21) of composite defect can be achieved with a fibula (Fig. 22) iliac crest or scapular free flap.

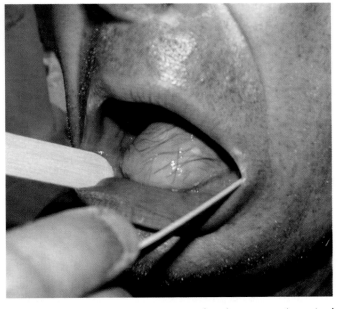

Fig. 17: Postoperative picture 8 months after surgery (marginal mandibulectomy). Reconstruction is performed by forearm fasciocutaneous microvascular flap

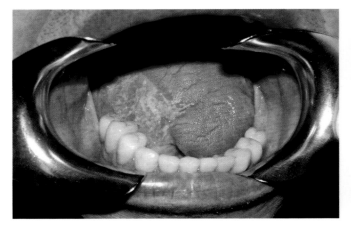

Fig. 18: Postoperative picture 8 months after surgery (pull-through resection). Reconstruction is performed by antebrachial fasciocutaneous microvascular flap

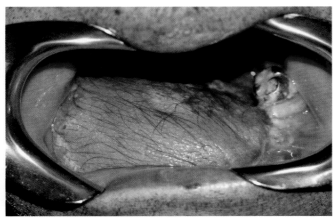

Fig. 19: Postoperative view of the floor of the mouth 3 months later

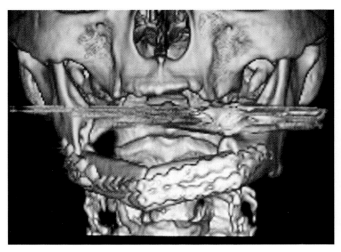

Fig. 20: Postoperative 3-D reconstruction CT scan

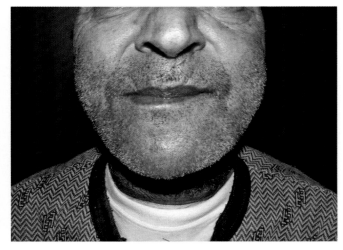

Fig. 21: Postoperative picture 3 months after surgery pull-through operation

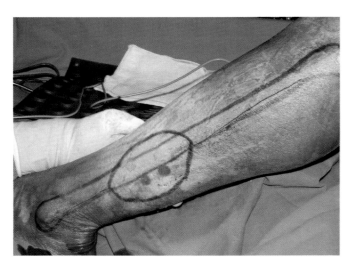

Fig. 22: Osteocutaneous fibula free flap designed with the skin perforator

HIGHLIGHTS

I. **Indications**
  • Transoral excision
    – T1-2, N0 tumors with limited deep infiltration (depth <3 mm)
  • Pull-through
    – T3-4a tumors independently to N stage (in case of T4 tumors, no massive bone infiltration has to be present so that a marginal mandibulectomy can be performed)
    – T1-T2 tumors with deep invasion (more than 3 mm) or cN+
  • Conservative transmandibular resection
    – Tumors with posterior extension to the tongue base, lateral oropharynx

- Anterior composite resection (segmental mandibular resection)
  - T4 tumors with extension to mandible, tongue and soft tissues.

II. Contraindications

- Transoral excision
  - cN+ tumors
- Pull-through
  - Bulky tumors
  - Infiltration of mandible (in which segmental mandibulectomy is required)
- Conservative transmandibular resection
  - Associated disease of the mandible (osteoradionecrosis post radiation, previous biphosphonate therapy)
  - Mandibular infiltration (cT4a-bone)
- Anterior composite resection (segmental mandibular resection)
  - Bad general conditions
  - Metastatic disease.

III. Special Preoperative Considerations

- Anterior composite resection (segmental mandibular resection)
  - Evaluate the denture state of the patient, eventually planning teeth extraction
  - Insert the nasogastric feeding tube after administering anesthesia
  - Use prophylactic antibiotic treatment to reduce infection.

IV. Special Intraoperative Considerations

- Anterior composite resection (segmental mandibular resection)
  - In case of partial glossectomy, suture can be performed between the mucosal margins and tongue intrinsic muscles to avoid tongue anchylosis.
  - In case of marginal mandibulectomy, preserve at least 10 mm of inferior border of the mandible as it provides integrity while mastication.
  - In case of conservative mandibulotomy, simple transverse osteotomy minimizes bone loss and is preferred to stair step osteotomy.

V. Special Postoperative Considerations

- Anterior composite resection (segmental mandibular resection)

- Do not start oral feeding before suture stabilization
- It is important to clean the oral cavity.

VI. Complications

- Transoral excision
  - Dehiscence of the oral suture
  - Infection, bleeding, tongue anchylosis
- Pull-through/Conservative transmandibular resection/Anterior or Lateral segmental resection
  - Orocervical salivary, bleeding, infections, complications related to neck dissection, tongue anchylosis
  - Flap necrosis
  - Teeth problems.

ADDITIONAL READING

1. Cilento BW, Izzard M, Weymuller EA, et al. Comparison of approaches for oral cavity cancer resection: lip-split versus visor flap. Otolaryngol Head Neck Surg. 2007;137(3):428-32.
2. Guerra MFM, Gìas LN, Campo FR, et al. Marginal and segmental mandibulectomy in patients with oral cancer: a statistical analysis of 106 cases. J Oral Maxillofac Surg. 2003;61(11):1289-96.
3. Myers EN (Ed). Operative Otolaryngology-Head and Neck Surgery, 2nd edition. Philadelphia: Saunders Elsevier; 2008. p. 241.
4. Pathak KA, Shah BC. Marginal mandibulectomy: 11 years of institutional experience. J Oral Maxillofac Surg. 2009;67(5):962-7.
5. Piantanida R, Ferrario F, Roselli R, et al. A free radial forearm flap in oral cavity reconstruction. Acta Otorhinolaryngol Ital. 1997;17(2):115-23.
6. Shah JP. Face, skull and neck. Color Atlas of Operative Techniques in Head and Neck Surgery. London: Wolfe Medical Publications Ltd; 1987.
7. Spiro RH, Huvos AG, Wong GY, et al. Predictive value of tumor thickness in squamous carcinoma confined to tongue and floor of the month. Am J Surg. 1986;152(4):345-50.
8. Spriano G, Bertoni F, Boschini P, et al. Treatment of carcinoma of the tongue: results of a retrospective study. Acta Otorhinolaryngol Ital. 1986;6(4):367-77.
9. Vidiri A, Ruscito P, Pichi B, et al. Oral cavity and base of the tongue tumors. Correlation between clinical, MRI and pathological staging of primary tumor. J Exp Cancer Res. 2007;26(4):575-82.

Chapter 44

Partial Pharyngectomy

Giuseppe Spriano, Paolo Ruscito, Barbara Pichi, Jacqueline Crupi

INTRODUCTION

Pharyngectomy is a surgical procedure, which may significantly impact the main functions of the upper aerodigestive tract namely: swallowing, respiration and phonation.

The oropharynx has a tubular conformation. The posterior and lateral walls are structured by the pharyngeal constrictor muscles, the anterior border is delineated by the soft palate and the root of the tongue muscles.

It takes part in the pharyngeal phase of deglutition, propulsion of the bolus into the hypopharynx that avoids spilling of food contents into the oral cavity and rhinopharynx. Closure of the glottis prevents aspiration into the airways. From the nasal and oral cavities, airflow enters the oropharynx and it is directed into the laryngeal lumen.

The pharynx contributes to phonation mainly by determining the resonance characteristics of the voice.

The relevant steps involved in the proper coordination of its activity and the possible impact of the surgery on the quality of life explain why more primary and salvage surgical procedures have been reported over the years with organ/function preservation intents.

A wide range of surgical procedures, from transoral tonsillectomy to transmandibular pharyngectomies, are still a valid oncologic approach to oropharyngeal tumors, which always consists of the treatment of the primary tumor and neck dissection (mono or bilateral). Surgery is reserved for the following cases (recommendation category 2A):

- Low stage tumors (T1, T2, N0-1)
  - Tumor excision (treatment of choice)
  - Surgical salvage, in case of residual disease after radiation or chemoradiation (selected N1 cases)
- High stage tumors (T3, T4a, N0-1; any T, N2-3)
  - Surgical salvage for residual disease following organ preservation protocols
  - Primary treatment
- Recurrent tumors.

Surgery for pharyngeal cancers must consider the complex pattern of spread of the neoplasms arising from this site particularly, the submucosal lymphatic diffusion, which may extend more than 1 cm away from the macroscopic margin of the tumor. Even the immunohistochemical and biological characteristic of the tumor, such as HPV and p16, as to be considered in treatment planning, as they are more and more important prognostic factors. Pharyngectomy, for oncological reasons, must always keep adequate free margins, at least 1.5 cm wide to prevent microscopic, residual disease (R1) at the tumor border.

Soft palate tumor treatment represents a particular challenge from a surgical point of view. Soft palate is anatomically structured by two mucosal layers among which the muscular layer forms a dynamic separation between oro- and rhinopharynx. The problems related to the surgical approach of this areas are oncological and functional as follows:

- Benign tumors are usually originating from minor salivary glands. In 25% of cases, malignant ones originate from minor salivary gland and in 75% of cases from pharyngeal mucosa (squamous cell carcinoma).
- High tendency of carcinoma to submucosal spread toward the palatine arch and the base of the tongue
- Synchronous tumor rate is about 10–15% higher than other oropharyngeal subsites. The risk of downstaging and consequently of inadequate treatment is therefore significant.

- High rate of nodal metastases related to squamous cell carcinoma, the most frequent histological type (80% of cases), in the lateral neck and retropharyngeal space (30–50% of cases); 15% of bilateral neck metastases.

Soft palate treatment options are represented by surgery or organ preservation protocols (radiotherapy or chemoradiation). Their oncological effectiveness is similar for low stage tumors (T1, T2), while multimodal treatments are generally indicated for the advanced ones. Surgical excision may require immediate reconstruction to avoid velopharyngeal insufficiency, which ranges from local flaps (in case of limited resections) to composite flap microsurgical transfers (in case of extended excisions). The functional results are generally poor despite the complexity of the reconstructive strategies. All these aspects, impacting the decision-making process for velopharyngeal tumors, determine the general attitude to nonsurgical treatment of the tumors of this site reserving the surgical approach as salvage procedure in case of (chemotherapy) radiation failure. Unlikely, quite a high rate of recurrence following organ preservation protocols, have been observed especially in case of locally advanced tumors.

Recent surgical mini-invasive, functional procedures have been introduced to treat selected oropharyngeal tumors radically, avoiding complex and invasive reconstructions. For all these reasons, it is possible to find many different treatment protocols in the literature. Clinical review evidenced high rate of recurrence of tumors involving the palatine arch, extended up to the base of the tongue and treated with radiation therapy.

Surgical techniques that involve the oropharynx may be categorized according to the surgical approach or the disease location [(subsite(s) involved)]. In the former category, three main ways to perform pharyngectomy are described:

1. *Transoral:* Surgical excision of the pharyngeal tumor through the oral cavity. This approach is reserved for limited benign disease or small, superficial tumors of the lateral, superior (soft palate) and posterior pharyngeal wall. Advances in technology, use of various devices, such as, laser devices and transoral robotic surgery (TORS) are extending even more indications to this procedure that may involve other subsites especially the base of the tongue, valleculae, or larger masses, which may be adequately exposed and safely excised in this manner.

2. *Transpharyngeal or transcervical:* Resection is achieved by a cervical, submandibular approach, which exposes the mass through a lateral and/or anterior pharyngotomy. This approach does not allow the wide exposure obtained by transmandibular surgery. Nevertheless, it guarantees en bloc tumor and neck dissection, preserving mandibular continuity.

3. *Transmandibular:* It defines all pharyngectomies achieved through the mandible. It may be preserved (mandibulotomy) or excised with the tumor via a composite resection

(mandibulectomy) depending on the stage (T4a bone) and/or the subsite of the tumor. The transmandibular approach allows wide exposure of the oropharyngeal lumen, from the base of the tongue to the tonsillar space and the posterior pharyngeal wall. Hence, the resection may be performed under direct visual control of the tumor, the carotid artery and/or internal jugular vein. Continuity may be maintained between the oropharyngeal resection and the neck dissection. The reconstruction is achieved by direct closure, using a pedicle or a microvascular, free flap.

Tracheostomy and nasogastric feeding tube are always required in transmandibular and transpharyngeal pharyngectomies cases but can be avoided in limited transoral procedures. After the excision, reconstruction by means of pedicled or free flaps is performed in a single stage procedure in order to:

- Divide the pharyngeal lumen from the neck spaces
- Restore organ function as much as possible
- Support wound healing with healthy tissue transposition or transfer in case of salvage surgery following radiation or chemoradiation.

PREOPERATIVE ASSESSMENT AND ANESTHESIA

The head and neck surgeon must perform a detailed history and physical inspection of the head and neck as the first step to a careful work-up for correct diagnosis, staging and treatment planning of an oropharyngeal tumor. This must include a bimanual palpation of the oral cavity, floor of the mouth and tongue, direct fiberoptic examination of the pharynx and laryngeal structures. Imaging examination includes computed tomography (CT) and magnetic resonance imaging (MRI) of the skull base and neck with and without contrast. Chest CT and/or PET/CT whole body scan is also required especially for tumor stages III and IV.

The patient is routinely prepared for blood and coagulation tests, urine test, electrocardiogram (ECG) and chest X-ray. The anesthesiologist evaluates the health conditions of the patient and the present risks to undergo surgery under general anesthesia. Any previous surgery or radiation to the area must be taken into consideration for adequate treatment planning. Blood units are either screened, typed and crossed or autologous blood is drawn if more than 500 cc of blood loss is estimated.

Effective prophylaxis is obtained by infusion of intravenous (IV) antibiotics (wide spectrum antibiotics) within 30 mins from the beginning of the surgical procedure. Nasotracheal or tracheal intubation may be considered, when tracheostomy is not required. If CO_2 laser surgery is being planned, precautions to laser setup are to be considered.

Surgical Procedures

TRANSORAL APPROACH

Surgical indications in the tonsillar region may differ considering the size and site of limited malignant lesions. It has been introduced at the beginning of the century for removal of tonsillar hypertrophy and since then, adapted for excisions of tumors involving this subsite. Despite the effectiveness of nonoperative organ preservation protocols for malignant lesions involving the tonsillar region, surgery remains a valid treatment with limited functional sequelae. Management of oropharyngeal cancer by transoral resection and elective neck dissection may spare the patient to adverse effect of full dose radiation therapy or chemoradiation. In addition, minimally invasive procedures using electrocautery, laser beams and recently proposed robotic surgery are being recognized as effective micromanipulation instruments over conventional procedures. The surgical anatomy of the oropharynx has to be outlined to comprehend the surgical approach to the tonsillar and faucial arches, soft palate complex. The extent of exposure of the transoral approach is clearly visualized in Figures 1A and B.

The transoral approach has advantages, but also has very strict limitations given by a narrow visual field of operation and an angled position of the lateral oropharyngeal wall during mouth opening.

Pros

- Avoid external incisions
- Early recovery of swallowing function with limited neural disability
- Reduced hospitalization time.

Cons

- Limited or inadequate visualization of lesion landmarks in case of bulky disease
- No visual control of deep neck vessels during the excision
- No possibility to perform en bloc resection of pharyngeal lesion and neck dissection.

TONSILLECTOMY

This procedure consists of transoral dissection of palatine tonsils. It is reserved to treat very small and superficial tumors, and to achieve adequate diagnostic samples for suspicious lymphoepithelial localization.

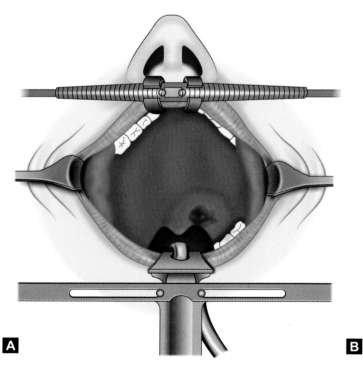

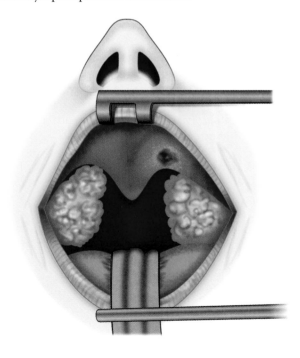

Figs 1A and B: The wider visualization of the soft palate is obtained by positioning of Dingman retractor mouth gag (A) than Crowe-Davis one (B) in case of soft palate tumor

Indications

- Superficial tumors (< 1 cm)
- Suspected lymphoma.

Contraindications

Treatment of any malignant lesions greater than 1 cm with radical purpose or infiltrating the tonsillar capsule.

Patient Position

The patient is intubated under general anesthesia and is kept supine in the operating room table. The Rose position may be used for surgery. A Crowe-Davis or Jennings mouth gag is suspended from the Mayo stand.

Surgical Procedure

The surgical field is exposed as mentioned above. A curved Allis clamp is used to grasp the tonsil in order to clearly visualize the inferior pole and retract it medially. The dissection margin is defined using an electrocautery, cold knife or other device (harmonic, plasma knife, etc.) to delineate the tonsillar capsule from the inferolateral margin to the superomedial tonsillar pillar. Once the capsule is well identified, blunt dissection of the tonsil is carried out away from its bed, paying careful attention to preserve the pharyngeal muscles. While dissection is taking place, the surgeon assures proper traction with the Allis clamp and orientation of the specimen while the assistant helps with local suction and cauterization as needed.

For a suspicious malignancy, such as lymphoma, the specimen is removed and kept under saline solution. At the end of tonsillectomy hemostasis is performed with bipolar or a simple electrocautery instrument. In selected cases, absorbable stitches may be positioned to achieve and guarantee adequate hemostasis especially at tonsillar poles.

Intraoperative Pearls

- The tonsillar capsule is a specialized portion of the pharyngobasilar fascia. In recurrent tonsillitis, the capsule becomes scarred and its septa that carry nerve and vessels remain firmly attached to the deep aspect of the tonsil. Dissection must be blunt and should progress slowly with careful cauterization of the encountered vessels.
- Dissection should be performed above the pharyngeal muscles to limit pain and bleeding for early recovery.
- Adherence of the triangular ligament to the tonsil (palatopharyngeal fibers below the midportion of the tonsil) may result in difficult tonsil enucleation and persistence of tonsillar tags.

EXTENDED TONSILLECTOMY (PHARYNGOTONSILLECTOMY)

This procedure was originally described by Huet and Pietrantoni. It consists of excision of the lateral wall of the oropharynx, comprehensive of the pharyngeal constrictor muscle. The tonsillar region is dissected en bloc with the anterior arch or glossopalatine fold and the posterior arch or pillar, formed by the palatopharyngeal muscle, part of the soft palate and the glossotonsillar sulcus. The excision at the deep margin of resection must include the pharyngeal constrictor muscles. It is indicated to treat limited neoplastic lesions of the tonsils.

Indications

- Limited (<4 cm, cT1/cT2) tonsillar tumors, not infiltrating the pharyngeal constrictor muscles
- T1, T2 tumors limited to the soft palate without extension to the lateral pharyngeal wall and/or the base of the tongue.

Contraindications

- Tumors of any size extending beyond the tonsillar fossa with invasion of the surrounding sites: laterally, toward the parapharyngeal space; inferiorly, toward the lateral pharyngeal wall and the glossotonsillar sulcus; anteriorly, toward the oral cavity. In particular, attention must be given to the extension to or beyond the constrictor muscle toward the parapharyngeal space.
- Soft palate tumors larger than 4 cms (>T2).
- Tumors, which cannot be widely exposed by transoral approach.

Surgical Procedure

Once the patient is positioned in the operating room table as mentioned for tonsillectomy, the oropharynx is exposed. Positioning of Dingman or Crochard mouth gag and the margins of resections are adequately visualized, retracting the cheek as in Figures 1A and B.

Palpation of the tumor will help to define the incision line, marked at least 1.5–2 cms away from the lesion border as in Figure 2.

Different devices may be used to dissect the lateral pharyngeal wall, such as electrocautery, harmonic scalpel and/or laser instruments. Suction should be available on the field to promptly take care of the bleeding.

In every case, the incision begins at the level of the inferior pole and at the glossotonsillar sulcus, as the area is difficult to expose once elevated. Once the anterior pillar is delineated

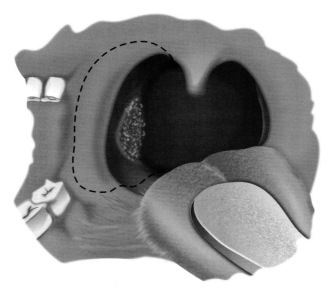

Fig. 2: Right tonsil carcinoma. The incision line of the soft palate and anterior tonsillar pillar (dotted)

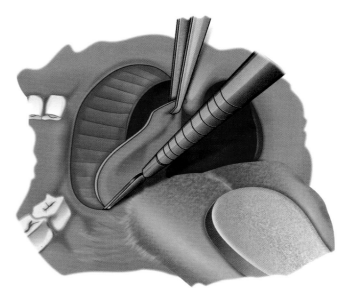

Fig. 3: The electrocautery dissection of the tonsillar fossa. The pharyngeal constrictor muscle is excised together with the tonsil

and dissected, the medial pterygoid muscles mark the level of the deep margin. By following the pterygoid plane, injury to the internal carotid artery is avoided. The dissection of the deep plane is performed under the pharyngeal constrictor muscle as in Figure 3.

Before tumor removal, a stitch is placed for orientation of the specimen. Frozen intraoperative examination of surgical margins is suggested. Accurate hemostasis is done throughout the dissection and at the end of the procedure to maintain a dry surgical field. If possible, in selected cases, 3-0 vicryl sutures may be used to approximate the tonsillar bed to limit postoperative pain and bleeding.

In case of soft palate tumor resection, direct closure may be achieved in most cases of limited tumors. Local pharyngeal flap may be used for slightly larger lesions, paying attention not to determine velopharyngeal patency, which could require a following surgical revision.

Once surgery is completed, the mouth gag is released from the Mayo stand and the surgical site is observed for further bleeding. A suction catheter is passed through the oral cavity to suction gastric contents prior to arousal.

Some authors have recommended external carotid ligation preoperatively to prevent bleeding from the ascending pharyngeal artery or descending palatal artery.

Elective or therapeutic neck dissection is done, as needed.

Intraoperative Pearls

Careful resection of the supratonsillar fold that is located in 40% of individuals on the upper pole of the tonsil is performed. Some stitches may be positioned in the upper pole of the surgical cavity to increase the tension of the soft palate in order to avoid nasopharyngeal reflux.

Postoperative Treatment

The patient is observed in recovery and medicated for any nausea/vomiting. The head of the bed is elevated at an angle of 30°. Humified air is given through a facial mask at 25% FIO2. Intravenous hydration is continued until the patient is ready for oral intake and discharge. Postoperative instructions include completion of the antibiotic course, clear liquid diet that is advanced to a soft diet for the first 2 weeks following surgery and light activity for at least 6 weeks.

Complications

Bleeding from the tonsillar bed may occur, perioperatively and up to 2 weeks following surgery due to fall of the eschar. When bleeding occurs, hospitalization is mandatory even if the hemorrhage stops by itself. Visualization or the artery pulsation in the oropharyngeal wall may alert a possible injury to the internal carotid artery, facial artery, ascending palatine and pharyngeal branches that may occur during surgery and must be promptly stopped in the operating room.

When the tonsillar fossa is violated, soft tissue edema may cause transitory pain or loss of taste at the posterior one-third of the tongue due to glossopharyngeal nerve injury. Extended tonsillectomy may require resection of the soft palate that may cause temporary or permanent swallowing and speech disorders due to open rhinolalia. Rarely, nasopharyngeal synechiae may occur that require surgical revision.

Least common events that occur 1–3 weeks following surgery are parapharyngeal wall infections or abscesses that must be treated aggressively through IV antibiotics and drainage. The patient may present with symptoms of fever, increasing dysphagia, hot potato voice with drooling and shortness of breath. Pain and neck stiffness with decrease lateral mobility may occur in presence of posterior pharyngeal space infections.

HIGHLIGHTS

I. Indications
- Small tumor (T1/2) of the tonsillar fossa
- T1, T2 tumors limited to the soft palate, without extension to the lateral pharyngeal wall and/or the base of the tongue.

II. Contraindications
- Lesions infiltrating the pharyngeal constrictor muscle
- Lesions extending massively to the soft palate
- Tumors extending to the parapharyngeal space
- Tumors extending toward the tongue base or the oral cavity.

III. Special Preoperative Considerations
- Pharyngeal constrictor muscle infiltration.

IV. Special Intraoperative Considerations
- Careful resection of the supratonsillar fold.

V. Special Postoperative Considerations
- Clinical evaluation between the 7th and 10th postoperative days.

VI. Complications
- Bleeding
- Hematoma
- Abscess.

Transoral Robotic Surgery (TORS)

In recent years, transoral robotic surgery (TORS) has been introduced to achieve transoral radical excision of pharyngeal and laryngeal tumors with the objective to improve functional and esthetic outcomes in selected cases, which would have required a transmandibular or transpharyngeal approach. TORS must be considered as an evolution of Transoral laser surgery (TOLS). It accomplishes a wider and frontal view of the surgical field thanks to the 0° and 30° mobile endoscope, which gives a 3D visualization of pharyngolaryngeal structures. Than it allows fine movements by mean of the 180° wristed 5 mm arms which can support instruments, such as DeBakey forceps, Maryland dissector, scissors, needle driver, monopolar cautery, laser devices, harmonic scalpel. These miniaturized tools mimic standard surgical instruments and the mobility of the arms, filtering any operator tremor.

Therefore, TORS allows transoral adequate exposition and radical excision of lesions, arising in oroparyngeal subsites, such as the base of the tongue, and the valleculae, which would result hidden to direct frontal vision, using "traditional" microscopic or endoscopic procedures.

For these reasons, even if TORS may be successfully applied to treat limited lesions of any oropharyngeal subsite, its main indications are:
- T1-T2 tumors of the base of the tongue and valleculae, independently from the N-stage.

In most cases tracheostomy is required. The indications to the elective or therapeutic treatment of the neck do not differ from those of other transoral, transmandibular or transpharyngeal approaches.

RESECTION OF POSTERIOR PHARYNGEAL WALL

This procedure consists of transoral excision of limited lesions to the posterior pharyngeal wall that do not involve the prevertebral fascia and do not reach the lateral pharyngeal wall. Adequate visualization is essential when choosing this route.

Indications
- Minor salivary gland tumors
- Limited tumors (≤ 3cm) not infiltrating the prevertebral fascia.

Contraindications
- Lesions infiltrating the prevertebral fascia
- Lesions extending to the rhinopharynx and/or to the hypopharynx
- Deep or bulky masses, difficult to be adequately exposed.

The preoperative evaluation includes a similar setup described for the tonsillar resection. The extent of the lesion must be evaluated by MRI for evidence of any prevertebral involvement. Staging will consider retropharyngeal lymph node involvement as well. The traditional cold knife excision is nowadays substituted by less bleeding devices, such as monopolar cauterization, coblation, radiofrequency ablation, CO_2 laser techniques, etc.

Surgical Technique

After tracheostomy, which is always suggested for airway safeness, the patient is placed in the Rose position and the lesion is visualized using a mouth gag. The margins of excision are delineated, according to the kind of affection (benign/malignant) which is going to be treated. The depth of the lesion is outlined and blunt dissection is performed and completed along the prevertebral fascia. Once the specimen is removed, frozen sections are sent to assure adequate free margins in case of tumoral lesions. Bleeding is controlled by electrocauterization, bipolar or other surgical tools (coblation, laser, etc.). The specimen is oriented for pathological examination.

If the defect is not reconstructed, purse-string stitches are placed between the borders of the resected area and the underlaying prevertebral fascia. In other cases, reconstruction is performed using split thickness skin grafts or transferring microvascular free flaps, such as the forearm radial free flap, which is anastomized with microsurgical technique to the neck host vessels, after bilateral neck dissection. Nasogastric feeding tube is positioned at the end of the procedure.

Complications

- Bleeding, hematoma formation, postoperative obstruction
- Poor healing, infection, deep abscess formation, sepsis
- Surgical revision is usually required only in case of gross involvement (hematoma, abscess) of the retropharyngeal space, especially when tracheostomy has been spared.

HIGHLIGHTS

I. **Indications**
- Benign mucosal and minor salivary gland diseases
- Limited (T1-T2) tumors (≤ 3 cms) not infiltrating the prevertebral fascia.

II. **Contraindications**
- Lesions infiltrating the prevertebral fascia
- Lesions extended to the rhinopharynx and/or to the hypopharynx
- Bulky masses, difficult to be adequately exposed.

III. **Special Preoperative Considerations**
- Prevertebral fascia infiltration.

IV. **Special Intraoperative Considerations**
- Always suture the remaining excision borders to the prevertebral fascia to the graft or flap
- Always perform a tracheostomy.

V. **Special Postoperative Considerations**
- Decannulation is achieved when there is no risk of airway obstruction and/or aspiration.

VI. **Complications**
- Bleeding
- Hematoma
- Abscess.

Transpharyngeal Approach

INTRODUCTION

It consists of a transcervical, submandibular pharyngectomy. It has been utilized as the standard approach to treat oropharyngeal tumors not involving the larynx or mandible. It is distinguished as median pharyngectomy via supra or subhyoid approach, and lateral pharyngectomy. The former is indicated to treat anterior wall oropharyngeal tumors, the latter to excise tonsillar and subtonsillar fossa neoplasms.

PREOPERATIVE EVALUATION AND ANESTHESIA

To determine whether transpharyngeal approach is indicated, all patients scheduled for surgery are evaluated preoperatively by the head and neck surgeon, anesthesiologist and speech pathologist. Physical examination, especially palpation and tongue motility, remains one of the most important aspects of the preoperative evaluation. Resectability of posterior pharyngeal wall lesions is determined by tumor size and

fixation. Endoscopy under general anesthesia, performed for bioptic mapping of the lesion is considered a mandatory procedure. Radiological evaluation of the patient includes MRI that proves to be the most sensitive modality for evaluating tumors involving the base of the tongue for well-known soft tissue dentition. Diagnosis of gross tissue invasion of the pre-epiglottic space and the depth of infiltration into the tongue base may be determined by obtaining sagittal MRI scans. The high signal intensity of the pre-epiglottic fat can usually be distinguished from the dense fibers of the hyoepiglottic ligament, tongue base musculature, lingual lymphoid tissue and cancer. A barium pharyngoesophagram can often assist in assessing mobility of these tumors.

Ultrasonography (US) of the neck is performed for complete the staging. Chest computed tomography (CT) or PET/CT whole body scan is also done in order to detect primary or metastatic pulmonary tumors. The structure of the oropharynx and hypopharynx plays a key role in swallowing. Temporary aspiration is a predictable postoperative occurrence. The patient's functional status, especially cardiopulmonary performance must be considered in patient selection. Patients with severe pulmonary disease may require laryngectomy to protect them from life-threatening postoperative aspiration and placement of percutaneous endoscopic gastrostomy (PEG).

It is recommended to routinely have a shower with chlorhexidine (Hibi Scrub®) on the morning of the operation. Broad-spectrum antibiotics are instituted perioperatively. All patients are operated in the supine position with a pillow under the shoulder to achieve head hyperextension. Tracheostomy is performed at the beginning of the operation and nasogastric feeding tube is positioned.

MEDIAN PHARYNGECTOMY

The surgical approach to the base of the tongue and to the posterior wall of the oropharynx is controversial because resection of isolated tumors may be associated with significant morbidity, primarily impaired speech and deglutition, which may at times also result in chronic aspiration. Carefully selected tumors arising in these anatomic sites may be surgically resected and reconstructed through a suprahyoid pharyngotomy approach with excellent opportunity for tumor control, little morbidity and very good cure rates.

Treatment results for tumors of the base of the tongue are measured in terms of speech and swallowing function, need for a gastrostomy or tracheostomy tube; local, regional and distant control and patient's quality of life.

The suprahyoid approach is a technique that allows adequate exposure of the tongue base and the posterior pharyngeal wall with complete tumor control, preservation of function and minimization of cosmetic deformity. The excellent exposure given to the oropharynx offers a precise macroscopic identification of tumor margins and minimizes possible injuries to vital neurovascular structures. The open wound can usually be closed primarily without the need of flap reconstruction.

Indications

- Limited, deep infiltrating (T1-T2 and selected T3) cancer of the tongue base
- Small tumors (T1, T2) of the posterior pharyngeal wall.

Contraindications

Tumors massively involving the supraglottic larynx.

Closure of the posterior pharyngeal wall stump may be achieved directly through internal stitches to the prevertebral fascia or through microvascular flap transfer. Some authors reported oncological success in treatment of T3 squamous cell carcinoma of the tongue base with this approach together with supraglottic laryngectomy.

Surgical Technique

The skin incision depends on the extension of the operation. A superiorly based apron flap or a horizontal linear skin incision, in a skin crease is outlined to perform bilateral neck dissections as in Figure 4.

After elevating the subplatysmal flap, a suprahyoid muscle flap is harvested and rotated downward, after its dissection from the the hyoid bone. The laryngopharyngeal complex is isolated to identify the vascular and neural structures. Care must be taken laterally around the greater cornu of the hyoid bone to avoid injury to the hypoglossal nerve when it is free from disease and lingual artery. Pre-epiglottic space is dissected keeping its connection to the hyoid bone. Lateral pharyngeal wall is exposed together to hypoglossal nerve and superior laryngeal vessels and nerves. Superior retraction of the separated suprahyoid tongue musculature will define the hyoepiglottic ligament, which extends from its broad hyoid origin to its narrow insertion into the epiglottis. Pharyngotomy represents the key point of the procedure. It must be performed far from the tumor to avoid residual disease and neoplastic intraoperative dissemination. When the tumor is placed close to the vallecula, laryngotomy in the supraglottic subsite represents a safe approach to the base of the tongue. In this case, epiglottis is removed together with hyoid bone and pre-epiglottic space. When there is no involvement of the vallecula, an incision through the mucosa just above the superior edge of hyoid bone provides entry into the pharynx as in Figures 5 to 8.

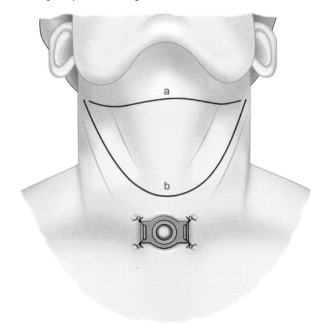

Fig. 4: Skin incision. Linear (a); Skin apron flap (b). In both cases, tracheostomy is kept separated

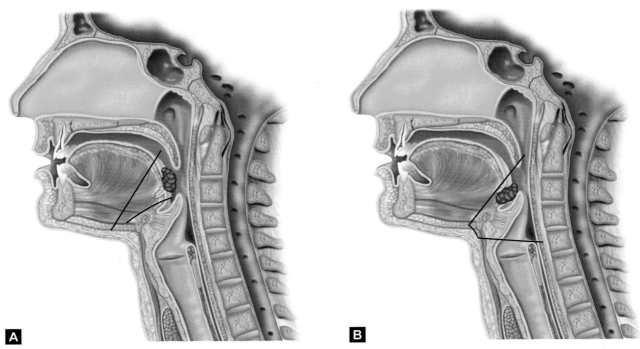

Figs 5A and B: Type of transpharyngeal resection. (A) Through the vallecula, when it is free or distant from the tumor; (B) Through the supraglottic space, when the vallecula is infiltrated by or close to the tumor

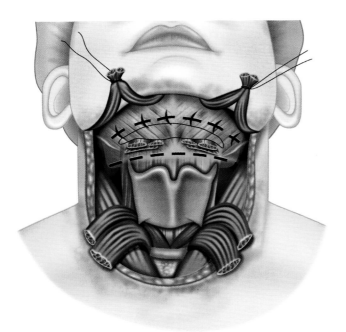

Fig. 6: Inferior pharyngotomy lines. Through the vallecula (++++); Through the supraglottic larynx (– – – –)

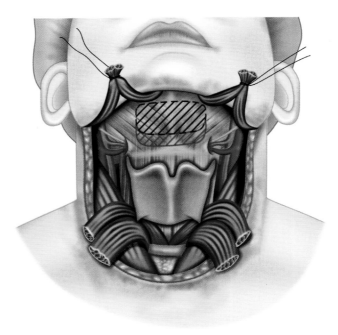

Fig. 7: Pharyngectomy. The supraglottic extension in case of vallecular involvement is marked blue

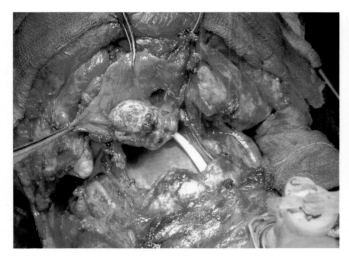

Fig. 8: Transpharyngeal resection through the supraglottic space. The excision is carried out under direct visual control from the superior edge of the thyroid cartilage to the lingual "V," after laryngotomy

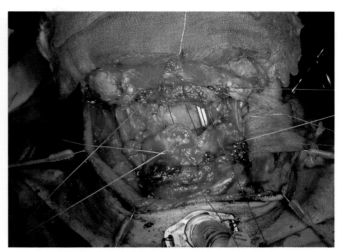

Fig. 9: Multiple separate stitches are positioned through the margins of the pharyngeal stump

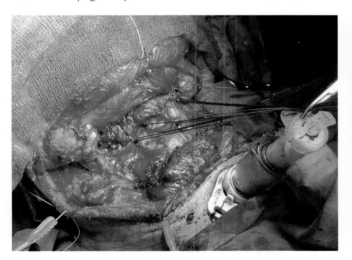

Fig. 10: Thyroglossopexy is completed

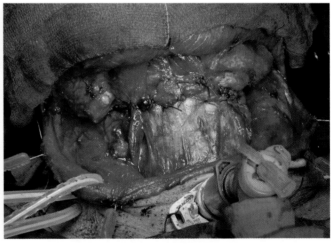

Fig. 11: Prelaryngeal muscle flap is rotated and sutured superiorly and laterally to cover and isolate the pexy

The hypoglossal nerve and lingual artery are identified and retracted laterally. A retractor is placed on the tongue base to draw it into the wound. When the tumor has been removed under direct visual control and adequacy of the resection has been verified by frozen section evaluation, thyroglossopexy is performed. It consists of the primary closure of the pharyngeal stump with multiple separate stitches as in Figures 9 and 10.

Prelaryngeal muscle flap is rotated and used to cover the pexy as in Figure 11.

The cervical wound is closed over drainage. Special attention must be paid to keep separate surgical fields between pharyngectomy and tracheostomy to prevent contamination of the cervical wound when the patient coughs and during drainage failure as in Figure 12.

The technique is modified in patients in whom the pharyngotomy is used to approach a lesion of the posterior pharyngeal wall. After the pharyngotomy is made at the level of the vallecula, the tumor is identified and excised from the posterior pharyngeal wall in order to reduce the risk of hypoglossal and superior laryngeal nerve damage. Frozen section control is carried out and hemostasis is obtained. There are several options for reconstruction of the defect as in transoral approach.

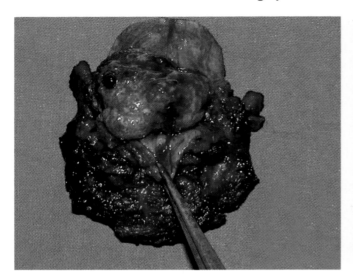

Fig. 12: The specimen composed by epiglottis, the pre-epiglottic space, the hyoid bone, the valleculae and the tongue base with the tumor

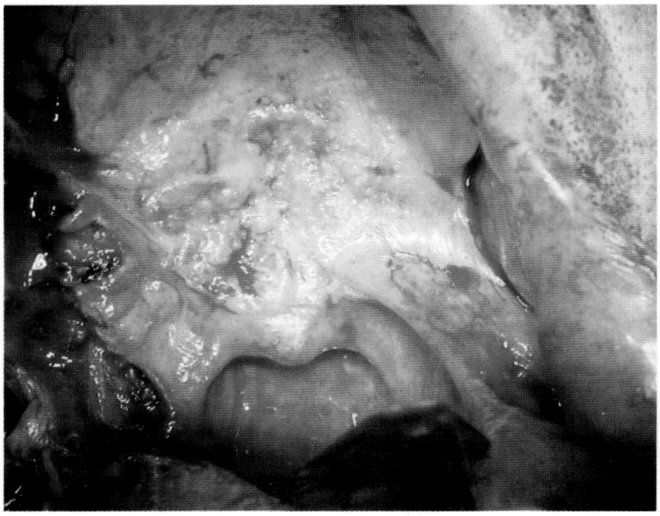

Fig.13: Soft palate carcinoma

LATERAL PHARYNGECTOMY

The surgical technique consists of en bloc resection of the tumor and the neck dissection via a lateral transpharyngeal approach, sparing the mandibular arch. It is indicated for small and mid-size tumors of this subsite without or limited extension to adjacent subsites, such as the tongue base or the posterior pharyngeal wall.

Indications

• T1-T2 tumors of the subtonsillar fossa, marginally extended to the tongue base or to the tonsillar fossa or to the posterior pharyngeal wall
• T2 and selected T3 tumors of the soft palate extended to the lateral pharyngeal wall or, marginally, to the base of the tongue.

Contraindications

• Tumors involving massively more than one subsite (tongue base or to the tonsillar fossa or to the posterior pharyngeal wall)
• Tumors infiltrating the mandible or pterygoid muscles
• Tumors massively invading the base of the tongue or the subtonsillar fossa.

Surgical Technique

Patient Position

• Supine position and neck extended and rotated contralaterally to the neck dissection, during the transcervical phase
• Supine position during the intraoral phase.

The line of incision is marked from the mastoid to the interdigastric joint. The flap is rotated and the neck dissection is completed. Internal carotid artery and jugular vein are isolated in the neck and in the parapharyngeal space, if necessary. Lingual artery is identified and ligated in the Farabeuf space, preserving the hypoglossal nerve, whenever possible. Superior thyroid artery may be ligated and sectioned too. Progressively, the omohyoid muscle is resected, then the sternohyoid ones and then the thyrohyoid ones. The pharyngolaryngeal complex is gently dissected from the prevertebral fascia. Pharyngotomy is performed as far as possible from the tumor, usually just above the superior edge of the thyroid cartilage. The resection continues ventrally toward the posterior pharyngeal wall or dorsally toward the hyoid bone in order to expose the subtonsillar and/or the tonsillar fossa from below and excise the tumor under direct visual control with adequate free margins. Frozen section examination completes the demolitive phase. In much selected cases, it is possible to combine the lateral transpharyngeal approach with the transoral approach, for tumors of the lateral pharyngeal wall. The excision may be extended to rim mandibulectomy. The specimen is dissected in the neck and removed en bloc via a pull-through maneuver. Direct closure is achieved by positioning stitches along the pharyngeal stump Alternative methods are represented by microvascular fasciocutaneous flap transfer, such as forearm free flap.

In case of soft palate tumor (Figs 13 and 14), the dissection of the tumor begins and is extended to the lateral pharyngeal wall. The lateral floor of the mouth is opened and the mylohyoid muscle is incised. In this way, the pharyngeal resection is extended to the base of the tongue and completed after its dissection in the neck. Closure requires

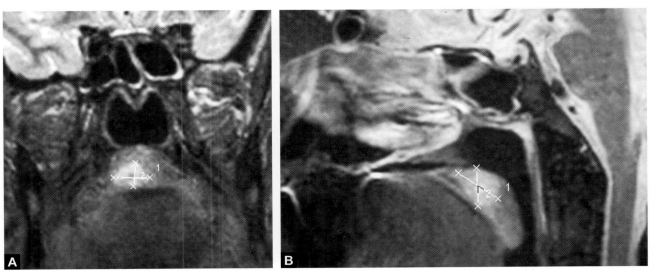

Figs 14A and B: Magnetic resonance imaging of the tumor (evidenced)

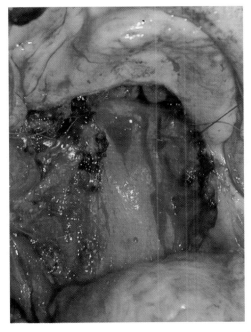

Fig.15: Surgical view at the end of resection. The whole soft palate has been excised, extended to two-thirds of the hard palate

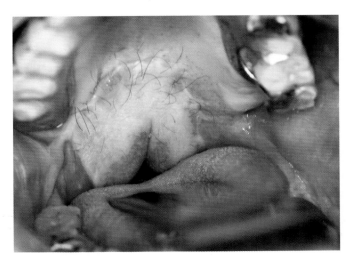

Fig.16: Postoperative pharyngeal view after reconstruction by means of a forearm free flap

the use of reconstruction flap to achieve separation of neck spaces from pharyngeal lumen and adequate protection of neck vessels.

Reconstruction of the soft palate is complex because its muscular architecture cannot be restored. Reconstruction of hemi-soft-palate defects after tumor resection is usually done by means of a regional flap, free tissue transfer or a prosthesis. Larger defects requires thin, elastic and light flaps,

whose goal is pharyngeal lumen separation from neck spaces and nose regurgitation prevention of the bolus, during swallowing; thanks to the closure of the velopharynx and the restoration of the valvular sphincteric function. In case of soft tissue defect, microvascular free flap transfer represents the first choice option. Among them fasciocutaneous flap are recommended (radial forearm, lateral arm) as in Figures 15 and 16.

More bulky flaps may be employed in case of huge resection of the base of the tongue (abdominis rectus, lateral thigh). Pedicled flaps are indicated in selected cases and must be considered as second choice option for reconstruction because of their poor functional results. Pectoralis major transposition is the most performed pedicled flap reconstruction in these cases.

Postoperative Treatment

All patients receive routine postoperative care for tracheostomy and for the cervical wound. Decannulation is achieved before removal of the nasogastric tube and initiation of oral feeding. Initial feedings take place under the guidance of our speech pathologist who evaluates the patient's readiness and instructs the patient in swallowing strategies. During this initial training of the swallowing act, the speech pathologist sits with the patient at mealtimes and helps the patient attain the technique necessary for swallowing.

HIGHLIGHTS

I. **Indications**
   - Early (T1-T2) cancer of the oropharynx
   - T2-T3 tumors of the soft palate extended to the lateral pharyngeal wall, to the base of the tongue
   - Small tumor of the posterior pharyngeal wall.

II. **Contraindications**
   - Tumor extends to the vallecula, tonsil or supraglottic larynx
   - Large tumor of the posterior pharyngeal wall.

III. **Special Preoperative Considerations**
   - Direct laryngoscopy
   - Imaging studies, particularly MRI (for detection of prevertebral fascia invasion) are fundamental.

IV. **Special Intraoperative Considerations**
   - Limited resection of tissue and preservation of both hypoglossal nerves leads to early return of functional deglutition without aspiration
   - The apron flap that is used for this procedure lends itself to the performance of bilateral neck dissection when appropriate.

V. **Special Postoperative Considerations**
   - Decannulation is achieved before removal of the nasogastric tube and initiation of oral feeding.

VI. **Complications**
   - Pharyngocutaneous fistula
   - Aspiration pneumonia.

Transmandibular Approach

INTRODUCTION

Transmandibular approaches are indicated in all those cases in which a wide exposition of the surgical field is required or when the mandibular arch is involved by primary tumor or nodal metastases. They are classically distinguished as "conservative" and "composite" transmandibular resections. The former consists of a pharyngectomy performed through mandibulotomy, the latter consists of a composite resection of soft tissue and a segment of mandible, infiltrated by or very close to the tumor. Leaving apart mandibulectomies, the main reasons for conservative transmandibular approaches are the following:

- En bloc excision of locally advanced primary tumors and neck dissection.
- Resection of primary tumor under visual control of internal carotid artery and internal jugular vein in the parapharyngeal space.
- Resection of primary tumors arising from the anterior pharyngeal wall (base of the tongue and valleculae) with anterior or lateral spread.
- Necessity to have wide exposition of the surgical field for reconstruction by means of pedicled or microvascularized free flaps.

Actually, the indications to open the mandible tend to be reduced more and more. Its healing is significantly longer than nontransmandibular resections. In fact, mandibulotomy is affected by a quite high rate of morbidity and possible postoperative complications and therefore it is either performed as a primary or salvage treatment. It requires the opening of the inferior lip and therefore frontal facial scar. It is usually performed in a paramedian position between the second incisive and canine dental element, to reduce the risk of injury to dental roots and preserve the anatomical integrity of the mandibular nerve (V3); nevertheless dental damages and trigeminal impairment may occur. Such position is due to distance mandibulotomy from irradiation postoperative field and to reduce the risk of infection and bone resorption around the osteosynthesis. In salvage surgery or chemoradiation failures, it is advisable not to split the lip but try to use a lateral visor flap.

The actual indications to conservative transmandibular approach are limited and are as follows:

- Tumors of the lateral pharyngeal wall massively invading the parapharyngeal space.
- Tumors involving both the anterior and the lateral wall of the oropharynx, for which the en bloc excision of the tumor and neck dissection is required, after the exposition of carotid artery and internal jugular vein and flap reconstruction is mandatory.
- Very selected cases of huge tumors of the posterior pharyngeal wall with involvement of the retropharyngeal space by the primary tumor or nodal metastases.

Considering that the wide majority of oropharyngeal tumors are surgically treated when they are locally advanced, they often require wide excisions through transmandibular approaches. The few cases of limited tumors (below 4 cms, T1-2) arising from the lateral, anterior and posterior pharyngeal wall, may be adequately resected through transoral approaches; "classical" or by robotic surgery, or through transcervical, transpharyngeal procedures. Transoral approaches are indicated for tumors not deeply infiltrating whereas the transpharyngeal ones (avoiding any mandibular injury) are reserved for cases of locally advanced tumors, deeply infiltrating and/or placed close to vessels or nerves to be preserved, which have to be excised en bloc with neck dissection and usually require flap reconstruction. In much selected cases, it is possible to combine partial pharyngectomy to rim mandibulectomy to excise tonsillar fossa tumor as described in the above transpharyngeal paragraph.

The different technical procedures of mandibulotomy considering the position, lines of osteotomy and osteosynthesis have been already described in the section dedicated to oral cavity tumor procedures. Therefore, in the present chapter they will be only briefly treated to explain their application to oropharyngeal procedures.

The transmandibular approaches are accomplished by:
- Conservative approach via mandibulotomy
- Radical approach through a segmental mandibulectomy.

SURGICAL TECHNIQUES

Tracheotomy is always necessary.

Conservative Transmandibular Pharyngectomy

It consists of a pharyngectomy performed through transcervical, transmandibular approach. The mandible and the muscles inserting into the mandible (pterygoid muscles) are not involved by the tumor, so segmental mandibular resection is not required. The osteotomy preserves the continuity of the bone by temporary separation (mandibular swing). Nowadays, the surgical approach is represented by paramedian conservative osteotomy approach between the second and third (canine) dental element. Midline conservative osteotomy via the symphysis is used as well, especially for midline translingual approach, as proposed by Trotter.

Paramedian Conservative Transmandibular Approach

Originally defined as "transmaxillary oropharyngectomy via symphysis osteotomy", it was described and elaborated by many authors (Piquet, Simon, Guerrier, Vandenbrouck, Dargent). It is indicated to treat tumors invading the anterior wall (base of the tongue) and the lateral wall (tonsillar fossa) of the oropharynx. Its main contraindications are mandible invasion and/or pterygoid muscle infiltration. In both these cases, mandibulectomy is required to achieve a radical excision of the tumor.

Skin and mucosal incision: The skin incision on the lip is midline, or incised in a stepwise fashion up to the midline. Then it reaches the underlining chin, which is surrounded to draw a curved line along the perimental line. A possible variant to mental skin incision is represented by a straight line in the middle. Once in the interdigastric space, it is prolonged variously in the neck depending on the type of neck dissection, which is required as in Figure 17.

Inside the mouth, the incision line reaches the incisor tooth socket between the second incisive and the canine dental element, passed through buccoalveolar sulcus. At this level, the gingiva is sectioned to skeletonize the mandibular alveolar ridge and prolonged intraorally along the floor of the mouth to obtain a good exposure of the tonsillar fossa and the base of tongue.

Skeletonization of the mandible: Once the neck dissection is completed, the soft tissues are dissected in the chin area to achieve the exposition of the mandible. The vestibule and buccal mucosa are incised through the socket of the lateral inferior incisor or the canine tooth. The mandible at this level is skeletonized using a Joseph dissector, and the mandibular nerve (V3) is identified and preserved at the mental foramen. At the end of this phase, a 5–6 cm long segment of mandible is exposed transcervically.

Mandibulotomy: The osteotomy line is drawn on the mandible. Preplating is performed prior to the osteotomy through titanium plates and hole drilling as in Figure 18.

By means of Gigli saw or sagittal saw osteotomy is done as planned. This can be performed in a linear or in a stepwise fashion to improve end to end approximation and contrast masticatory muscle traction. Bipolar cauterization and/or bone wax positioning controls bleeding from the mandibular sections.

The mandibular swing allows visualization of the floor of the mouth, which is sectioned to achieve the complete exposition of the pharyngeal tumor (Fig. 19). It is advisable to maintain the mucosa attached to the mandible, in order to facilitate the closure by stitch positioning at the end of the procedures.

Resection of the tumor: To obtain an en bloc resection of the tumor and neck dissection, the mylohyoid muscles are sectioned, and the stylohyoid and posterior digastric muscle plane is followed to elevate the contents of the neck dissection previously performed and the tumor excision is carried out (Fig. 20). The structures of the neck, which must be preserved, are identified and gently isolated, such as carotid artery, internal jugular vein, hypoglossal nerve, etc.

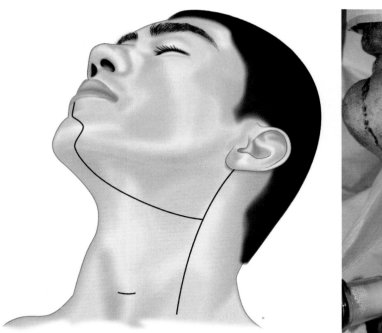
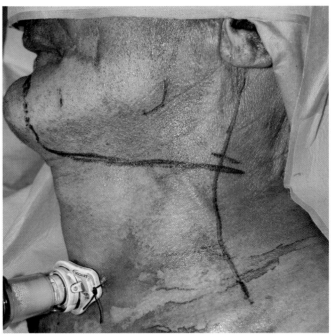

Fig. 17: Incision line. The submandibular branch of this incision must be drawn 2 cm below the inferior mandibular border to avoid facial nerve injury

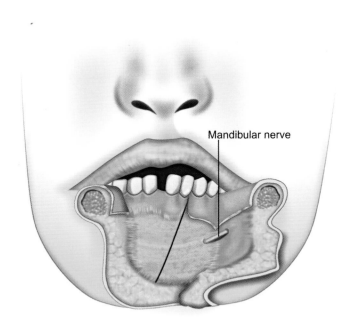

Mandibular nerve

Fig. 18: Mandibulotomy line. The holes, drilled during the preplating phase, are placed in order to avoid possible injury to V3 nerve by two plates and the screws

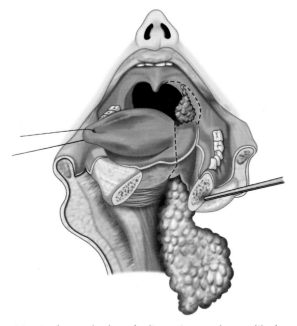

Fig. 19: At the end of neck dissection and mandibulotomy, mandibular swing permits the wide exposure of the tumor in the pharyngeal lumen and its safe en bloc excision

The dissection is performed under direct visual and palpatory control. The excision line is drawn intraorally, keeping 1.5–2.0 cms of healthy mucosa from the tumor edge and the resection is completed both intraorally and transcervically, through the mandibular swing. In case of glossectomy, one side of lingual artery may be ligated in the Farabeuf space to reduce bleeding. At least one hypoglossal nerve must be spared to guarantee adequate swallowing

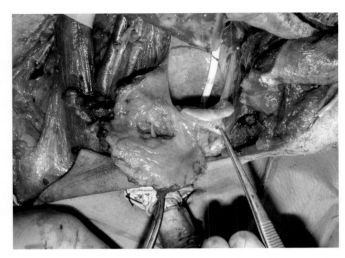

Fig. 20: Tumor excision is almost carried out. The tumor is located on the right side of the tongue base and vallecula

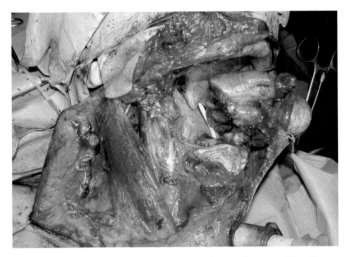

Fig. 22: Surgical view. The tongue base, the tonsillar fossa, part of the soft palate and the epiglottis have been removed. Such a wide excision requires flap reconstruction

rehabilitation. Resected mucosal margins, soft tissues and nerve fragments are examined intraoperatively to evidence any residual disease or spread of the tumor as in Figures 21 and 22.

Reconstruction: The reconstruction of tumors of the oropharynx is related to two main goals:

1. Anatomical separation of the pharynx lumen from the neck spaces.
2. Functional reconstruction of the pharynx.

Flap reconstruction must be reserved to those cases, in which direct reconstruction is not achievable.

Direct closure: Direct closure consists of multiple separate absorbable stitches, which are positioned on different layers

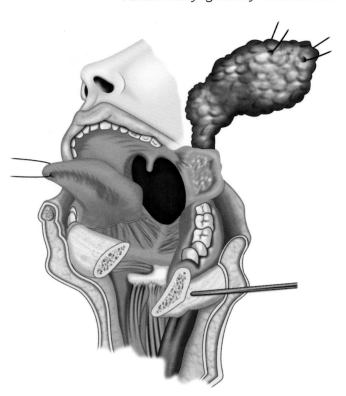

Fig. 21: Surgical view at the end of conservative transmandibular pharyngectomy

intraorally and transcervically. It is possible to perform direct reconstruction in case of:

- Resection of the base of the tongue (less than 50%)
- Limited resection of the lateral pharyngeal wall.

Flap reconstruction: It is indicated in all cases in which direct closure is not possible or risky for severe anatomical or functional complications or sequelae. It is required whenever neck spaces and structures communicate with the pharyngeal lumen. Therefore, it must be performed in the following cases:

- Base of the tongue resection (more than 50%)
- Base of the tongue resection (less than 50%), extended to the lateral pharyngeal wall (tonsillar fossa, subtonsillar fossa)
- Extended full thickness resection of the lateral pharyngeal wall.

The problems related to the flap reconstruction are mainly functional. The ideal reconstruction should guarantee the same volume of soft tissue (base of the tongue), motility and above all sensitivity. Although the reconstruction procedures through microvascular flap transfer are more and more improving, pharyngeal reconstruction hardly ever succeeds in functional recovery; very often achieves good anatomical, static reparation of the organ. Therefore, swallowing rehabilitation tends to improve the sensory and motor activity of the residual pharynx.

Another indication for flap reconstruction is salvage surgery after chemo/radiation treatment. Free tissue transfer or transposition guarantees safer and better healing due to the positioning of healthy tissues.

Nowadays, flap reconstruction comprehends microvascular flap transfer as first option, pedicled flap as second option, particularly in case of salvage treatment after radiation or chemo/radiation and in patients with poor performance status. The former permits the choice of different kind of flaps, considering their thickness, extension, lack of bulky pedicle, possibility of sensory harvesting. The latter guarantees adequate cover and anatomical reconstruction by the transposition of soft tissue paddle.

The first choice flap for primary reconstruction is microvascular: the base of the tongue requires a flap, which fills the soft tissue defect determined by glossectomy avoiding residual empty spaces, which could determine bolus stagnation and the risk of post swallowing aspiration. It must guarantee adequate mobility of the residual tongue too. Whenever possible it should be sensorized. Forearm, transverse rectus abdominis myocutaneous (TRAM) free flaps represent the most frequently performed flaps. The use of "perforator flaps" such as the deep inferior epigastric (DIEP) flap, lateral thigh and anterolateral thigh flap (ALT), superficial inferior epigastric artery (SIEA) flap have served to further decrease donor site morbidity as in Figures 23A and B.

Pedicled flaps are second choice flaps in primary treatments, but may be the only possible reconstruction in cases unsuitable for free flaps. It is represented mainly by pectoralis major myocutaneous flap. Other cervical pedicled flaps reported in the literature, such as infrahyoid muscle pedicled or arterialized flaps are hardly ever used, preferring microvascular free flaps and are considered oncologically risky,

because their pedicle harvesting may reduce the radicality of the II level neck dissection. Finally, they cannot be used in case of salvage treatment because they are placed in a previously irradiated and/or dissected area.

Osteosynthesis and closure: Mandible continuity is obtained via osteosynthesis using titanium plates and screws, secured in the previously prepared holes at the bone ends. Approximation of the buccal mucosa in the gingivobuccal sulcus, the vermilion border and the skin is performed for final closure. Cervical drains are positioned in the neck, far from the mucosal sutures to avoid direct aspiration of oral cavity secretions as in Figure 24.

Postoperative course: Parenteral hydration is given during the first 24–48 hours together with broad-spectrum intravenous antibiotics. The patient is medicated daily with special attention to the pooling of secretions in the oral cavity and the oropharygeal region.

Tracheotomy tube is usually kept for 5–7 days. Progressive advancement of nasogastric feeding occurs till swallowing rehabilitation is achieved.

Complications: Postoperative complications may be distinguished as local and general; the former are mainly represented by infections. Infections may be secondary due to poor oral hygiene, metabolic disease (diabetes, hepatitis) circulatory disease dehabilitation. Tissue dehiscence may occur at the level of the oral pelvis, where suture tension is more common, due to the traction of the residual tongue and secretions tend to filter among stitches. Infections and dehiscence may determine: the formation of fistula between the oral cavity and the neck, usually along the cervical incision in the second level; mandibular infection at the level of the osteotomy line and the screw holes represents one of the

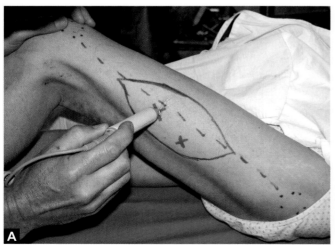
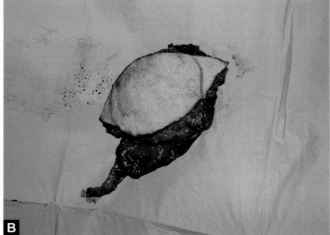

Figs 23A and B: (A) Lateral thigh (LT) flap is drawn around the perforating vessels;
(B) Harvested LT flap immediately before its transfer

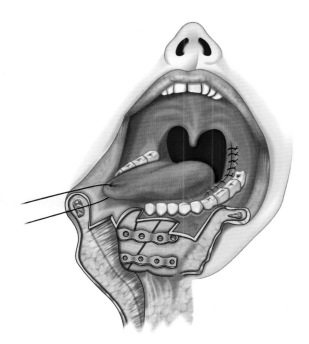

Fig. 24: Direct closure following pharyngectomy. Two plates restore mandibular continuity

most serious complications of this procedure. Medications, surgical treatment of tissue dehiscence, nasogastric tube feeding and antibiotic therapy are the main tools to treat them.

HIGHLIGHTS

I. Indications
- Locally advanced tumors (T3, T4a) of the lateral pharyngeal wall extended to the parapharyngeal space.
- Locally advanced tumors (T3, T4a) of the anterior and lateral wall of the oropharynx.
- Tumors (T3, T4a) of the posterior pharyngeal wall with involvement of the retropharyngeal space by the primary tumor or nodal metastases.

II. Contraindications
- Tumor attached or infiltrating the mandible.

III. Special Preoperative Considerations
- Imaging studies, particularly MRI/CT to detect mandibular infiltration or distance between the tumor and the mandible.

IV. Special Intraoperative Considerations
- Preserve dental roots during mandibulotomy
- Avoid V3 injuries.

V. Special Postoperative Considerations
- Antibiotic prophylaxis (penicillin and clavulanic acid, adjunctive IV metronidazole, 500 mg × 2).

VI. Complications
- Osteomyelitis
- Bone necrosis
- Malocclusion
- Teeth lesions
- Pseudarthrosis.

COMPOSITE TRANSMANDIBULAR PHARYNGECTOMY

Segmental mandibulectomy, generally named "COMMANDO operation", acronym for Combined Mandibulectomy and Neck Dissection Operation consists of the segmental mandible removal, performed in the setting of a composite resection, in continuity with the oropharyngeal cancer.

Excision of the mandible, as performed nowadays, was reported by Slaughter and colleagues, and then by Ward and Robben half a century ago, and the main step of the procedure did not change. Cancer arising in the lateral or anterior wall of the oropharynx may infiltrate the mandible. Mandibulectomy is indicated in case of mandibular infiltration or in those cases, in which the tumor is so close to the mandible that its excision is at risk of residual disease, if bone is preserved. For pharyngeal tumors, it mostly occurs when there is a pterygoid muscle infiltration.

In addition to careful examination under anesthesia by bimanual palpation, radiographic evaluation of the mandible should be available for satisfactory treatment planning.

Patient Position and Tracheostomy

The patient is positioned in supine position with a pillow under the shoulder to achieve adequate head hyperextension.

Temporary tracheotomy is mandatory to guarantee adequate air flow and prevent postoperative aspiration of secretions. It must be performed at the beginning of the procedure to allow the removal of the endotracheal tube and expose all the oropharyngeal lumen.

Skin Incision and Cervical Flap

According to the type of neck dissection and the extension of the operation, a visor flap (an upper neck incision 2–4 cm below the mandible) or a lip-splitting incision are performed. Whenever it is possible, any facial and particularly labial incision should be avoided especially in case of salvage surgery for radiation/chemoradiation failures as in Figures 25 and 26.

Skeletonization of the Mandible and Pharyngectomy

After neck dissection is completed, the inferior mandibular ridge is exposed and a subperiosteal dissection of the external

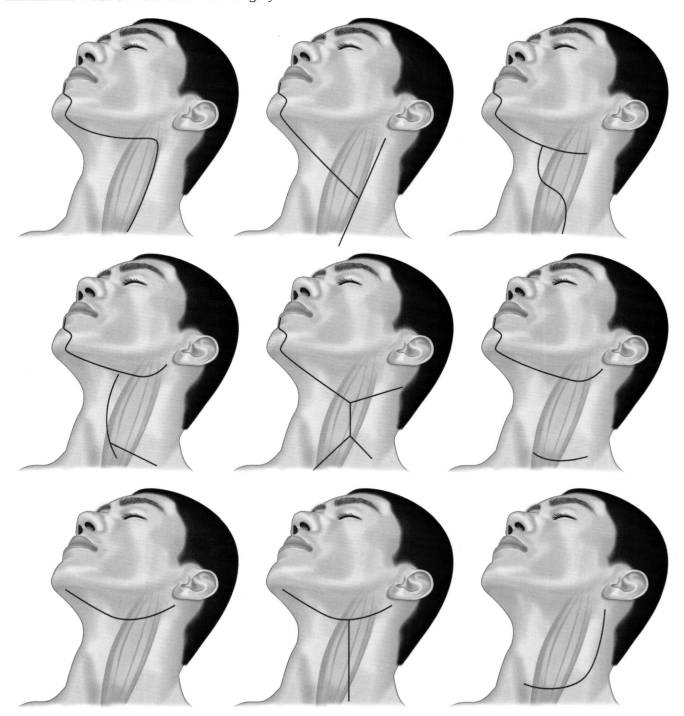

Fig. 25: Skin incisions for composite resection and neck dissection

cortical side is completed, sectioning the masticatory muscles and displacing the parotid gland up to the coronoid process.

The endoral phase of the procedure must consider the site of the oropharyngeal tumor. So the mucosal incision of the gingivobuccal sulcus, which should be performed close to the gingival ridge, must be performed at least 2 cms far from the tumor border. Now the cheek flap may be elevated exposing the segment of the mandible and the oropharyngeal lumen. The dissection of the soft tissue part of the tumor continues under direct visual control. Using electrocautery,

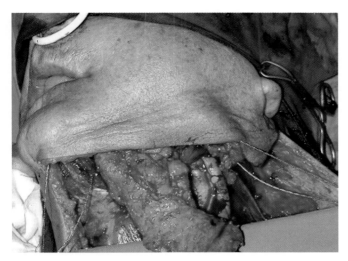

Fig. 26: Lip sparing skin incision for composite resection and neck dissection. It is possible to see two Gigli saw positioned at the mandibular resection extremities and neck dissection

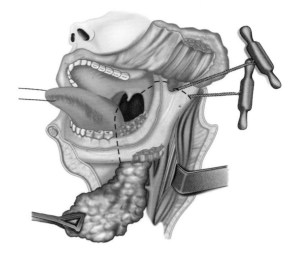

Fig. 27: Mandibulectomy by means of Gigli saw. It is performed when neck dissection has been completed. In the present view, lip-split approach is represented for iconographic reasons

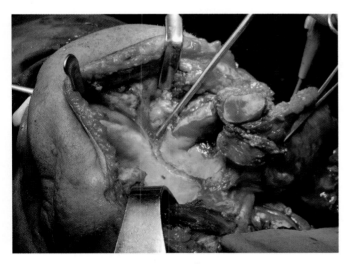

Fig. 28: Composite pharyngectomy through lip sparing incision

the mandible is completely isolated from soft tissues along the two osteotomy lines, both in its external and internal sides.

Mandibulectomy and Composite Resection

The segmental mandibulectomy must include the mandibular channel and its ostium at the the level of the spina mandibulae, to achieve the radical excision of the mandibular nerve lymphatics. It must be performed as far as possible from mandibular infiltration. This is why the mandibular resection, comprehensive of the whole ascending branch up to the condilum, may be required. Osteotomy may be per-

formed by means of Gigli saw, oscillating or sagittal saw as in Figures 27 and 28.

The excision of the soft tissue part of tumor is now completed transcervically under direct visual control, displacing and tractioning the mandibular segment. At the end of the excision phase, the specimen is composed of the tumor, the mandibular segment and the neck dissection as in Figures 29 and 30.

Reconstruction

The most difficult decision-making, regarding segmental resection of the mandible, is its reconstruction. It must be planned preoperatively to achieve adequate functional and esthetical results. The reconstruction at the end of a composite resection must consider either soft tissue or bone continuity restoration. With the advent of microvascular surgery, composite free tissue transfer represents the first option. Fibula, iliac crest osteomuscular microvascular free flap represent the preferred procedures in the literature, in relation to anatomical, esthetical and functional outcome, and donor site morbidity.

Decision regarding reconstruction should be based on the patient's age, dentition, previous treatments, expectations, etc. Reconstruction of defects, involving the mandible posterior to the mental foramen, is still debated. Komisar demonstrated that these patients do not benefit functionally from the reconstructive efforts that are required to reconstitute bone continuity. Urken reported that reconstruction is warranted to facilitate dental prosthetic rehabilitation with osseointegrated fixation devices placed in vascularized bone. Nonetheless, substantial morbidity rate accompanies these

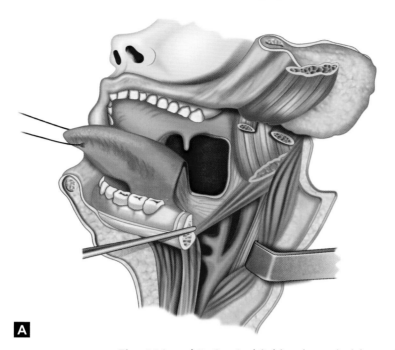

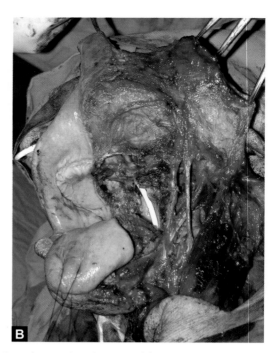

Figs 29A and B: Surgical field at the end of the excision phase. The pharyngeal lumen is in continuity with the neck and parapharyngeal spaces

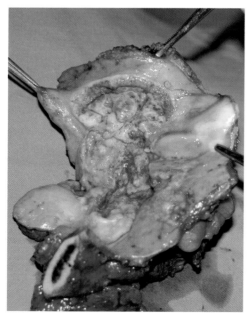

Fig. 30: The specimen of a T4a tumor of the oropharynx infiltrating the mandible

reconstructive procedures, so the surgeon must not decide *"What is best,"* but *"what is best for the determinate patient."* A composite flap is necessary in order to substitute bone and soft tissue. If fibula is used, an overlaid skin paddle is harvested to fill the soft tissue loss.

Postoperative Management

Careful nursing management of the drains and tracheal suction are necessary. If a free flap has been used, monitoring of its blood supply by the nursing staff is critical for success. Blood pressure must be monitored after free flap, skin paddle of flap is monitored by nurse every one hour, at the same time suction drains vacuum must be evaluated.

The authors did not use dressing in patients who have undergone flap reconstruction (either pedicled or free flap microvascular) for fear that the dressing could lead to venous congestion of the flap and result in tissue ischemia and necrosis. To avoid infection, in association with penicillin and clavulanic acid, adjunctive intravenous metronidazole (500 mg × 2) can be administered.

Tracheotomy is removed between the 7th and 14th postoperative day, when there is not any reasonable risk of surgical revision and swallowing rehabilitation has begun. In order to identify an orocervical fistula a methylene blue diluted solution can be administered orally so that it can be detected in the neck drainage (within 24 hours) or through a cervical dehiscence.

The patient kept on nasogastric tube feeding till soft tissue healing allows swallowing rehabilitation. Initial feedings take place under the control of a speech pathologist. Some patients require placement of percutaneous endoscopic gastrostomy (PEG) depending on the amount of base of tongue removed in the composite operation. Soft food is recommended until approximately the 6th postoperative month after the outpatient physical therapy (OPT) control.

HIGHLIGHTS

I. Indications
- Gross invasion by oral oropharyngeal cancer
- Primary bone tumor of the mandible
- Metastatic tumor to the mandible
- Invasion of inferior alveolar nerve or canal by tumor
- Massive soft tissue disease adjacent to the mandible.

II. Contraindications
- Poor performance status
- Metastatic disease.

III. Special Preoperative Considerations
- Adequate assessment of the mandible invasion by tumor. In addition to careful examination under anesthesia by bimanual palpation, radiographic evaluation of the mandible should be available for satisfactory treatment planning.

IV. Special Intraoperative Considerations
- Preplating the mandible before resection can assist in accurate reconstruction and occlusion
- Frozen section analysis of bone margins is not a possibility, so a generous margin of bone must be taken to avoid positive margins.

V. Special Postoperative Considerations
- The success of free flap reconstruction depends on excellent nursing care.

VI. Complications
- Flap failure
- Reconstruction plate exposition
- Permanent dysphagia
- Aspiration pneumonia.

ADDITIONAL READING

1. Blassingame CD. The suprahyoid approach to surgical lesions at the base of the tongue. Ann Otol Rhinol Laryngol. 1952;61(2):483-9.

2. Gopalan KN, Primuharsa Putra SH, Kenali MS. Suprahyoid pharyngotomy for base of tongue carcinoma. Med J Malysia. 2003;58(4):617-20.

3. Komisar A. The functional result of mandibular reconstruction. Laryngoscope. 1990;100(4):364-74.

4. Moore DM, Calcaterra TC. Cancer of the tongue base treated by a transpharyngeal approach. Ann Otol Rhinol Laryngol. 1990;99(4 Pt 1):300-3.

5. Rethi A. A new method of transverse pharyngotomy. J Laryngol Otol. 1948;62(7):440-6.

6. Sadeghi N, Panje WR. Cancer of the soft palate. In: TJ Saclarides, KV Millikan, CV Godellas (Eds). Surgical Oncology. An algorithmic approach. New York: Springer; 2003. pp. 32-9.

7. Seikaly H, Rieger J, Zalmanowitz J, et al. Functional soft palate reconstruction: a comprehensive surgical approach. Head Neck. 2008;30(12):1615-23.

8. Sessions DB. Surgical resection and reconstruction for cancer of the base of the tongue. Otolaryngol Clin North Am. 1983;16(2):309-29.

9. Slaughter DP, Roeser EH, Smejkal WF. Excision of the mandible for neoplastic disease: indications and techniques. Surgery. 1949;26(3):507-22.

10. Sofferman RA. Soft-palate reconstruction with the modified pharyngeal flap. Head Neck Surgery. 2006;1(6):505-11.

11. TNM. AJCC Cancer Staging handbook, 2002.

12. Urken ML, Buchbinder D, Weinberg H, et al. Functional evaluation following microvascular oromandibular reconstruction of the oral cancer patient. a comparative of reconstructed nonrecontructed patients. Laryngoscope. 1991;101(9):935-50.

13. Vidiri A, Ruscito P, Pichi B, et al. Oral cavity and base of the tongue tumors. Correlation between clinical, MRI and pathological staging of primary tumor. J Exp Cancer Res. 2007;26(4):575-82.

14. Ward GE, Robben JO. A composite operation for radical neck dissection and removal of cancer of the mouth. Cancer. 1951;4(1):98-109.

15. Weber PC, Johnson JT, Myers EN. The suprahyoid approach for squamous cell carcinoma of the base of the tongue. Laryngoscope. 1992;102(6):637-40.

16. Zeitels SM, Kim J. Soft-palate reconstruction with a "SCARF" superior-constrictor advancement-rotation flap. Laryngoscope. 1998;108(8 Pt 1):1136-40.

Chapter 45

Horizontal Supraglottic Laryngectomy

Giuseppe Spriano, Raul Pellini, Paolo Ruscito, Valentina Manciocco, Giuseppe Mercante

INTRODUCTION

Horizontal supraglottic laryngectomy (HSL) is a partial resection of the portion of larynx placed above the glottis, including epiglottis, ventricular folds, superior part of Morgagni ventricles and corresponding supraglottic spaces. It can be variously enlarged depending on the tumor extension; anteriorly to the oropharynx (valleculae or base of the tongue), laterally to the hypopharynx (pyriform sinus), posteriorly to the arytenoids and inferiorly to the vocal cord. In these cases, the procedure is called extended horizontal supraglottic laryngectomy (EHSL). These operations are always associated with bilateral neck dissection.

The rationale of supraglottic horizontal laryngectomy is that a tumor arising in the supraglottic portion of the larynx, originating from the third and fourth visceral arches (buccopharyngeal origin), tends to be an "ascending tumor" growing toward the pharynx. This attitude has been explained embryologically, considering the barrier of the glottic plane, coming from the sixth visceral arch of tracheopulmonary origin to downward tumor extension. The high incidence of lymphatic spread related to this tumor determines the necessity to dissect bilaterally the neck node levels at risk for elective purpose or all the levels for therapeutic purpose.

PREOPERATIVE EVALUATION

In order to select a candidate for HSL, specific diagnostic work-up is suggested. Patients have to be submitted to flexible endoscopy under local anesthesia to evaluate the tumor extension and vocal cord mobility.

During the surgical session, direct laryngoscopy using rigid fiberoptic 0°, 30°, 70 is recommended. In order to define the tumor extension, attention is given to critical points, such as, the distance of the tumor from the anterior commissure, the involvement of arytenoids, ventricles and the spread outside the limit of supraglottic site.

Computed tomography (CT) scan or magnetic resonance imaging (MRI) is used to check the deep infiltration of tumor and the involvement of laryngeal skeleton. In advanced stage tumors, CT scan of the chest is suggested.

Horizontal supraglottic laryngectomy is indicated for excision of most of the supraglottic tumors that are clinically staged as T1, T2 and selected T3 (only for pre-epiglottic space involvement). The resection can be extended outside the classical limits of HSL. In this case, the procedure is called extended HSL. The tumor spreads out of the supraglottic larynx; superiorly to the valleculae or base of the tongue, laterally to the medial wall of pyriform sinus, inferiorly to the ventricle.[1,2] It is indicated to treat primary tumors and in selected cases, limited local recurrences after radiation or chemoradiation.

Contraindications may be distinguished in local and general forms. The former is represented by thyroid cartilage infiltration, anterior commissure involvement, vocal cord mobility impairment related to paraglottic space invasion, bilateral arytenoid infiltration, pyriform apex and postcricoid mucosa involvement. Massive involvement of cervical lymph node may be considered as a relative contraindication because the necessity of adjuvant concurrent chemotheradio-therapy; this is related with more frequent local morbidity and pulmonary complications, if postoperative meal aspiration occurs. The latter is still a matter of discussion.

Advanced age do not represent an absolute contraindication by itself, but is individually related to the patient performance status. Out of all organic and psychological disease, the pulmonary impairment is the most important one. Low pulmonary reserve evaluated by spirometric function tests, impaired cough reflex, stroke victims and low arterial oxygen concentration, may contraindicate supraglottic laryngectomy. From a practical point of view, the ability to tolerate physical exercise is generally admitted as the most reliable parameter to be evaluated, in order to select candidates. "If the patient can climb stairs of two floors, he will probably be eligible for partial laryngectomy."

SURGICAL TECHNIQUE

Patient Position

The position of the patient is supine with horizontally oriented shoulder roll. The patient's neck is extended to perform laryngectomy and the head is rotated away from the operative side during bilateral neck dissection. The table can be kept straight with the anesthesia machine placed on the left side of the patient to allow positioning of two assistants, on the opposite side and at the head of the table respectively. Prophylactic antibiotics are necessary to cover aerodigestive flora.

Tracheostomy

Tracheostomy is usually performed under local anesthesia (Fig. 1), through a 3 cm skin incision below thyroid gland isthmus, at the second and the third tracheal ring, isolated from the laryngectomy incision. This can reduce the rate of postoperative subcutaneous emphysema. The tracheal opening is obtained by means of an opposite "U" shaped tracheal incision to obtain a small tracheal flap, which is sutured with separate stitches to the inferior skin border to protect great vessels of anterior upper mediastinum (Björk procedure) and to facilitate the tube replacement in postoperative period. A cuffed tracheostomy tube is positioned (number 8 or 7 for men, number 6 for women) and connected to an anesthesia machine. Nasogastric feeding tube is also inserted.

Skin Incision

It should preferentially be separated from the tracheostomy incision. In case of bilateral selective neck dissection, a curved skin incision is marked in the skin crease connecting the anterior borders of sternocleidomastoid muscles of both the sides, through the inferior edge of cricoid cartilage. When modified radical neck dissection is required, a wider skin incision (apron incision) can be drawn to the mastoid process tip on the both sides.

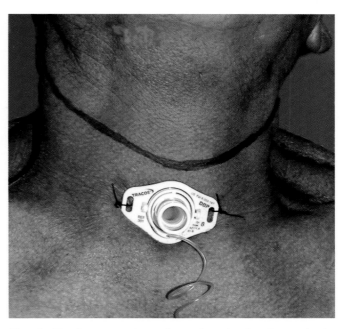

Fig. 1: Tracheostomy is performed under local anesthesia. Continuous line indicates the skin incision in case of bilateral neck dissection and horizontal supraglottic laryngectomy

The maintenance of two separate surgical fields: the tracheostomy and the laryngectomy, reduces the risk of aspiration drainage failure, due to the connection of the neck space to the external outer one and contamination by aerodigestive flora from the tracheal opening. Another advantage could be an easier recovery of laryngeal motility during swallowing after tracheostomy tube removal.

Some surgeons propose a unique single incision and in such a case, preparation of a temporary circumferential stoma is required.

The shape and width of the cervical skin flap does not depend on laryngectomy but on the type of neck dissection, which is required in relation to the status of lateral neck nodes. In case of clinical N0 neck, bilateral selective neck dissection of levels II–IV can be achieved even through a skin incision marked at the level of cricoid cartilage to avoid skin suture line overlapping the pexia.

The incision is continued through the subcutaneous fat and the platysma muscle up to the superficial cervical fascia, which must be preserved. It can be performed either by means of a scalpel or by electrocautery with a thin tip. The cervical skin flap harvesting is achieved by blunt dissection through the poorly vascularized plane of the cervical superficial fascia, just below the platysma muscle. The dissection upward reaches the level of the hyoid bone and digastric muscles. Laterally, it depends on the type of neck dissection. It will be limited to the anterior edge of sternocleidomastoid muscle in case of selected neck dissection (levels II–IV), paying attention to external jugular vein and great auricular nerve preservation. Extension should be done posteriorly and superiorly in order to reach the edge of the trapezium muscle and the mandible inferior border, in case of modified radical neck dissection (levels I–V), indicated for clinical N+ status.

The apron flap is rotated upward and elevated downward the inferior flap to obtain a wide exposure of the central and bilateral neck. Once, the bilateral neck dissection has been completed the laryngectomy procedure begins.

Laryngeal Skeletonization

The hyoid bone and the infrahyoid strap muscles are isolated by electrocautery (Fig. 2). In case of tumors limited to the supraglottic larynx without pre-epiglottic space invasion, an omo and sternohyoid muscles flap is harvested, resecting it about 1 cm below the hyoid bone. Then, this muscle flap is gently dissected and rotated downward to expose the laryngotracheal complex.

In case of pre-epiglottic space involvement, the removal of strap muscles is suggested en bloc with the laryngeal and bilateral neck dissection specimen for oncological safety. Similarly, the thyrohyoid muscles are resected.

The inferior border of the hyoid bone is skeletonized sectioning the thyrohyoid membrane and ligaments, paying attention not to damage the lingual arteries and the hypoglossal nerves. The pre-epiglottic space is dissected (Fig. 3) and the content is pulled downward. The superior laryngeal vascular pedicles are isolated and sectioned bilaterally, after

the identification of the superior laryngeal nerves, which are located in a deeper plane than superior laryngeal vessels and must be carefully preserved. The external perichondrium of the thyroid cartilage is sectioned along the superior edge and gently dissected downward to harvest a perichondrial flap, which is kept attached to the inferior third of thyroid cartilage and reflected (Fig. 4).

The superior constrictor muscle is bilaterally sectioned along its thyroid cartilage attachment and dissected to preserve pyriform sinuses from excision.

Some authors prefer to remove the hyoid bone in all cases, in order to achieve a wider excision of pre-epiglottic space. If the tumor invasion is not massive, the authors prefer to spare the hyoid bone in order to avoid the risk of injury to the lingual artery and hypoglossal nerve, and to achieve a better and stable matching of the pexy.

Laryngectomy

Thyroid chondrotomy requires the location of the projection point of the anterior commissure on the line connecting the thyroid notch and the inferior edge of the thyroid cartilage. It is mandatory not to cut at the level of the glottic plane. Then, the cartilage incision may be performed following different incision lines, passing over this point in order to enter the ventricles. The thyroid cartilage may be resected about half way between the thyroid notch and its inferior edge determining this point location considering its distance from the thyroid notch that ranges between 3.5 mm and

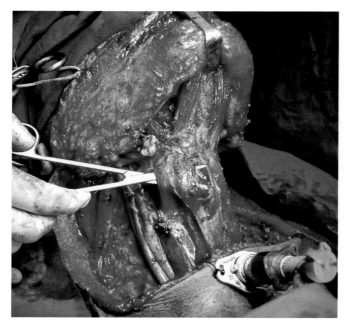

Fig. 2: Cutting of the infrahyoid strap muscles, just 1 cm below the insertion to the hyoid bone to expose the thyroid cartilage (after bilateral neck dissection)

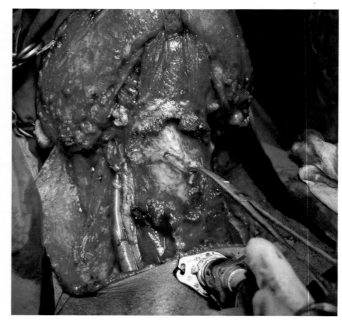

Fig. 3: After the exposure of the thyroid cartilage pre-epiglottic space is cleared

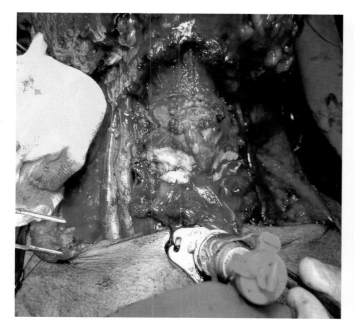

Fig. 4: The external perichondrium of the thyroid cartilage is incised along the superior border of the thyroid cartilage and reflected inferiorly. The inferior attachment is preserved and the flap is used for reconstruction

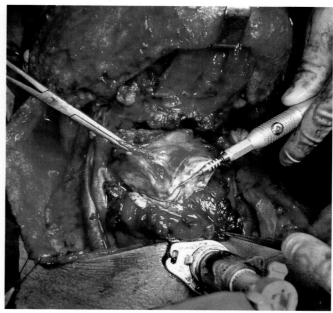

Fig. 5: The thyroid cartilage is divided horizontally. The incision line passes midway between the thyroid notch and the inferior border of the thyroid cartilage. The cut can be performed by oscillating saw, scalpel or scissors

The incision line may differ in relation to the tumor extent and the hyoid bone preservation. The thyroid cartilage may be cut horizontally (removing both superior cornu) or in different fashions ("V" or "L" shaped incisions) related to the site of the tumor as in Figure 5.

Curved line incisions were generally performed when supraglottic laryngectomy included the hyoid bone excision and thyroglossopexy was performed. Nowadays, hyoid bone is usually preserved and therefore, horizontal linear thyroid cartilage incision is preferred to achieve better matching of the laryngeal and pharyngeal stumps after thyrohyoidpexy.

In case of intrinsic tumors of the larynx, pharyngotomy is carried out at the level of the vallecula. In this way, the epiglottis may be tractioned and rotated outward to provide adequate view of the laryngeal lumen and the tumor extension (Fig. 6). At this step, the surgeon moves to the head of the patient. The laryngectomy continues under direct visual control, along the aryepiglottic folds up to the anterior edge of the arytenoids, which are preserved when not involved by the tumor (Fig. 7). Usually, the surgeon cuts the aryepiglottic folds vertically. Then, the surgeon rotates the scissors at 90° cutting horizontally along the floor of the ventricles and reaching the area of insertion of the epiglottis petiole. Then, the supraglottic laryngectomy is completed. The entire removal of the supraglottic larynx must be achieved by preserving the connection between the external skeleton of the supraglottic larynx and its soft tissues to avoid

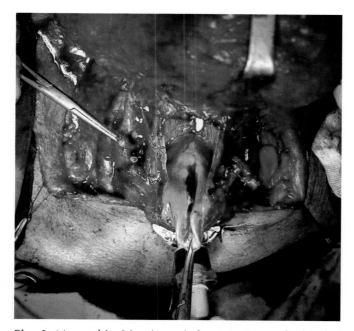

Fig. 6: Mucosal incision is carried out starting at the level of the vallecula. The epiglottis is tractioned and rotated outward to provide adequate view of the laryngeal lumen and tumor extension

6.0 mm in man and between 3.0 mm and 5.0 mm in woman.[3] Chondrotomy can be achieved by means of oscillating saw, scalpel or scissors.

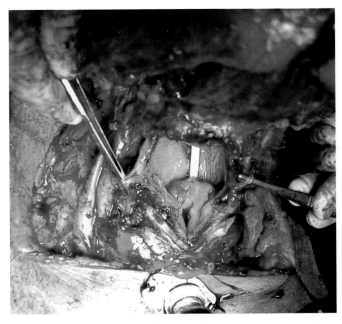

Fig. 7: Under direct visual control, the incisions run along the aryepiglottic folds up to the anterior edge of arytenoids, which are preserved when not involved by the tumor. Then, the incision is carried along the ventricles to complete supraglottic laryngectomy

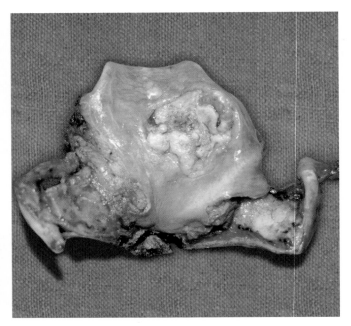

Fig. 8: Specimen after supraglottic laryngectomy. Frozen section of the limits of the resection is routinely taken

oncological spread. The specimen is carefully examined by the surgeon, who opens the piece of larynx, fracturing its cartilaginous framework and examining accurately the complete removal of the tumor and the adequate width of the free margins.

Intraoperative frozen sections of the mucosal margins taken from the residual larynx, completes the excision phase of the procedure (Fig. 8). Hemostasis is usually performed by means of bipolar coagulation along the mucosal edge of the pharyngolaryngeal stump with special regard to the base of the tongue.

Reconstruction

Laryngeal reconstruction is achieved through thyrohyoidpexy by the positioning of various separate stitches, which determines the approximation of the oropharyngeal stump to the glottis. These stitches may be positioned by either passing through the cartilage or by surrounding its inferior border.

The external perichondrial flap, which has been previously harvested and preserved (originally used for its strongness), is used to complete the defect. The authors prefer to rotate it inward to cover the thyroid cartilage cut edge and fixed with 4-0 absorbable stitches to the inner glottic larynx (usually to the internal perichondrium).

In this way, it is possible to protect the cartilage and to interpose a soft tissue layer between the chondrial edge of the laryngeal stump and the osseous border (hyoid bone) of the oropharyngeal one.

On the other hand, some authors use this chondrial flap to cover the thyrohyoidpexy externally suturing it to the suprahyoid muscles, in order to get a better isolation of the laryngeal lumen from the neck space, preventing or reducing the risk of neck emphysema.[4]

The pexy is achieved by approximating the base of the tongue and the glottic portion of the residual larynx. In this phase, the removal of the shoulder roll and the following reduction of the neck extension facilitate the matching of the two stumps.

Three to five thick, separate stitches (n#2) are generally used to perform thyrohyoidpexy. The stitches must pass through or around the residual thyroid cartilage avoiding the involvement of the vocal cords. They are introduced in the base of the tongue first and then, surround the hyoid bone passing through the suprahyoid muscles (Fig. 9). If the hyoid bone has been removed, it is suggested to surround a larger amount of base of the tongue. The stitches are positioned at a distance of about 1 cm from each other, beginning from the central one, corresponding at the commissural vertical line. The positioning of pharyngeal suture is not necessary but can be done.

While an assistant keeps the patient's head flexed in order to reduce tension, the stitches are tied synchronously on the two opposite sides beginning from the lateral ones

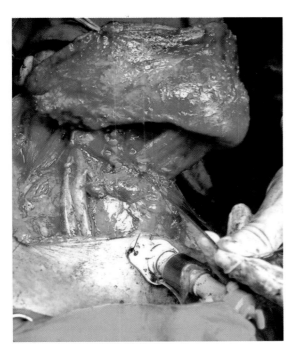

Fig. 9: Reconstruction is achieved through approximation of the base of tongue/hyoid bone to the residual thyroid cartilage stump with five separate stitches in reabsorbable suture. The external perichondrial flap is approximated to the base of the tongue with nonabsorbable suture. More laterally the mucosa of the pyriform sinus can be closed to the lateral portion of the base of the tongue to avoid air leakage

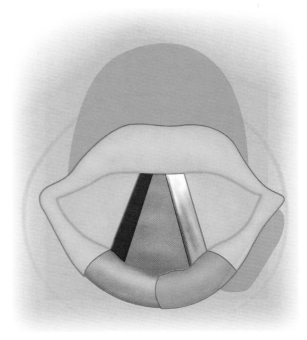

Fig. 10: The figure shows the possible extension of classical supraglottic laryngectomy (yellow), base of tongue (blue), arytenoid cartilage (green), pyriform sinus (orange), vocal cord (brown)

and ending with the median stitch, in order to avoid cartilage fracture. Perichondrial flap is positioned and sutured in those cases in which it is not used to cover the cartilaginous cut line. Prelaryngeal muscle flap is rotated to cover the pexy and fixed to suprahyoid muscles.

Closure

Two different suction drains are positioned. One suction drain is positioned in each lateral neck, where node dissection has been performed.

The skin is closed in layers. Compressive dressing is reserved for those cases, in which subcutaneous emphysema cannot be completely avoided by the action of the central compartment suction drain. Maintaining the open view is useful in order to monitor the postoperative healing.

Extended Horizontal Supraglottic Laryngectomy

Classical HSL can be extended to other laryngeal subsites or regions (Fig. 10). In these cases, the procedure is called EHSL and the denominations are comprehensive of the site/structure to which the laryngectomy has been extended to as follows:

- In case of upward spread of the tumor to the valleculae and/or to the base of the tongue, HSL extended to the base of the tongue or to the oropharynx can be done. In this case, the infiltration of the base of the tongue must be limited because the resection cannot exceed lingual V, in order to avoid intractable aspiration.

- In case of lateral spread of the tumor to the pyriform sinus, HSL extended to the pyriform sinus or to the hypopharynx will be necessary. In the previous cases, the denomination of partial laryngopharyngectomy may be correctly used, referring generally to the kind and site of resection.

- If the tumor goes downward involving the Morgagni's ventricle, HSL will be extended to the vocal cord of that side, in order to achieve the en bloc excision of the ventricle and its surrounding structures. This procedure is called three-quarter laryngectomy by Ogura (1965), but many other denominations have been used: five-sixth laryngectomy, vertical subtotal laryngectomy, extended horizontal resection, subtotal laryngectomy, extended hemilaryngectomy.

- Finally, in case of limited mucosal infiltration of the arytenoid mucosa for tumors spreading backward, without cricoarytenoid junction involvement, HSL will be extended to the arytenoid.

In all cases of partial pharyngolaryngectomies, the mucosal free margins of the pharyngeal edge will have to be wider than the laryngeal ones, i.e. more than 1 cm. This is done to avoid microscopic residual disease because of the submucosal lymphatic spread of the tumor in its pharynx portion.

Horizontal Supraglottic Laryngectomy Extended to the Base of the Tongue

If the tumor involves the vallecula or the base of the tongue, for an extension of no more than 1.5 cm, the en bloc resection is achieved by extended HSL to the base of the tongue.[5] The procedure consists of HSL together with partial glossectomy. The excision requires the removal of the hyoid bone. The lingual limit of resection is represented by the vallate papillae line.

Contraindications to extended HSL consist of massive involvement of the base of the tongue by the tumor, reaching the foramen cecum and the vallate papillae or its spread to the lateral oropharyngeal wall.

The initial phases of the procedure are the same as HSL up to laryngectomy. In this case, the laryngectomy does not begin at the level of the valleculae for the tumor presence, but opening the lateral pharyngeal wall of the less involved side. So laryngectomy may be carried out under direct visual and palpatory control at the level of the base of the tongue, it is mandatory to preserve at least one hypoglossal nerve and one lingual artery. The thyroid cartilage cut, whose shape is linear in case of HSL with the hyoid bone preservation, may be curved, sparing part of supraglottic thyroid cartilage at the level of the less interested side by the tumor.

The pexy is achieved using five stitches passing through the suprahyoid muscles of the residual tongue by the same material mentioned before. Attention has to be paid in order to include a large amount of lingual tissue in the suture line.

Horizontal Supraglottic Laryngectomy Extended to the Pyriform Sinus

This technique is indicated in case of tumors, which are extended laterally to involve a limited (<1 cm) portion of medial wall of the pyriform sinus.

The main contraindications consist of lateral wall invasion and/or when the apex of pyriform sinus is interested by the disease, as the tumor is spread below the ventricle plane.

The procedure allows the entire removal of laryngopharyngeal tumors through an HSL and a partial lateral pharyngectomy.

The initial steps of the procedure are the same as HSL: (i) tracheostomy; (ii) skin incision and; (iii) laryngeal skeletonization must be performed as previously described.

Laryngectomy phase remains the same till thyroid chondrotomy. Pharyngotomy is carried out at the level of the vallecula opposite to the tumor. The epiglottis is pulled outward to expose the laryngeal lumen and tumor. The excision continues under direct visual control along the aryepiglottic fold, contralateral to the tumor up to the anterior edge of arytenoid. Then, the resection follows the ventricles from the healthy side to the affected one. Finally, the specimen remains connected to the hypopharynx only through the tumoral aryepiglottic fold, which is resected at the end of the procedure, preserving or not the arytenoid and keeping at least 1 cm of mucosal free margin. Some 4-0 absorbable stitches are positioned on the side of the pharyngeal stump, in order to reduce the hypopharyngeal defect. The pexy completes the procedure and is similar to HSL.

Horizontal Supraglottic Laryngectomy Extended to the Arytenoids

Horizontal supraglottic laryngectomy may be extended posteriorly to the arytenoids (Figs 11 and 12), in case of its mucosal involvement. The mucosal infiltration must be limited to the anteromedial and anterolateral aspect without any involvement of the retrocricoid area and cricoarytenoid junction.

The initial steps of the procedure are the same as HSL up to laryngectomy. Then, the resection is carried out behind the arytenoids involved by the tumor, preserving the posterior mucosae free of disease, cutting the insertion of posterior and

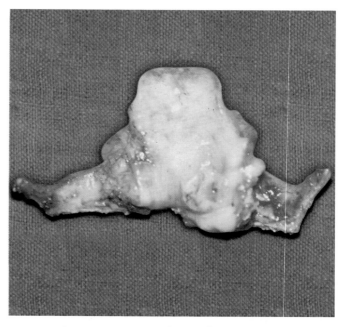

Fig. 11: Specimen of supraglottic extended to right arytenoid cartilage

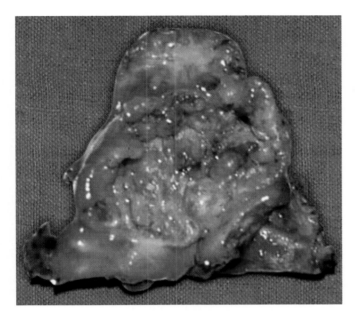

Fig. 12: Specimen of supraglottic extended to left arytenoid cartilage and base of the tongue

lateral cricoarytenoid muscles, as well as the interarytenoid muscle and then passing through the cricoarytenoid junction and the upper edge of the cricoid cartilage, to surround and remove the arytenoid. The true vocal cord disconnected from the vocal process of the arytenoid is preserved and sutured with absorbable stitches to the cricoid edge in a paramedian position to avoid its retraction. The residual mucosa of the hypopharyngeal side of the arytenoid is sutured to cover the cartilaginous edge of the cricoid with 4-0 absorbable stitches. The pexy is performed in the usual way.

Horizontal Supraglottic Laryngectomy Extended to One Vocal Cord (Three-Quarter Laryngectomy)

When a supraglottic tumor spreads inferiorly to involve one ventricle and/or the true vocal cord[6] or when even the vocal cord and the paraglottic space are involved, it is necessary to switch to a supracricoid laryngectomy. If the tumor extension is posterior, one arytenoid can be removed as well. In case of unilateral extension, a three-quarter laryngectomy can be performed.

The procedure resembles to the HSL. On the affected side, the thyroid cartilage excision is extended below the glottic level while, on the opposite side, it is done at the Morgagni ventricle level. The cartilage incision is step-shaped. Soft tissue excision includes the vocal cord and often the arytenoid cartilage. Lacking completely the glottis of one side, to achieve a complete approximation of the laryngeal and pharyngeal stumps through pexis, a myochondrial flap

represented by the thyrohyoid muscle is rotated inward to interpose a soft tissue layer in order to line up the irregular chondrial edge of laryngectomy and the inferior border of the hyoid bone.

Pexy is achieved by separate nonabsorbable stitches connecting the hyoid bone to the laryngeal stump; the stitches have to surround the inferior border of the thyroid cartilage. Two or more of these extensions can be variably associated.

POSTOPERATIVE TREATMENT

Supraglottic laryngectomy determines the opening of a visceral lumen colonized by germs and its communication with sterile neck spaces in which nerves, vessels are placed.

This procedure impact significantly to swallowing and breathing functions determining aspiration that is massive in the first postoperative period, mild during rehabilitation training and sometimes, residual after its completion.

The draining tubes are removed, when the secretions become serous and lower than 20–30 ml a day. Neck dressing is usually not positioned to avoid discomfort to the patient and have an immediate and easier visual control of the neck status.

Compressive dressing may be required, especially when subcutaneous emphysema is observed in the first postoperative days, due to air passing from the laryngeal lumen into the neck spaces or through the pexy.

Tracheostomy tube is kept cuffed during the first two postoperative days; then, it is removed and a new noncuffed tracheostomy tube is positioned to avoid damages to the tracheal wall by the pressured cuff.

Wide-spectrum prophylactic antibiotics are administered for the first 10–15 postoperative days, till wound healing is achieved and swallowing rehabilitation is close to be completed.

In case of infection, the antibiotic therapy will be tailored, depending on the results of the antibiogram of tracheal and/or wound secretions and kept till its resolution.

Stitches are removed between the 7th and the 10th postoperative day, in case of primary treatment and later, (between the 10th and 15th postoperative day) in case of salvage surgery after radiation[7] failures.

The rehabilitation training of the HSL is essentially meant for the swallowing function recovery.[8] It is achieved thanks to the work of a dedicated team of specialized doctors and therapists.

The tracheostomy tube is removed when the edema is reduced enough to restore normal breathing. It usually occurs between 7th and 14th day postoperatively. In this way, the patient do not suffer from the foreign body sensation and the mobility impairment during swallowing, determined by the tube in his neck. Early decannulation, when possible, helps a fast swallowing recovery. Swallowing rehabilitation starts within 12–14 days postoperatively along with consultation with a speech pathologist. Usually, oral uptake begins by using solid food because the aspiration is less compared to fluids. The nasogastric feeding tube is removed when the aspirations episodes are rare, especially following fluid swallowing.

Swallowing rehabilitation includes stimulating exercises, retraining the tongue base and arytenoid to contact each other to shut the airway tube and avoid or reduce aspiration. It requires usually 2–4 weeks in case of primary HSL and more in case of extended HSL. If the surgical procedure is extended to include a part of the vocal fold(s) or the tongue base, the time of rehabilitation is significantly prolonged. Functional total laryngectomy for massive and persisting aspiration, hardly ever is required. It could be necessary, following large pharyngeal resections together with HSL. When not accepted by the patient, it is possible to perform percutaneous endoscopic gastrostomy to give a safe way for food consumption.

Laryngeal postoperative stenosis is a rare event, usually due to scar tissue. Its treatment is usually an endoscopic resection. The recovery of voice is usually good and spontaneous; out of few cases mostly related to extended procedures.

HIGHLIGHTS

I. Indications
- Horizontal supraglottic laryngectomy
  - Tumor with normal cords mobility limited to one or more of the following sites:
    - Epiglottis
    - False cords
    - Aryepiglottic folds, with or without pre-epiglottic space invasion.
- Extended horizontal supraglottic laryngectomy
  - Tumor of the supraglottis extended to:
    - Arytenoid with conserved mobility (EHSL to arytenoid)
    - Valleculae or base of tongue (1 cm from the circumvallate papillae, EHSL to base of tongue)
    - Medial wall of the pyriform sinus without invasion of the apex (ESHL to pyriform sinus)
    - Morgagni ventricle (EHSL to vocal cord).

II. Contraindications
- Bilateral massive cervical lymph node involvement (relative contraindication)

- Patient with poor cardiopulmonary reserve (low tolerance to exercise)
- True vocal cord involvement
- Both arytenoids involvement
- Anterior and/or lateral wall of pyriform sinus involvement
- Thyroid cartilage invasion
- Extensive involvement of the base of the tongue.

III. Special Preoperative Considerations
- Tumor board to discuss alternative to surgery
- Preoperative evaluation
  - Computed tomography of the larynx and neck, chest CT
  - Tumor mapping and biopsy under microscopic direct laryngoscopy
  - Assessment of cardiopulmonary function (internal medicine consultation, pulmonary function tests).

IV. Special Intraoperative Considerations
- Place a shoulder roll to extent the neck
- Perform tracheotomy under local anesthesia using a small skin incision separate from the incision necessary for the main procedure
- Preserve the external thyroid perichondrium in order to reinforce the suture between the thyroid cartilage stump and the base of the tongue/hyoid bone
- Enter vallecula on uninvolved side and perform the resection under direct vision of the glottic plane
- Suture the base of tongue to overhang the laryngeal introitus
- The procedure can be extended to oropharynx, arytenoids, medial wall of pyriform sinus and vocal cord.

V. Special Postoperative Considerations
- Swallowing rehabilitation starts within 12–14 days postoperatively along with consultation with a speech pathologist. In case of recurrence after radiotherapy, rehabilitation starts at least 1 week later.
- Perform full decannulation when patient is able to maintain the completely closed cannula for at least 24 consecutive hours and is able to sleep in supine position with the cannula closed.

VI. Complications
- Bleeding
- Infection
- Loss of voice
- Aspiration with inability to swallow
- Persistent necessity of tracheostomy
- Potential need for subsequent total laryngectomy to address intractable aspiration.

REFERENCES

1. Ogura JH. Supraglottic subtotal laryngectomy and radical neck dissection for carcinoma of the epiglottis. Laryngoscope. 1958;68(6):983-1003.
2. Spriano G, Antognoni P, Piantanida R, et al. Conservative management of T1-T2N0 supraglottic cancer: a retrospective study. Am J Otolaryngol. 1997;18(5):299-305.
3. Gurr E. Z Laryngol Rhinol Otol. 1948;1(1):71.
4. Silva N, Lore JM. Partial horizontal supraglottic laryngectomy. A method of reconstruction. Laryngoscope. 1977;87(7): 1165-8.
5. Suarez C, Rodrigo JP, Herranz J, et al. Extended supraglottic laryngectomy for primary base of tongue carcinomas. Clin Otolaryngol Allied Sci. 1996;21(1):37-41.
6. Ogura J. Personal experience with three-quarter laryngectomy. Tumori. 1974;60(6):527-9.
7. Spriano G, Antognoni P, Sanguineti G, et al. Laryngeal long-term morbidity after supraglottic laryngectomy and postoperative radiation therapy. Am J Otolaryngol. 2000;21(1):14-21.
8. Wasserman T, Murry T, Johnson JT, et al. Management of swallowing in supraglottic and extended supraglottic laryngectomy patients. Head Neck. 2001;23(12):1043-8.

Chapter 46

Tracheal and Cricotracheal Resection and Anastomosis in Adults

Cesare Piazza, Giorgio Peretti, Piero Nicolai

INTRODUCTION

Tracheal and cricotracheal resection and anastomosis (TRA and CTRA respectively) are single-stage surgical procedures aimed at treating airway stenoses of the subglottic larynx and upper half (cervical) trachea that are not amenable to endoscopic management. First described by Gerwat and Bryce in 1974[1] and later by Pearson and colleagues in 1975,[2] these surgical techniques were subsequently refined, extensively applied and popularized by Grillo and coworkers.[3]

Even though the vast majority of TRA/CTRA are performed for management of acquired cicatricial (mainly post-intubation and post-tracheotomy) tracheal or cricotracheal stenoses (Figs 1A and B),[4-6] a number of series have reported their application for primary subglottic and/or tracheal tumors (Figs 2A and B)[7,8] as well as for advanced thyroid cancers infiltrating the airway as in Figure 3.[9,10]

The single most important advantage of TRA/CTRA is the possibility to circumferentially resect the pathologic tract of the airway and to re-establish its continuity in a single step by performing a direct anastomosis between the healthy proximal and distal stumps. Postoperative tracheotomy and/or endoluminal stents are usually not needed (except in case of local and/or systemic complications), thus allowing a fast recovery and regaining of a normal (even though shortened) airway. The impact of this surgery on swallowing, when performed properly, is virtually nonexistent, while vocal parameters, particularly after CTRA can be impaired in terms of lowering of vocal pitch due to removal of the cricoid arch and cricothyroid muscles with an ensuing lack of vocal cord tension.

Even though in more recent series the final success rate of TRA/CTRA has been reported to be as high as 96%, they should be always regarded as major surgical procedures with potential mortality and a non-negligible prevalence of complications.[3-10] Therefore, meticulous patient selection is always mandatory to reduce the rates of both failure and complications.

PREOPERATIVE EVALUATION AND ANESTHESIA

Cardiopulmonary function must be adequately evaluated before TRA/CTRA, as in every patient needing partial laryngeal surgery. In case of neurologic sequelae from neurotrauma or previous prolonged comatose state from other causes, swallowing should be accurately assessed by endoscopic and/or videofluoroscopic examinations. Indeed, major aspiration during swallowing represents an absolute contraindication for TRA/CTRA. If major constraints to the patient's mobilization are present at the time of diagnosis (traumatic sequelae of the spine and/or limbs), adequate physiotherapy should be planned before TRA/CTRA in order to minimize the need for postoperative stay in bed. In this sense, tetraplegia should be considered an absolute contraindication to a major surgical procedure on the airway.

The cornerstone in evaluation of the stenotic airway still remains endoscopy, either by flexible video endoscopy under local anesthesia and/or by rigid endoscopy (possibly associated with a biopsy in case of idiopathic subglottic stenosis, vasculitis related stenosis or tumors) under general

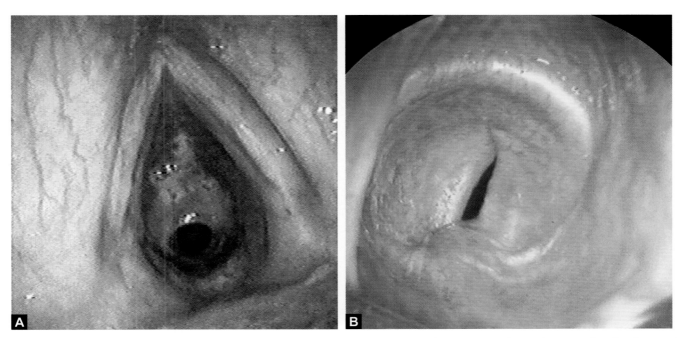

Figs 1A and B: (A) Flexible fiberoptic endoscopy of postintubation cricotracheal stenosis involving the cricoid arch, plate and first two tracheal rings; (B) Endoscopy by 0° rigid telescope under general anesthesia of post-tracheotomy stenosis of the first tracheal ring

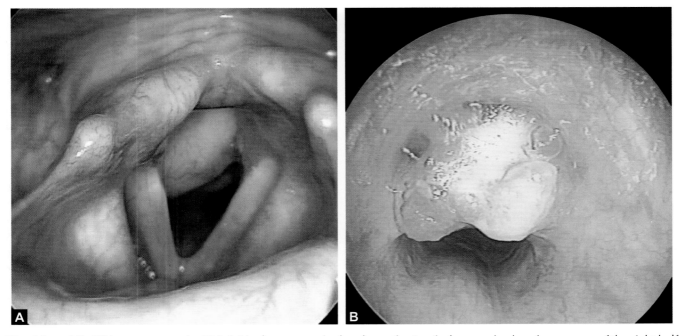

Figs 2A and B: (A) Laryngoscopy by 70° rigid telescope under local anesthesia of a low-grade chondrosarcoma of the right half of the cricoid plate; (B) Endoscopy by 0° rigid telescope under general anesthesia of a low-grade mucoepidermoid carcinoma of the third and fourth tracheal rings

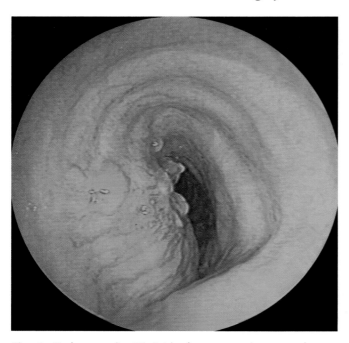

Fig. 3: Endoscopy by 0° rigid telescope under general anesthesia of a papillary thyroid cancer infiltrating the left aspect of the first six tracheal rings

anesthesia. Vocal cords mobility and laryngeal/hypopharyngeal sensation should be assessed. It is worth mentioning that even though unilateral recurrent/vagal palsy does not represent *per se* an absolute contraindication to TRA/CTRA, it may increase the risk of airway related complications during the postoperative course. Moreover, during endoscopy, the type and extent of stenosis must be accurately evaluated. Short (<1 cm), cicatricial, web-like stenoses without evidence of cartilaginous collapse or malacia represents an ideal indication for a first endoscopic attempt of laser-assisted dilation (Figs 4A and B). On the other hand, a good indication for TRA/CTRA is a long (1.0–5.5 cm), complex (subglottic and tracheal) stenosis with profound alterations of the laryngotracheal cartilaginous framework and an ensuing malacia of the airway. TRA/CTRA should never be planned before stenosis is stabilized and mature, without florid granulation tissue, edema, and hyperemia or superimposed infection. In fact, these unfavorable conditions may impair healing of the anastomosis and expose the patient to a high probability of dehiscence and/or restenosis.

Adequate antibiotic therapy must be started well before surgery, while topical or systemic corticosteroids should be avoided for at least 2 weeks before TRA/CTRA. In case of pending respiratory distress, effort should be made to

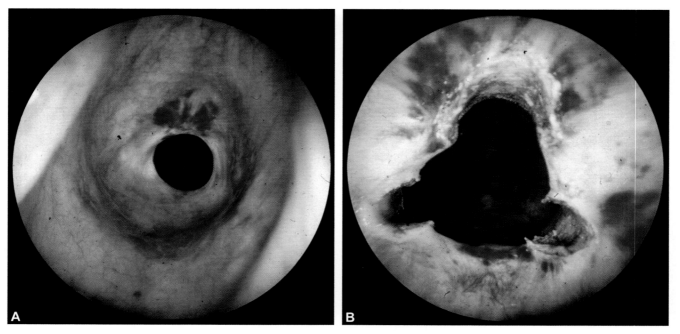

Figs 4A and B: (A) Endoscopy by 0° rigid telescope under general anesthesia of a short, web-like postintubation stenosis of the first tracheal ring without involvement of the cricoid; (B) Same view after Nd-YAG laser-assisted radial incisions

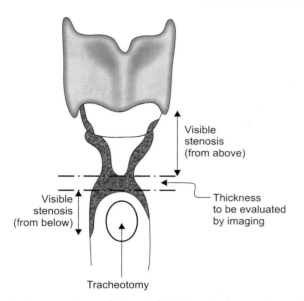

Fig. 5: In case of complete subglottic/tracheal stenosis, multislice CT scan can be useful in quantifying the vertical height (thickness) of cicatricial tissue between the most caudal portion of the airway visible through the nose and the tracheotomy site. This can be either a subtle diaphragm of few millimeters or a thick scar of 2 cm or more. The precise measurement of this length is of fundamental importance in the accurate planning of TRA/CTRA, particularly in long stenoses approximating the ideal limit of 5.5 cm

perform tracheotomy in an elective scenario in order to open the airway in the middle of the stenotic tract and limit damage to the adjacent proximal and distal healthy tracheal rings.

Indications for preoperative radiologic imaging are usually limited and in no case can it replace proper endoscopic assessment. Specific issues to be addressed by multislice computed tomography (CT) scan are the precise length of stenosis in case of complete airway obstruction above the tracheotomy (Fig. 5) and the presence of major alterations of the laryngeal framework (fractures, chondritis or chondronecrosis of the cricoid cartilage and sequelae of previous open neck surgical procedures on the airway) as in Figures 6A and B. Magnetic resonance imaging is undoubtedly superior to CT in evaluation of cricoid and/or tracheal primary tumors (Figs 7A to C), as well as in the assessment of thyroid malignancies involving the upper aerodigestive tract (Figs 8A and B). In this respect, the radiologic check list must include accurate measurement of the craniocaudal invasion of the airway, assessment of the cricoarytenoid joint(s), thyroid cartilage, hypopharynx/esophagus and evaluation of regional lymph node status.

Nasogastric feeding tube is usually not needed before or after TRA/CTRA. Even in case of anticipated dysphagia, its use should be avoided in favor of total parenteral nutrition through a central venous catheter until sufficient oral intake is resumed.

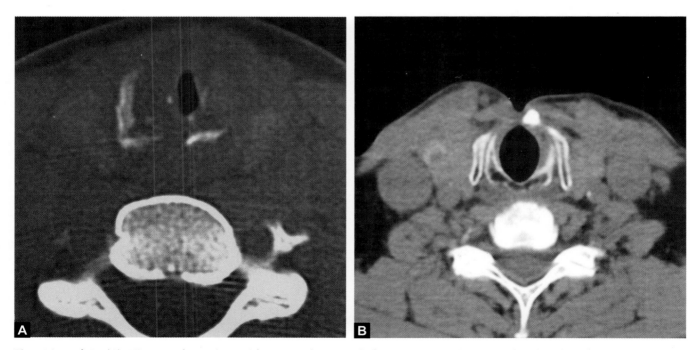

Figs 6A and B: (A) CT scan of a patient with postintubation subglottic stenosis after major head and neck trauma. Imaging showing a misdiagnosed cricoid plate fracture due to blunt trauma on the anterior portion of the neck; (B) CT scan of a patient with recurrent tracheal stenosis after failure of a previous open neck laryngotracheoplasty with anterior costal graft interposition performed elsewhere

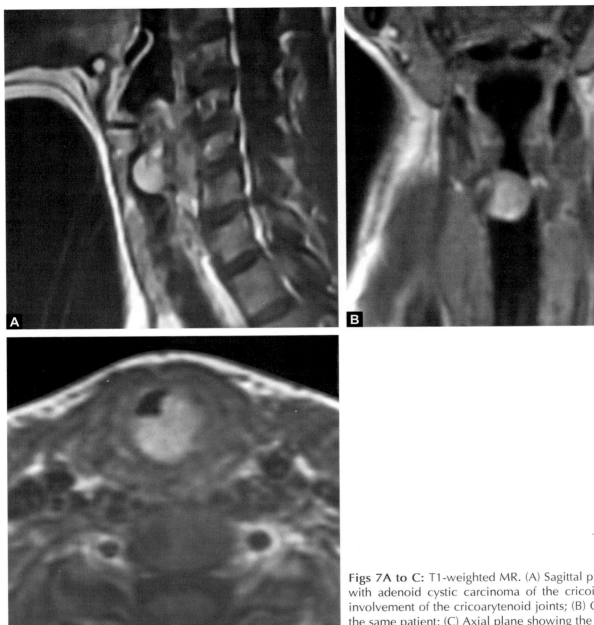

Figs 7A to C: T1-weighted MR. (A) Sagittal plane of a patient with adenoid cystic carcinoma of the cricoid plate without involvement of the cricoarytenoid joints; (B) Coronal plane of the same patient; (C) Axial plane showing the small pedicle of the tumor at the level of the left part of the cricoid plate, without extension to the extralaryngeal tissues

Anesthesia for TRA/CTRA certainly represents a major task for anesthesiologists. Close co-operation between a restricted numbers of specialists in difficult airway management is an essential prerequisite for safely performing this type of surgery. If the patient is not already tracheotomized, an attempt for avoiding preoperative opening of the airway (especially, in an emergency situation) should be made. This implies a progressive dilation of the stenotic airway by bougies or uncuffed tubes up to a caliber, sufficient enough to pass the definitive endotracheal reinforced cuffed tube (Fig. 9). During this phase, the most experienced surgeon available in the theater should be ready to perform an emergency tracheotomy in the middle of the stenotic airway tract. Further details of anesthesiology airway management during TRA/CTRA and after surgery will be discussed in the next paragraph.

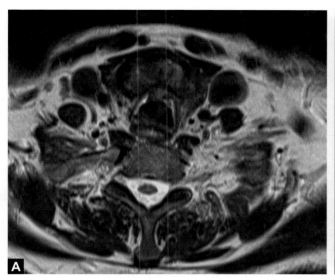

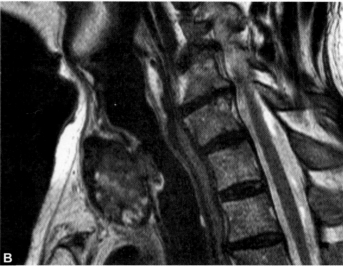

Figs 8A and B: T1-weighted MR. (A) Axial plane of a patient with giant cell tumor of the thyroid gland infiltrating the airway from the second to the fifth tracheal ring; (B) Sagittal plane of the same patient

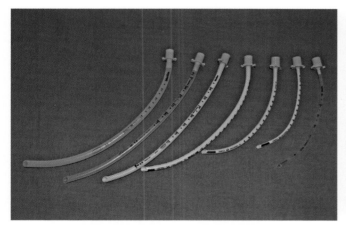

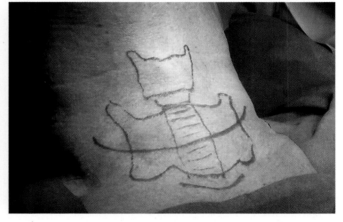

Fig. 9: Series of uncuffed tubes (ID ranging from 2 to 8) used for progressive dilation of cicatricial stenoses before definitive endotracheal intubation by a reinforced cuffed tube of adequate caliber

Fig. 10: Collar incision used for TRA in a case of giant cell tumor of the thyroid gland infiltrating from the second to the fifth tracheal ring. In this patient, neck dissection was limited to the central compartment (level VI and recurrent lymph nodes) due to the specific biological behavior of this low-grade malignancy

SURGICAL TECHNIQUE

After the induction of anesthesia and endotracheal intubation, the patient's neck and upper thorax are scrubbed and draped with sterile towels. Proper attention should be paid to leave the extremity of the endotracheal tube easily accessible to an anesthesiologist during the entire procedure. The patient's position for most part of the TRA/CTRA is similar to that of every surgical procedure on the larynx with the neck extended by placing a sandbag or a rolled towel under the shoulders.

A collar incision is carried out according to that usually required for thyroidectomy (Fig. 10). It can be adjusted

case by case according to the site of stenosis, patient's body habitus, presence of a tracheotomy (to be included into the incision line), scars from previous open neck procedures or the need for simultaneous neck dissection (as in case of thyroid malignancies infiltrating the airway). Quite rarely (only 1 out of 121 patients in our series), an additional stenotomy is needed to address a stenosis of the midportion of the trachea. This can be required either by the presence of a very short and obese neck with the cricoid cartilage at the level of the sternal notch or by the cicatricial sequelae of a previous thoracic (mainly cardiosurgical) intervention, which limits mobilization of the mediastinal stump of the trachea. This rare situation is beyond the scope of this chapter.

After subplatysmal elevation of the superior and inferior skin flaps, the superficial cervical fascia is opened along the midline, paying attention to the ligation of large or crossing over anterior jugular veins. Strap muscles are separated along the midline from the cricoid to the sternal notch in case of TRA, up to the thyroid notch in case of CTRA.

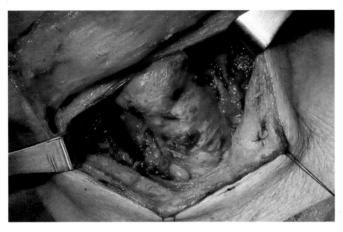

Fig. 11: Image of the same patient as shown in Figure 10, after total thyroidectomy and central compartment neck dissection. Please note the presence of a component of thyroid tumor infiltrating the central part of the third and fourth tracheal ring. Any attempt to remove it en bloc with the involved portion of the trachea should be avoided

In case of thyroid cancer infiltrating the airway, thyroidectomy with central compartment neck dissection is performed in a standard fashion by carefully identifying and preserving the parathyroid glands and recurrent nerves, whose sacrifice is justified only in case of preoperative palsy or massive involvement by the tumor. This maneuver should be always attempted, whenever peeling off the tumor from the nerve is feasible without leaving gross neoplastic residues around it. En bloc resection of a thyroid tumor infiltrating the airway together with the involved tract of cricoid and/or trachea should be never performed. In fact, en bloc resection carries an undue high-risk of recurrent nerve damage and inappropriate evaluation of the proximal and distal airway stumps. In such a scenario, cutting at the level of the tumor-airway interface allows proper assessment of craniocaudal neoplastic involvement of the larynx and/or trachea before starting the TRA/CTRA as in Figure 11.

When TRA/CTRA is not performed for thyroid cancer, the isthmus of the thyroid gland must be separated on the midline and the first tracheal rings should be completely exposed up to the tracheoesophageal groove bilaterally (Fig. 12). In this setting, recurrent nerves are usually not identified and remain lateral and deep with respect to the divided thyroid lobes. Moreover, if tracheal isolation is performed with meticulous hemostasis and strict adherence to the external perichondrium of the airway, no major risk of recurrent lesions is encountered.

When the full length of the stenotic airway has been exposed, it is usually opened in the middle of stenosis (Fig. 13). This maneuver must be performed with caution in order not to damage the cuff of the endotracheal tube,

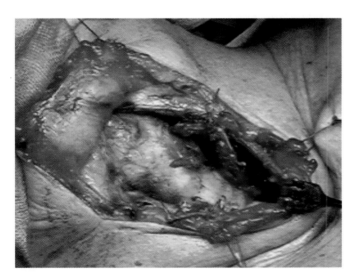

Fig. 12: Separation of the thyroid isthmus along the midline and exposure of the cricoid arch and first tracheal rings

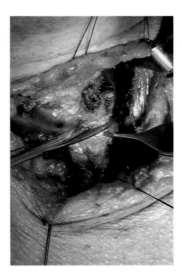

Fig. 13: Opening of the stenotic airway at the level of the cricotracheal membrane

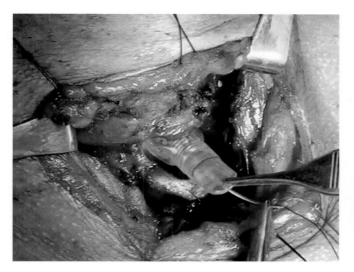

Fig. 14: Withdrawal of the orotracheal tube, fixed by a stitch for later retrieval

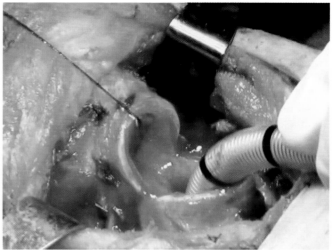

Fig. 15: Endotracheal intubation through the distal airway stump (note the stitch anchored to the proximal tube previously withdrawn up into the larynx)

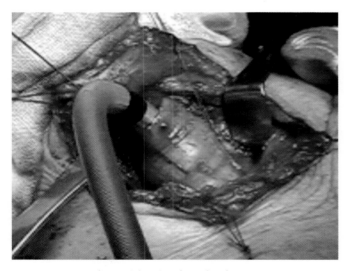

Fig. 16: Beveling of the distal tracheal stump in a patient treated by CTRA with removal of the anterior cricoid arch

which is then withdrawn up to the level of the cricoid or vocal cords, fixed with a stitch for later retrieval (Fig. 14) and substituted by another reinforced cuff tube that is passed into the distal stump of the airway (Fig. 15). This latter tube is used for ventilation from now up to the time of anastomosis. At this point, the tracheal resection is completed transecting the airway at the level of the first distal healthy tracheal ring. In case of TRA with an intact cricoid cartilage, the distal resection line can be made in a standard fashion following the intra-annular ligament between the two rings. When CTRA is performed due to the involvement of the cricoid

arch and/or cricoid plate, the distal resection line should be accomplished beveling the first residual tracheal ring from a high point in the anterior midline to the lower margin of that ring posteriorly on either side (Fig. 16). The membranous wall of the trachea will be cut straight across in case of TRA and with an inverted U shape during CTRA for covering the cricoid plate if its mucosa, submucosa and part of the cartilaginous structure have been removed.

The resection is then completed at the proximal level, which usually represents the most complex step of the entire procedure. If the cricoid is not involved by the stenosis, cutting the airway at the cricotracheal junction is an easy and straightforward maneuver. In contrast, if the cricoid is involved, its resection must be performed taking into account the position of the vocal cords above (<1 cm from the inferior border of the thyroid cartilage) and of the recurrent nerves laterally and posteriorly. Cricoid arch removal is safe whenever performed between the cricothyroid joints (Fig. 17), while partial removal of the cricoid plate must be carried out leaving a posterior shield of cartilage in front of the perichondrium and posterior cricoarytenoid muscles, where the nerve enters the larynx (Fig. 18). The mucosal and submucosal layers covering the cricoid plate can be safely removed up to the level of the cricoarytenoid joints. However, the involvement of the posterior commissure by scar tissue usually needs to be addressed by adding a median thyrotomy, which allows better visualization and management of this difficult area. When stenosis involves the entire glottic and/or supraglottic plane, median thyrotomy is needed to position either a posterior and/or cartilaginous (costal) graft. However, this is usually not a single-stage procedure and implies the use of an endoluminal stent with temporary

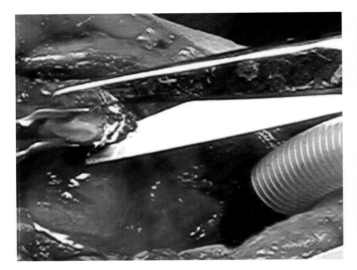

Fig. 17: Cricoid arch removal (performed by scissors) in between the two cricothyroid joints

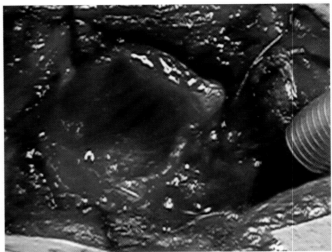

Fig. 18: Subtotal removal of the cricoid plate in a patient affected by low-grade chondrosarcoma of the cricoid cartilage. Note resection of mucosa, submucosa and cartilage from the cricoarytenoid joints superiorly to the inferior border of the plate inferiorly and up to the external perichondrium posteriorly

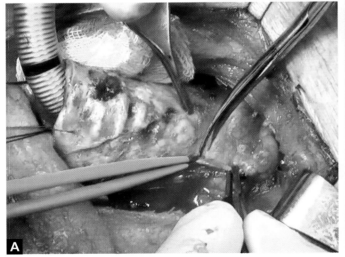

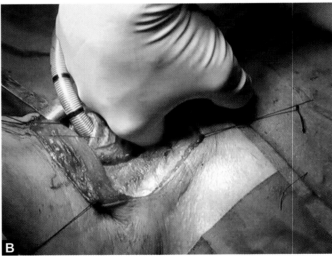

Figs 19A and B: (A) Sharp removal of fatty tissue surrounding the mediastinal portion of the distal tracheal stump; (B) Blunt dissection of the pretracheal plane up to the innominate artery and carina to gain complete tracheal release

tracheotomy and possible subsequent endoscopic refinements. Fortunately, such supraglottic, glottic, subglottic and tracheal stenoses are not very common, and their complex management is therefore not discussed further in this chapter.

Once the resection of the entire stenotic airway has been accomplished, frozen sections must be performed on the proximal and distal stumps of the larynx and the trachea in case of neoplastic lesions. On the other hand, when faced with inflammatory stenoses, the state of the endoluminal mucosa and cartilaginous framework must be carefully

checked in order to exclude the presence of residual scar tissue, chondritis or malacia.

In any case, before starting the anastomosis the distal tracheal stump must be adequately mobilized from the surrounding fat tissue of the tracheoesophageal groove and upper/anterior mediastinum by careful, blunt dissection (Figs 19A and B). For airway resection up to 3.0–3.5 cm in length, this type of inferior (tracheal) releasing maneuver is usually sufficient. In case of longer resections or in older patients with inelastic tracheal rings, an adjunctive superior (laryngeal) release is sometimes needed to drop down the cricoid and perform a tension free anastomosis. Even though different techniques of laryngeal release have been described,[11,12] the authors currently prefer infrahyoid muscle division along the superior border of the thyroid cartilage. Separation of the thyroid cornua, thyrohyoid ligaments and membrane can be also accomplished. However, careful attention must be paid to not injure the superior laryngeal pedicles and to minimize the bleeding occurring during this phase. Moreover, the surgeon should always keep in mind that aggressive laryngeal release maneuvers might be associated with postoperative dysphagia (usually of mild entity and short duration).

The anastomotic time starts by placing two "stay sutures" (2-0 vicryl) at the level of the distal tracheal stump, encircling a ring (including mucosa) at least one cartilage distal to the most proximal complete ring (Figs 20A to C). The same is done at the proximal airway stump. If residual tracheal rings are present below the cricoid, this maneuver is carried out in the same way as described above. If the entire cricoid is present, the upper "stay sutures" must be placed through the substance of the cricoid arch, paying attention to remain in a submucosal plane (Fig. 21A). If the cricoid arch has been removed up to the thyrocricoid joints, then the upper "stay sutures" must be passed through the inferior half of the thyroid alae (Fig. 21B). In any case, the upper and lower "stay sutures" must be placed at corresponding points along the circumference of the airway.

Anastomosis preparation is then completed by passing five 4-0 vicryl stitches between the posterior tracheal wall below and the trachea or posterior cricoid mucosa above (Fig. 22). A number of (from 12 to 15, using 2-0 and 3-0

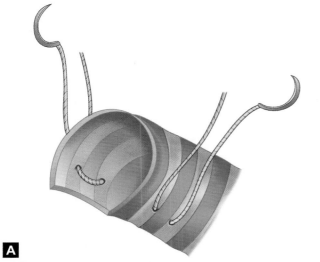

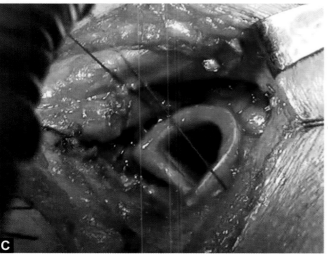

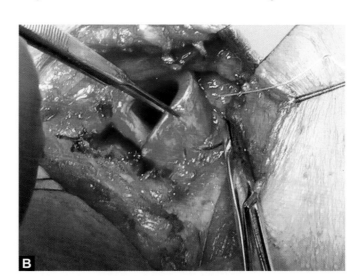

Figs 20A to C: (A) Diagram showing details of distal "stay sutures"; (B) Right distal "stay suture" by 2-0 vicryl; (C) Distal tracheal stump after placement of the left and right "stay sutures"

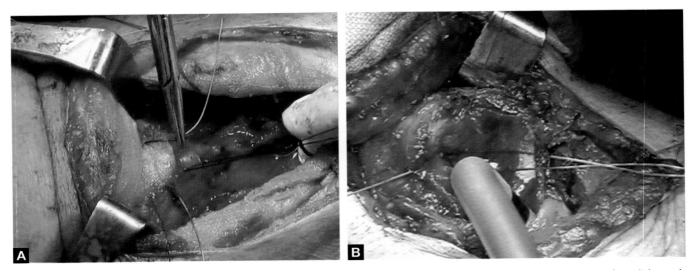

Figs 21A and B: (A) In case of TRA with entire cricoid cartilage preservation, two upper "stay sutures" must be placed through the substance of the cricoid arch, paying attention to remain in a submucosal plane; (B) If CTRA must be performed with excision of the entire cricoid arch up to the thyrocricoid joints, the upper "stay sutures" must be passed through the inferior half of the thyroid alae

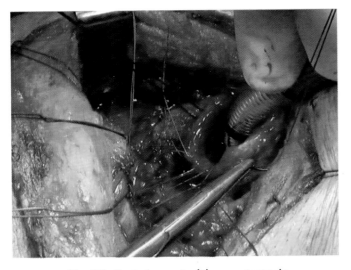

Fig. 22: Posterior part of the anastomosis by 4-0 vicryl stitches

vicryl sutures) stitches are then passed around the entire anterolateral circumference of the trachea below and cricoid arch or thyroid laminae above (Figs 23A and B). All sutures must be made in a precise and ordinate manner making sure that the subsequent knots will be placed outside the airway as in Figure 24.

At this point, the endotracheal tube in the distal airway stump is removed and the former (previously withdrawn up at the glottic level) is pushed down again into the residual trachea. The head is slightly flexed by putting a cushion under the occiput in order to further reduce the tension at the anastomotic level. Anastomosis is then accomplished by tying the knots in a sequential fashion starting from the "stay sutures" and subsequently from the posterior to the anterior portion of the airway circumference. This maneuver is carried out simultaneously by two surgeons, working on both the sides of the neck as in Figures 25A and B.

Closure of the isthmus, prelaryngeal muscles and superficial cervical fascia on the midline is then performed. Suction drainage is usually placed superficial to the prelaryngeal muscles in order not to interfere with the healing process of the anastomotic line. Skin is closed in the usual fashion and 2-0 silk "guardian sutures" are passed from chin to chest, thus forcing the patient to maintain the flexed position of the neck, obtained during anastomosis and needed for its proper healing for at least 8 days after TRA/CTRA as in Figure 26.

The surgeon follows the awakening of the patient under flexible laryngoscopy through the nose, in order to aspirate secretions above the endotracheal cuffed tube, exclude arytenoids and/or vocal cords edema and assess recurrent nerve function (Fig. 27). Lastly, the endotracheal tube is withdrawn and breathing is assisted with an oxygen mask. Patients are usually transferred to the department except in case of respiratory distress. In the latter case, intensive care unit (ICU) monitoring for the first postoperative day and/or reintubation with subsequent endoscopic re-evaluation can be considered on a case-to-case basis. In case of failure of further extubation or cardiopulmonary complications,

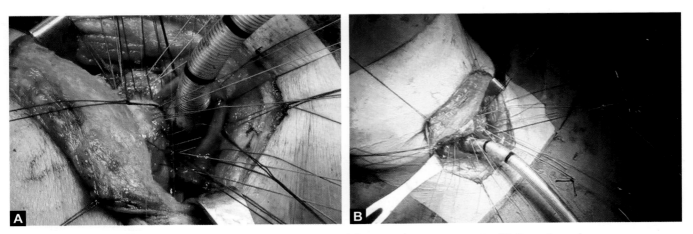

Figs 23A and B: (A) Anterolateral portion of the complete anastomosis; (B) Overview of the surgical field before starting to tie each single knot

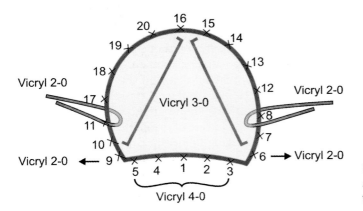

Fig. 24: Diagram showing the sequence of stitches placed along the anastomosis. The same order will be followed for tying them

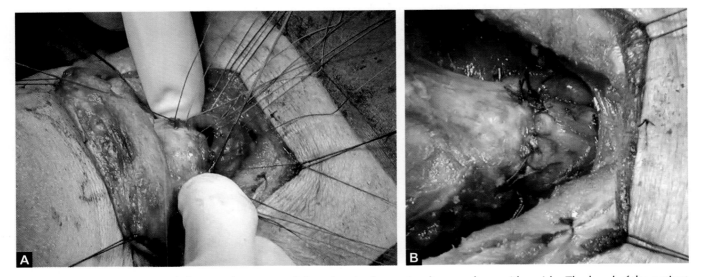

Figs 25A and B: (A) Accomplishment of anastomosis by tying the knots simultaneously on either side. The head of the patient in this phase is slightly flexed to reduce the degree of tension at the anastomotic level; (B) Completion of anastomosis

tracheotomy should be performed two tracheal rings below the anastomotic line using the smallest cannula available. This should be removed as soon as possible in order to limit its potential damage to the anastomosis and the distal airway.

POSTOPERATIVE TREATMENT

The wound is kept clean by rinsing it once a day in a standard fashion. Pain control does not usually represent a major concern and is obtained by nonsteroidal anti-inflammatory drugs (while corticosteroids should be strictly avoided for their known propensity to interfere with anastomotic

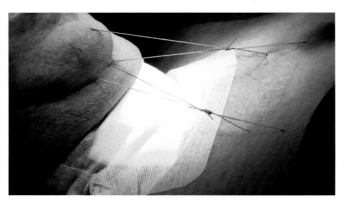

Fig. 26: "Guardian sutures" with the head in a flexed position

healing). Broad-spectrum antibiotic therapy is administered for at least 2 weeks after surgery. Anticough and antiemetic medications may be administered to reduce the risk of neck emphysema. If present, this should be always carefully evaluated to rule out major anastomotic dehiscences (usually observed in the first 5 days after TRA/CTRA). Chin to chest "guardian sutures" are responsible for major discomfort to the patient, which can be significantly reduced by the administration of myorelaxants. Adequate antiepileptic drugs (in previously neurotraumatized patients) must be administered due to the potentially devastating effects of such a crisis on the anastomotic line in spite of the most robust "guardian sutures."

A normal oral diet is usually started on the second postoperative day. Endoscopic follow-up is performed by flexible video endoscopy. Usually, no radiologic imaging is needed except for chest X-ray in case of fever of possible pulmonary origin. Suction drainage is removed on the 4th, "guardian sutures" on the 8th and cutaneous stitches on the 10th postoperative day respectively. Patients are usually discharged on the 11th–12th postoperative day.

One month after surgery, an endoscopic control under local anesthesia is scheduled for all the patients (Fig. 28) and repeated three months later. In case of inflammatory stenoses, if control visits are negative, no further follow-up is required. However, in case of neoplastic stenoses, periodic endoscopic and imaging follow-up is performed according to the histotype and stage of the lesion.

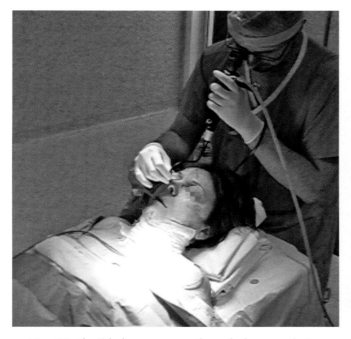

Fig. 27: Flexible laryngoscopy through the nose during awakening of the patient in the operating theater

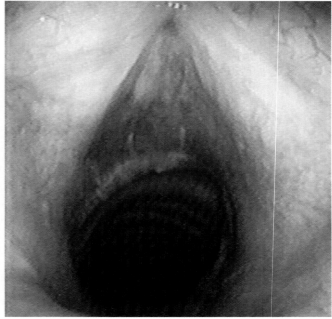

Fig. 28: Postoperative flexible fiberoptic control, 1 month after CTRA for papillary thyroid cancer infiltrating the airway

HIGHLIGHTS

I. Indications
- Long (1.0–5.5 cm), complex (subglottic and tracheal) inflammatory stenoses with alterations of the laryngotracheal cartilaginous framework and malacia of the airway.
- Primary tumors of the cricoid (mainly chondroma/chondrosarcoma and minor salivary gland tumors) and cervical trachea (minor salivary gland tumors and other rare histotypes).
- Thyroid tumors infiltrating the airway beyond the external perichondrium.

II. Contraindications
- Major cardiopulmonary and neurologic comorbidities
- Stenoses longer than 5.5 cm, even though older patients can be exposed to the risk of an excessive tension at the level of the anastomotic line even after shorter resections.
- Major aspiration during swallowing
- Bilateral recurrent/vagal palsy
- In case of tumors, involvement of the glottic plane and/or thyroid cartilage, one cricoarytenoid joint, full thickness of the hypopharynx/esophagus, unresectable regional or mediastinal lymph nodes, distant metastasis (even though the latter is usually not an absolute contraindication in case of well-differentiated thyroid cancer).

III. Special Preoperative Considerations
- Endoscopically evaluate the patient by state-of-the-art technique
- In selected cases, CT and/or MRI can also be required after endoscopy
- Operate only stable, mature inflammatory stenoses
- Avoid preoperative corticosteroids for at least 2 weeks before surgery
- Share a common algorithm of difficult airway management with an anesthesiologist.

IV. Special Intraoperative Considerations
- Perform accurate hemostasis
- Maintain a plane of dissection as close as possible to the external perichondrium of the cricoid and trachea.
- Remove the cricoid arch between the cricothyroid joints up to the inferior border of the thyroid laminae
- Remove the cricoid plate from inside to outside, leaving a shell of cartilage in front of the posterior perichondrium and the posterior cricoarytenoid muscles.
- Always perform tracheal release maneuvers.
- Limit laryngeal release maneuvers to only long stenoses
- Anastomosis done in an ordinate and scrupulous way
- Always put chin to chest "guardian sutures" (leave them for at least 8 days after surgery).

V. Special Postoperative Considerations
- Extubate the patient immediately after surgery in the operating theater under flexible fiberoptic control through the nose (not through the endotracheal tube) and transfer him/her to the department.
- Reintubate or send the patient for ICU monitoring in case of postoperative respiratory distress.
- Re-evaluate the situation 24–48 hours later: if further extubation failures are encountered, perform tracheotomy two rings below the anastomotic line and remove it as soon as possible.
- Avoid corticosteroids for at least 2 weeks after surgery.

VI. Complications
- Uni- or bilateral, transient or permanent recurrent nerve palsy.
- Laryngeal edema (in case of bilateral neck dissection for thyroid cancer)
- Postoperative bleeding with ensuing laryngopharyngeal edema.
- Minor (with neck emphysema only) and major anastomotic dehiscences (with restenosis of the airway and need for a redo anastomosis)
- Granuloma formation along the anastomotic line for inappropriate alignment of the proximal and distal airway stumps or persistent inflammation.
- Pneumothorax for lesion of the mediastinal pleura (particularly after previous thoracic surgery or radiotherapy on the mediastinum).
- Tracheoesophageal fistula.

REFERENCES

1. Gerwat J, Bryce DP. The management of subglottic laryngeal stenosis by resection and direct anastomosis. Laryngoscope. 1974;84(6):940-57.
2. Pearson FG, Cooper JD, Nelems JM, et al. Primary tracheal anastomosis after resection of the cricoid cartilage with preservation of recurrent laryngeal nerves. J Thorac Cardiovasc Surg. 1975;70(5):806-16.

3. Grillo HC. Development of tracheal surgery: a historical review. In: Grillo HC (Ed). Surgery of the Trachea and Bronchi. Hamilton, London: BC Decker Inc; 2004.

4. Bisson A, Bonnette P, el Kadi B, et al. Tracheal sleeve resection for iatrogenic stenosis (subglottic laryngeal and tracheal). J Thorac Cardiovasc Surg. 1992;104(4):882-7.

5. Couraud L, Jougon J, Velly JF, et al. Sténoses iatrogênes de la voie respiratoire. Evolution des indications thérapeutiques. Ann Chir Thorac Cardiovasc. 1994;48:277-83.

6. Grillo HC, Donahue DM, Mathisen DJ, et al. Post intubation tracheal stenosis. Treatment and results. J Thorac Cardiovasc Surg. 1995;109(3):486-93.

7. Grillo HC, Mathisen DJ. Primary tracheal tumors: treatment and results. Ann Thorac Surg. 1990;49(1):69-77.

8. Perelman MI, Koroleva N, Birjukov J, et al. Primary tracheal tumors. Sem Thorac Cardiovasc Surg. 1996;8(4):400-2.

9. Ishihara T, Kobayashi K, Kikuchi J, et al. Surgical treatment of advanced thyroid carcinoma invading the trachea. J Thorac Cardiovasc Surg. 1991;102(5):717-20.

10. Grillo HC, Suen HC, Mathisen DJ, et al. Resectional management of thyroid carcinoma invading the airway. Ann Thorac Surg 1992;54(1):3-10.

11. Dedo HH, Fishman NH. Laryngeal release and sleeve resection for tracheal stenosis. Ann Otol Rhinol Laryngol. 1969;78(2): 285-96.

12. Montgomery WW. Suprahyoid release for tracheal anastomosis. Arch Otolaryngol. 1974;99:255-60.

Chapter 47 Anterolateral Thigh Perforator Flaps in Head and Neck Reconstruction—Indications and Surgical Technique

Arik Zaretski, Eyal Gur, Fu Chan Wei

INTRODUCTION

Microsurgical free tissue transfer has revolutionized head and neck reconstructive surgery. It gives oncologic surgeons more freedom to perform radical tumor resections because single-stage reconstructive solutions are now available for the majority of defects.[1-4] Patients who were previously thought inoperable, such as those with locally advanced or recurrent disease, can now be considered candidates for surgical treatment.[2,4,5] Ablative surgery in such a complex anatomical site can cause severe impairments for the patient. An ideal reconstruction preserves both function and esthetic appearance without compromising the principles of cancer surgery. In recent practice, the authors have selected three workhorse free flaps for head and neck reconstruction: (i) the anterolateral thigh (ALT), (ii) fibula, and (iii) radial forearm flaps.[3-9]

The ALT flap has only recently gained popularity because its original description preceded the development of perforator flap surgery. Song et al. in 1984, described the ALT flap as being supplied by septocutaneous vessels originating from the descending branch of the lateral circumflex femoral artery.[10] This was later demonstrated only to be true in 15% of cases, with the outstanding 85% (majority) supplied by a musculocutaneous perforator.[3,11-13] Developments in intramuscular perforator and retrograde dissection techniques laid the foundations for the harvest of muscle-sparing ALT flaps.[2,14,15] Koshima et al. were the first to describe the use of the ALT flap to reconstruct head and neck defects.[16,17] Since then, others have reported their experience, establishing the ALT flap as one of the major workhorse flaps used for head and neck reconstruction.[1,3,9,18-26]

RELATED ANATOMY

The ALT flap is supplied by the descending branch of the lateral circumflex femoral artery; the largest branch of the profunda femoris system. Its artery, usually associated with two concomitant veins, traverses obliquely with the nerve to vastus lateralis within the groove formed between the rectus femoris and vastus lateralis muscles.[12,13,27,28] The anterior branch of the lateral cutaneous nerve of the thigh can be included to create a sensory flap.[29] The pedicle terminates near the knee joint in the vastus lateralis muscle after having provided septocutaneous vessels that pierce the fascia to access the ALT skin and perforators to the rectus femoris and vastus lateralis muscles. It is usually these musculocutaneous perforators that are encountered and dissected when harvesting a cutaneous or fasciocutaneous flap. Anterolateral thigh flap of pedicle length between 8 cm and 16 cm and vessel diameters of at least 2 mm are quite adequate for anastomoses [12,13,27,28] as in Figure 1.

VARIOUS TYPES OF ANTEROLATERAL THIGH FLAP

The unique anatomy of the thigh permits several methods of harvesting the ALT flap. The types of tissue to be included in the flap can be selected according to the defect to be reconstructed. The ALT flap can be harvested at the suprafascial level to include just skin and subcutaneous fat, useful for when a thin flap is desired.[3,12,27,28,30-33] When harvested at the subfascial level, the flap can bring additional tissue bulk including the fascia lata on the deep surface. The

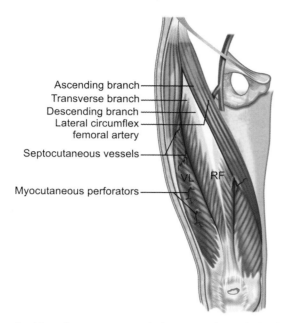

Fig. 1: Vascular anatomy of the anterolateral thigh flap. Note the skin flap supplied by either septocutaneous vessels or myocutaneous perforators from the descending branch of the circumflex femoral vessel

fascia is particularly useful in a number of situations, such as when repairing dural or tendon defects, and when creating a sling to support the oral commissure.[2,9,30,34,35] A musculocutaneous flap can be harvested by including part of the vastus lateralis muscle.[3,12,17,27,28] The muscle can be attached to the overlying skin or splayed out on a separate vascular branch that arises from the same vascular pedicle to create a chimeric flap.[3,35]

SURGICAL TECHNIQUES FOR HARVESTING THE ANTEROLATERAL THIGH FLAP

The cutaneous vessels can be mapped out with a handheld pencil Doppler probe placed at the midpoint between the anterosuperior iliac spine and the superolateral corner of the patella.[1,3,30,36] The majority of skin vessels are located in the inferolateral quadrant of a circle with a 3 cm radius centered on this same midpoint, but they can also be located elsewhere.[1,3,30,36] The flap should be centered over these vessels and designed with its long axis parallel to that of the thigh. A simultaneous two team approach can be achieved with the patient supine, as this usually allows the operation to be completed without altering the patient's position.

Elevation of a Cutaneous Flap without Fascia (Suprafascial Dissection)

The first incision is placed on the medial side of the designed flap outline and continued down to just above the fascia lata. Skin and subcutaneous tissues are then gently dissected away from the fascia laterally until the vessels to the skin are revealed. The identified skin vessel is dissected back to the main pedicle, leaving a small piece of fascia encircling the vessel. Intramuscular dissection proceeds if the vessel is a musculocutaneous perforator. Such vessels always give several branches from their lateral and posterior aspects to supply the neighboring vastus lateralis muscle, with fewer arising anteriorly. The musculocutaneous perforator can therefore be easily traced by incising the muscle over the perforator and ligating each branch to the muscle arising laterally and posteriorly. Dissection is even easier, if instead, the skin vessel is septocutaneous and is performed between the vastus lateralis and rectus femoris muscles back to the main pedicle. It is possible to elevate a cutaneous flap as thin as 3–5 mm, however, excessive thinning should be avoided in less experienced hands to avoid marginal necrosis.[3,33,37]

Elevation of a Fasciocutaneous Flap

The skin is incised down to the fascia lata, which is included in the flap. The cutaneous vessel from the lateral circumflex femoral artery system is identified beneath the fascia. Flap elevation proceeds similarly as described for suprafascial dissection.

Elevation of a Musculocutaneous Flap

Dissection of the perforator or septocutaneous vessel is not necessary when elevating a musculocutaneous flap, because the portion of vastus lateralis muscle within which the skin perforator travels is included. The necessary portion of vastus lateralis muscle is divided away whilst paying attention to the intramuscular branches that require ligation. Again, the main pedicle is dissected as before.

Elevation of a Chimeric Anterolateral Thigh Flap

Numerous chimeric ALT flap combinations are possible because the lateral circumflex artery provides lateral, medial and descending branches. Most involve an ALT flap in combination with rectus femoris muscle, tensor fascia lata, anteromedial thigh skin or the vastus lateralis muscle. Thus, chimeric ALT flaps can be musculocutaneous, fasciocutaneous or cutaneous only with more than one skin island.[35] Chimeric ALT flaps are a versatile choice for reconstructing three-dimensional defects because two or more separate tissues can be harvested on one pedicle, which maximizes the flexibility of the flap inset (Fig. 2).[35]

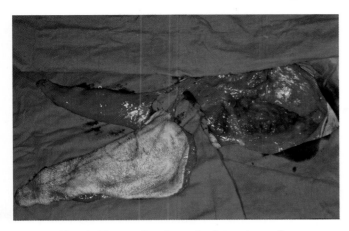

Fig. 2: Descending branch of the circumflex femoral vessel provides chimeric flaps

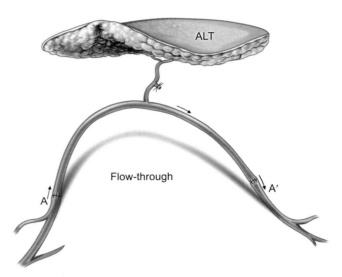

Fig. 3: Scheme of flow-through anterolateral thigh flap

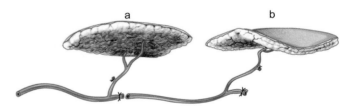

Fig. 4: Schematic diagram demonstrating the harvest of two independent flaps (a and b) from the same pedicle. Note the site of pedicle division for the second flap (b)

Elevation of a Flow-through Flap

Usually, the pedicle terminates distally into the vastus lateralis muscle by branching into cutaneous vessels. This distal end of the pedicle can be dissected to the required length clear of the vastus lateralis muscle, in order to serve as recipient vessels for a second free flap (Fig. 3).[3,38]

Elevation of Two Independent Cutaneous Flaps from the Same Pedicle

As the descending branch of the lateral circumflex femoral artery provides multiple septocutaneous vessels and myocutaneous perforators to the thigh, two independent skin flaps can be harvested from the same donor site, reducing both the total time of flap harvests and overall donor site morbidity. Two separate cutaneous vessels are required for this and each needs to be dissected back to the main pedicle. If longer or wider vessels are needed, the dissection can be continued to reach the descending branch of the lateral circumflex femoral artery. In order to maximize the length of the pedicle for the distal flap, its origin should be defined as being located immediately distal to the origin of the branch supplying the proximal flap (Fig. 4).

ANTEROLATERAL THIGH FLAP FOR HEAD AND NECK RECONSTRUCTION

The vascular anatomy of the thigh allows considerable flexibility when designing an ALT flap for a given defect in the head and neck. It can be harvested as thinly as the radial forearm flap or augmented by inclusion of subcutaneous tissue, fascia lata or the vastus lateralis muscle.[3,9] Chimeric ALT flaps are available for defects demanding reconstruction in even greater than three dimensions. Although the flap size can range from just a few centimeters up to the length of the thigh, its width should be limited to between 8 cm and 13 cm if primary donor site closure is to be achieved, as larger donor sites usually necessitate skin grafting.[1,3,6,30]

TONGUE RECONSTRUCTION

The tongue is one of the sites most frequently affected by oral cancer. Invasion into the floor of the mouth, oropharynx and hypopharynx is common.[39,40] A thin ALT flap is the first choice in our center for reconstructing defects smaller than that of a hemitongue. For larger defects, such as a total glossectomy, more tissue is readily available.[3,9] Muscle inclusion facilitates obliteration of dead space, such as in the submandibular and neck regions following neck dissection. Furthermore, the flap can be de-epithelialized and folded for extra volume and sensation can be provided by inclusion of the lateral cutaneous nerve of the thigh.[3] The ALT flap can provide as much tissue volume as the rectus abdominis myocutaneous flap, however, it is easier to inset, because it can be harvested with two separate skin islands or with a separate mass of muscle based on the same pedicle (Figs 5A and B) and it causes less donor site morbidity.[30]

RECONSTRUCTION OF BUCCAL AND THROUGH AND THROUGH CHEEK DEFECTS

Buccal defects created from cancer ablation can be divided into two major categories: (i) those that are partial; and (ii) those that are of full thickness. The ALT flap can be safely thinned intraoperatively, making it applicable for reconstructing partial thickness cheek defects.[3,30,37] Although the radial forearm flap is also good in this setting, the ALT flap leaves a less conspicuous donor site with less morbidity. Full thickness cheek defects, which involve the oral lining, buccal fat, masseter muscle and facial skin are more challenging to

reconstruct, particularly, if the oral commissure is involved. Reconstruction of such defects with the radial forearm flap usually results in inadequate functional and esthetic outcomes. When the oral commissure is not involved, the folded ALT flap is the authors' preferred option. Again, a segment of vastus lateralis muscle can be included for additional volume. Involvement of the oral commissure calls for a well designed chimeric ALT flap to increase the flexibility of the flap inset, resulting in improved oral continence and quality of speech (Figs 6A to D).[3,35]

RECONSTRUCTION OF COMPOSITE DEFECTS OF THE MANDIBLE

Composite mandibular defects are ideally reconstructed with an autogenous bone flap, most commonly the vascularized osteoseptocutaneous fibula flap.[41-43] Another option is to bridge the bony gap with a reconstruction plate and gain

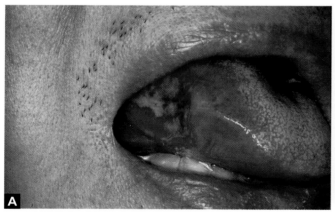
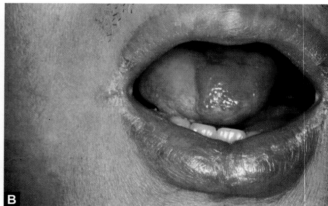

Figs 5A and B: Reconstruction of the hemiglossectomy defect with an anterolateral thigh flap.
(A) Preoperative cancer lesion; (B) Postoperative appearance

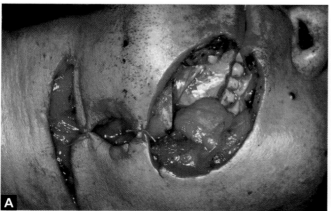
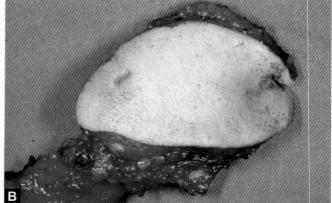

Figs 6A and B

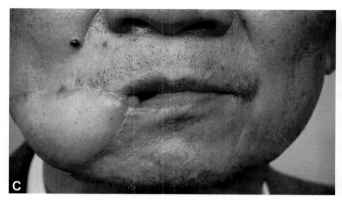
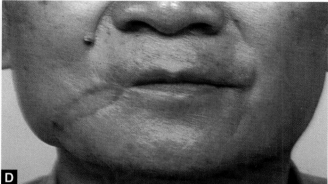

Figs 6A to D: Reconstruction of a through and through cheek defect with an anterolateral thigh flap. (A) Through and through cheek defect including oral commissure; (B) Excised surgical specimen; (C) Appearance after reconstruction with a folded anterolateral thigh cutaneous flap; (D) Appearance after excision of the external face skin flap

coverage with a soft tissue flap.[44,45] This is usually indicated for short or lateral mandibular segmental defects, older patients or patients with a poor prognosis.[46]

From the authors' experience and the work of others the ALT flap is the first choice for the soft tissue reconstruction.[3,4,30,35] Radical treatment for extensive T3 and T4 cancers creates large composite defects requiring both bone and extensive soft tissues for reconstruction.[46,47] Although a composite vascularized osteoseptocutaneous fibula flap can provide intraoral and external coverage, its volume is usually inadequate for larger resections or for through and through cheek defects. The simultaneous use of a second free flap has been advocated by several authors as a means of overcoming this soft tissue deficiency.[4,5,48-50] The second flap can obliterate the dead space resulting from resection of the masticator muscles, buccal fat and parotid gland, and prevents the accumulation of fluid that leads to secondary infection or an orocutaneous fistula.[4,5] Adequate volume and quality of soft tissue is important to prevent bone and plate exposure, especially in patients scheduled for radiation therapy.[4,5]

A particular advantage of the ALT flap is that it provides a good contour for the face. Although it may have a bulky appearance at first, it will usually shrink after radiotherapy (Figs 7A to E).

MIDFACE RECONSTRUCTION

Reconstruction of the midface can be challenging since the defect is usually three-dimensional and involves more than one tissue type.[9] The flaps most commonly described for midface reconstruction are the radial forearm for small and the rectus abdominis or latissimus dorsi for larger defects. However, the ALT flap is suitable for a range of defect sizes.[9] A cutaneous or fasciocutaneous ALT is suitable for reconstructing small defects, however, an almost unlimited area of the skin is available for larger defects and the vastus lateralis

muscle can be included as necessary for bulk. The muscle component is useful for obliterating the maxillary sinus and for providing well vascularized coverage for bone grafts used when reconstructing the orbital floor (Figs 8A and B).

SCALP RECONSTRUCTION

When only the exposed calvarium needs coverage, a large ALT flap can be harvested.[30,31] The flap can be thin and provide good quality skin without excessive bulk, unlike when myocutaneous flaps, such as the rectus abdominis or latissimus dorsi are used.[9,51] The skin quality of the ALT flap is superior to a muscle flap covered with split thickness skin graft. Furthermore, the functional impairment related to muscle harvest is avoided. For defects involving both the calvarium and dura, fascia lata can be included to reconstruct the dura and seal against cerebrospinal fluid leakage (Figs 9A to C).

DISCUSSION

Radical tumor ablations in the head and neck region can significantly impair function and esthetics, and usually require complex reconstructions. In the past, options for soft tissue coverage were limited only to pedicled flaps. Traditional free flaps were either too thin or too bulky, or were not ideal for texture matching. The introduction of perforator-based flap harvest and the chimeric flap concept allowed the surgeon to choose a more accurate single-stage reconstruction that could both restore good function and achieve an esthetically acceptable result in the majority of patients.

During the recent 10 years, the authors at Chang Gung Memorial Hospital, Taipei, Taiwan, have performed more than 2,600 cases of ALT flaps; 70% of which were for head and neck reconstruction. The authors have found that the

ALT flap possesses many of the important properties that make a flap ideal for head and neck reconstruction, namely: (i) anatomically constant with a long and sizeable pedicle; (ii) good match for recipient site tissue characteristics; (iii) flexibility of tissue volume, be that thick, bulky or thin and pliable; (iv) flexibility in design, including the availability of different tissue types for harvesting on the same pedicle, as in a chimeric flap; (v) the option to harvest two separate flaps from the same site; (vi) insignificant donor site morbidity; (vii) simultaneous flap harvest and tumor ablation afforded by a two team approach; and (viii) the option for sensory reinnervation.[3,6,8,9] The authors have only rarely encountered cases that required vein grafts, even when reconstructing cases following recurrent cancer, difficult neck dissections or when having to turn to the contralateral neck to find suitable recipient vessels. A particularly important advantage of the ALT flap is the relatively low donor site morbidity that accompanies even a substantial flap

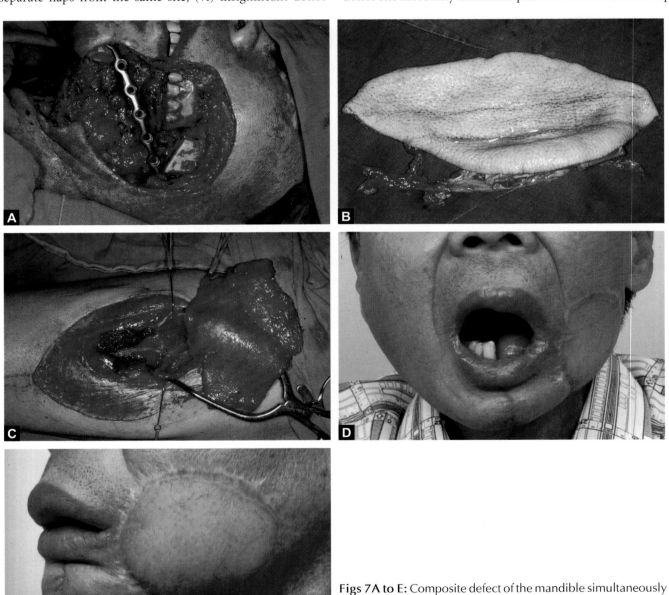

Figs 7A to E: Composite defect of the mandible simultaneously reconstructed with fibula osteoseptocutaneous flap for oral lining and mandible, and an anterolateral thigh flap for external face and cheek bulk. (A) Composite mandibular defect; (B) A fibula osteoseptocutaneous flap; (C) Anterolateral thigh flap; (D) Appearance 2 years after surgery; (E) Closeup lateral view 3 years after surgery

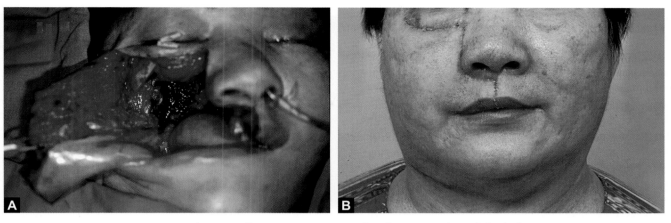

Figs 8A and B: Maxillectomy reconstructed with an anterolateral thigh flap. (A) Maxillectomy defect; (B) Postoperative appearance after reconstruction

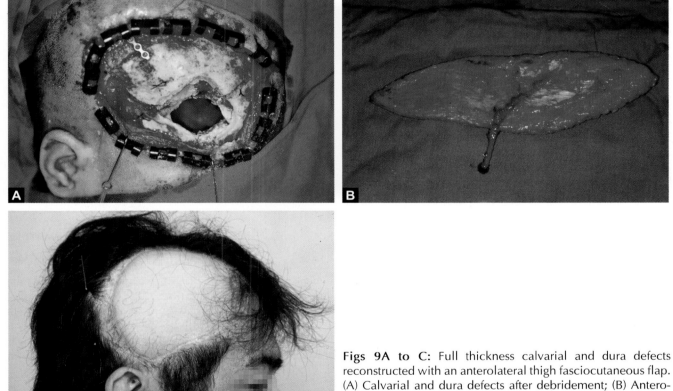

Figs 9A to C: Full thickness calvarial and dura defects reconstructed with an anterolateral thigh fasciocutaneous flap. (A) Calvarial and dura defects after debridement; (B) Antero-lateral thigh fasciocutaneous flap. Note the fascia lata for dura repair; (C) Appearance after reconstruction

harvest. An increase in the size of a cutaneous flap does not appear to cause a proportional increase in donor site morbidity. Dissection and protection of the nerve to the vastus lateralis muscle should be performed carefully to preserve maximal quadriceps function when harvesting a cutaneous ALT flap. The inclusion of a segment of the vastus lateralis muscle might be expected to increase donor site morbidity, however, it was objectively demonstrated at long-term follow-up with a kinetic communicator machine that only a minimal weakness of the thigh results.[52] In authors' experience, no significant functional deficits were noted either by the patient or examining physician.

CONCLUSION

Although numerous other soft tissue flaps have been described, most are less useful than the ALT flap for head and neck reconstruction, because they variably fail to offer a sufficient number of these advantages. The diversity that the ALT flap offers allows its use for most indications in head and neck reconstruction, including those of the intraoral, tongue, buccal, midface and scalp regions. Resultant donor site morbidity is low when compared with other available flaps.

REFERENCES

1. Demirkan F, Chen HC, Wei FC, et al. The versatile anterolateral thigh flap: a musculocutaneous flap in disguise in head and neck reconstruction. Br J Plast Surg. 2000;53:30-6.
2. Jeng SF, Kuo YR, Wei FC, et al. Reconstruction of extensive composite mandibular defects with large lip involvement by using double free flaps and fascia lata grafts for oral sphincters. Plast Reconstr Surg. 2005;115:1830-6.
3. Wei FC, Jain V, Celik N, et al. Have we found an ideal soft-tissue flap? An experience with 672 anterolateral thigh flaps. Plast Reconstr Surg. 2002;109:2219-26.
4. Wei FC, Celik N, Chen HC, et al. Combined anterolateral thigh flap and vascularized fibula osteoseptocutaneous flap in reconstruction of extensive composite mandibular defects. Plast Reconst Surg. 2002;109:45-52.
5. Wei FC, Demirkan F, Chen HC, et al. Double free flaps in reconstruction of extensive composite mandibular defects in head and neck cancer. Plast Reconstr Surg. 1999;103:39-47.
6. Lutz BS, Wei FC. Microsurgical workhorse flaps in head and neck reconstruction. Clin Plast Sur.2005;32:421-30, vii.
7. Santamaria E, Wei FC, Chen HC. Fibula osteoseptocutaneous flap for reconstruction of osteoradionecrosis of the mandible. Plast Reconstr Surg. 1998;101:921-9.
8. Gedebou TM, Wei FC, Lin CH. Clinical experience of 1284 free anterolateral thigh flaps. Handchir Mikrochir Plast Chir. 2002;34:239-44.
9. Chana JS, Wei FC. A review of the advantages of the anterolateral thigh flap in head and neck reconstruction. Br J Plast Surg. 2004;57:603-9.
10. Song YG, Chen GZ, Song YL. The free thigh flap: a new free flap concept based on the septocutaneous artery. Br J Plast Surg 1984;37:149-59.
11. Ao M, Uno K, Maeta M, et al. De-epithelialised anterior (anterolateral and anteromedial) thigh flaps for dead space filling and contour correction in head and neck reconstruction. Br. J. Plast. Surg. 1999;52:261-7.
12. Kimata Y, Uchiyama K, Ebihara S, et al. Anatomic variations and technical problems of the anterolateral thigh flap: a report of 74 cases. Plast Reconstr Surg. 1998;102:1517-23.
13. Xu DC, Zhong SZ, Kong JM, et al. Applied anatomy of the anterolateral femoral flap. Plast Reconstr Surg. 1988;82:305-10.
14. Mardini S, Tsai FC, Wei FC. The thigh as a model for free style free flaps. Clin Plast Surg. 2003;30:473-80.
15. Wei FC, Silverman RT, Hsu WM. Retrograde dissection of the vascular pedicle in toe harvest. Plast Reconstr Surg. 1995;96: 1211-4.
16. Koshima I, Yamamoto H, Hosoda M, et al. Free combined composite flaps using the lateral circumflex femoral system for repair of massive defects of the head and neck regions: an introduction to the chimeric flap principle. Plast Reconstr Surg. 1993;92:411-20.
17. Koshima I, Fukuda H, Yamamoto H, et al. Free anterolateral thigh flaps for reconstruction of head and neck defects. Plast Reconstr Surg. 1993;92:421-8.
18. Chen CM, Chen CH, Lai SH, et al. Anterolateral thigh flaps for reconstruction of head and neck defects. J Oral Maxillofac Surg. 2005;63:948-52.
19. Lyons AJ. Perforator flaps in head and neck surgery. Int J Oral Maxillofac Surg. 2006;35:199-207.
20. Chana JS, Wei FC. A review of the advantages of the anterolateral thigh flap in head and neck reconstruction. Br J Plast Surg. 2004;57:603-9.
21. Lin DT, Coppit GL, Burkey BB. Use of the anterolateral thigh flap for reconstruction of the head and neck. Curr Opin Otolaryngol Head Neck Surg. 2004;12:300-4.
22. Makitie AA, Beasley NJ, Neligan PC, et al. Head and neck reconstruction with anterolateral thigh flap. Otolaryngol Head Neck Surg. 2003;129:547-55.
23. Nakayama B, Hyodo I, Hasegawa F, et al. Role of the anterolateral thigh flap in head and neck reconstruction: advantages of moderate skin and subcutaneous thickness. J Reconstr Microsurg. 2002;18:141-6.
24. Hayden RE, Deschler DG. Lateral thigh free flap for head and neck reconstruction. Laryngoscope. 1999;109:1490-4.
25. Truelson JM, Leach JL. Lateral thigh flap reconstruction in the head and neck. Otolaryngol Head Neck Surg. 1998;118: 203-10.
26. Miller MJ, Reece GP, Marchi M, et al. Lateral thigh free flap in head and neck reconstruction. Plast Reconstr Sur. 1995;96:334-40.
27. Kuo YR, Seng-Feng J, Kuo FM, et al. Versatility of the free anterolateral thigh flap for reconstruction of soft-tissue defects: review of 140 cases. Ann. Plast. Surg. 2002;48:161-6.
28. Zhou G, Qiao Q, Chen GY, et al. Clinical experience and surgical anatomy of 32 free anterolateral thigh flap transplantations. Br J Plast Surg. 1991;44:91-6.
29. Luo S, Raffoul W, Luo J, et al. Anterolateral thigh flap: a review of 168 cases. Microsurgery. 1999;19:232-8.
30. Chen HC, Tang YB. Anterolateral thigh flap: an ideal soft tissue flap. Clin Plast Surg. 2003;30:383-401.
31. Shieh SJ, Chiu HY, Yu JC, et al. Free anterolateral thigh flap for reconstruction of head and neck defects following cancer ablation. Plast Reconstr Surg. 2000;105:2349-57.
32. Wolff KD, Plath T, Hoffmeister B. Primary thinning of the myocutaneous vastus lateralis flap. Int J Oral Maxillofac Surg. 2000;29:272-6.

33. Celik N, Wei FC. Technical tips in perforator flap harvest. Clin Plast Surg. 2003;30:469-72.

34. Heller F, Hsu CM, Chuang CC, et al. Anterolateral thigh fasciocutaneous flap for simultaneous reconstruction of refractory scalp and dural defects. Report of two cases. J Neurosurg. 2004;100;1094-7.

35. Huang WC, Chen HC, Jain V, et al. Reconstruction of through-and-through cheek defects involving the oral commissure, using chimeric flaps from the thigh lateral femoral circumflex system. Plast Reconstr Sur. 2002;109:433-41.

36. Celik N, Wei FC, Lin CH, et al. Technique and strategy in anterolateral thigh perforator flap surgery, based on an analysis of 15 complete and partial failures in 439 cases. Plast Reconstr Surg. 2002;109:2211-6.

37. Kimura N, Satoh K. Consideration of a thin flap as an entity and clinical applications of the thin anterolateral thigh flap. Plast Reconstr Surg 1996;97:985-92.

38. Pribaz JJ, Orgill DP, Epstein MD, et al. Anterolateral thigh free flap. Ann Plast Surg. 1995;34:585-92.

39. Haughey BH. Tongue reconstruction: concepts and practice. Laryngoscope. 1993;103:1132-41.

40. Ildstad ST, Bigelow ME, Remensnyder JP. Squamous cell carcinoma of the tongue: a comparison of the anterior two-thirds of the tongue with its base. Am J Surg. 1983;146:456-61.

41. Hidalgo DA. Fibula free flap: a new method of mandible reconstruction. Plast Reconstr Surg. 1989;84:71-9.

42. Wei FC, Chen HC, Chuang CC, et al. Fibular osteoseptocutaneous flap: anatomic study and clinical application. Plast Reconstr Surg. 1986;78:191-200.

43. Wei FC, Seah CS, Tsai YC, et al. Fibula osteoseptocutaneous flap for reconstruction of composite mandibular defects. Plast Reconstr Surg. 1994;93:294-304.

44. Raveh J, Stich H, Sutter F, et al. Use of the titanium-coated hollow screw and reconstruction plate system in bridging of lower jaw defects. J Oral Maxillofac Surg. 1984;42:281-94.

45. Raveh J, Sutter F, Hellem S. Surgical procedures for reconstruction of the lower jaw using the titanium-coated hollow-screw reconstruction plate system: bridging of defects. Otolaryngol Clin North Am. 1987;20:535-58.

46. Mariani PB, Kowalski LP, Magrin J. Reconstruction of large defects postmandibulectomy for oral cancer using plates and myocutaneous flaps: a long-term follow-up. Int J Oral Maxillofac Surg. 2006;35:427-32.

47. Urken ML, Weinberg H, Vickery C, et al. Oromandibular reconstruction using microvascular composite free flaps. Report of 71 cases and a new classification scheme for bony, soft-tissue and neurologic defects. Arch Otolaryngol. Head Neck Surg. 1991;117:733-44.

48. Blackwell KE, Buchbinder D, Biller HF, et al. Reconstruction of massive defects in the head and neck: the role of simultaneous distant and regional flaps. Head Neck. 1997;19:620-8.

49. Koshima I, Fukuda H, Soeda S. Free combined anterolateral thigh flap and vascularized iliac bone graft with double vascular pedicle. J Reconstr Microsurg. 1989;5:55-61.

50. Urken ML, Weinberg H, Vickery C, et al. The combined sensate radical forearm and iliac crest free flaps for reconstruction of significant glossectomy-mandibulectomy defects. Laryngoscope. 1992;102:543-58.

51. Lutz BS. Aesthetic and functional advantages of the anterolateral thigh flap in reconstruction of tumor-related scalp defects. Microsurgery. 2002;22:258-64.

52. Kuo YR, Jeng SF, Kuo MH, et al. Free anterolateral thigh flap for extremity reconstruction: clinical experience and functional assessment of donor site. Plast Reconstr Surg. 2001;107:1766-71.

Chapter 48

Ear Reconstruction

Moshe Kon, Eyal Gur, David Leshem

INTRODUCTION

Microtia is a relatively rare disorder. There are several types of microtia, classified according to their appearance by Nagata.[1,2] They are: (i) lobular type; (ii) concha type; (iii) small concha type; (iv) anotia (no or minimal remnants of ear) or atypical microtia as in Figures 1A to C.

Microtia is more common in males than in females, with ratios varying from 2 to 3 times as often in males. The right to left to bilateral ratio is estimated at 4:2:1 and 3:2:1.

In Asians and Hispanics, microtia is more common than in whites and blacks. Risk factors include the use of Roaccutane® (isotretinoïne) and antiepileptic drugs during pregnancy.[3-5] The auricle malformation often appears with malformations of the jaw and hemifacial microsomia.[6]

Tanzer was the first to introduce autologous costal cartilage grafts for auricular reconstruction in 1959[7,8] and since then authors, such as Brent,[9] Nagata,[1,2] Park and Firmin have introduced modifications to improve outcome.

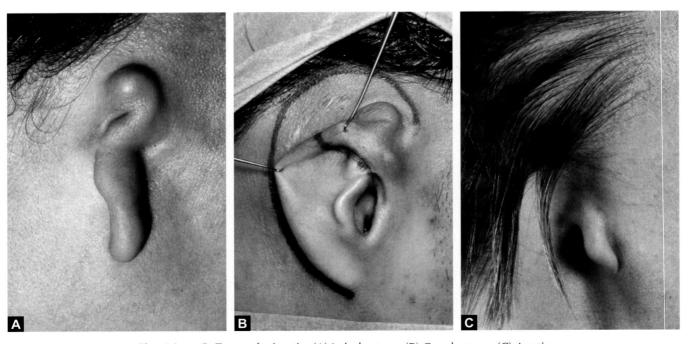

Figs 1A to C: Types of microtia. (A) Lobular type; (B) Concha type; (C) Anotia

The most important modification was the change from a four-stage reconstruction (Brent) to a two-stage reconstruction (Nagata) with transposition of the lobule and placement of the costal cartilage frame at the same time in the first stage. Alloplastic materials are only used by few surgeons because of the chances of extrusion.[10,11]

PREOPERATIVE EVALUATION AND ANESTHESIA

Timing of surgery is between 8 years and 10 years of age in order to be able to harvest sufficient costal cartilage from a stable ribcage. At this age, the ear has reached almost the size of an adult ear, which allows us to use a template from the contralateral healthy ear. Also, better patient cooperation and motivation can be expected. Endotracheal intubation is used for the procedure.

SURGICAL TECHNIQUE

First Stage

Using a transparent film, a template of the contralateral healthy ear is made, including landmarks for positioning the ear in the right anatomical place. The landmarks used are lateral canthus and lobule position of the contralateral side.

Costal cartilage is harvested from sixth rib to eighth rib (Fig. 2), from the ipsilateral side (Nagata), although it can be harvested from the contralateral side as well (Brent). The perichondrium is preserved and after harvest, it is approximated to allow reshaping of the rib by neocartilage formation.

On a side table, the cartilage is carved using carving instruments. The cartilage from the sixth rib and the seventh rib are used for the base of the framework, the tragus and antihelix, while the eighth rib is usually used for carving the helix. The framework is designed according to the template taken from the contralateral ear (Fig. 3).

The different cartilage parts are sutured together with stainless steel sutures and the ends are buried into the cartilage to avoid extrusion.

Using the transparent film template, the recipient site is marked and the skin is incised. A pocket is created and the ear cartilage remnants are removed. Sometimes a subcutaneous pedicle is left intact for better circulation of the skin.[12] The lobule, if present, is transposed as in Figure 4A.

After inserting the framework (Fig. 4B) into the pocket, one or two small vacuum drains are positioned in such a way that it achieves good skin draping and definition of the framework.

Skin closure is performed with 5-0 resorbable sutures and meticulous dressing is applied using Vaseline gauze and soft padding.

A piece of cartilage is banked under the chest donor site incision for the second stage outsetting.

Postoperative Treatment

The dressing is left in place for 4–5 days, during which the vacuum is maintained in order to achieve adequate skin draping. After the dressing is removed, instructions for good hygiene are given.

Second Stage

The second stage is the outsetting of the reconstructed ear and takes place around 6 months after the first stage.

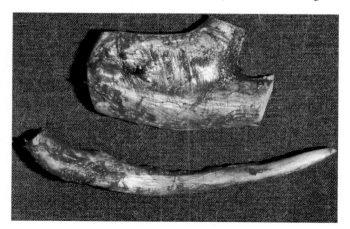

Fig. 2: Costal cartilage

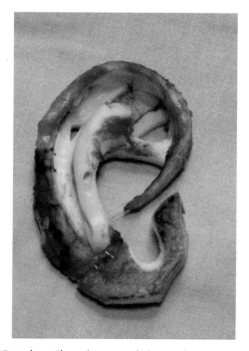

Fig. 3: Costal cartilage framework for total ear reconstruction

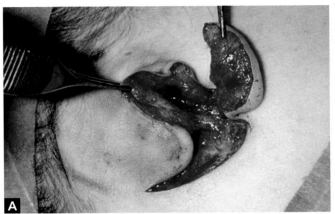

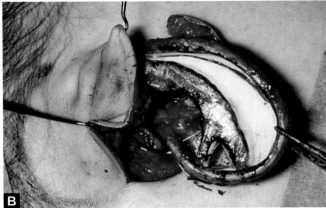

Figs 4A and B: (A) Transposition of earlobe; and (B) Insertion cartilage frame

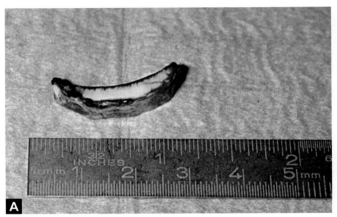

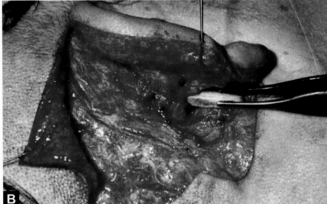

Figs 5A and B: Second stage. (A) Moon-shaped cartilage block; (B) Insertion into a subfacial tunnel

The banked rib cartilage is harvested from the chest wall and cut into a moon-shaped block as in Figure 5A.

An incision is performed along the helical rim. In cases where the post auricular tissue is of substantial quality, a tunnel is made under the cartilage framework and the fascia (Fig. 5B). The cartilage is inserted and fixed tightly with nonabsorbable sutures.

A full thickness skin graft is harvested from the groin and applied to the post auricular area and sutured using absorbable sutures. A tie over dressing is applied.

In cases that do not have sufficient soft tissue coverage over the cartilage block after mobilization, a temporoparietal fascia (TPF) flap is turned down for coverage of the posterior side of the ear and cartilage block. A split thickness skin graft is draped over the TPF and a loose tie over dressing is applied.

Postoperative Treatment

The dressing is left in place for about 5 days. After the removal of the bandage cleaning instructions are given.

Additional Procedures

In order to achieve a good groove definition, injection of steroids can be administered into these areas. Minor surgeries can be done for lobule refinement or deepening of the tragus-concha area. Till good end results are obtained as in Figures 6 and 7.

A low hairline requires laser epilation prior to reconstructive surgery or a few months after surgery. Another option for this problem is the use of TPF for the framework coverage and a skin graft as in Figures 8A to C.

Partial Ear Reconstruction

In partial defects, the same surgical technique can be used as for total ear reconstruction. In small defects, conchal cartilage from the ipsilateral or the contralateral side can be sufficient. In larger defects, costal cartilage has to be used (Figs 9A to C). The posterior auricular skin or the TPF are used for

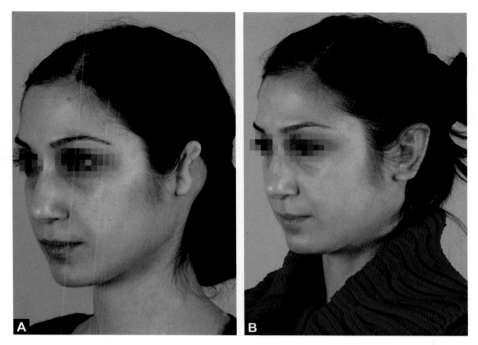

Figs 6A and B: Lobular type microtia. Pre- and postoperative

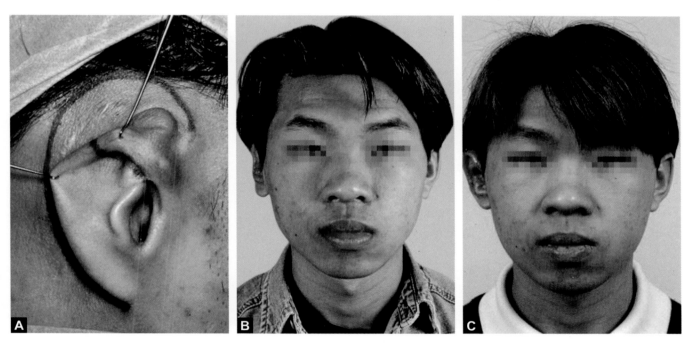

Figs 7A to C: Concha type microtia right side. After first stage and after second stage (mobilization)

cover of the cartilage framework and a second operation is often needed for mobilization of the ear. When the lobule is amputated, it can be reconstructed with a bilobed flap using costal or conchal cartilage for support. In case the patient wants to wear earrings, during reconstruction holes can be made in the cartilage frame before insertion to prevent piercing of the cartilage at a later stage as in Figures 10A and B.

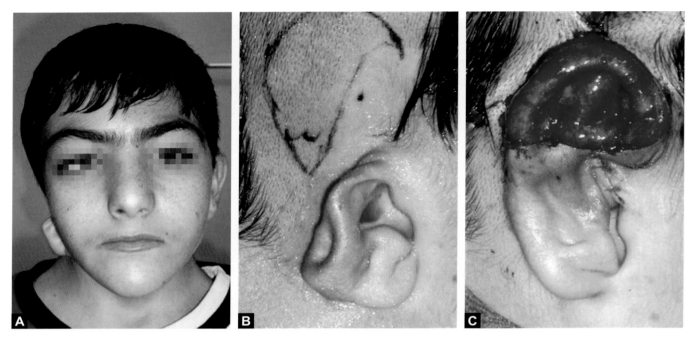

Figs 8A to C: (A) Low hairline and low ear implant; (B) Excision of hairy skin and;
(C) Use of temporoparietal fascia (before application of skingraft)

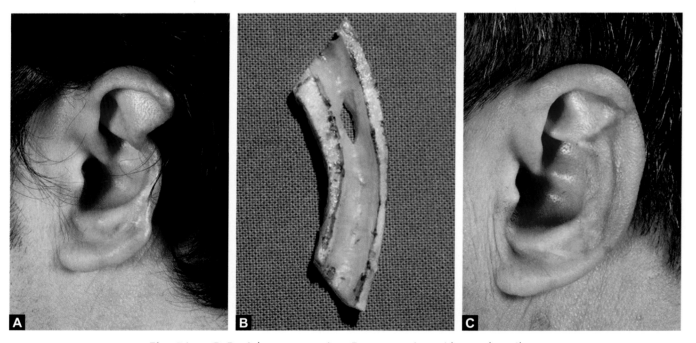

Figs 9A to C: Partial ear amputation. Reconstruction with costal cartilage

CONTRAINDICATIONS

Unrealistic expectations of patients, in case of unacceptable outcomes after earlier reconstruction attempts, need to be addressed carefully. When the area is much scarred, the temporoparietal fascia is not available and the temporal vessels are damaged, prosthetic solutions are advisable.

The elderly patient with an ear amputation for cancer is also a good candidate for prosthesis.

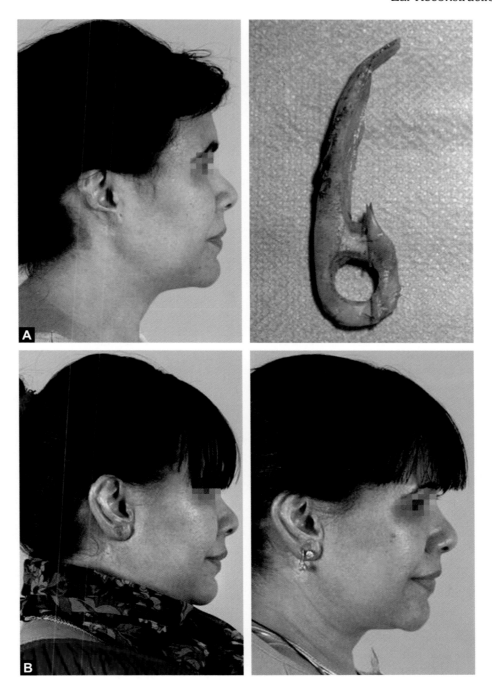

Figs 10A and B: (A) Partial ear reconstruction with costal cartilage; (B) Earlobe reconstruction and cartilage hole for ear rings

COMPLICATIONS

Infections after ear reconstruction are not frequent. Thorough cleaning of the area before reconstruction, pre- and postoperative antibiotic treatment, and gently handling of the tissues during operation decreases the chances of infection.

It is necessary to instruct the patient about skin damage due to pressure or related problems. Skin necrosis and cartilage exposure need immediate surgical treatment. Depending on the size of the skin defect local transposition flaps or the use of the TPF is advisable.

Insufficient definition caused by fibrosis or scar tissue can be treated by local steroid injections.

HIGHLIGHTS

I. Indications
- Microtia
- Anotia
- Traumatic ear defects.

II. Contraindications
- Unrealistic expectations
- Noncooperative patient.

III. Complications
- Infection
- Skin necrosis
- Cartilage exposure
- Insufficient definition.

REFERENCES

1. Nagata S. Modification of the stages in total reconstruction of the auricle: Part I–IV. Plastic Reconstructive Surgery. 1994;93(2):221-53, discussion 267-8.
2. Nagata S. Microtia: auricular reconstruction. In: Achauer BM, Eriksson E (Eds). Plastic Surgery: Indication, Operations and Outcomes. London: Mosby Inc; 2000. pp. 1023-5.
3. Harris J, Källén B, Robert B. The epidemiology of anotia and microtia. J Med Genet. 1996;33(10):809-13.
4. Mastroiacovo P, Corchia C, Botto LD, et al. Epidemiology and genetics of microtia-anotia: a registry based study on over one million births. J Med Genet. 1995;32(6):453-7.
5. Wu J, Zhang R, Zhang Q, et al. Epidemiological analysis of microtia: a retrospective study in 345 patients in China. Int J of Pediatr Otorhinolaryngol. 2009;33(4):528-2.
6. Kearns GJ, Padwa BL, Mulliken JB, et al. Progression of facial asymmetry in hemifacial microsomia. Plastic Reconstr Surg Transplant Bull. 2000;105(2):492-8.
7. Tanzer RC. Total reconstruction of the external ear. Plastic Reconstr Surg. Transplant Bull. 1959;23(1):1-15.
8. Dupertuis SM, Musgrave RM. Experiences with the reconstruction of the congenitally deformed ear. Plastic Reconstr Surg Transplant Bull. 1959;23(4):361-73.
9. Brent B. Microtia repair with rib cartilage grafts: a review of personal experience with 1000 cases. Clin in Plastic Surg. 2002;29(2):257-71,vii.
10. Cronin TD, Greenberg RL, Brauer RO. Follow-up study of silastic frame for reconstruction of the external ear. Plast Reconstr Surg. 1968;42(6):522-9.
11. Yang SL, Zheng JH, Ding Z, et al. Combined fascial flap and expanded skin flap for enveloping medpor framework in microtia reconstruction. Aesthetic Plast Surg. 2009;33(4):518-22.
12. Ishikura N, Kawkami S, Yoshida J, et al. Vascular supply of the subcutaneous pedicle in Nagata's method of microtia reconstruction. Br J Plast Surg. 2004;57(8):780-4.

Chapter 49

Local Flaps in Facial Reconstruction

Ehud Miller, Eyal Gur

INTRODUCTION

Facial defects are caused by trauma or more commonly after removal of skin tumors. The method of choice of removing skin tumors is the Mohs technique with minimal recurrence rate as compared to other methods and maximal preservation of the healthy tissue.

Defects can be reconstructed by several methods according to the reconstruction ladder. Primary closure is the first choice and the simplest one. In several locations, secondary healing gives a fair result, such as in the medial canthus, the concha of the ear and the upper forehead, as in cases of forehead flap donor site.

Skin graft is also an option, preferably full-thickness grafts harvested from above the clavicle, for better color and texture match. Local flaps are the workhorse of reconstruction of many facial defects. The use of local flaps and for larger defects, regional flaps, has been studied for many years. Great improvement has been achieved in understanding flap design and the forces influencing the flap, the wound and the donor site.

The arrival of microsurgery and free tissue transfer opened doors for reconstruction of complicated and large defects. Still, most defects can be closed using local tissue. The surgeon should always consider simple reconstruction methods before using complicated reconstruction methods. The reconstruction choice should be tailored to each patient after studying the defect, tissue availability and the advantages and disadvantages of each method.

In this chapter, the author introduces some of the more common local flaps used for reconstruction of facial defects.

BILOBED FLAP

First described by Esser in 1918,[1] this transposition random pattern flap is used for distal nasal defects; 1–1.5 cm in diameter (Figs 1A to D). The flap enables to transfer loose proximal nasal skin to cover lesions in the distal most sebaceous area of the nose. The flap has a primary lobe that covers the initial defect and a secondary lobe that fits into the secondary defect. The donor site of the second lobe is closed primarily. The flap should be carefully designed.

The first lobe should be of equal size to that of the defect. A too small lobe might cause the alar rim to be pulled upwards. A too large lobe is more prone to pincushioning and might push the alar rim downwards. The second lobe should be 80–85% of the first lobe in diameter and should be able to close primarily.[2] It is better to place it perpendicular to the axis of the alar rim in order to minimize any vector that could pull the rim upwards.[3] The whole flap should rotate/transpose around 90–100°.[3] Before raising the flap, one should evaluate the defect, rigidity of the alar rim and the nasal skin type. A nonfirm alar rim might benefit conchal cartilage graft.

Sebaceous, rhinophema-type of skin might not suit this flap. The flap mobility is limited and there are greater chances of pin cushioning. The flap should be raised in

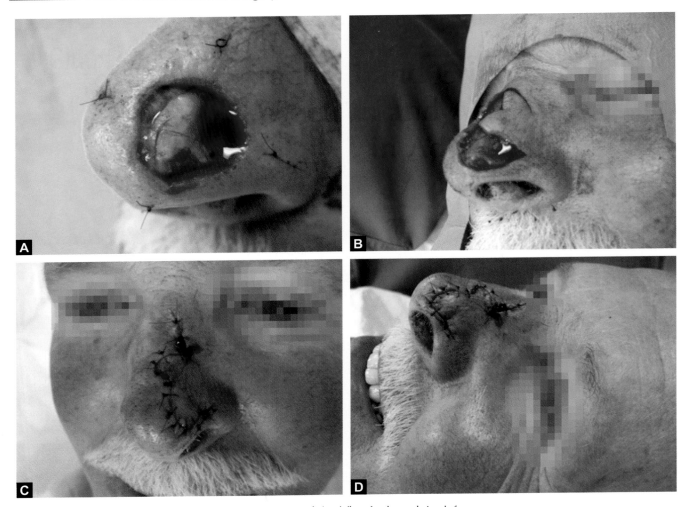

Figs 1A to D: Bilobed flap for lateral tip defect

the submuscular layer. The dog-ear at the lower part of the defect is removed before raising the flap for easier rotation. The area surrounding the flap and the defect should be well undermined. Flap is sutured without tension, with skin only interrupted sutures that will be removed in 7 days.

NASOLABIAL FLAP

The nasolabial flap (Figs 2 to 5) is a versatile flap. It can be used for reconstruction of the nasal sidewall, ala, columella, nasal tip, nasal lining and also intraoral and lip reconstructions.

The flap can be raised based on a superior or inferior pedicle as a transposition or an interpolation flap. The flap is traditionally considered as an axial flap based on muscular perforants of the facial artery via the angular artery. Some authors claim that the blood supply is random based on a

subcutaneous and subdermal network.[4,5] In any case, the flap is reliable and with the exception of smoker could be thinned and manipulated with very little risk. The size of the flap is based on the size of the defect and the laxity of the cheek. Usually, it is a good option for defects of the nasal ala and sidewall of up to 2 cm in height.[6] It is not a good option for patients with a poorly defined nasolabial fold and modest cheek laxity.[7]

Cartilage support graft should be considered for defects close to the alar rim. The nasolabial fold is first marked and then the defect is measured using a foil template. The flap is raised from distal to proximal. While the distal part can be thinned to the level of the dermis, the proximal aspect should be more deeper. The flap is sutured with skin only stitches. Donor site is closed in layers. The flap tends to pincushion and might need revisions. Using the interpolation flap, the pedicle is divided within 3–4 weeks. Donor site is closed primarily.

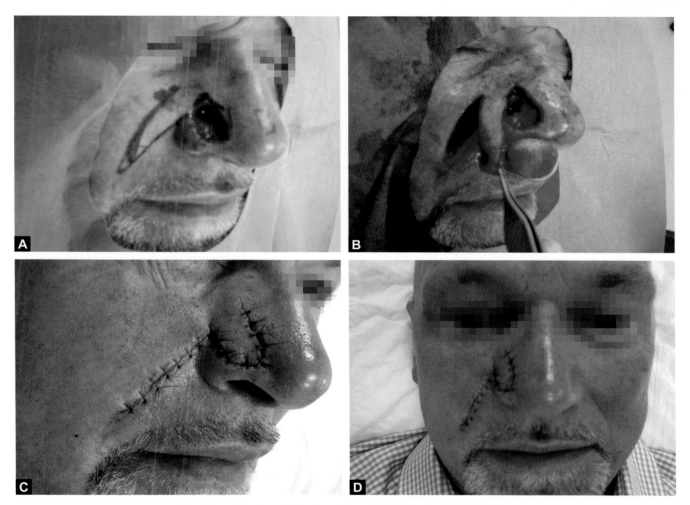

Figs 2A to D: Superiorly-based nasolabial flap for lobule defect

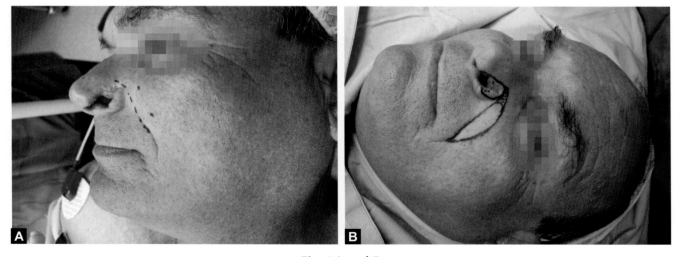

Figs 3A and B

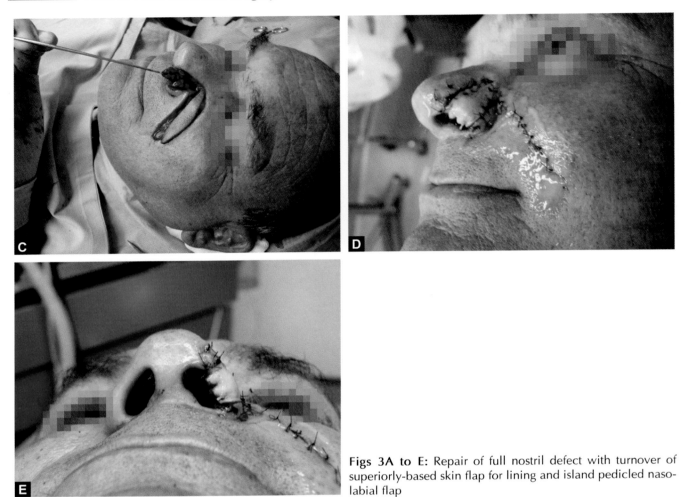

Figs 3A to E: Repair of full nostril defect with turnover of superiorly-based skin flap for lining and island pedicled naso-labial flap

Figs 4A and B

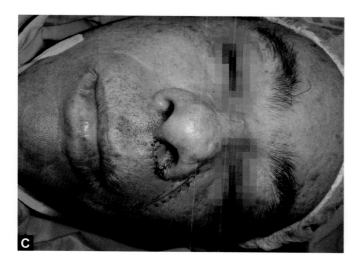

Figs 4A to C: Repair of nostril base with island pedicled nasolabial flap. A release of the nostril seal was performed for insetting

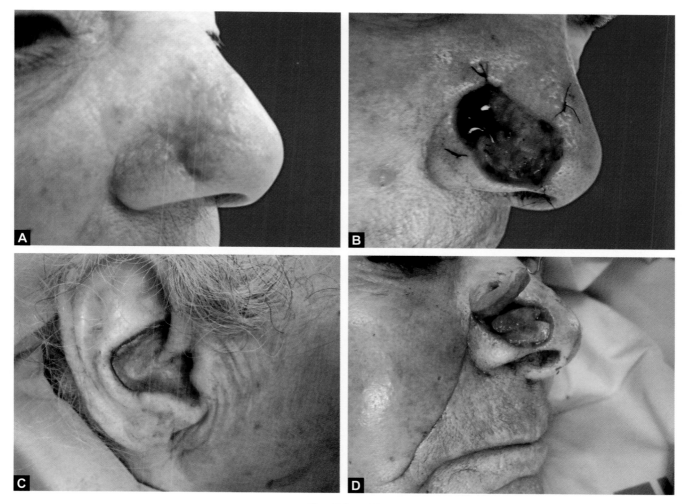

Figs 5A to D

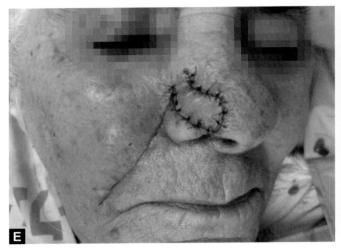

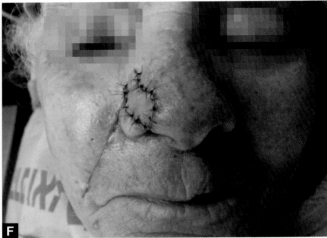

Figs 5A to F: Incompletely excised basal cell carcinoma and the defect after three rounds of Mohs surgery. Conchal support graft was harvested from the anterior side and a superiorly nasolabial flap was used

FOREHEAD FLAP

The use of the forehead flap goes back to the "Indian" flap, about a thousand years ago. The flap has been studied and evolved greatly with Millard, and later Burget and Menick contributing to its esthetic and functional results.[8]

The forehead flap (Figs 6 and 7) is the workhorse of nasal reconstruction. It is used to cover defects greater than 2 cm in diameter up to a whole nose replacement including lining. It provides similar color and texture, it is a reliable flap and the donor site scar is acceptable.

The flap has an axial blood supply through the supratrochlear artery. The flap is supplied by a network of vessels rather than a single one and there is no need for Doppler identification of the supratrochlear vessel. It is usually transferred in two stages. The flap is thinned at its distal end at the first stage, and 3–4 weeks later, the pedicle is divided.

For large complicated lesions, lesions that require nasal lining, Menick has introduced the three-stage technique. The flap is raised including the frontalis muscle throughout its length without any thinning. Four weeks later, the flap is raised off its recipient site at the subcutaneous layer, the nose surface is sculptured and the flap is sutured back. Four weeks later, the pedicle is divided. This procedure is especially beneficial for smokers that have the greatest risk for complications.[8,9] The procedure is best performed under general anesthesia.

Lesion is evaluated for size, esthetic units involved and need of cartilage support. A lesion involving more than 50% of an esthetic unit is best enlarged to the size of the whole unit.

The defect is measured using foil template. The forehead midline is drawn and the template is drawn vertically on the ipsilateral side at a measured distance to the defect.

1.2 cm off the midline at the height of the glabella, mark the middle of the pedicle. 0.5 cm to each side, mark the pedicle's borders. Actually, due to the rich network of blood vessels at that region any 1 cm wide pedicle between the midline and 2 cm laterally will be safe. If needed, the flap can be elongated toward the hair on the distal part or toward the medial canthus at its proximal part.

The flap is raised from distant toward the pedicle with or without muscle and the dissection deepens as we approach the pedicle.

Cartilage is grafted and placed for support if needed.

The flap is sutured into place with one layer of nylon sutures, the donor site is closed in layers, while its upper portion might be left for secondary healing. Quilting sutures can be used for better contour defining.

MUSTARDE AND CHEEK/ CERVICOFACIAL FLAPS

Skin of the lower eyelid is the thinnest in the body and one should replace it with skin of similar texture, thickness and color.

The best choice for that is the mustarde (Figs 8A and B) or rotation advancement cheek flap. The flap brings tissue from the lateral area toward the eyelid.[10] Its blood supply is random based on branches of the facial artery. Large flaps should be avoided if possible in smokers. Delay procedure should be considered in these cases.

The flap is raised with the subcutaneous fat above the SMAS. The superior border of the flap should lie above the height of the lateral canthus in order to avoid downwards pull of the eyelid.

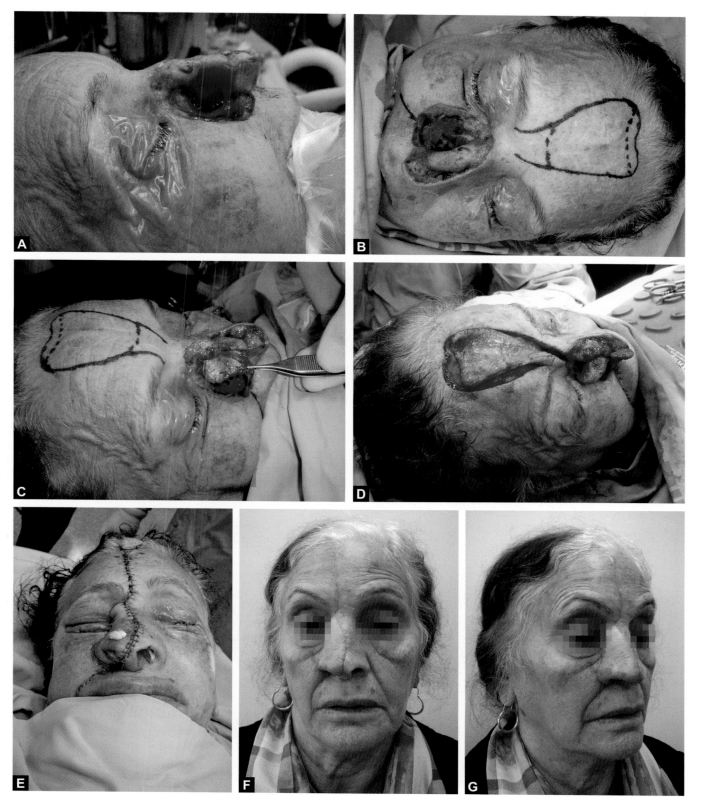

Figs 6A to G: Forehead flap for hemi-nose defect. Contralateral mucosal flap was used for lining. A nasolabial flap and conchal cartilage graft were used for support

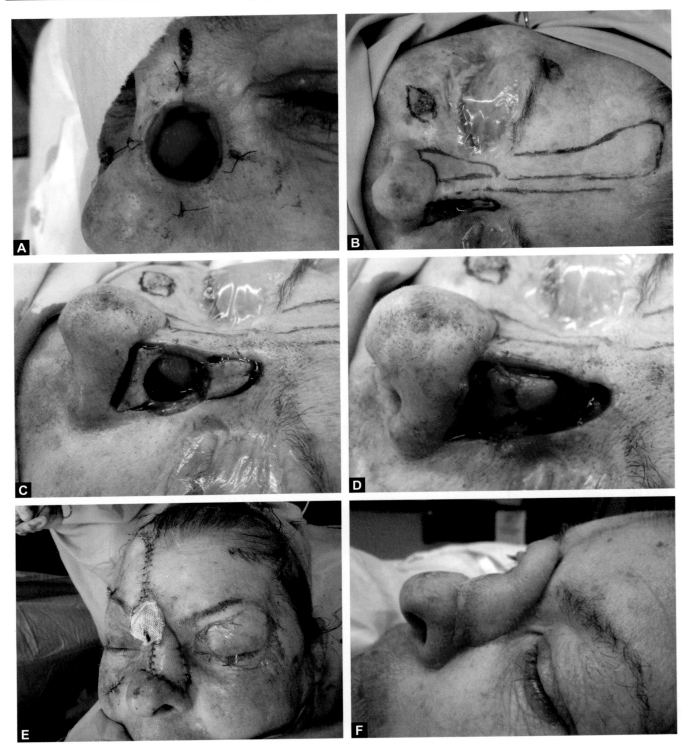

Figs 7A to F

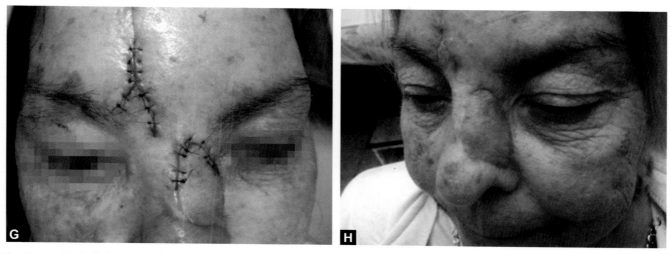

Figs 7A to H: Full-thickness defect of the nasal sidewall after Mohs excision for squamous cell carcinoma. Lining was restored with turnover flaps that defined the esthetic sidewall unit. Figure 7F shows the flap 4 weeks later, just before division of the pedicle. Figure 7H shows the result 4 weeks after division

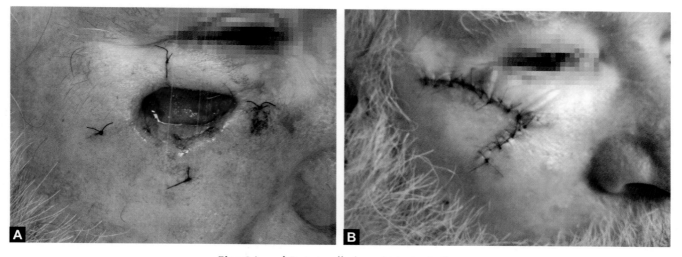

Figs 8A and B: Laterally-based Mustarde flap

Tarsus is replaced if needed with upper lid graft or flap, or nasal septal mucochondral graft.

The cheek flap (Figs 9 and 10) is a good solution for defects in the whole midface region.

The cheek/cervico facial flap can be extended to the pre-auricular, postauricular and the neck region and go down as far as the chest. The blood supply then arrives also from branches of the submental and transverse cervical artery. Flaps that extend to the chest are further supplied by perforants of the internal mammary artery. A cut at the nasolabial fold can be added for better advancement and hide of the "dog ear" formed by the rotation. Tension should be avoided in the medial canthus and lower eyelid regions.

ANTIA-BUCH FLAP

First introduced by Antia and Buch in 1967, this chondro-cutaneous flap is the flap of choice for reconstruction of 1–2 cm defects of the helical rim (Figs 11 and 12).[11]

It is a rotation-advancement random flap. Its blood supply arrives from branches of the posterior auricular and occipital arteries that supply the posterior ear.

The flap is raised at the caudal part of the defect and the mobility of the lobule enables us to cover most of the defects. When needed, the superior part can be released too with a V-Y advancement of the helical root. The posterior skin pedicle should be well-separated from the concha. The

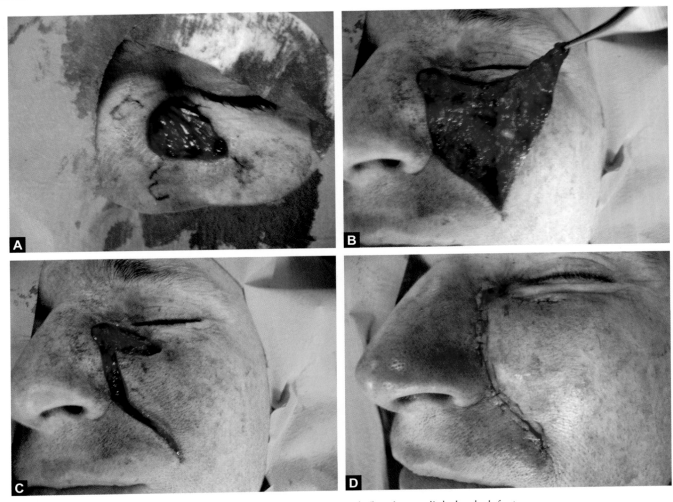

Figs 9A to D: Inferiorly-based cheek flap for medial cheek defect

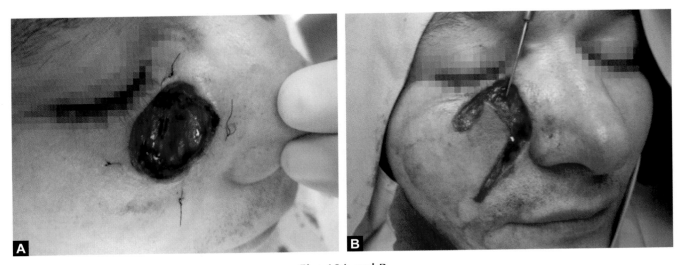

Figs 10A and B

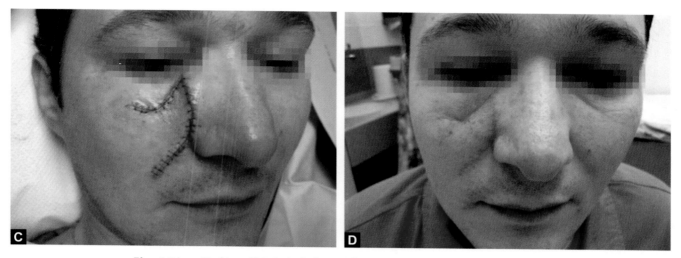

Figs 10A to D: (A to C) Inferiorly-based flap after four rounds of Mohs surgery for basal cell carcinoma; (D) Picture was taken 6 weeks after the operation

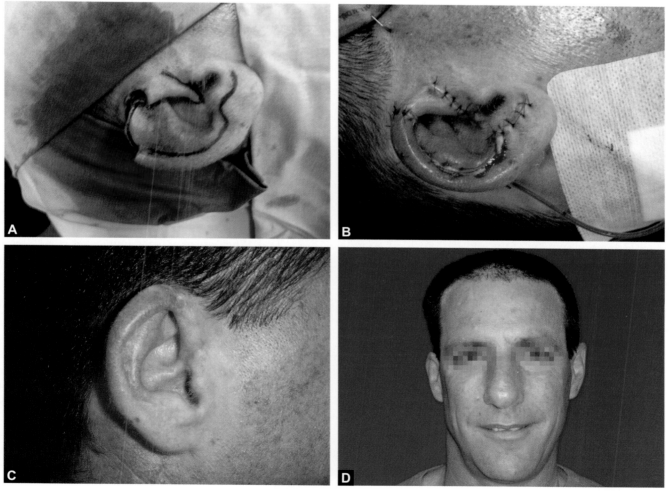

Figs 11A to D: Antia-Buch flap for helical defect, after wide excision of malignant melanoma. The lower and the upper flaps were used

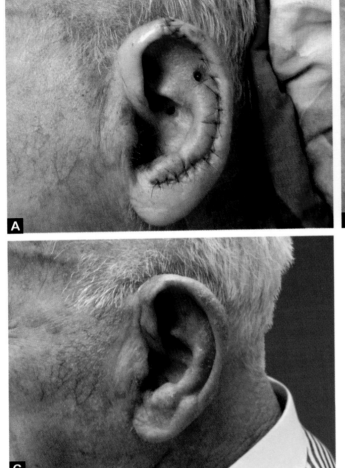

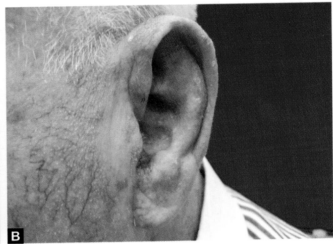

Figs 12A to C: (A) Antia-Buch flap at the end of the operation; and (B and C) Two months later

perimeter of the antihelix might need to be reduced in order to avoid anterior cupping of the ear. Scars are hidden in the interhelical groove.

HIGHLIGHTS

I. Indications
- Facial defects due to tumor resections or trauma
- Defects that cannot be closed primarily
- Most defects can be reconstructed by local tissue.

II. Contraindications
- Absence of tumor free margins. Free margins are best achieved by Mohs surgery.
- Questionable viability of tissue, mainly after trauma. It is better to wait for clear demarcation between viable and dead tissue.

- Anticoagulation treatment is a relative contraindication. When use of a flap is anticipated, it is better to adjust or stop anticoagulants with approval of the appropriate specialist.

III. Complications
- Immediate and early bleeding should be prevented by thorough control. Exploration should be considered liberally.
- Infections are best prevented by proper surgical technique. Antibiotics should be considered when encountering oral or nasal mucosa, when there is use of free cartilage graft and patients condition, such as diabetes or risk of SBE.
- Flap ischemia and necrosis are quite rare and could be attributed to poor design of flap or patient factors, such as smoking or vascular disease. When ischemia is anticipated, surgeon should consider

delaying the flap by suturing it back at the donor site and insetting it 2–3 weeks later.

- Each flap has its specific design considerations as mentioned before for avoiding asymmetry and esthetic misshapes.

IV. Special Considerations

- When in doubt, it is always better to postpone the reconstruction. In most cases, wounds can be left open for days.
- General anesthesia should be considered for large or complicated reconstructions.

REFERENCES

1. Esser JFS. Gestielite Lokale Nasenplastik mit Zweizipfligem Lappen, Deckung des Sekundaren Defektes vom Ersten Zipfel durch den Zweiten. Dtsch Z Chir. 1918;143:385-90.
2. Zitelli JA. The bilobed flap for nasal reconstruction. Arch Dermatol. 1989;125:957-9.
3. Moy RL, Grossfeld JS, Baum M, et al. Reconstruction of the nose utilizing a bilobed flap. Int J Dermatol. 1994;33:657-60.
4. Barron JN, Emmett AJJ. Subcutaneous pedicle flaps. Br J Plast Surg. 1965;18:51.
5. Hagerty RF, Smith W. The nasolabial cheek flap. 1958;24:506.
6. Rohrich R, Connard MH. The superiorly based nasolabial flap for simultaneous alar and cheek reconstruction. Plast Reconstruct Surg. 2001;108:1727-30.
7. Thornton JF, Weathers WM. Nasolabial flap for nasal tip reconstruction. Plast Reconst Surg. 2008;122:775-81.
8. Menick FJ. Nasal reconstruction with a forehead flap. Clin Plast Surg. 2009;36(3):443-59.
9. Little SC, Hughley BB, Park SS. Complications with forehead flaps in nasal reconstruction. Laryngoscope. 2009;119(6):1093-9.
10. Mustarde JC. The use of flaps in the orbital region. Plast Reconst Surg. 1970;45(2):146-50.
11. Antia NH, Buch MS. Chondrocutaneous advancement flap for the marginal defect of the ear. Plast Reconst Surg. 1967;39(5):472-7.

Chapter **50**

Pectoralis Major Pedicled Flap for Head and Neck Reconstruction

Yoav Barnea, Eyal Gur, Aharon Amir

INTRODUCTION

The pectoralis major pedicled flap based on the thoraco-acromial artery was first described by Ariyan in 1979. Its utility in soft tissue reconstruction was quickly recognized and it developed into the "workhorse" flap for head and neck reconstruction, abandoning the previous deltopectoral flap. Its advantages include a readily identifiable and reliable blood supply, relative ease of harvest, low donor site morbidity, and proximity to the head and neck, with no need to change the patient's position. Its relative bulk can prove advantageous in filling large defects or protecting vital structures in the head and neck and its large skin island can cover large defects or defects involving two epithelial surfaces.

In recent years, the refinement of microsurgical techniques has allowed for the increasing use of free tissue transfer for head and neck reconstruction. Nevertheless, the pectoralis major pedicled flap remains the reconstructive technique of choice in selected patients and may offer particular advantages in salvage reconstruction. Furthermore, the scope of reconstructive options is greatly expanded with the use of simultaneous free-tissue transfer and pedicled pectoralis flap.

ANATOMY

The pectoralis major is a large and fan-shaped muscle with two proximal heads: (i) the clavicular; and (ii) sternocostal (Fig. 1). The origin of the muscle is from the medial half of the clavicle (clavicular head) and the anterior surface of the sternum, superior six costal cartilages, and the aponeurosis of the external oblique muscle (sternocostal head). It inserts into the intertubercular groove of humerus. The thoraco-acromial artery provides its major blood supply entering the muscle at the midclavicular point, while the intercostal perforators arising from the internal mammary artery provide a segmental blood supply. The medial and lateral anterior thoracic nerves provide innervation for the muscle entering posteriorly and laterally. The action of the pectoralis major is to flex, adduct and rotate the arm medially.

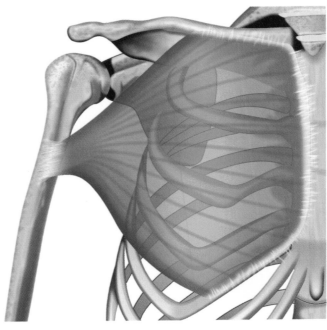

Fig. 1: Schematic drawing of the pectoralis major muscle

FLAP TYPES

Muscle Flap

Muscle flap—harvesting the muscle only, for coverage of vital head and neck structures. The flap can be buried or externally insetted, covered with a skin graft. Skin incisions commonly used are inframammary with or without accompanying superior incision and also lateral incision. All incisions avoid the medial skin at the level of 2nd–4th ribs preserving the internal mammary perforators for future deltopectoral skin flap (Figs 2A to C). When used, superior skin incision facilitates vascular pedicle dissection and easy mobilization of the flap during its transfer to the head and neck area.

Myocutaneous Flap

Myocutaneous flap comprising a single or double skin paddle over the muscle for the reconstruction of oral mucosa, skin or both (Figs 3A to C). The skin paddle is outlined caudally from the fourth costal cartilage level and along the inframammary fold, to facilitate the flap arc of rotation and preserve upper medial skin (see the surgical technique). Blood supply to the anterior chest skin inferior to the fourth costal cartilage is mainly through perforating vessels derived from the internal thoracic artery and its anterior intercostal branches on the fourth, fifth and sixth intercostal spaces. During flap harvest, the perforating vessels are divided off the chest wall thereby opening choke vessels inside the muscle. This facilitates blood flow from the vascular pedicle (pectoral branch of the thoracoacromial artery) to skin perforating vessels inferior to the fourth intercostal space level.

Osteomyocutaneous

Osteomyocutaneous—harvesting the muscle with a segment of rib or the sternum. The bone is supplied by vessels from the muscle to the overlying periosteum.

Combination

Combination—combining the pectoralis muscle flap with other flaps, mainly free flaps, or regional flaps, e.g. deltopectoral flap, trapezius flap (Figs 4A and B). The pectoralis

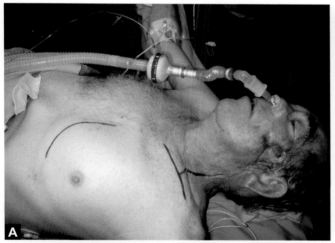

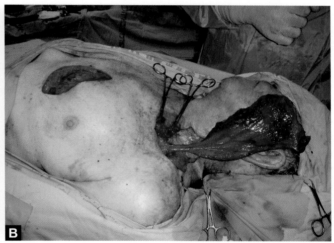

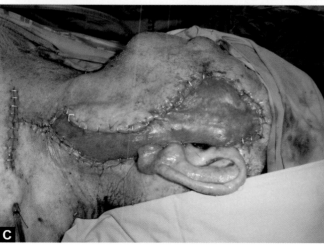

Figs 2A to C: Pectoralis major muscle flap. (A) Upper and lower skin incisions; (B) Harvest of the flap with vascular pedicle dissection; (C) Inset of the flap with split-thickness skin graft coverage

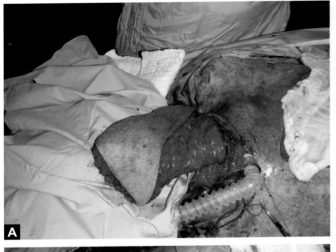

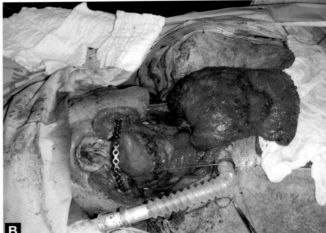

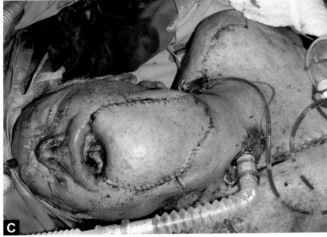

Figs 3A to C: Pectoralis major myocutaneous flap. (A) Harvest of the flap; (B) Defect including mandible with surgical plate, oral mucosa, and skin of lower lip, chin and neck; (C) Inset of the flap with a large skin paddle

flap offers large and pliable soft tissue component to a large defect, providing protection to major vessels at risk of rupture and preventing possible breakdown with the additional skin paddle.

SURGICAL TECHNIQUE

Pectoralis Myocutaneous Flap

Skin paddle is outlined in an area comprising superiorly the fourth costal cartilage, inferiorly the seventh costal cartilage, medially the outer edge of the sternum and laterally 2–3 cm from the edge of the pectoralis major muscle. In practice, skin incision or skin paddle are marked at the inframammary fold extending cephalad to the fourth costal level and 2–3 cm lateral to the muscle edge. The skin paddle marking is designed to the defect size (Fig. 5A) and is shaped as gull wings at its lateral aspect to match inframammary side length and facilitate closure (Fig. 5B). Skin paddle dissection

is carried with attention being taken to bevel the incision outward, mainly upward over the muscle to include more perforators arising from the muscle. The skin may be sutured to the underlying muscle to prevent its shearing. Dissection is commenced at the areolar plane over the muscle, i.e. superficially up to the clavicle exposing the lateral margins of the muscle and preserving 2nd–4th perforators medially. The inferior edge of muscle is identified by blunt or monopolar cautery dissection, and the muscle is detached from its sternocostal attachments using monopolar cautery (Fig. 5C). This allows visual identification of the vascular pedicles (lateral thoracic and thoracoacromial arteries) on the undersurface of the muscle. Blunt dissection and monopolar cautery are used to dissect the muscle from the chest wall. A crease can be noted between the clavicular and sternocostal heads of the muscle and at this level the vascular pedicle is dissected off the muscle (Fig. 5D). The sternocostal head is divided first laterally at a line lateral to the pedicle and medially lateral to the internal mammary perforators to the

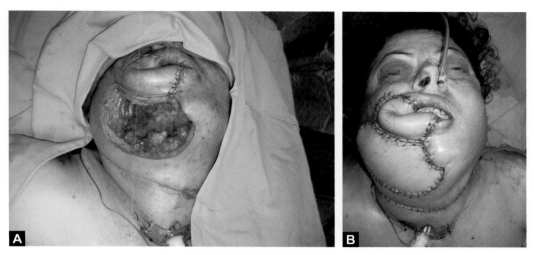

Figs 4A and B: Flap combination for large and complex defects. (A) Upper and lower lip reconstruction using a free radial forearm flap; (B) Combining a pectoralis major myocutaneous flap for neck skin defect and coverage of the vessels in the neck

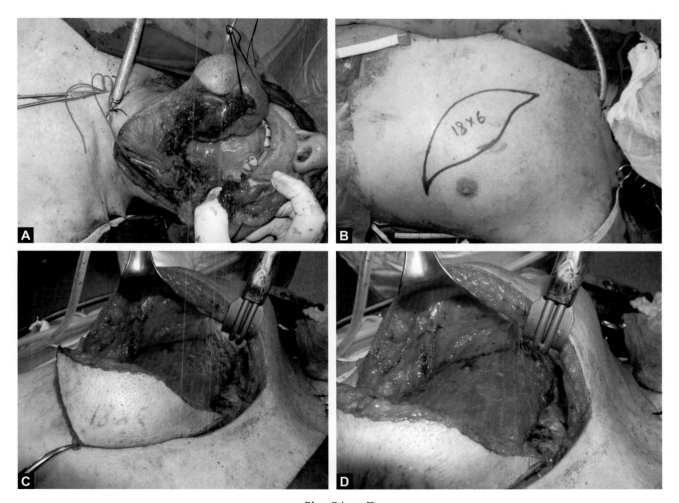

Figs 5A to D

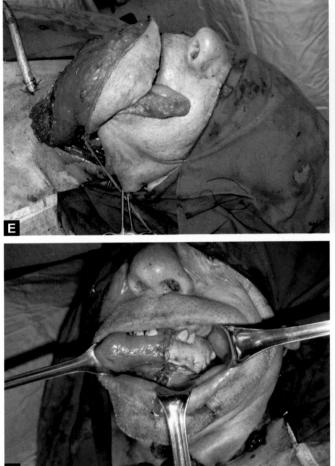

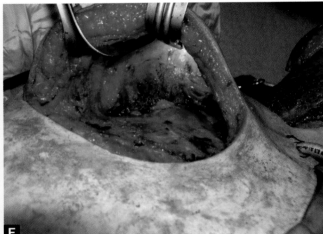

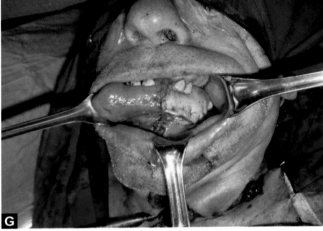

Figs 5A to G: Surgical technique harvesting pectoralis major myocutaneous flap. (A) Measuring the skin defect at the recipient site; (B) Marking the skin paddle accordingly, in a gull-wing fashion; (C) Harvest of the flap; (D) Dissection of the pedicle off the clavicular pectoral head; (E) Skeletonization of the pedicle for pedicle length gain; (F) Subcutaneous tunneling over the clavicle for flap delivery; (G) Insetting of the flap

intact skin over 2nd–4th ribs avoiding unnecessary muscle bulk in the neck. The clavicular head is detached medially off the chest wall and the clavicle exposing the pedicle underneath. The pedicle is further dissected bluntly and with scissors up to the clavicle allowing adequate mobilization. Clavicular head may be left attached to the chest wall with the flap passed under it after incising its attachments to the clavicle. Further mobilization allows the identification of the motor nerve to the pectoralis muscle. The nerve is divided to reduce tethering and avoid later annoying muscular activity. Skeletonization of the pectoral branch of the thoracoacromial vessels to the branching off point permits further gain in pedicle length. A subcutaneous tunnel is created over the clavicle and is assisted from the neck side, enlarged using monopolar cautery allowing the passage of the flap (Fig. 5E). The flap is then delivered through the tunnel and insetted (Figs 5F and G). Further debulking of the muscle after transposition over the clavicle

can be done at this time if necessary to reduce muscular bulge. A closed suction drain is placed both at the chest donor area and at the recipient site.

HIGHLIGHTS

I. Indications
- Primary head and neck reconstruction (buried flap, single skin paddle, double skin paddle)
- Salvage reconstructive procedure
- Combined with free flap
- Poor recipient vessels.

II. Operative Technique
- Skin paddle design
- Pedicle dissection and flap mobilization
- Delivery to the recipient site and insetting.

III. Complications
- Donor site morbidity (infection, bleeding, seroma, hematoma, wound breakdown)
- Flap necrosis (partial/total skin and/or muscle)
- Recipient site morbidity (dehiscence, fistula, hematoma, infection).

ADDITIONAL READING

1. Ariyan S. The pectoralis major myocutaneous flap. A versatile flap for reconstruction in the head and neck. Plast Reconstr Surg. 1979;63(1):73-81.
2. Chepeha DB, Annich G, Pynnonen MA, et al. Pectoralis major myocutaneous flap vs revascularized free tissue transfer: complications, gastrostomy tube dependence and hospitalization. Arch Otolaryngol Head Neck Surg. 2004;130(2):181-6.
3. Dedivitis RA, Guimarães AV. Pectoralis major musculocutaneous flap in head and neck cancer reconstruction. World J Surg. 2002;26(1):67-71.
4. Joseph CA, Gregor RT, Davidge-Pitts KJ, et al. The versatility of the pectoralis major myocutaneous flap. Head Neck Surg. 1985;7(5):365-8.
5. Kroll SS, Evans GR, Goldberg D, et al. A comparison of resource costs for head and neck reconstruction with free and pectoralis major flaps. Plast Reconstr Surg. 1997;99(5):1282-6.
6. Liu R, Gullane P, Brown D, et al. Pectoralis major myocutaneous pedicled flap in head and neck reconstruction: retrospective review of indications and results in 244 consecutive cases at the Toronto General Hospital. J Otolaryngol. 2001;30(1):34-40.
7. Mehrhof AI, Rosenstock A, Neifeld JP, et al. The pectoralis major myocutaneous flap in head and neck reconstruction. Analysis of complications. Am J Surg. 1983;146(4):478-82.
8. Milenović A, Virag M, Uglesić V, et al. The pectoralis major flap in head and neck reconstruction: first 500 patients. J Craniomaxillofac Surg. 2006;34(6):340-3. Epub 2006 Jul 24.
9. Righi PD, Weisberger EC, Slakes SR, et al. The pectoralis major myofascial flap: clinical applications in head and neck reconstruction. Am J Otolaryngol. 1998;19(2):96-101.
10. Vartanian JG, Carvalho AL, Carvalho SM, et al. Pectoralis major and other myofascial/myocutaneous flaps in head and neck cancer reconstruction: experience with 437 cases at a single institution. Head Neck. 2004;26(12):1018-23.
11. Zbar RI, Funk GF, McCulloch TM, et al. Pectoralis major myofascial flap: a valuable tool in contemporary head and neck reconstruction. Head Neck. 1997;19(5):412-8.

Chapter **51**

Facial Paralysis Reconstruction
Focus on Long-lasting Facial Paralysis, Cross-face Nerve Grafting and Free Gracilis Muscle Transfer

Eyal Gur, Ron Zuker, Ehud Arad

INTRODUCTION

Paralysis of the facial mimetic muscles causes loss of voluntary facial movement, loss of involuntary facial expression and dysfunction in facial tone. It is a devastating condition with profound functional, aesthetic and psychological consequences. Symptoms include ocular dryness and tearing, speech difficulties, oral incontinence, impairment in mastication and obstruction of nasal airway. Significant emotional distress is the result of facial disfigurement, impaired communication and social dysfunction.

Facial paralysis manifests as a spectrum of conditions, presenting as either unilateral or bilateral and ranging from partial to complete weakness. Etiology is either congenital or acquired, the latter including neoplasms, trauma, infection, iatrogenic and idiopathic causes.

Reanimation of the paralyzed face focuses on restoration of form and function; it is an immense reconstructive challenge necessitating multidisciplinary management. The goals are to achieve protection of the eye, facial symmetry at rest, voluntary symmetric-facial movement and to restore involuntary mimetic facial expression. Perhaps the most significant unit for reconstruction, from a functional and esthetic perspective, is the buccal-zygomatic muscle complex (BZMC) which is responsible for smiling and for tone of cheeks.

PREOPERATIVE EVALUATION AND THE RELEVANT SURGICAL OPTIONS

Static Correction of Facial Asymmetry

Static procedures aim to correct asymmetry at rest. A combination of procedures is commonly used. Fascial slings are used to achieve symmetry and correct oral incontinence. Fascia lata or various tendons are harvested and are placed between the orbicularis oris muscle and the temporal fascia, suspending the commissure at a desired position. This is done in conjunction with face lift. Asymmetry can also be balanced by brow lift, blepharoplasty (of lower and upper eyelids), fat injection or suction, and nasolabial accentuation.

Dynamic Reanimation of the Paralyzed Face

Dynamic reanimation attempts to restore symmetry both at rest and while smiling. Three elements are required for the formation of a smile: neural input, a functional muscle innervated by the nerve and proper muscle arrangement.

Reconstructive modalities can be classified by two basic criteria—whether reconstruction is based on the facial nerve or on a different cranial nerve, and whether the working muscle unit is the original BZMC or a transferred muscle flap.

Facial nerve-based reanimation can be based on either an ipsilateral or contralateral facial nerve, depending on the presence of a functional branch or stump. Duration of paralysis is the principal determinant for the need for muscle transfer; if duration is less than 12 months, the BZMC is assumed to be viable. Muscles become near-irreversibly atrophic by 24 months, in which case muscle transfer is indicated.

Acute or Recent Facial Nerve Paralysis Reconstruction

Primary facial nerve repair is possible in cases of recent trauma to the facial nerve. Within 72 hours from injury, direct suturing of the stumps may be achieved; otherwise, a sural cable nerve graft is used to interconnect the distal stumps of the zygomatico-buccal facial branches with an ipsilateral trunk of the facial nerve.

In cases of recent paralysis in which a functional facial nerve branch is available only on the contralateral face, a cross-face sural nerve graft is used to relay facial nerve input across the face to the BZMC. Axons from the contralateral facial nerve regenerate through the sheath of the graft and innervate the muscle over 4–6 months. Since muscle atrophy can develop while the facial nerve regenerates, an ipsilateral motor nerve (either masseter or hypoglossal) is transposed to serve as a temporary innervator ("baby-sitter") to the muscle (Fig. 1). Thus, muscle tone is preserved while spontaneous smiling is to be restored.

Long-Lasting Facial Paralysis

Nonmicrosurgical facial reanimation: Patients that are unsuitable or do not wish to undergo a microsurgical procedures may be reconstructed by transfer of local muscles flaps, namely the temporalis or masseter muscles. This is a simple, one-stage procedure, which usually achieves fare static and dynamic results. However, it does not provide for a spontaneous smile and donor-site morbidity may be significant.

Free gracilis muscle connected to ipsilateral facial nerve stump: Facial nerve-based reanimation for long-lasting paralysis necessitates both reinnervation and muscle transfer. When an ipsilateral nerve is available, a one-stage free gracilis muscle flap transfer is performed. An innervated-free gracilis muscle flap is harvested from the thigh and transferred to the paralyzed side of the face. The flap is inset subcutaneously in the paralyzed cheek. The blood vessels of the flap are anastomosed to facial vessels and its motor nerves sutured to the available ipsilateral facial nerve branch.

Free gracilis muscle flap connected to masseter nerve (cranial nerve V— trigeminal): Nonfacial nerve reanimation is based either on the ipsilateral motor nerve to the masseter or on the ipsilateral hypoglossal nerve. Thus, the stimulus to create smiling movement depends on voluntary actions such as teeth clenching or movement of the tongue. These efforts may become more natural over time. The need for muscle transfer is dependent on duration of paralysis. In cases of recent paralysis, a sural cable nerve graft can connect these nerves to the BZMC nerve stump. For long-lasting paralysis, one stage free gracilis muscle transfer to masseter motor branch is performed.

Cross-Face Nerve Grafting and Free Gracilis Muscle Transfer

When a functional facial branch is only available on the other cheek, a two-stage cross-face sural nerve graft and free gracilis muscle transfer (two-stage procedure) is conducted. In the first stage, a sural nerve graft is harvested from the calf , coapted to a contralateral facial branch responsible for smiling stimulus, tunneled across the face to the paralyzed side and banked in the upper buccal sulcus (Fig. 2).

The second stage is scheduled 9 months later, and consists of free gracilis muscle flap transfer (see procedure technique below), but in this case the nerve is coapted to the cross-face graft. Reinnervation of the muscle commences after 4 months and reaches full capacity within a year.

CROSS-FACE NERVE GRAFTING AND FREE GRACILIS MUSCLE TRANSFER

Operative Technique

First Stage

Sural nerve harvest (Fig. 3): The sural nerve comes out from the tibial nerve at the popleteal region. It goes deep in between the two heads of the gastrocnemius muscle, emerges superficially along their course to the heal and is directed subcutaneously to the posterior aspect of the lateral malleolus. Around the malleolus, it splits into several small branches that give sensation the lateral aspect of the foot up to two-thirds the distance to the toes.

Dissection starts with a 1.5 horizontal or longitudinal incision about 3 cm from the popliteal fossa. The nerve is detected usually with the lesser saphenous vein escorting it along its course. The nerve is transected proximally and a dull edge vein stripper is introduced and bluntly dissects the nerve to a branching point where another skin opening is taken. The process is repeated until adequate nerve length is achieved (usually 11–14 cm).

Through a modified face lift incision extending slightly to the neck, superficial dissection of the superficial muscular aponeurotic system (SMAS) is taken until the anterior border of the parotid gland is reached. At that point, the dissection goes deeper to the thin fascia that covers the masseter muscle. Dissection of facial nerve branches at that level is limited to the space between the lower border of the zygoma to the Stenson duct.

Using a nerve stimulator, two relatively large facial nerve branches responsible for the motion of the BZMC will be identified (Fig. 4). The one with less intense stimulus on the BZMC and less effect on the orbicularis oculi will be sacrificed and serve as the donor motor nerve branch for the cross-face graft.

The sural nerve graft is then tunneled in a subcutaneous level across the cheek and upper lip to the contralateral upper buccal sulcus right above the canine tooth (Figs 5A and B). Through a buccal sulcus incision, it is verified that the nerve

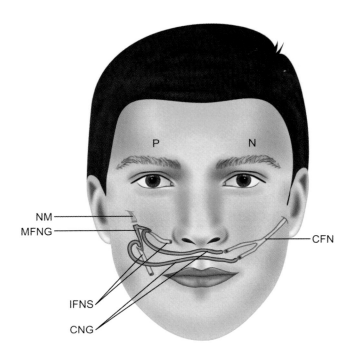

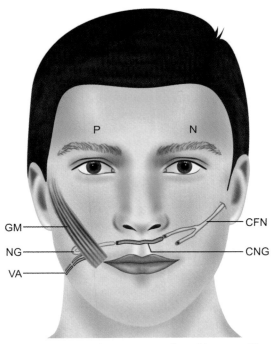

Fig. 1: The "baby-sitter" procedure: two cross face cable grafts together with cable graft from motor master nerve to facial nerve

P: Paralyzed; N: Normal; NM: Nerve to masseter; MFNG: Masseter to facial nerve grafts; CFN: Contralateral facial nerve; CNG: Cross face nerve graft; IFNS: Ipsilateral facial nerve stumps

Fig. 2: Two stage cross face nerve graft and free gracilis muscle transfer shown at the end of the process

P: Paralyzed; N: Normal; GM: Gracilis muscle; NG: Nerve of gracilis (part of obturator nerve); VA: Venous and arterial anastomoses; CFN: Contralateral facial nerve; CNG: Cross face nerve graft

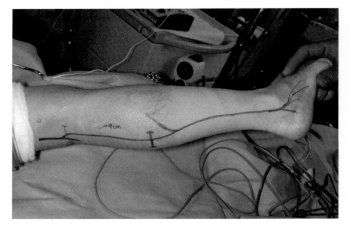

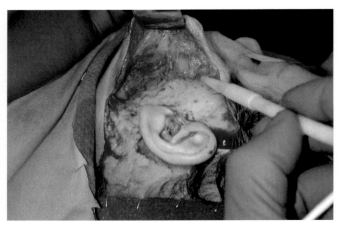

Fig. 3: Surface landmarks for sural nerve harvest

Fig. 4: Mapping and identification of the normal contralateral facial nerve branch to be sacrificed

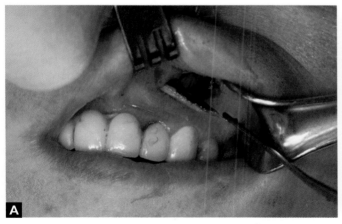

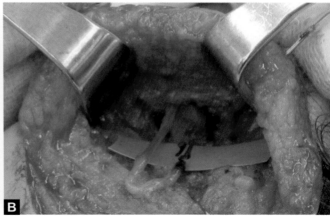

Figs 5A and B: Anastomosing and tunneling of the sural nerve graft to the paralyzed side upper buccal sulcus

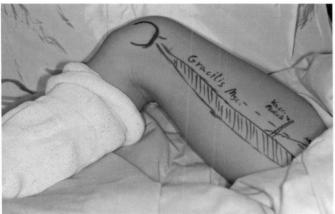

Fig. 6: Surface landmarks for gracilis muscle harvest

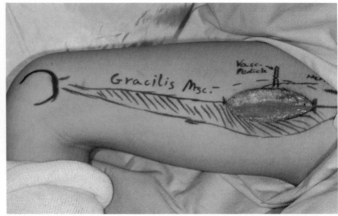

Fig. 7: Identification of the gracilis muscle in the thigh

graft reached its place and is marked with a 3/0 blue nylon suture. Under the operating microscope the sural nerve is anastomosed to the facial nerve branch in an interfascicular fashion and the incisions are closed over a Penrose drain.

Second Stage (Takes Place 8–9 Months after the First Stage)

Surface landmarks for gracilis muscle harvest (Fig. 6): A line is drawn in the medial side of the thigh, from the pubic tubercle to the medial chondyle of the femur. The gracilis muscle lies 3 cm posteriorly to that line. The neurovascular pedicle should be found about 8 cm from the tubercle.

An 8–10 cm incision is performed on the assumed location of the muscle. After the superficial and deep fascias of the thigh are incised longitudinally, the muscle should be present right under, with several perforating vessels coming from its surface to the skin (Fig. 7). The muscle is dissected lengthwise and the fascia between the gracilis and the adductor longus is incised.

Right behind that fascia, the neurovascular pedicle is identified and serves to identify and verify the gracilis muscle.

At that stage, the nerve is dissected to its origin from the obturator foramen and then transected to give the longest nerve pedicle as possible. The gracilis vascular pedicle is then dissected between the adductor longus and the adductor magnus up to its origin to the profunda femoris vessels (Fig. 8).

The gracilis muscle is further dissected and freed 360°. The muscle is then tailored by splitting it longitudinally to fit the narrow space of the cheek (Fig. 9). The muscle strip

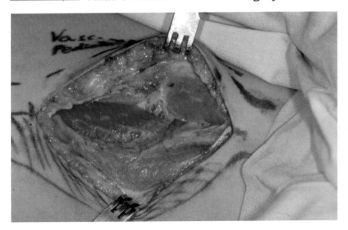

Fig. 8: Dissection of the neurovascular pedicle

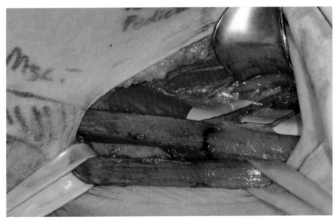

Fig. 9: Tailoring of the gracilis muscle

that is harvested may occasionally weight no more than 10 gm. The length of the needed muscle unit is measured in the cheek from the oral modiolus to the superficial temporal fascia superior to the auricular helix take-off and marked in the thigh when the knee is stretched. The knee is then flexed. And the muscle transected caudally and cephalically.

Along the transected muscle edge to be sutured to the modiolus, five 4/0 vicryl sutures are aligned to create a blocking point to the main stitches that will later connect the muscle to the modiolus. Only when the cheek recipient vessels are fully dissected and flow verified, the gracilis vessels are transected (Fig. 10).

A modified face lift incision is marked with an upward extension of 5 cm superior to the helix take-off and a short 2 cm curved neck extension about 1 cm caudal to the mandible angle (Fig. 11A). The incision line is infiltrated with lidocaine 2% - adrenalin 1:100,000 solution.

Subcutaneous dissection is carried out, leaving thin fatty layer under the skin flap (Fig. 11B). The dissection area covers a fan-shaped space from the full length of the skin incision to the modiolus and 1.5 cm along the upper and lower lips. It is important to notice the facial/angular artery near the oral commissure as a landmark for the appropriateness of the level of dissection.

At that stage, the facial artery and vein are dissected at their cross over point with the mandible where the artery will usually go anteriorly toward the commissure and the vein cephalically toward the anterior border of the masseter muscle. By compressing the cheek bulk from the inside the buccal fat pad is identified, dissected and resected to free space for the gracilis (Figs 11C and D).

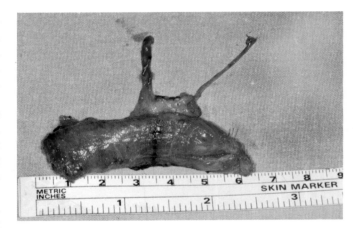

Fig. 10: Flap vessels are transected following placement of blocking stitches along muscle edge

Four 0 white vicryl sutures are looped through the remnants and fibrotic layer of the orbicularis oris: one at the modiolus, two (0.5 apart) at the upper lip and one at the lower lip. Careful placement of those stitches will determine the right natural pull of the mouth at motion and the accurate creation of the nasolabial fold (Fig. 12).

The intraoral upper buccal sulcus old scar from the cross-face procedure is reincised carefully revealing the marking stitch and the nerve ending of the cross-face nerve graft (Figs 13A and B). The very end of the cross-face graft is transected and sent for frozen section identification of viable peripheral nerve axons. A tunnel is created between the facial to the intraoral dissections and a vessel loop is transferred from one space to the other.

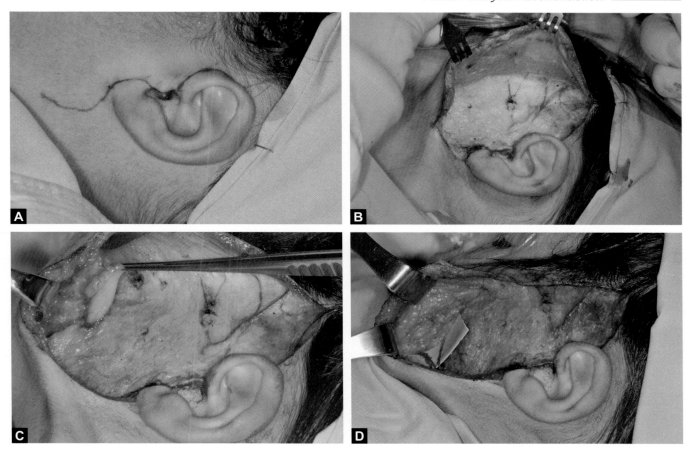

Figs 11A to D: Dissection of recipient paralyzed cheek. (A) Incision landmarks;
(B) Subcutaneous flap dissection; (C) Resection of fat pad; (D) Facial vessels dissected

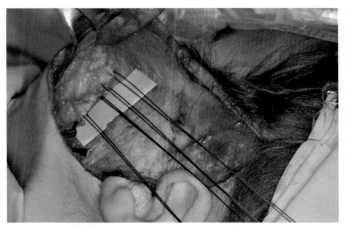

Fig. 12: Placement of anchoring
vicryl sutures at the modiolus

The gracilis muscle after detached from the thigh is transferred to the face. The 0 vicryl sutures are looped twice through it and through the old orbicularis to serve as a pulley that will help in mobilizing the flap to the modiolus and for securing it properly into place.

Only after arterial and venous anastomosis in the face and neural anastomosis in the buccal sulcus, the muscle is stretched to reach its origin in the temporal region above the auricle (Figs 14 and 15). It is secured by 4–5, 0 vicryl sutures that are placed by pulling the muscle and fixating the muscle at the point where the lip or modiolus move just slightly with the muscle pull. At the end of that part the oral commissure should be slightly pulled obliquely and upwards exposing the lateral upper teeth (Figs 16A and B).

At the end of the procedure, a Penrose drain is left in the operated cheek and a vacuum drain in the donor site in the thigh (Fig. 17).

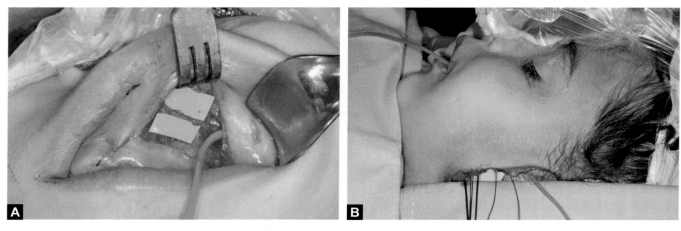

Figs 13A and B: Dissection of the cross-face nerve graft

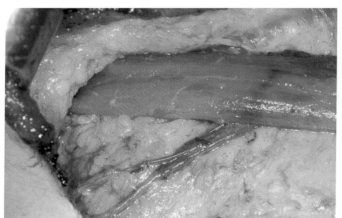

Fig. 14: Vessels and
nerve anastomosis

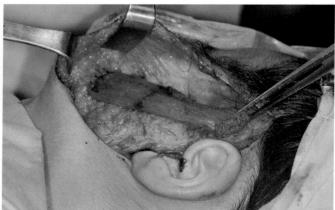

Fig. 15: Positioning and tension measurement
of the gracilis muscle

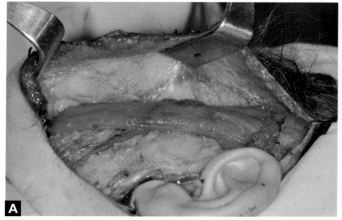

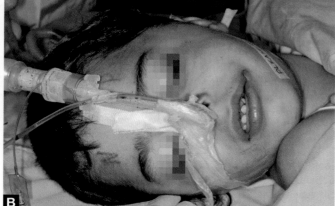

Figs 16A and B: Muscle flap secured with correct tension

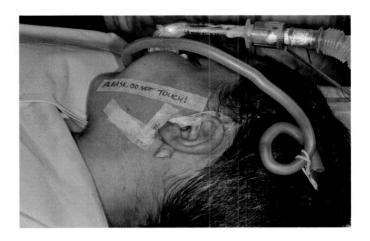

Fig. 17: A Penrose drain is left in the operated cheek

PRE- AND POSTOPERATIVE PHOTOS

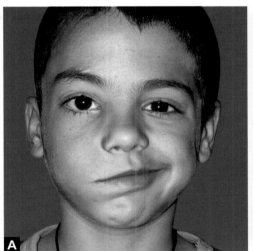

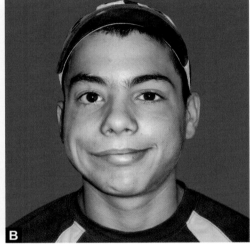

Figs 18A and B: Patient 1—congenital right complete facial paralysis

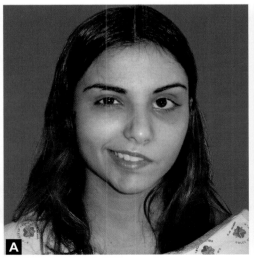

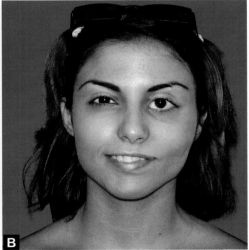

Figs 19A and B: Patient 2—facial paralysis due to AV malformation and intracranial hemorrhage

The skin is closed meticulously and a protecting sticker and a hook-splint is sutured to the patient's scalp and its hook is inserted to the oral commissure to protect the new muscle from sliding through the stitches and to protect the cheek from extra external pressure.

HIGHLIGHTS

I. Indications
- Acute or long-standing facial paralysis
- Acute facial paralysis should be reconstructed within 72 hours from injury onset, if proximal and distal facial nerve stumps are present on the paralyzed side
- Subacute facial paralysis reconstruction should be managed not later than a year after injury onset (before muscle atrophy occurred) whether ipsi- or contralateral facial nerve stumps (Babysitter procedure) are used. For patients over 50 years, a cross-face nerve graft should not be used and the masseter motor nerve should be connected to the distal, ipsilateral, facial nerve stump
- Long-standing facial paralysis scan be reconstructed at any time using the staged cross-face nerve graft and free gracilis transfer for patients younger than 50 years
- Long-standing facial paralysis scan be reconstructed at any time using the free gracilis transfer connected to a viable ipsilateral facial nerve stump (if present) at any age
- Long-standing facial paralysis scan be reconstructed at any time using free gracilis transfer connected to the masseter motor nerve for patients older than 50 years or for bilateral facial paralysis (including Möbius syndrome) patients.

II. Contraindications
- Current oncologic disease
- Medical status not permitting long anesthesia
- Major depression
- Unrealistic expectations.

III. Complications
- Injury to functioning facial nerve
- Recipient or donor site wound infection
- Recipient or donor site hematoma
- Failure to achieve facial motion or symmetry
- Facial bulge over gracilis muscle
- Inadequate motion or spastic transplanted muscle.

IV. Special Preoperative Considerations
- Assess whether there is a viable facial nerve stump on the paralyzed side
- If there is no viable ipsilateral facial nerve, is there a functioning facial nerve on the contralateral side

- Assess whether there is a viable facial muscles on the paralyzed side
- Choose the appropriate surgical approach for patients over 50 years
- Assure that the patient understands the nature of those long procedures and the long time lag until the final result shows. Assure reasonable expectations of the final results.

V. Special Intraoperative Considerations
- At first stage—cross-face nerve graft: pick a reasonably large nerve branch, but assure it does have a stronger nerve that does the same action
- Assure that the selected normal branch to be sacrificed does not play a major role in orbicularis oculi action
- Bank the cross-face nerve stump in a constant location and mark it with a thick (3/0) nylon suture—for the ease of retrieving it at the second stage
- At the second stage—treat the muscle gently and preserve its epimysium. Tailor the muscle to be transferred, to make it as thin, gentle and long as possible and needed, while not compromising the neurovascular pedicle that penetrates it
- Place the muscle obliquely from the modiolus to the fascia superior to the auricle.

VI. Special Postoperative Considerations
- Immediate extubation
- Do not use any vasopressor therapy even when blood pressure is low
- Admit the patient to a step down unit for 24 hours after surgery
- Protect the operated cheek by proper signaling and the designated splint
- When motion starts, several months after the procedure, the patient should practice daily, in front of a mirror, to strengthen the muscle action and create more symmetry with the healthy side smile.

ADDITIONAL READING

1. Aviv JE, Urken ML. Management of the paralyzed face with microneurovascular free muscle transfer. Arch Otolaryngol Head Neck Surg. 1992;118:909-12.
2. Bae YC, Zuker RM, Manktelow RT, et al. A comparison of commissure excursion following gracilis muscle transplantation for facial paralysis using a cross-face nerve graft versus the motor nerve to the masseter nerve. Plast Reconstr Surg. 2006;117:2407-13.
3. Braam MJ, Nicolai JP. Axonal regeneration rate through cross-face nerve grafts. Microsurgery. 1993;14:589-91.

4. Ferreira MC, Marques de Faria JC. Result of microvascular gracilis transplantation for facial paralysis – personal series. Clin Plastic Surg. 2002;29:515-22.

5. Harrison DH. The treatment of unilateral and bilateral facial palsy using free muscle transfers. Clin Plastic Surg. 2002;29:539-49.

6. Kumar PA, Hassan KM. Cross-face nerve graft with free-muscle transfer for reanimation of the paralyzed face: a comparative study of the single-stage and two-stage procedures. Plast Reconstr Surg. 2002;109:451-62.

7. Manktelow RT, Tomat LR, Zuker RM, et al. Smile reconstruction in adults with free muscle transfer innervated by the masseter motor nerve: effectiveness and cerebral adaptation. Plast Reconstr Surg. 2006;118:885-99.

8. Rose EH. Autogenous fascia lata grafts: clinical applications in reanimation of the totally or partially paralyzed face. Plast Reconstr Surg. 2005;116:20-32. (discussion 33-5)

9. Takushima A, Harii K, Asato H, et al. Revisional operations improve results of neurovascular free muscle transfer for treatment of facial paralysis. Plast Reconstr Surg. 2005;116:371-80.

10. Tate JR, Tollefson TT. Advances in facial reanimation. Curr Opin Otolaryngol Head Neck Surg. 2006;14:242-8.

11. Terzis JK, Noah EM. Dynamic restoration in Möbius and Möbius-like patients. Plast Reconstr Surg. 2003;111:40-55.

12. Terzis JK, Noah EM. Analysis of 100 cases of free-muscle transplantation for facial paralysis. Plast Reconstr Surg. 1997;99(7):1905-21.

13. Terzis JK, Olivares FS. Long-term outcomes of free-muscle transfer for smile restoration in adults. Plast Reconstr Surg. 2009;123:877-88.

14. Ueda K, Harii K, Asato H, et al. Neurovascular free muscle transfer combined with cross-face nerve grafting for the treatment of facial paralysis in children. Plast Reconstr Surg. 1998;101:1765-73.

15. Yoleri L, Songur E, Mavioglu H, et al. Cross-facial nerve grafting as an adjunct to hypoglossal-facial nerve crossover in reanimation of early facial paralysis: clinical and electrophysiological evaluation. Ann Plast Surg. 2001;46:301-7.

Chapter **52**

Surgical Approaches for Oral Cavity Cancer

Jatin Shah

INTRODUCTION

Surgery is the preferred and most frequently used treatment for oral cavity cancers. It is employed as a single modality for early stage cancers. In advanced stage cancers, surgery is generally followed by postoperative radiation or chemoradiation. The goals of treating a primary oral cavity tumor are durable local control, preservation or restoration of form and function, and minimizing the sequela of treatment. Therefore, selecting the appropriate surgical approach is important for achieving these goals.

PREOPERATIVE EVALUATION AND ANESTHESIA

Preoperative evaluation of an oral cavity cancer should include either biopsy of the tumor or a review of the slides from a previous biopsy, if one has already been performed. Pathologic assessment should include the tumor histology, grade and depth of invasion, if depth is evaluable from the biopsy. Along with a review of the tumor pathology, careful physical examination is the most important and informative aspect of preoperative evaluation. Inspection and palpation of the tumor is done to document its size, location, involvement of adjacent structures, as well as its depth and extension to other sites within the oral cavity. These factors are used to determine the T stage as well as the surgical approach needed for successful tumor removal. Examination of the entire upper aerodigestive tract should be performed to look for synchronous lesions. Either indirect mirror examination or flexible laryngoscopy in the office is a necessary part of a comprehensive head and neck examination in these patients.

Examination of the tumor is again carried out under anesthesia at the time of surgery, and in appropriate cases, endoscopy should also be performed for adequate assessment of the tumor, and other parts of the upper aerodigestive tract.

Determining the need for surgical management of the mandible and/or maxilla is a critical part of the preoperative evaluation. Tumor involvement of these structures is assessed first during the physical examination in the office. Adequate uninvolved soft tissue between the tumor and the mandible or the maxilla indicates that these structures do not need to be resected. If the tumor is adjacent or adherent to the bone, then imaging is indicated to assess the extent of invasion. If there is no cortical bone invasion, then an en bloc marginal mandibulectomy or partial maxillectomy is oncologically safe in order to obtain clear margins around the tumor. If there is cortical bone invasion, then segmental resection of the mandible or infrastructure maxillectomy is necessary to achieve safe margins.

Radiological imaging of small primary oral cavity tumors, such as T1 or T2 tumors, is generally not indicated. Although, neck imaging may be required depending on the status of cervical lymph nodes and the depth and size of the primary tumor. Larger tumors and tumors that clinically involve the mandible or maxilla, however, should be imaged. If the neck is being evaluated with a contrast enhanced CT scan, the scan should be extended superiorly to include the oral cavity. Cortex erosion seen on bone windows of a computed tomography (CT) scan has high specificity for tumor invasion. A panoramic X-ray of the mandible is useful for evaluation of the alveolar process as well as the tooth roots and for planning mandibulotomy or mandibulectomy sites between the roots. Magnetic resonance imaging (MRI) is good for assessing spread within the bone, if there is known cortical invasion. MRI is also useful for assessing soft tissue extension into the base of the tongue and perineural invasion of larger (named) nerves, particularly when this is clinically suspected. Patients with trismus due to fibrosis from prior treatment, such as radiation or due to tumor invasion into the pterygoid space or from other pathology, such as submucous fibrosis can all limit access for examination. If physical assessment of the tumor is limited due to trismus, then imaging, use of fiberoptic endoscopy in the office and examination under anesthesia are needed.

Nasotracheal intubation should be used routinely for anesthesia, since it improves access and exposure during surgery, except when an upper cheek flap or maxillary resection is being performed. Full paralysis under general anesthesia is helpful for obtaining the best exposure possible for posteriorly located tumors and also reduces bothersome muscle contraction while using an electrocautery.

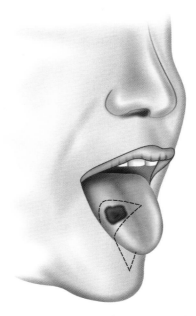

Fig. 1: Peroral approach can be used for most small oral cavity tumors

SURGICAL TECHNIQUE

The surgical approach selected for excision of tumors of the oral cavity depends on the size of the tumor (T stage), location (anterior vs posterior), proximity to bone (mandible or maxilla) and the need to perform neck dissection. The most commonly employed approaches are as follows:
- Peroral
- Lower cheek flap
- Mandibulotomy
- Visor flap
- Upper cheek flap.

Peroral

Most early-stage tumors (T1 and T2 tumors) of the oral cavity including the mobile tongue, floor of mouth, buccal mucosa and, upper and lower gum can be safely excised and reconstructed through a peroral approach. The obvious advantage of operating through the mouth is that there are no external incisions. The esthetic and functional consequences of peroral resection are generally quite minimal, once healing is complete.

Oncologically effective surgery requires obtaining adequate margins in all dimensions around the tumor. This requires continuous assessment of the tumor margins with palpation and inspection during surgery. Frozen sections should be obtained from the margins of the surgical defect to ensure oncologically complete resection. A self-retaining retractor placed on the contralateral molars is helpful to keep the mouth open. The tongue can be grasped with an Adair clamp or with a large stitch, such as a 2-0 silk and retracted to one side or the other side. Small Richardson retractors are used to retract the cheeks. For mobile tongue tumors, a transverse wedge excision is generally preferred over longitudinally oriented excisions (Fig. 1). A guarded tip should be used for electrocautery and the patient's lips should be carefully protected from secondary cautery burn injury. Resections that are anterior and include a small portion of bone, such as an alveolectomy or limited partial maxillectomy can also be performed using the peroral approach. Careful assessment of the mouth opening for adequacy of exposure is critical to successful peroral resection.

Lower Cheek Flap

Tumors requiring resection of any part of the mandible or large posterolateral tumors that cannot be accessed via a peroral approach can be adequately exposed and excised using a lower cheek flap. As with peroral resection, nasotracheal intubation improves exposure in these cases. An orotracheal tube also has the disadvantage of distorting the lip and mouth anatomy making it difficult to perform an esthetic midline incision and closure.

A lower midline lip-splitting incision is performed through the skin, orbicularis oris muscle and mucosa. The skin is incised with a scalpel but the rest of the procedure is carried out with the electrocautery. During subsequent use of the electrocautery, care is taken to avoid injury to the skin of the chin and lip. Dissection is carried down to the periosteum of the mandible anteriorly. The incision can be extended down into the neck if a neck dissection is

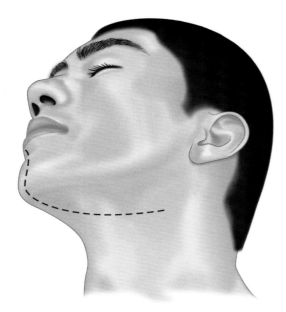

Fig. 2: A midline lip-splitting incision
is used for raising a lower cheek flap

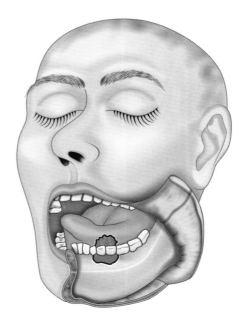

Fig. 3: Reflecting the lower cheek flap laterally exposes
the mandible and the posterior oral cavity

to be performed (Fig. 2). A midline incision over the chin generally gives the best cosmetic outcome. The periosteum should be left intact on the mandible as it is an important source of blood supply and will facilitate bone healing. A mucosal incision is performed in the gingivobuccal sulcus on the side where the flap is being raised. A cuff of mucosa of at least 1 cm should be left on the gingival side when making this incision so that there is adequate mucosa to suture to, while closing. The cheek flap is elevated off the mandible, working laterally (Fig. 3). The mental branch of the inferior alveolar nerve, as it exits from the mental foramen inferior to the second premolar tooth, has to be divided to permit elevation of the lower cheek flap posteriorly. If the cheek flap is extended to the neck for exposure of the inferior or posterior mandible or for performing a neck dissection, attention should be given to identifying and preserving the marginal mandibular branch of the facial nerve. Loss of lip sensation from division of the mental nerve and lip depression resulting from injury to the marginal mandibular branch of the facial nerve can affect the oral competence and result in cosmetic deformity respectively. While sacrifice of the mental nerve is unavoidable when raising a lower cheek flap, extreme care should be exercised in protecting and preserving the marginal branch of the facial nerve to avoid its functional and esthetic deformity.

After raising a cheek flap, there is an excellent exposure of the mandible and if necessary, a marginal or segmental mandibulectomy can be performed for resection of the tumor with surrounding mucosa, soft tissue and involved

underlying bone in an en bloc fashion. The techniques for marginal and segmental mandibulectomy are described in separate chapters. Raising a cheek flap gives good exposure to the posterior oral cavity and resection of tumors of the tongue, floor of mouth, buccal mucosa, upper or lower gum, retromolar trigone and soft palate can be performed through this approach. It also allows good access for insetting a flap for reconstruction of the surgical defect in these areas, if one is needed.

Mandibulotomy

Larger lesions of the posterior oral cavity, such as those of the posterior floor of the mouth, bulky tumors of the middle and posterior third of the tongue and tumors that involve the base of the tongue, pharyngeal wall and tonsil can be exposed through mandibulotomy. It is critical however to ensure that the mandible is neither involved, nor require resection, before planning a mandibulotomy, for example, if the mandible is divided anteriorly for mandibulotomy and subsequently it is resected laterally by performing either a marginal or segmental mandibulectomy, the intervening bone will not be viable and will result in unnecessary mandible loss. As with a cheek flap, a midline lip-splitting incision is performed through the skin, orbicularis oris muscle and labial mucosa in order to expose the mandible. A short cheek flap is elevated on the side of the paramedian mandibulotomy by dissection laterally to further expose the mandible and the mandibulotomy site. The flap is elevated up to the mental foramen and the mental nerve is preserved.

Mandibulotomy should be performed in a paramedian location, usually between the lateral incisor and canine teeth. The lateral incisor and canine tooth roots usually diverge and provide adequate space for dividing the mandible without removing any teeth, while also avoiding exposure of the tooth roots with the bone cut. Having a preoperative panorex image in the operating room allows visualization of the tooth roots, as well as any pathology such as infected teeth, so that they can be avoided when selecting the mandibulotomy site.

The mandible should be exposed on either side of the planned mandibulotomy before cutting the bone in order to allow for preplating. Bending the plates for fixation of the mandible, and drilling screw holes prior to cutting the mandible aids in correct alignment of the mandible during closure. This is especially important for maintaining proper occlusion in dentate patients. The mandible should be fixed with two-plane fixation (two plates) and each plate should have two or more screws on either side of the mandibulotomy site. The lateral plate is positioned below the site of the teeth roots so that they are not injured by the screws. The second plate is placed along the inferior edge of the mandible. Once the mandible is cut, a mucosal incision is made along the lingual side of the mandible on the floor of mouth allowing the mandible to be retracted laterally. At least 1 cm of mucosa should be left on the lingual side of the mandible to allow adequate closure. In order to swing the mandible further laterally, the anterior belly of the digastric muscle and the mylohyoid muscle are

transected. Mandibulotomy provides wide exposure of the oral cavity and oropharynx permitting satisfactory resection of large and posterior tumors with adequate margins. It also facilitates exposure for reconstruction with free or pedicled flaps as needed (Fig. 4). An elective temporary tracheostomy is usually recommended when performing mandibulotomy. If a flap is used to reconstruct the defect, then a tracheostomy is necessary to maintain an adequate airway until swelling subsides.

Visor Flap

Larger lesions of the anterior oral cavity involving the anterior floor of mouth and lower gum that are not amenable to a peroral approach can sometimes be accessed using a visor flap. This approach avoids the need for a lower lip-splitting incision but has the disadvantage of causing anesthesia of the skin of the chin and lower lip because of sacrifice of the mental nerves. Anesthesia of the lower lip can affect oral competence and is a bothersome postoperative sequela. A visor flap (Fig. 5) allows wide exposure to the anterior lesions, but does not provide good access to tumors that extend to the middle or posterior oral cavity. A mucosal incision is made along the gingivobuccal sulcus on one side and extended all the way across the gingivolabial sulcus to the contralateral gingivobuccal sulcus. A cuff of mucosa, at least 1 cm wide should be left on the mandible, except where dictated by the need for margins around the tumor. Dissection is carried down to the mandible and the soft tissues on the anterior

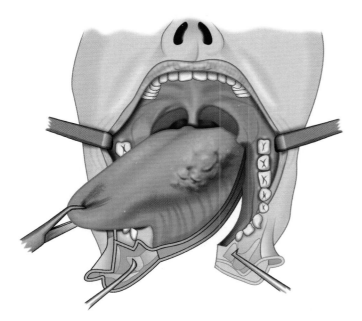

Fig. 4: Mandibulotomy exposes large posterior tumors that cannot be accessed with a peroral or lower cheek flap approach

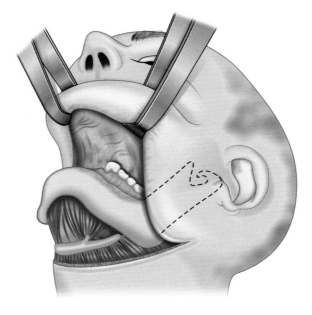

Fig. 5: A visor flap approach is useful for the anterior most tumors and avoids a lip-splitting incision

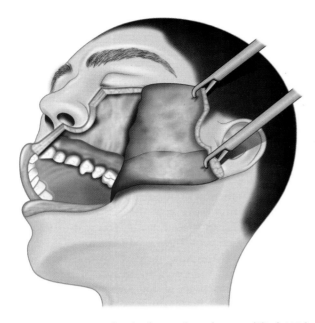

Fig. 6: An upper cheek flap using the modified Weber-Ferguson incision, either alone or with a subciliary extension, exposes the infra- and suprastructure of the maxilla

and lateral surface of the mandible, which are mobilized leaving the periosteum intact to preserve its blood supply. A transverse incision is made in the neck skin from below the mastoid tip on one side to the same location contralaterally. Subplatysmal flaps are elevated superiorly through this incision and connected with the intraoral dissection. This incision can also be used to access the upper neck for neck dissection. Care should be taken to preserve the marginal mandibular branch of the facial nerve on both sides. Once the skin and soft tissue is mobilized off the mandible, this can be retracted superiorly exposing the mandible through the neck incision (Fig. 5). With this exposure, the anterior most oral cavity tumors can be safely resected. If needed, an anterior marginal or segmental mandibulotomy, as described in Chapter 26 can be performed. If necessary, there is also good anterior exposure for insetting a flap.

Upper Cheek Flap

An upper cheek flap approach is required for tumors of the hard palate, upper gum, upper gingivobuccal sulcus and anterior soft palate that cannot be adequately accessed perorally. Small lesions that require a limited partial maxillectomy can often be adequately accessed through the open mouth. When greater exposure is necessary, the entire lateral aspect of the maxilla can be exposed using a Weber-Ferguson incision with a subciliary extension as shown in Figure 6.

When the resection is limited to the hard palate or upper gum, usually a Weber-Ferguson incision or lateral rhinotomy incision alone provides adequate exposure. An orotracheal tube should be used and a nasotracheal tube should be avoided as it will distort the anatomy of the nose and philtrum during the incision and closure of these areas.

A midline upper lip-splitting incision is made through the skin, orbicularis oris muscle and mucosa of the upper lip. At the columella, the incision turns laterally along the columella to the floor of the nasal cavity. Careful placement of the Weber-Ferguson incision is critical to its esthetic outcome. The incision is carried a bit further in the floor of the nasal cavity, and then out of the nasal cavity following the curve of the ala up onto the nasal dorsum, following the nasal subunit of the ala. This is extended up to bulb and the side of the nose along the lateral nasal wall respecting the lateral wall and the nasal dorsum subunits. The skin is incised with a scalpel and then electrocautery is used to transect the orbicularis oris and musculature deep to the ala of the left nostril.

Dissection is carried down onto the anterior face of the maxilla. The angular branches of the facial vessels frequently require ligation. A mucosal incision is made along the gingivobuccal sulcus leaving an adequate cuff of mucosa on the maxilla for closure, if required, except where dictated by tumor margins. The cheek flap is elevated off the anterior maxilla working from medial to lateral in the subperiosteal plane. Attention is given to identifying and preserving the infraorbital nerve and vessels. These should be preserved, unless they are involved by tumor or if transection is necessary for wider exposure or for securing margins. Elevation of the upper cheek flap provides adequate access for most infrastructure maxillectomy, as described in Chapter 29. Use of subciliary extension exposes the maxillary suprastructure.

POSTOPERATIVE TREATMENT

Patients with complex reconstruction or major suture lines in the oral cavity should be maintained with enteral tube feeds via a small-bore nasogastric tube placed during surgery. Nothing is given orally for a period of up to 1 week or longer to allow the healing with a watertight seal. It is important to maintain adequate nutrition during this period. Routine perioperative antibiotics are given for 48 hours, but can be stopped after that if there is no sign of infection and the wounds are all closed.

HIGHLIGHTS

I. Indications
- Oral cavity tumors

II. Contraindications

- Tumor surrounding the internal carotid artery
- Tumor involving the base of skull
- Anterior mandibulotomy should not be performed if posterior mandible is involved by tumor, as the intervening mandible will be unnecessarily lost.

III. Special Preoperative Considerations

- Computed tomography scan imaging, when indicated clinically, should be used to assess for bone involvement.
- Magnetic resonance imaging is useful to assess the extent of base of tongue involvement and perineural invasion of named nerves, if either of these are clinically suspected.
- A panoramic X-ray of the mandible (orthopantomogram) is required prior to mandibulotomy or marginal mandibulectomy to assess the status of the bone (alveolar process) and the roots of the teeth.

IV. Special Intraoperative Considerations

- Nasotracheal tube should be used for mandible or other lower oral cavity surgeries.
- Orotracheal tube should be used for maxillary or superior oral cavity surgeries.
- Complete paralysis with muscle relaxants during anesthesia improves exposure with all approaches.
- Tracheostomy should be performed, if there is a large resection or a flap is being used for reconstruction, or when potential airway compromise is suspected.

V. Special Postoperative Considerations

- Maintain patient's NPO for a period based on extent of resection and closure.
- Supplement nutrition with the help of tube feedings, if patient remains NPO for more than 24 hours.

VI. Complications

- Inadequate exposure will result in inadequate resection if the appropriate approach is not used.

ADDITIONAL READING

1. Carvalho AL, Singh B, Spiro RH, et al. Cancer of the oral cavity: a comparison between institutions in a developing and a developed nation. Head Neck. 2004;26(1):31-8.
2. Gross ND, Patel SG, Carvalho AL, et al. Nomogram for deciding adjuvant treatment after surgery for oral cavity squamous cell carcinoma. Head Neck. 2008;30(10):1352-60.
3. Lin K, Patel SG, Chu PY, et al. Second primary malignancy of the aerodigestive tract in patients treated for cancer of the oral cavity and larynx. Head Neck. 2005;27(12):1042-8.
4. Shah JP, Gil Z. Current concepts in management of oral cancer—surgery. Oral Oncol. 2009;45(4-5):394-401.
5. Shah J, Patel S, Singh B. Head and Neck Surgery and Oncology, 4th Edition. Elsevier; 2012.
6. Shah JP, Singh B. Keynote comment: why the lack of progress for oral cancer? Lancet Oncol. 2006;7(5):356-7.
7. Shah JP. The role of marginal mandibulectomy in the surgical management of oral cancer. Arch Otolaryngol Head Neck Surg. 2002;128(5):604-5.

Chapter **53**

Thyroidectomy and Neck Dissection

Jatin Shah

INTRODUCTION

The majority of well-differentiated thyroid carcinomas are confined to the thyroid gland at the time of initial presentation. Intrathyroidal tumors are removed with either thyroid lobectomy or total thyroidectomy depending upon the size, and extent of the tumor and the status of the contralateral lobe. The main objectives of surgery are: (i) complete removal of the entire lobe or the whole gland in an extracapsular fashion, containing the tumor without leaving any thyroid tissue behind; (ii) preservation of the parathyroid glands and their blood supply; and (iii) prevention of injury to the superior and recurrent laryngeal nerves. A secondary goal is an esthetically acceptable skin incision. Well-differentiated thyroid carcinoma can invade into the soft tissues and structures surrounding the thyroid gland. Anterior extension into the perithyroidal adipose tissue or sternothyroid muscle (T3 tumors) is treated with total thyroidectomy, but with en bloc excision of the involved tissues. Less commonly, well-differentiated thyroid carcinomas invade posteriorly into the more critical structures, such as the larynx, trachea, esophagus or recurrent laryngeal nerve (T4a tumors). The primary management of advanced extrathyroidal disease requires special considerations and resection of all involved structures, to remove all gross disease and whatever structures are necessary to achieve complete excision.

When there is clinically apparent spread of well differentiated thyroid cancer to lymph nodes in the neck, as commonly occurs with papillary thyroid cancer, the lymph nodes contained in the soft tissues in the affected compartment of the neck should be removed with a therapeutic neck dissection. Elective neck dissection of the central or lateral neck in the absence of grossly evident metastasis is not beneficial for well-differentiated thyroid cancers and therefore is not recommended.

PREOPERATIVE EVALUATION AND ANESTHESIA

A patient referred with a biopsy, diagnostic or suggestive of thyroid cancer frequently has undergone anatomic imaging of the thyroid gland and neck, most commonly with an ultrasound. If not, then imaging of the thyroid gland and neck should be obtained to determine whether there are additional nodules or tumors in the contralateral thyroid lobe, whether there is gross extrathyroidal extension and whether there is evidence of regional metastatic disease. If gross extra thyroid extension is suspected clinically, or retrosternal extension is suspected, then a contrast enhanced CT scan of the neck and mediastinum is desirable. Administration of the iodine contrast dye, may delay postoperative administration of radioactive iodine by a couple of months. However, accurate demonstration of the extent of disease is crucial for the conduct of a safe and oncologically complete operation. This information is important in planning appropriate surgery for each patient. All patients should also undergo assessment of their vocal cord function with either indirect mirror examination or fiberoptic nasolaryngoscopy. Preoperative vocal cord paralysis, whether secondary to the thyroid pathology or due to some other cause is an important information to document and to accurately assess the extent and stage of the disease and for intraoperative decision-making. No special anesthesia technique is required for thyroidectomy or neck dissection, although maintaining a slightly hypotensive blood pressure during and immediately after surgery is important for both a safe operation and to avoid perioperative hematoma. If, however, intraoperative nerve monitoring is planned, then a special endotracheal tube equipped with contact electrodes is required. However, nerve monitoring is not employed routinely in most centers. A small endotracheal tube, such as a #6.0 or 6.5 will reduce mechanical trauma to the vocal cords and larynx during surgery. Topical lidocaine administered by the anesthesiologist via the endotracheal tube 15 or 30 minutes before waking the patient, facilitates emergence from anesthesia without violent coughing or "bucking." Antibiotics have not been shown to improve outcomes in thyroid surgery and should not be used routinely.

SURGICAL TECHNIQUE

Thyroidectomy

The incision should be designed firstly to provide adequate exposure for the safe and effective removal of the tumor and thyroid gland and secondly, to provide the best cosmetic result. A transverse cervical incision in an existing skin crease most commonly fulfills these criteria (Fig. 1). Generally, a skin crease overlying the region of the cricoid cartilage is preferred. Similarly, a higher skin crease near or at the cricoid cartilage is preferred over a lower skin crease. Marking the skin incision, with the patient awake and sitting up can be helpful. The planned incision should take into account the length and width of the patient's neck, the size of the thyroid gland and

tumor, the need to perform lymphadenectomy as a part of the procedure, as well as any previous neck scars or incisions. A long neck may dictate a higher incision to enable adequate exposure of the superior poles of the thyroid. Alternately, a longer incision will also enable superior pole exposure. In females, breast size is an important consideration as larger breasts will pull the neck skin down over the manubrium. This is especially true, if the incision is marked when the patient is supine on the operation room table. Incisions that get pulled down over the sternum due to the heavy weight of large breast are more likely to develop hypertrophic scar and less likely to have a good cosmetic outcome. In males, a low skin incision can be used intentionally to hide the scar below the collar line, and in the chest hair. After induction of anesthesia, the patient is positioned supine on the operating table. The top of the patient's head should be positioned at the top edge of the table and the head is stabilized by placing it on a donut cushion. The reverse Trendelenburg position used in combination with neck extension improves neck exposure. Care should be taken with older patients and patients with cervical spine disease not to overextend their neck to an extent that will cause injury or postoperative discomfort.

The skin incision is made sharply with a scalpel. Electrocautery is not used until the skin has been completely divided through the dermis, with the scalpel in order to avoid thermal trauma to the skin edges, which can result in more scarring. The platysma muscle is divided but the underlying anterior jugular veins are left intact. Subplatysmal flaps are elevated superiorly up to the thyroid notch and inferiorly to the sternum (Fig. 2). The anterior jugular veins are left down

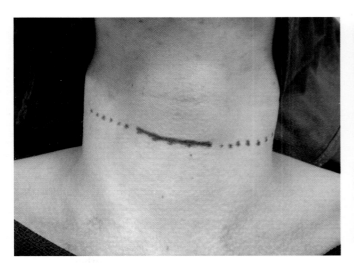

Fig. 1: A transverse neck incision should be carefully placed taking into consideration the patient's neck, an existing skin crease and thyroid anatomy, location and size of the tumor, as well as possible need for a neck dissection

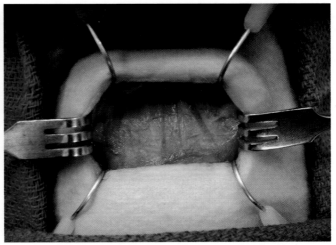

Fig. 2: Subplatysmal flaps are elevated superiorly and inferiorly exposing the strap muscles

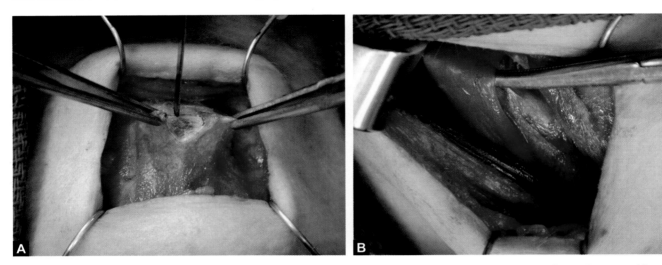

Figs 3A and B: The strap muscles are separated through an incision in the fascia along the median raphe and retracted laterally to expose the thyroid gland. The sternothyroid muscle can be divided along its superior attachment to expose the superior pole vessels

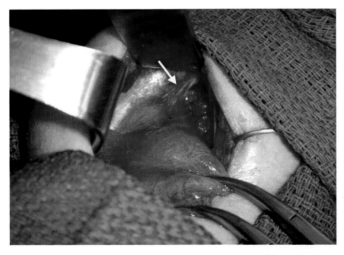

Fig. 4: Adequate exposure of the superior pole allows ligation of the superior pole vessels, individually and often helps in identification of the external branch of the superior laryngeal nerve

on the superficial layer of the deep cervical fascia, which covers the strap muscles. Elevation of subplatysmal flaps exposes the strap muscles lying over the thyroid gland. The right and left sternohyoid muscles are separated from one another along the avascular median raphe, which runs vertically between them (Figs 3A and B). Occasionally, one of the anterior jugular veins crosses the midline and must be ligated and divided. Separating the sternohyoid and sternothyroid muscles exposes the underlying thyroid isthmus. The sternohyoid

muscle is elevated off the sternothyroid muscle and retracted laterally. The sternothyroid muscle is then carefully elevated off of the anterior surface of the thyroid gland. The superior attachment of the sternothyroid muscle can be divided to provide better access to the superior pole of the thyroid gland. Once the sternohyoid and sternothyroid muscles are retracted laterally, additional superior retraction will expose the superior thyroid pole and the superior pole vessels (Fig. 4). The external branch of the superior laryngeal nerve crosses from lateral to medial in this region on its course from the vagus nerve to the larynx. The nerve follows the course of the superior thyroid artery and is located posteromedial to the artery. The superior pole vessels (terminal branches of the superior thyroid artery) should be individually ligated and divided distal to the medial take off, of the external laryngeal branch of the superior laryngeal nerve. Careful search for the external branch of the superior laryngeal nerve should be made before dividing these vessels. It is however, not necessary to search exhaustively for the nerve and inflict dissection trauma. If the nerve is not seen, ligate the branches of the inferior thyroid artery individually as close to the thyroid capsule as possible. The external branch of the superior laryngeal nerve often turns medially, and out of the way as the superior pole vessels are divided and the thyroid lobe is retracted inferiorly. After the superior pole vessels are divided, the gland can be grasped with a clamp and retracted inferiorly and medially. Careful dissection along the lateral border of the gland over the capsular plane, starting from the superior pole will allow the gland to be rotated further medially. Monopolar electrocautery should not be used after

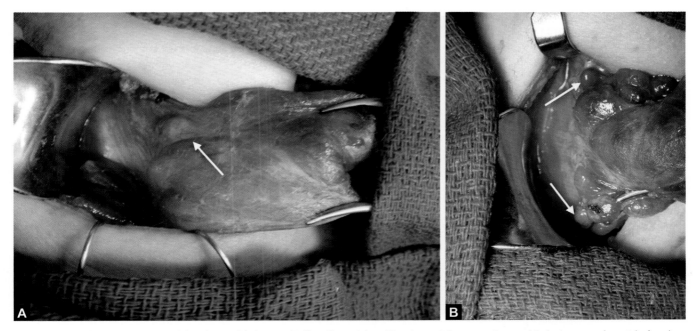

Figs 5A and B: Retraction of the thyroid lobe medially allows identification of the superior and inferior parathyroid glands

rotating the gland, as transmission of the current as well as thermal injury can traumatize the parathyroid glands, their blood supply and the recurrent laryngeal nerve. Rotation of the gland and meticulous dissection over the capsule of the thyroid gland will expose the superior parathyroid gland, which is usually seen first and then the inferior parathyroid gland, when the thyroid lobe is rotated further medially (Figs 5A and B). By staying over the capsular plane and giving careful attention, the parathyroid glands and their vascular pedicle will be exposed. The location of the parathyroids is variable but the superior parathyroid gland is commonly located on the posterior surface of the upper pole of the thyroid gland. The parathyroid glands are carefully dissected away from the thyroid gland, while preserving their blood supply. If a parathyroid gland is devascularized it will change to a dark caramel color and have a congested appearance. If the supplying vessels have been inadvertently divided, the parathyroid should be removed, frozen section of a small fragment of the gland should be performed for confirmation and the remaining gland should be reimplanted in a neck muscle. The gland is minced with a scalpel before placing it in a pocket within the sternocleidomastoid muscle at the conclusion of the case. Nonabsorbable sutures are used to mark the location of reimplantation so that it can be found in the future in the unlikely event that additional parathyroid surgery is required. Additional retraction of the thyroid

gland medially will expose the tracheoesophageal groove and the tuberculum of Zuckerkandl (Fig. 6). It is not necessary to dissect laterally in the tracheoesophageal groove in order to identify the recurrent laryngeal nerve. After identification and dissection of the parathyroid glands, retracting them away from the thyroid gland, a plane is maintained over the capsule of the thyroid gland, as it is carefully rotated away from the trachea. The recurrent laryngeal nerve will be visualized as it passes underneath the thyroid gland and enters the larynx. Usually, the nerve lies underneath the tuberculum of Zuckerkandl although; it can also course laterally around the tuberculum or even run medial to it. Once the nerve is identified, the remaining inferior and lateral vessels supplying the thyroid can be safely ligated. Also, with the nerve under visualization, the attachment of the thyroid gland to the trachea at the ligament of Berry can be divided allowing the thyroid to be mobilized off the trachea. If a lobectomy is being performed, the isthmus is clamped, divided and oversewn with a chromic stitch to secure hemostasis in the remaining thyroid lobe. If total thyroidectomy is being performed, the same technique is used to mobilize the contralateral thyroid lobe. In either case, attention should be paid to include the pyramidal lobe, which can extend superiorly from the thyroid isthmus. This is a frequently overlooked area where residual thyroid tissue is left following surgery. Following lobectomy or total

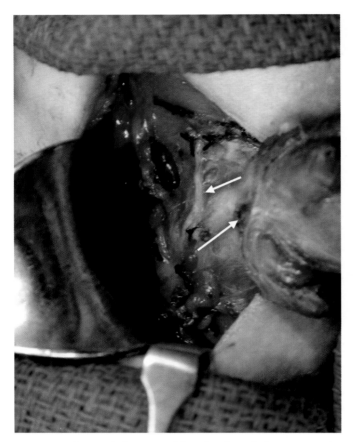

Fig. 6: Further mobilization of the gland medially exposes the tubercle of Zuckerkandl and allows identification of the recurrent laryngeal nerve

thyroidectomy, the strap muscles are reapproximated in the midline. A Penrose drain is inserted if excessive amount of oozing is observed or if extensive central compartment surgery is performed. The platysma is reapproximated with 3-0 chromic suture and the skin is approximated with 5-0 nylon suture.

When there is gross extrathyroidal extension of tumor, this should be resected en bloc with the thyroid gland (Fig. 7). Anterior extension usually involves perithyroidal adipose tissue or the strap muscles (T3) and very rarely, the skin. These structures can be resected en bloc with the tumor with little or no functional sequelae for the patient. The same technique described for thyroidectomy can be used with relatively minor modification. If the sternothyroid muscle is adherent to the gland, it should be divided at its superior insertion on the thyroid cartilage and its inferior insertion on the sternum. In this way, it is removed in an en bloc fashion. The other strap muscles can be treated in a similar fashion. If, however, the tumor extends posteriorly, a more significant surgical resection is necessary with much higher functional sequelae for the patient. Thyroid tumors that invade posteriorly can involve the trachea, larynx, esophagus or recurrent laryngeal nerve (T4a). Minor tracheal adhesion can be treated with submucosal resection or "shave" of the cartilage in order to obtain a clear margin. Deeply invasive tumors require a sleeve resection of the trachea. Similarly, minor invasion of the esophagus can be treated with submucosal resection, while deep invasion necessitates full-thickness resection and closure or reconstruction. When the larynx is invaded, partial laryngeal resection is indicated

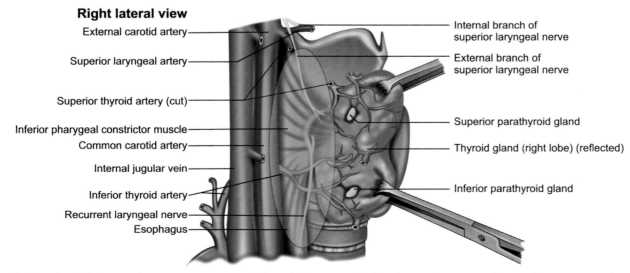

Fig. 7: Extrathyroidal extension can occur anteriorly, which generally involves minor extension to the strap muscles, and achieve an en bloc resection. Posterior extrathyroid extension may involve, trachea, cricoid, thyroid, pharynx, esophagus or recurrent laryngeal nerves, and will need major resection to achieve a complete excision

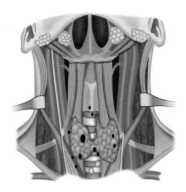

Primary site
Thyroid

**First echelon
lymph nodes**
• Perithyroid nodes
• Tracheoesophageal groove
• Level VI

Fig. 8: The central compartment lymph nodes are contained in the fatty tissue between the trachea medially and the carotid artery laterally, and extends from the hyoid superiorly to the upper border of the innominate artery inferiorly

where this is possible. Preoperative recurrent laryngeal nerve paralysis is an ominous sign, and requires very careful surgical planning and intraoperative judgment, to achieve an oncologically complete resection, keeping the functional sequela in mind.

Intraoperatively, the invaded nonfunctioning nerve should be included with the resection, taking into consideration, the contralateral vocal cord function. When the vocal cord is mobile preoperatively, every effort should be made to dissect a well-differentiated thyroid tumor off the nerve, although there are circumstances when this is not feasible.

Neck Dissection

Thyroid cancer metastatic to lymph nodes in the central compartment of the neck is treated with central compartment node dissection. The central compartment is comprised of neck levels VI and VII. Level VI includes lymph node bearing tissue between the carotid arteries laterally, the hyoid bone superiorly and the suprasternal notch inferiorly. Level VII is below level VI and includes the anterior superior mediastinal tissues that are above the innominate artery (Fig. 8). Clinically evident metastatic disease in the central compartment is treated with removal of all of the lymph node containing tissue in this compartment. Elective dissection of the central compartment has not been shown to affect the prognosis and is not recommended. In fact, it may increase the morbidity of iatrogenic hypoparathyroidism with no benefit to the patient. Generally, the same incision used for total thyroidectomy is adequate for central compartment node dissection in most patients, but in some patients, lateral extension may be necessary (Fig. 1). The important structures contained within the central compartment that require meticulous dissection and preservation are the parathyroid glands and their vascular supply and the recurrent laryngeal

nerves. Laterally, the central compartment tissues should be dissected off the carotid artery from the level of the thyroid cartilage to the innominate artery on the right. Rarely, there is lymph node containing tissue in the central compartment above the level of the thyroid cartilage laterally, although careful inspection should be performed in this area. Minimizing the dissection in this area facilitates preservation of the superior parathyroid gland and its vascular supply. The inferior parathyroid gland can be preserved if it is not involved in bulky nodal disease and if its blood supply is not compromised during the dissection necessary to mobilize the fibroadipose tissue containing the lymph nodes in inferior level VI. The recurrent laryngeal nerve should be carefully mobilized along its course in the central compartment. The lymph node containing tissue is pulled underneath the nerve toward the trachea. Once free of the parathyroid glands and the nerve, the remaining attachments to the deep neck and trachea can be divided so that the specimen is free. Sometimes, there are lymph nodes located posterior and medial to the recurrent laryngeal nerves. They should be meticulously dissected out. After removal of the specimen, careful attention should be given to the parathyroid glands. If any of them are devascularized, they should be reimplanted as described earlier in the section on thyroidectomy, including the use of frozen section to confirm the histology. For reoperative cases, where the patient has already undergone thyroidectomy or there is recurrence following prior dissection of the neck, the sternothyroid muscle can be excised as part of the specimen, which will improve access and exposure and also clear the anterior margin in the previously operated and potentially contaminated field. After central compartment node dissection, the remaining strap muscles are reapproximated along the midline after a Penrose drain is placed in the surgical site.

The indications for dissection of the lateral neck is the same as that for the central neck, i.e. clinically apparent metastatic disease to lymph nodes in this compartment of the neck. Similarly, elective dissection of the lateral neck has not been shown to affect the prognosis and should not be performed for well-differentiated thyroid cancer. If a lateral neck dissection is being performed at the same time as thyroidectomy, the neck incision for thyroidectomy should be placed at the level of the cricoid or higher and extended laterally in a skin crease or relaxed tension line (Fig. 1). If thyroidectomy has already been performed in the past, then the old scar is excised. Otherwise, the same incision used for thyroidectomy is extended laterally. However, this will require a longer incision to obtain sufficient superior access. There is no need to extend the incision superiorly in the shape of the letter "U". Such extension produces and unpleasant scar. If additional exposure is required, simply extend the incision further laterally, along the same skin crease. The postoperative

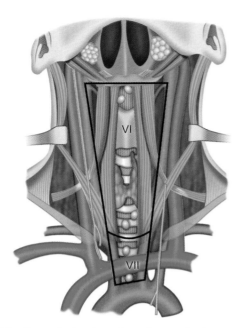

Fig. 9: The first echelon lymph nodes are in the central compartment at levels VI and VII. The second echelon lymph nodes include level II, III, IV and V in the lateral neck

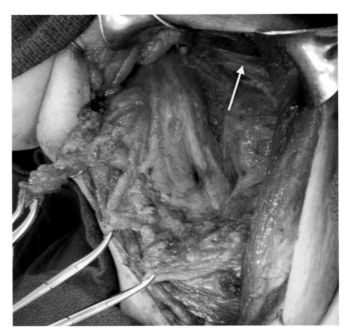

Fig. 10: A subplatysmal flap is elevated and lymph node dissection is carried out by retraction of the sternomastoid muscle laterally, to expose the spinal accessory nerve in the posterior triangle, which serves as the superior and lateral extent of lymph node dissection

appearance of laterally extended incision along a skin crease is much superior to a "hockey stick" incision that curves up toward the mastoid tip. When lateral metastatic adenopathy is present, the lymph node containing tissues in level IIA, III, IV and V should be removed routinely (Fig. 9). If metastatic disease is present in other levels of the neck, then these should also be included in the dissection. Subplatysmal skin flaps should be elevated inferiorly to the clavicle and superiorly to expose the digastric muscle. As the flaps are elevated laterally, the platysma will be absent and the flaps are elevated in the plane of the fascia of the sternocleidomastoid muscle. The great auricular nerve and the external jugular veins are left intact on the muscle during flap elevation. Posterior to the sternocleidomastoid muscle, the spinal accessory nerve can be quite superficial and care should be taken while elevating the flap in this area. Once the anterior border of the trapezius muscle is exposed, the spinal accessory nerve is identified just superior to where the great auricular nerve crosses the posterior edge of the sternocleidomastoid muscle at Erb's point. The spinal accessory nerve is then followed until it reaches the trapezius muscle (Fig. 10). Lymph node containing tissues below and medial to the spinal accessory nerve are dissected away from the trapezius and off the deep muscles of the neck. The posterior belly of the omohyoid muscle is encountered, transected and included in the specimen. The specimen is retracted anteriorly and dissected off the floor of the neck leaving the fascia overlying the

brachial plexus, scalene muscles and phrenic nerve intact. The transverse cervical vessels may be encountered and are ligated. Cutaneous branches of the cervical nerve roots are encountered over the prevertebral muscles. The lymph node bearing tissue is dissected off from the cervical plexus, which is preserved.

The fascia at the anterior border of the sternocleidomastoid muscle is incised and the dissection of level II lymph nodes begins by retracting the sternocleidomastoid muscle laterally. At this juncture, the spinal accessory nerve is identified as it courses through level II. The nerve is traced superiorly until it passes underneath the posterior belly of the digastric muscle. The sternocleidomastoid muscle is retracted posteriorly exposing levels II, III and IV. It is not necessary to remove the contents of IIB unless grossly involved metastatic disease is present at level IIA. However, the tissue in level IIA, which is inferior and anterior to the spinal accessory nerve, is always included. The posterior border of the sternocleidomastoid muscle is dissected and the muscle is mobilized from the underlying tissues. The specimen of the posterior triangle lymph node is passed underneath the muscle and is retracted anteriorly. The inferior attachments of the specimen between the phrenic nerve and the jugular vein should be carefully clamped and ligated to avoid a chyle leak either from the thoracic duct on the left or accessory chyle channels on the right. Further mobilization of the specimen off the floor of the neck will expose the contents of the carotid sheath including the carotid artery, vagus nerve and jugular vein. Attachments to these structures are transected with care. In level II the fascia overlying the hypoglossal nerve and the common facial vein should be left intact. Finally, the medial attachment of the specimen at the strap muscles is encountered and the specimen is freed by transecting the anterior attachment of the omohyoid muscle. Suction drains are necessary after lateral neck dissection. The platysma is reapproximated and the skin is closed using either interrupted nylon suture or staples.

POSTOPERATIVE TREATMENT

The acute postoperative care following thyroidectomy includes monitoring the patient for surgical complications, such as hematoma, hypocalcemia or laryngeal nerve injury. Hematoma is an uncommon complication that is best avoided with careful surgical technique. Small or stable hematomas can be managed with needle aspiration. Large or rapidly expanding hematomas are potentially life-threatening and should be treated with expeditious wound exploration in the operating room. Patients experiencing airway compromise should have emergent bedside hematoma evacuation prior to re-exploration in the operating room. Hypocalcemia is temporary, unless all parathyroid glands have been inadvertently removed. Oral calcium supplementation is usually sufficient and once the serum calcium is stable or increasing on calcium supplementation, the patient can be discharged and calcium supplements can be continued at home. Vocal cord paralysis is temporary unless the recurrent laryngeal nerve has to be sacrificed because of tumor involvement or is inadvertently transected. As long as the patient has an adequate voice for their daily needs, they can be observed for restoration of the function. If the vocal cord is still not functional, a temporary vocal cord medialization can be performed with percutaneous injection of fat, gelfoam or other inert injectable substances. Permanant medialization of the paralyzed vocal cord may require open thyroplasty.

HIGHLIGHTS

I. Indications
- Thyroid lobectomy for low-risk tumors (unifocal or multifocal and intrathyroidal, confined to one lobe) in young patients
- Total thyroidectomy for tumors contained within the thyroid with bilobe involvement, or with contralateral nodules.

- Extended thyroidectomy for en bloc resection of extrathyroidal extension
- Appropriate neck dissection for clinically apparent metastatic disease in any compartment of the neck.

II. Contraindications
- Elective neck dissection is not indicated for well-differentiated thyroid cancer.

III. Special Preoperative Considerations
- Evaluation for regional metastasis prior to surgery
- Assessment of vocal cord functioning preoperatively.

IV. Special Intraoperative Considerations
- Divide superior pole vessels individually while looking for the external branch of the superior laryngeal nerve.
- Careful dissection over the thyroid capsule to facilitate identification and preservation of the parathyroid glands and their vascular supply.
- Identification of the recurrent laryngeal nerve, as it travels toward its insertion in the larynx, rather than laterally in the tracheoesophageal groove.

V. Special Postoperative Considerations
- Monitor patients for postoperative hypocalcemia
- Monitor patients for postoperative hematoma
- Replace calcium for significant hypocalcemia or symptomatic patients
- Suction drains used for lateral neck dissection or very large tumors
- Penrose drain used for thyroid and central compartment neck dissection.

VI. Complications
- External branch of the superior laryngeal nerve injury (temporary or permanent)
- Recurrent laryngeal nerve injury (temporary or permanent)
- Hypoparathyroidism (temporary or permanent)
- Hematoma.

ADDITIONAL READING

1. Attie JN, Khafif RA. Preservation of parathyroid glands during total thyroidectomy. Am J Surg. 1975;130:399-404.
2. Ellenhorn JD, Shah JP, Brennan MF. The impact of therapeutic regional lymph node dissection for medullary carcinoma of the thyroid . Surgery. 1993;114:1078-82.
3. Gil Z, Patel SG. Surgery for thyroid cancer. Surg Oncol Clin N Am. 2008;17:93-120, viii.
4. Hay ID, Grant CS, Taylor WF, et al. Ipsilateral lobectomy versus bilateral lobar resection in papillary thyroid carcinoma: a retrospective analysis of surgical outcome using a novel prognostic scoring system. Surgery. 1987;102: 1088-95.
5. Hughes CJ, Shaha AR, Shah JP, et al. Impact of lymph node metastases in differentiated carcinoma of the thyroid: a matched pair analysis. Head Neck. 1996;18:127-32.

6. Ibrahimpasic T, Nixon IJ, Patel SG, et al. Undetectable thyroglobulin following total thyroidectomy in patients with low risk and intermediate risk papillary thyroid cancer—is there a need for RAI? Surgery; 2012.

7. Iyer NG, Kumar A, Nixon IJ, et al. Incidence and significance of delphian node metastasis in papillary thyroid cancer. Ann Surg; 2011. Impact factor 7.9. PMID: 21372688.

8. Lore JM. Practical anatomical considerations in thyroid tumor surgery. Arch Otolaryngol. 1983;109:568-74.

9. Nixon IJ, Ganly I, Patel S, et al. Changing trends in incidence, histological distribution, clinical management and outcomes of well differentiated thyroid carcinoma over eight decades in one institution. International Journal of Surgery.

10. Nixon IJ, Ganly I, Patel S, et al. The impact of microscopic extrathyroid extension on outcome in patients with clinically T1 and T2 well differentiated thyroid cancer surgery. 2011;150 (6):1242-9.

11. Nixon IJ, Ganly I, Patel S, et al. Thyroid lobectomy for treatment of well differentiated intrathyroid malignancy. Surgery; 2011.

12. Nixon IJ, Palmer FL, Whitcher MM, et al. Thyroid isthmusectomy for well-differentiated thyroid cancer. Ann Surg Oncol. 2011;18(3):767-70. PMID 21046263 Impact factor 4.1

13. Nixon IJ, Whitcher M, Glick J, et al. Surgical management of metastases to the thyroid gland. Ann Surg Oncol. 2011;18(3): 800-4. PMID: 21046263.

14. Shaha AR, Shah JP, Loree TR. Patterns of nodal and distant metastasis based on histologic varieties in differentiated carcinoma of the thyroid . Am J Surg. 1996;172:692-4 .

15. Shah JP, Loree TR, Dharker D, et al. Lobectomy vs total thyroidectomy for differentiated carcinoma of the thyroid. A matched pair analysis . Am J Surg. 1993;166:331-5.

16. Shah JP, Loree T, Dharker D, et al. Prognostic factors in differentiated carcinoma of the thyroid. Am J Surg. 1992;164:658-61.

17. Shah JP. Management of regional metastases in salivary and thyroid cancer. In: Larson DL, Ballantyne AJ, Guillamondegui OM (Eds). Cancer in the neck—evaluation and treatment. New York: Macmillan; 1986.pp.253-8.

18. Stojadinovic A, Shoup M, Ghossein RA, et al. The role of operations for distantly metastatic well-differentiated thyroid carcinoma. Surgery. 2002;131:636-43.

Index

Page numbers followed by *f* refer to figure and *t* refer to table